Medical Disorders in Pregnancy

Medical Disorders in Pregnancy

Medical Disorders in Pregnancy:
A Manual for Midwives

Edited by

S. Elizabeth Robson
MSc RGN RM ADM Cert(A)Ed MTD FHEA
Senior Lecturer in Midwifery
De Montfort University

and

Jason Waugh
BSc(Hons) MB BS DA MRCOG
Consultant in Obstetrics and Maternal Medicine
Royal Victoria Infirmary
Newcastle-upon-Tyne
Honorary Senior Lecturer
University of Newcastle-upon-Tyne
Honorary Senior Lecturer
University of Leicester

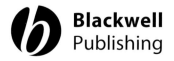

Library of Congress Cataloging-in-Publication Data

Medical disorders in pregnancy : a manual for midwives / edited by S. Elizabeth Robson and Jason Waugh.
    p. ; cm.
  Includes bibliographical references and index.
  ISBN-13: 978-1-4051-5168-9 (pbk. : alk. paper)
  ISBN-10: 1-4051-5168-4 (pbk. : alk. paper)   1. Pregnancy–Complications–Handbooks, manuals, etc.
  2. Midwifery–Handbooks, manuals, etc.   I. Robson, S. Elizabeth.   II. Waugh, Jason.
  [DNLM: 1. Pregnancy Complications–Handbooks.   2. Midwifery–Handbooks.
  3. Prenatal Care–methods–Handbooks. WQ 39 M4878 2008]
  RG571.M433 2008
  618.2—dc22

2007042416

A catalogue record for this book is available from the British Library.

Set in 9/11pt Palatino by Graphicraft Limited, Hong Kong
Printed in Singapore by C.O.S. Printers Pte Ltd

1   2008

Contents

Contributors

EDITORS

S. Elizabeth Robson RGN RM ADM Cert(A)Ed MTD MSc FHEA
Senior Lecturer in Midwifery and Admissions Tutor at De Montfort University

After staff nurse experience on medical and gynaecological wards in Cambridge, Elizabeth qualified as a midwife and had five years of hospital experience. After winning the Jack Kerr Memorial Award for Trent Regional Health Authority she entered midwifery education. Her ADM was attained in Bristol, educational qualifications from Nottingham University, an MSc in research methods from Loughborough University. With 20 years' experience as a midwifery lecturer, she leads a module on medical disorders for student midwives with a particular interest in immunology. Her link lecturer areas comprise a high-risk maternity ward and community team. She has presented nationally, and has a number of publications.

Jason Waugh BSc (Hons) DA MB BS MRCOG
Consultant/Honorary Senior Lecturer Obstetrics and Maternal Medicine at the Royal Victoria Infirmary, Newcastle-upon-Tyne

Jason trained in maternal medicine in Sheffield, New Zealand and Leicester before working as a consultant in Leicester for five years. He is now lead consultant for maternal medicine in Newcastle-upon-Tyne and has established maternal medicine training programmes for obstetricians in both cities. His current research interests are hypertension in pregnancy and renal and cardiovascular disease in pregnancy and he has published extensively in these fields as well as producing national guidelines for the management of pre-eclampsia and renal disease. He was recently made president of the UK's Macdonald Obstetric Medicine Society.

MEDICAL AUTHORS

Christopher Brightling BSc (Hons) MBBS MRCP PhD FCCP
MRC Clinician Scientist and Honorary Consultant Respiratory Physician, UHL NHS Trust, Leicester

Chris Brightling trained in London and Leicester and in 2002 was appointed Senior Lecturer and Honorary Consultant in Respiratory Medicine at Glenfield Hospital. His major research interests are the utilisation of inflammatory markers in the management of airway diseases and mast cell/airway smooth muscle interactions in the pathophysiology of asthma. He has authored over 50 peer-reviewed papers.

Professor Nigel J Brunskill MB ChB PhD FRCP
Nephrologist at Leicester General Hospital and Professor at the University of Leicester

After training as a Nephrologist in Sheffield, St. Louis, Missouri, USA and Leicester, Nigel became a Consultant

Nephrologist in 1997. As a clinical academic, in addition to clinical responsibilities, he supervises a laboratory team investigating cellular mechanisms of kidney disease. His particular clinical interests include proteinuria, progressive renal disease and management of renal disease in pregnancy. He has published widely in the field of kidney disease.

Frances A Bu'Lock MD FRCP
Consultant Paediatric Cardiologist at Glenfield Hospital, Leicester

Frances graduated from Cambridge and Oxford, and trained in Congenital Heart Disease in Bristol, Birmingham and Liverpool before coming to Leicester in 1999. Her main clinical interests are in fetal and adult congenital heart disease, which fit remarkably well together. She is the Cardiology Associate Editor for Archives of Diseases in Childhood and has written extensively in the field of congenital and fetal heart disease. She is currently co-investigator for a large study into the genetics of Congenital Heart Disease funded by the British Heart Foundation.

Catherine Gittins BM MRCGP DCH DRCOG DFFP DPD
General Practitioner and GPSI (GP with a Special Interest) in dermatology

From 1996–1998 Catherine worked as a staff grade in dermatology. She passed the Diploma in Practical Dermatology (DPD) with distinction in 1999. She has nine years' experience as a GP and has continued with her special interest in dermatology. Between 2005 and 2007 as well as being a GP she was a GPSI (GP with a Special Interest) for South Leicester PCT. Since relocating to Newcastle-upon-Tyne Catherine has continued working as a GP and is setting up a GPSI dermatology service in the area. She is a member of the Primary Care Dermatology Society.

Julie Goddard MBBS DFFP MRCOG
Specialist Registrar Obstetrics and Gynaecology, Royal Victoria Infirmary, Newcastle-upon-Tyne

Julie graduated in medicine from the University of Newcastle-upon-Tyne in 1998. Having completed training posts in Sunderland, Durham and Gateshead she is currently working as a senior registrar in Obstetrics and Gynaecology at the Royal Victoria Infirmary in Newcastle-upon-Tyne. Her interests are in high-risk obstetrics, intrapartum care and maternal medicine. She has completed Special Skills Modules in Management of the Labour Ward and Maternal Medicine.

Robert Gregory BA MB BS DM FRCP
Consultant Physician and Head of Service Metabolic Medicine at University Hospitals of Leicester NHS Trust

Rob undertook research in the immunology of diabetes at University Hospital, where he developed an interest in the medical problems of pregnancy and in the management of diabetes in pregnancy in particular. In 1992 he published a controversial article questioning the value of pre-pregnancy counselling clinics for women with diabetes. He researched metabolic aspects of gestational diabetes in Cambridge. Since moving to Leicester he works in multiprofessional diabetic antenatal clinics. The team visited San Antonio in 1996 thanks to a Trent Regional Quality Travel Award to study the management of gestational diabetes in Hispanic women.

Sheena Hodgett BMedSci BM BS MRCOG
Consultant Obstetrician and Gynaecologist, University Hospitals of Leicester

Sheena was appointed to this post in 2000 after completing her training in the West Midlands where she developed a special interest in high-risk pregnancy and obstetric ultrasound, gaining the RCOG/RCR Diploma. She is a member of a multi-disciplinary team of obstetricians, physicians, specialist midwives and nurses providing care for women with medical problems in pregnancy at Leicester General Hospital.

Edmund S Howarth MB ChB MRCOG
Consultant in Maternal and Fetal Medicine, and Head of Service, at the University Hospitals of Leicester NHS Trust

General training in Obstetrics and Gynaecology followed by sub-specialty training in maternal and fetal medicine. Provides tertiary level service for both maternal medical problems and fetal problems. Well-established service for management of neurological problems in pregnancy in conjunction with the local neurology service.

Javed Iqbal BSc MSc (Hons) FRCPath FRCP
Consultant in Biochemical Medicine

Javed Iqbal qualified with commendation from the University of Dundee Medical School. Whilst a Senior Registrar at the Royal Liverpool University Hospital he developed an interest in metabolic bone disease which continues to be the main area of his clinical and laboratory practise. He has a special interest in clinical aspects of disorders of vitamin D metabolism.

Manjiri M Khare MRCOG MD FCPS DNB Diploma in obstetric ultrasound
Consultant in Maternal–Fetal Medicine at the University Hospitals of Leicester NHS Trust

Manjiri has completed sub-specialty training in maternal–fetal medicine in Leicester after training in Obstetrics and Gynaecology as a South East Thames trainee. She has special interests in managing multiple pregnancies, high-risk mothers with medical problems, infection in pregnancy and prenatal diagnosis. She has contributed to substantive textbooks in her field.

Renuka Lazarus MBBS MD MRCPsych
Consultant Liaison Psychiatrist and Clinical Lead for Perinatal Psychiatry

After training in the Charing Cross rotation in London, Dr Lazarus completed her higher training in Psychiatry in Leicester. She took up her consultant post in Liaison Psychiatry in 2002. She is the clinical lead for the Perinatal Psychiatry Service in Leicestershire. She runs a weekly specialist perinatal psychiatry clinic based in the Antenatal Clinic at the Leicester Royal Infirmary; in-patient care is provided in a specialist Mother and Baby Unit. She is involved in teaching

medical and midwifery students and is a clinical supervisor for psychiatry trainees. She has organised training sessions for midwives and obstetricians. She is actively involved in research and audit. She is on the Expert Advisory Committee for the East Midlands Perinatal Psychiatry Clinical Network.

Christina Oppenheimer MB BS FRCS FRCOG Consultant in Obstetrics and Gynaecology, Leicester Royal Infirmary and Honorary Senior Lecturer in Medical Education

Christina qualified from Cambridge and London and pursued a broad-based surgical background prior to settling in Obstetrics and Gynaecology. Her particular interests are in obstetric haematology, hands-on high-risk intrapartum care with emphasis on multi-professional care and training, paediatric gynaecology and pastoral aspects of medical education. She has published in both obstetric haematology and using qualitative research techniques in obstetrics. Team-working and multi-disciplinary care is a particular passion.

Sue Pavord MB ChB FRCP FRCPath
Consultant Haematologist and Honorary Senior Lecturer in Medical Education at the University Hospitals of Leicester NHS Trust

Sue was appointed to this post in 1998. Her specialist clinical interests are obstetric haematology and haemostasis and thrombosis. In collaboration with obstetricians and specialist nurses, she established and has continued to develop a comprehensive obstetric haematology service with a heavy throughput of patients. She also runs a large Haemostasis Thrombosis Unit and is Haemophilia Comprehensive Care Centre Director. She is co-founder of the national Obstetric Haematology Group and established a postgraduate certificate course for health care workers in the field of obstetric haematology.

Tanu Singhal MRCOG
Consultant Obstetrician at University Hospitals of Leicester

After obtaining a medical degree in India, Tanu trained extensively in the field of Obstetrics and Gynaecology before coming to the UK in 1996. She trained further in her chosen field developing her special interest in high-risk obstetrics. She obtained the Advanced Diploma in Obstetric Ultrasound Scanning under the joint auspices of Royal Colleges of Radiology (RCR) and Obstetrics and Gynaecology (RCOG). Tanu was among the first few trainees to complete the RCOG Special Skills module in High-Risk Obstetrics.

Karen Watkins MB ChB(Hons) MRCOG
Lead Obstetrician for Intrapartum Care and Maternal Medicine at The Royal Cornwall Hospital, Truro

Karen graduated in 1993 with honours. She completed her basic training in Obstetrics and Gynaecology then in 1998 she became Clinical Research Fellow for the Magpie Trial, a large international randomised trial investigating magnesium sulphate and its role in preventing eclampsia. Following this, Karen worked for a number of years in Australia and during this time was awarded 'Best of Free Communications' at the RANZCOG Annual Scientific Meeting, June 2000 for research she had undertaken whilst in Australia. Karen completed the RCOG Maternal Medicine Module in May 2005 and spent a further year gaining additional training in maternal and fetal medicine.

MIDWIFERY AND NURSING AUTHORS

Abena Addo MA PDGE BSc RGN RM
Senior Lecturer in Midwifery and Midwifery Programme Leader at De Montfort University

After staff nurse experience in general surgery at the Royal Masonic Hospital in London, Abena trained as a midwife in Surrey, followed by a period of work in the antenatal clinic at the Royal Free Hospital. Whilst working mainly in a midwifery-led environment, Abena developed an interest in the care of women with sickle cell anaemia in pregnancy and their coping strategies. Abena then undertook a BSc at the University of Westminster University followed by an MA in teaching health care ethics. With ten years' experience as a midwifery lecturer she teaches ethics and contemporary midwifery practice with a keen interest in global midwifery issues.

Trudy Boyce RGN RM MBE
Recently Specialist Midwife in Hypertension at the University Hospitals of Leicester NHS Trust

Trudy worked as a midwife for 40 years in all areas of midwifery care including ten in the community. For the last 15 years of her career she dedicated herself to the care of women and their families who had experienced the hypertensive disorders of pregnancy. She was involved in setting up the Leicester Hypertension Clinic and founded the Leicester branch of the APEC support group. Trudy was awarded an MBE in 2005 for her outstanding services to the NHS and midwifery.

Eleanor Burns-Kent RM BSc (Hons)
Midwife at the University Hospitals of Leicester NHS Trust

Eleanor has worked full time in all aspects of midwifery within the hospital setting since qualification in 2000. For the past five years she has worked in a high-risk delivery suite setting with a passion for trying to normalise childbirth for the high-risk pregnant woman.

Claire Dodd RGN BA (Hons) RM BSc (Hons)
Specialist Midwife in Hypertension at the University Hospitals of Leicester NHS Trust

Claire worked as a staff nurse in haematology before undertaking her midwifery training in 1997. With a keen interest in the hypertensive disorders of pregnancy since 1999 she has been involved in a number of research projects including the Magpie Trial and GOPEC. She has been a specialist midwife since 2006.

Rowena Doughty MSc PGDE BA(Hons) RGN RM ADM FHEA
Senior Lecturer in Midwifery and Programme Leader at De Montfort University

After staff nurse experience in general medicine and gerontology, the author qualified as a midwife and accrued 12 years' full-time experience in all aspects of midwifery care, before her lectureship with De Montfort University in 1997. Her specialist interests include promoting normality in midwifery, breast-feeding, resuscitation and metabolic disorders. She has published on the latter. She is also an Intermediate Responder (IHCD qualified) providing initial treatment and management to victims of emergencies in her local and very rural community prior to the arrival of the Ambulance Services.

Daksha Elliott RGN RSCN
Specialist Nurse for Obstetric Haematology at the University Hospitals of Leicester

Daksha has been working in the field of haemostasis and thrombosis since 1999, with her previous clinical background being paediatric nursing. The haematology/obstetric service provides shared patient management of high-risk patients who have a haematological problem including those with inherited coagulation disorders and patients with haemoglobinopathies. Her current role involves working as part of a multi-disciplinary team to provide education, support and co-ordination of care of these women to improve the outcome of the pregnancy.

Caroline Farrar RGN RM BSc(Hons) PGDipEd MSC
Senior Lecturer in Midwifery and Programme Leader at De Montfort University

After working as a staff nurse in burns and plastic surgery Caroline qualified as a midwife and experienced all areas of midwifery including integration of midwifery practice. Her enthusiasm was clearly within the delivery suite environment and thus she studied an MSc in midwifery which in turn focused her energy into becoming a midwifery lecturer.

Michelle Goldie RM
Specialist Midwife, UHL NHS Trust, Leicester

Michelle Goldie trained as a midwife in Leicester and currently works as a specialist midwife in substance and alcohol misuse at the University Hospitals NHS Trust, Leicester. In addition, she works in the maternal medicine clinic, has a research interest in respiratory disease and pregnancy and has published research presented at the American Thoracic Society.

Andrea Goodlife RGN RM DipRenalNursing
Specialist Midwife in Renal Disease at the University Hospitals of Leicester NHS Trust

After two years as a nephrology unit staff nurse, the author trained as a midwife and has practised as a midwife since 1988, in the antenatal clinic and pregnancy assessment area for the past 13 years. A combined renal/obstetric clinic was set up in 1998. With her previous nursing experience Andrea is the lead midwife for the clinic.

Kathryn Gutteridge RGN RM SoM MSc PGDip Counselling & Psychotherapy, elected RCM Council member
Consultant Midwife Sandwell and West Birmingham Hospitals NHS Trust

In her early midwifery career Kathryn founded a group for women with postnatal illness in Tamworth that is still offering therapeutic support; this project was highly commended in the RCM Centenary Awards. During this time Kathryn began her postgraduate training in integrative psychotherapy culminating in research into psychodynamic transition to motherhood. In Leicester Kathryn worked in developing midwifery-led care and latterly in supporting women's mental health and wellbeing. She is involved with education and clinical support in providing assessment and individualised care plans for women with emotional and mental health problems. Kathryn is regarded as an expert advisor in women survivors of sexual abuse and the impact this has during childbirth; she regularly presents on this subject. Kathryn is a member of the Expert Advisory Committee for the East Midlands Perinatal Psychiatry Clinical Network.

Marie Halliday RGN RM
Specialist Midwife – Diabetes at University Hospitals of Leicester NHS Trust

After nursing training at Whipps Cross Hospital, London, Marie qualified as a midwife at Princess Margaret Hospital, Swindon in 1976. She has worked as a midwife ever since, more recently as a Diabetes Specialist Midwife in Leicester. She has acted as a CEMACH panellist and undertakes regular audits of the diabetes antenatal clinics in Leicester. She has co-authored several published abstracts describing aspects of the service.

Miranda Hayer MSc RGN RM
Consultant Midwife, Teenage Pregnancy and Sexual Health, Honorary Senior Lecturer at De Montfort University

Miranda trained as a nurse in 1985 and as a midwife in 1990. She has worked in a number of hospital and community midwifery settings before completing her MSc in Midwifery at Nottingham University. The post of Consultant Midwife in Leicester has enabled Miranda to concentrate on providing specialised services for particularly vulnerable groups and lecture on public health, teenage pregnancy and vulnerable groups, drugs and alcohol abuse, sexual health and child protection.

Juliet Houghton MSc Dip RGN RSCN ENB:934
Recently the Child and Family HIV/Hepatitis Specialist Nurse at UHL NHS Trust, and now the Coordinator of the CHIVA/KZN Support and Mentoring Initiative based in Durban, South Africa

Juliet worked on neonatal units and a paediatric oncology ward before qualifying in HIV nursing. She then attained a Diploma in Tropical Nursing at the London School of Hygiene and Tropical Medicine. More recently, she has graduated from Brunel University with an MSc in the Social Anthropology of Children and Child Development. Juliet won the medical category of the Barnardo's Children's Champion award for 2005.

Veronica Johnson-Roffey BA(Hons) RGN RM RHV FETC DipInfection Control
Infection Control Lead Nurse, Northamptonshire NHS Trust

Veronica has worked in the NHS for 30 years. After general nurse training she trained and practised as a midwife and later health visitor and consequently has worked both in hospital and the community. During her career she has also worked at Great Ormond Street Children's Hospital and also specialised in cancer genetics, public health and infection control. While a public health nurse she undertook her honours degree in Health and Social Policy at Warwick University. Currently she is lead nurse for infection control.

Rosemary Lydall RGN RM BA(Hons)
Education and Practice Development Facilitator – Women's Perinatal and Sexual Health Directorate, University Hospitals of Leicester

After working as a staff nurse in orthopaedics, Rosemary trained as a midwife in 1985. Rosemary is experienced in all areas of midwifery within the hospital setting, and has an interest in gastrointestinal disorders. In 2000, Rosemary became a Supervisor of Midwives at the University Hospitals of Leicester, which enhances her current role as Education and Practice Development Facilitator for Midwifery. This educational role provides support and education for midwives, medical staff and midwifery care assistants, in the classroom and the working environment.

Jo Matharu BA(Hons) PsychAdv DipHEMidwifery PGradCertMidwifery RM
Specialist Midwife – Hypertension, University Hospitals of Leicester LRIMH

Since qualifying in Nottingham, Jo's midwifery roles have included Community Midwife, Fetal Assessment Midwife, Delivery Suite Coordinator and Obstetric Triage Lead. The experience gained within these posts has allowed Jo to develop her passion for caring for women with high-risk pregnancies and teaching and extending colleagues' knowledge of women with medical disorders.

Moira McLean RGN RM ADM ENB:402 PGCEA MTD PGDip SoM
Senior Lecturer in Midwifery and Programme Leader at De Montfort University

Moira trained as a nurse and midwife in Scotland. After ten years midwifery practice in Cambridge she moved into education and has been teaching student midwives for over 20 years. She has specialist interest in normal midwifery, all intrapartum care issues, fetal heart monitoring, bereavement care and neonatal resuscitation. She is an external examiner to two centres, and in 2005 was short-listed for excellence in teaching by the RCM. Until recently she maintained a caseload of mothers in clinical practice, and is currently a voluntary breast-feeding advisor and Bank Midwife at Rosie Hospital, Cambridge.

Marian Parrish RGN RM DMS
Ward Manager at the University Hospitals of Leicester NHS Trust

Marian completed her general nurse training in Trafford General Hospital and was a staff nurse in a rehabilitation unit before undertaking midwifery training in Shropshire. She now manages a 32-bed antenatal and postnatal ward for complicated pregnancies at Leicester General Maternity Hospital. She has recently completed a post-graduate Diploma in Management Studies.

Jane Scullion BA(Hons) RGN MSc
Respiratory Nurse Consultant at University Hospitals of Leicester NHS Trust; Honorary Senior Lecturer at De Montfort University; Clinical Research Fellow at Aberdeen University

Jane Scullion is a Respiratory Nurse Consultant working across the interface of primary and secondary care with patients with chronic respiratory diseases and developing respiratory services. She has published widely and presented both nationally and internationally.

Diane Todd BSc(Hons) DipHE RM RGN
Specialist Midwife – Diabetes at the University Hospitals of Leicester NHS Trust

Diane trained as a staff nurse in 1984 and gained several years experience in surgical speciality and intensive care nursing, after which she chose a career in midwifery. Qualifying in 1992 much of her practice has focused on high-risk pregnancies, in particular those women who have diabetes. As part of a multi-disciplinary team she has further developed the care and service offered to these women, winning a Trent Travel Award in 1995, for a Leicester team to visit Edinburgh Royal Infirmary to learn more about pre-conception clinics and actively participating in the recent CEMACH Diabetes in pregnancy study. She has also undertaken specific courses to enhance her knowledge and skills and has presented at national and international levels.

Foreword

Despite the considerable advances in maternity care, and world-class maternity services provided by highly trained and motivated health care professionals, good maternal health is not a given or a universal right even in countries with high quality functioning maternity services with their attendant very low maternal mortality and morbidity rates. And whilst we would all hope that pregnancy, birth and the early weeks of parenthood would be enjoyable and relatively comfortable experiences for new mothers, babies and families we know, sadly, that this is not always the case.

Not all mothers start pregnancy in the best of health, and others develop problems as they go along. The latest Confidential Enquiry into Maternal Deaths Report for 2003–2005, Saving Mothers' Lives, shows that more of our mothers died from pre-existing, or new, medical conditions aggravated by pregnancy than from the big obstetric killers of the past such as haemorrhage, sepsis and pre-eclampsia. These so-called 'indirect' maternal deaths have outnumbered those from causes directly related to pregnancy for more than 10 years. And each death is just the tip of the iceberg of severe morbidity and complications. In the last Saving Mothers' Lives report more women died from cardiac disease than from any other cause, including the leading 'directly' associated cause thrombo-embolism, and deaths from acquired heart disease brought on by unhealthy lifestyles and obesity are increasing at an alarming rate. These findings show that whilst the lessons for the management of common obstetric conditions have clearly had an impact in the past, maternity professionals need to be more aware of the impact of, and identification and management of medical conditions affecting pregnancy before conception and during and after pregnancy. This is what this book aims to achieve.

A number of factors have led to the increase in the proportion of pregnant women or new mothers who have more medically complex pregnancies. They include rising numbers of older or obese mothers, women whose lifestyles put them at risk of poorer health and a growing proportion of women with serious underlying medical conditions who would not have chosen, or have been able to become pregnant in the past. The rising numbers of births to women born outside the UK also affects the underlying general level of maternal health as these mothers often have more complicated pregnancies, more serious underlying medical conditions or may be in poorer general health.

This publication is therefore extremely timely. Its authors are to be congratulated for developing a highly readable, informative and practical book each chapter of which, in the best traditions of maternity care, has been written jointly by a midwife and obstetrician. Such partnership working is emphasised throughout the book, with a clear focus on each other's respective roles and responsibilities within the clinical team. The need for pre-pregnancy counselling and preparation for women living with conditions that are adversely affected by pregnancy, or which ideally require a change in treatment or medication prior to conception is also rightly highlighted as an important, but often overlooked aspect of obstetric medicine. Midwives, obstetricians and all other maternity team members together with those with a general interest in pregnancy and birth should find this book informative and easy to read. Acting on the important messages continued within each chapter should help lead to wider improvements in the understanding and management of mothers who need extra care to ensure they have as healthy and happy pregnancies, birth and babies as possible.

Gwyneth Lewis MBBS, MSc, MRCGP, FFPHM, FRCOG
National Director for Maternal Health, England
Director of the United Kingdom Confidential Enquiries
into Maternal Deaths

Preface

Midwives are practising in a rapidly changing world with advances in technology, increasing expectations of mothers and pressure to provide a cost-effective service in state-funded health sectors. A modern maternity service that is flexible and adaptable with midwives open to both learning and change is advocated[1]. Innovative schemes of care have been developed, such as case-holding midwifery, concentrating on normal childbearing that foster autonomy in the midwife's practice.

The nature of the child-bearing woman is also changing, with women delaying pregnancy until their thirties and forties and sometimes beyond[2]. Whilst fertility and obstetrical aspects of such a delay are well documented, the association with medical disorders warrants attention. Advancing maternal age increases risk of chronic medical conditions[3]. A medical disorder can subsequently complicate pregnancy, or it can present for the first time in pregnancy[4].

Knowledge of medical conditions is therefore necessary, first to avoid mothers being booked inappropriately for low-risk midwifery care schemes, and second for midwives to recognise the signs of deterioration in order to take principled action. The *Why Mothers Die* report found *'some midwives and junior obstetricians failed to pick up and act upon warning signs of common medical conditions unrelated to pregnancy'*[5]. Associations between medical conditions and mortality are outlined in Appendix 1.1.

Ironically, a midwife is increasingly likely to encounter women with a medical disorder at a time when the pool of dual-qualified nurse-midwives is diminishing in the UK. This should place emphasis on inclusion of medical disorders within midwifery direct entry education programmes, although curriculum guidelines place emphasis on normality[6]. Indeed, the value of medical placements for student midwives was established[7] in 1996, and individual British midwifery courses may run a module covering medical disorders sometimes addressed as 'altered health states'.

Until 2008, no textbook on pre-existing medical disorders written *specifically for midwives* existed. Our experience in Leicester found student midwives unenthusiastic about standard medical textbooks, due to the lack of midwifery emphasis, and they resorted to home internet use with inherent risk of simplistic understanding. Poor computer and internet access for midwives and lack of confidence with accessing the NHSnet is well identified[8] as are concerns about the reliability and credibility of some medical information on the internet[9].

This led to the decision to create a book specifically for midwives and student midwives, using local and national expertise from midwives, obstetricians and physicians. In Leicester and other parts of the UK there is a well-developed system of high-risk specialist antenatal services to provide care for women with potential medical complications in pregnancy. Care in these clinics is multi-disciplinary, and care pathways are tailored to individual maternal needs.

The multi-professional authorship suits the current ethos for *'educating for professional pluralism to minimise arrogance and dominance without diluting professional uniqueness'*.[10] Necessity for an inter-professional culture has already been established[11] with a need to improve teamwork in the maternity services[12]. It is the aim of this book to contribute towards this.

Such a book may invite scrutiny, as midwives are identified as being practitioners of normality. Midwives interested in complicated pregnancy might find themselves dubbed 'medwife' rather than midwife! However, midwifery responsibilities include *'Maximising normality for women in high dependency care'* and *'Recognising deviations from normal. Making appropriate referral and working as equal partners in a multi-disciplinary team.'*[1]

With the midwifery emphasis, there are some differences from traditional medical textbooks. In particular, differential diagnosis has not been addressed as this is very much the art of medicine. We have taken the stance that most women will already have had their medical disorder diagnosed when she meets the midwife at the booking appointment.

The book is divided into chapters, then into sections using a template for each medical condition. The first page of each is predominately non-pregnancy, giving an explanation of the condition (which might include investigations), complications and non-pregnancy treatment, and then preconception care is addressed. The second page identifies key issues pertinent to the ante-, intra- and postpartum periods in the left-hand column. Then in the right-hand column the management and care by both midwife and doctor is outlined. This allows a midwife to go quickly to the access point, for all the conditions, which often suits pressurised practice circumstances. Each chapter has its own appendix which addresses additional factors that did not fit the template concept. This text concentrates on facts and essential action, so midwives will need to consult more substantial texts for in-depth understanding.

Risk scoring is complicated[13] but the terms low- and high-risk are used daily, so each section identifies risk as low, variable, high or life-threatening. This allows a midwife to recognise the potential severity of a condition immediately, which will influence decisions at the booking interview.

We could not cover all conditions, and some inclusions are not strictly speaking medical disorders, e.g. alcohol and drug abuse. However Appendix 16.1 showing associations with infant death should make the reasons behind their inclusion apparent.

The book is intended for midwives practising on British and European Union influenced models, where the midwife is part of a multi-disciplinary team referring mothers with problems to a doctor and assisting the latter where appropriate[14]. Therefore, midwives in the EU, UK and British Commonwealth should find the book beneficial, with appropriate allowances for national differences.

Acknowledgements

In addition to the sterling work of the contributors we have received assistance and guidance from the practitioners below, who have been generous with their time and advice in relation to specialist subjects. We are truly indebted to:

Alison Kinder MRCP MB BS BMedSci
Consultant Rheumatologist at the University Hospitals of Leicester NHS Trust

Sue Dyson RGN RM BSc EdE MSc PhD
Principal Lecturer in Nursing at De Montfort University, and Research Associate at the Unit for Social Study of Thalassaemia and Sickle Cell

Barbara Howard RGN RM BSc ENB:405,904,998
Neonatal Lecturer–Practitioner at the University Hospitals of Leicester NHS Trust

Jean Johnson MCSP
Service Lead of the Women's Health Physiotherapy Team at University Hospitals of Leicester NHS Trust

Debbie Frost RGN RM BSc(Hons)
Midwifery Practice Development Facilitator at the University Hospitals of Leicester NHS Trust

Jo Smith RGN RM
Midwife at Leicester Royal Infirmary

Alison Sheppard RGN MSc BSc(Hons)
Tutor in Health/Social Care at Gateway College, Leicester

We would like to extend our gratitude to the many colleagues at the Universities Hospitals of Leicester and De Montfort University who have answered queries and given advice and moral support.

Furthermore we would like to thank the associations and institutions addressed in the appendices for giving their assistance, and in all cases have waived a copyright fee for reproducing their material enabling the book to be kept at an affordable price for students and midwives.

Editing of the book had considerable impact upon domestic life, and completion would not have been possible without significant spousal support. We are truly appreciative of Kate Waugh for all her forbearance and support, and Matthew Broughton for his endless patience, editing exercises and repeated proofreading.

Acronyms and Abbreviations

Abbreviations in the main narrative, or in daily use

ABO	A, B and O blood groups
ABU	Asymptomatic Bacteruria
aCL	Anticardiolipin Antibodies
ADHD	Attention Deficiency Hyperactive Disorder
AFP	Alpha Feto-protein
Ag	Antigen
AIDS	Acquired Immune Deficiency Syndrome
ALT	Alanine Transaminase (a liver enzyme)
ANA	Antinuclear Antibody
ANC	Antenatal (prenatal) Clinic or Care
Anti-Ro/La	Lupus antibodies Ro and La
APA	Antiphospholipid Antibodies
APAH	Associated Pulmonary Arterial Hypertension
APH	Antepartum Haemorrhage
APS	Antiphospholipid (Hughes) Syndrome
AR	Aortic Regurgitation
ARDS	Acute Respiratory Distress Syndrome
ARM	Artificial Rupture of Membranes
AS	Aortic Stenosis
ASD	Atrial Septal Defect
AST	Aspartate Transaminase (a liver enzyme)
BMD	Bone Mineral (measurement) Density
BMI	Body Mass Index (formally Quetelet Scale)
BP	Blood Pressure
C1,2,etc.	Cervical vertebrae number one, two, etc.
C1,2,etc.	Complement one, two, etc. levels
CAM	Complementary and Alternative Medicine
CAPS	Catastrophic Antiphospholipid Syndrome
CAT/CT	Computerised Axial Tomography (scan)
CD	Crohn's Disease
CF	Cystic Fibrosis
CHB	Congenital Heart Block
CHD	Coronary Heart Disease
CHF/CCF	Congestive Heart Failure (Cardiac)
CHT	Chronic Hypertension
CJD	Creutzfeldt–Jakob Disease
CKD	Chronic Kidney Disease
CMV	Cytomegalovirus
CNS	Central Nervous System
CO	Cardiac Output
CPR	Cardiopulmonary Resuscitation
CREST	Calcinosis, Raynaud's, Oesophageal dysmotility, Sclerodactyly & Telangiectasia
CRP	C-Reactive Protein
CTG	Cardiotocograph
CTPA	Computed Tomographic Pulmonary Angiography
CVA	Cerebrovascular Accident
CVP	Central Venous Pressure
DIC	Disseminated Intravascular Coagulation
DLE	Discoid Lupus Erythematosus
DNA	Deoxyribonucleic Acid
DOE	Dyspnoea On Exertion
DVT	Deep Vein Thrombosis
ECG	Electrocardiograph
EDD	Expected Date of Delivery/confinement
EEG	Electroencephalogram
EF	Ejection Fraction (heart)
EFM	Electronic Fetal Monitoring (of fetal heart)
EPDS	Edinburgh Postnatal Depression Scale
ERCP	Endoscopic Retrograde Cholangiopancreatography
ERPC	Evacuate Retained Products of Conception
ESR	Erythrocyte Sedimentation Rate
FAE	Fetal Alcohol Effects
FAS	Fetal Alcohol Syndrome
FBC	Full Blood Count
FFP	Fresh Frozen Plasma
FH	Fetal Heart
FHR	Fetal Heart Rate
FMAIT	Feto-Maternal Alloimmune Thrombocytopenia
FPAH	Familial Pulmonary Arterial Hypertension
FSE	Fetal Scalp Electrode
fT3	Free Tri-iodothyronine (a thyroid hormone)
fT4	Free Throxine (a thyroid hormone)
FVL	Factor V Leiden (a clotting factor)
FVS	Fetal Varicella Syndrome
GD	Graves' Disease
GDM	Gestational Diabetes Mellitus
GFD	Gluten Free Diet
GFR	Glomerular Filtration Rate
GH	Genital Herpes (infection)
GnRH	Gonadotropin Releasing Hormone
GO	Graves' Ophthalmopathy
GORD	Gastro-oesophageal Reflux Disease
GTD	Gestational Trophoblastic Disease
GTT	Glucose Tolerance Test
GVH	Graft Versus Host (disease)
HAV, HBV	Hepatitis Virus type A, type B, etc.
Hb	Haemoglobin
HbA1c	Haemoglobin A1c (monitor blood glucose)
HBIG	Hepatitis B Immune Globulin
HCG	Human Chorionic Gonadotrophin
HD	Haemodialysis
HDU	High Dependency Unit
HELLP	Haemolysis, Elevated Liver enzymes Low Platelets
HF	Heart Failure
HIV	Human Immunodeficiency Virus
HRT	Hormone Replacement Therapy
HSV	Herpes Simplex Virus
IBD	Inflammatory Bowel Disease
IBS	Irritable Bowel Syndrome
ICD	Intracardiac Device
ICP	Intrahepatic Cholestasis of Pregnancy
Ig	Immunoglobulin (types A, E, D, G and M)
INR	International Normalized Ratio
IPAH	Idiopathic Pulmonary Arterial Hypertension
IQ	Intelligence Quotient
ITP	Immune Thrombocytopenic Purpura
IUCD	Intrauterine Contraceptive Device
IUFD	Intrauterine Fetal Death
IUGR	Intrauterine Growth Restriction/retardation
IUS	Intrauterine System (contraception)
JIA	Juvenile Idiopathic Arthritis
JRH	Juvenile Rheumatoid Arthritis

L1,2, etc.	Lumber vertebrae one, two, etc.
LA	Lupus Anticoagulants
LDH	Lactate Dehydrogenase
LFT	Liver Function Test
LHRH	Luteinizing Hormone Releasing Hormone
LSCS	Lower Section Caesarean Section
LV	Left Ventricle
MCM	Major Congenital Malformations
MCV	Mean Cell Volume
MRI	Magnetic Resonance Image (scan)
MS	Multiple Sclerosis
MS	Mitral Stenosis
MSU	or MSSU – Midstream Specimen of Urine
MVA	Mitral Valve Area
MVP	Mitral Valve Prolapse
NAS	Neonatal Abstinence Syndrome
OASI	Obstetric Anal Sphincter Injury
OC	Obstetric Cholestasis
OGTT	Oral Glucose Tolerance Test
PAH	Pulmonary Arterial Hypertension
PAPS	Primary Antiphospholipid Syndrome
PD	Peritoneal Dialysis
PDA	Patent Ductus Arteriosus (heart)
PE	Pulmonary Embolism
PEA	Pulseless Electrical Activity (heart)
PET	Pre-eclamptic Toxaemia
pH	Potential Hydrogen (measure acid/alkaline)
PH	Pulmonary Hypertension
PIH	Pregnancy Induced Hypertension
PKU	Phenylketonuria
PM	Pacemaker
PND	Paroxysmal Nocturnal Dyspnoea
PPH	Postpartum Haemorrhage
PS	Pulmonary Stenosis
PUVA	Psoralen with Ultraviolet A light
PVD	Pulmonary Vascular Disease
RA	Rheumatoid Arthritis
RBC	Red Blood Cell (erythrocyte)
RCT	Randomised Control Trial
Rh	Rhesus Factor (positive or negative)
SAH	Sub-arachnoid Haemorrhage
SAPS	Secondary Antiphospholipid Syndrome
SB	Serum Bilirubin
SCD	Sickle Cell Disease
SIDS	Sudden Infant Death Syndrome
SLE	Systemic Lupus Erythematosus
SRM	Spontaneous Rupture of Membranes
STI	Sexually Transmitted Infection
SV	Stroke Volume (heart)
T1DM	Type 1 Diabetes Mellitus
T2DM	Type 2 Diabetes Mellitus
T3	Tri-iodothyronine (a thyroid hormone)
T4	Throxine (a thyroid hormone)
TA	Truncus Arteriosus
TB	Tuberculosis
TED	Thromboembolic Disease
TEDS	Thromboembolic Disease Stockings
TENS	Transcutaneous Electrical Nerve Stimulation
TGA	Transposition of the Great Arteries
TIA	Transient Ischaemic Attack
ToF	Tetralogy of Fallot
ToP	Termination of Pregnancy
TPO	Thyroid Peroxidase
TRALI	Transfusion Related Acute Lung Injury
TSH	Thyroid Stimulating Hormone
TSHR	Thyroid Stimulating Hormone Receptor

TSIg	Thyroid Stimulating Immunoglobulin
UC	Ulcerative Colitis
U&E	Urea and Electrolyte (analysis)
USS	Ultrasound Scan
UTI	Urinary Tract Infection
UVA,B,C	Ultraviolet A or B or C waves
VDRL	Venereal Disease Research Laboratory
VF	Ventricular Fibrillation
VQ	Ventilation Perfusion
VSD	Ventricular Septal Defect (of heart)
VTE	Venous Thrombo-embolism
VWD	Von Willebrand's Disease
WBC	White Blood Cell (leucocyte)
Xa	Clotting Factor Ten, sub-set A

Abbreviations of Practitioners and Institutions

BHS	British Hypertension Society
BTS	British Thoracic Society
CEMACH	Confidential Enquiry Maternal Child Health
DoH	Department of Health (UK)
FSA	Food Standards Agency (UK)
GMC	General Medical Council (UK)
GP	General Practitioner
HV	Health Visitor/Public Health Nurse
ITU	Intensive Therapy Unit
MDT	Multi-disciplinary Team
NHS	National Health Service (UK)
NICE	National Institute for Clinical Excellence (UK)
NMC	Nursing and Midwifery Council (UK)
NNU	Neonatal Unit
NTIS	National Teratology Information System (UK)
NYHA	New York Heart Association (USA)
RCM	Royal College of Midwives
RCOG	Royal College of Obstetricians & Gynaecologists
SHOT	Serious Hazards of Transfusion
SIGN	Scottish Intercollegiate Guidelines Network
WHO	World Health Organisation

Drug Administration Abbreviations (Latin in *italics*)

bd	Twice a day	(*Bis die*)
tds	Three times a day	(*Ter die sumendus*)
qds	Four times a day	(*Quatre die sumendus*)
prn	As necessary	(*Pro re nata*)
po	By mouth	(*Per orum*)
pr	Rectally	(*Per rectum*)
pv	Vaginally	(*Per vaginum*)
im	Intramuscular	
iv	Intravenous	
IVI	Intravenous infusion	
nocte	At night	
sc	Subcutaneous	
stat	At once	

Measurement Abbreviations

FL	Fluid
fl	Femtolitre
g/dl	Grams per decilitre
IU	International Units
IU/l	International Units per litre
kg	Kilogram
mg	Milligrams
mg/l	Milligrams per litre
ml	Millilitre
mmHg	Millimetres of Mercury
mmol/l	Millimoles per litre

| ng/ml | Nanograms per millilitre |
| nM/l | Nanograms per litre |

Drug and Immunisation Abbreviations

6MP	Six-Mercaptopurine
ACEI	Angiotensin Converting Enzyme Inhibitors
AED	Antiepileptic Drug
ARB	Angiotensin Receptor Blockers
ARV	Anti-Retroviral drug
AZT	Azidothymidine
BCG	Immunisation to prevent tuberculosis
CBZ	Carbimazole
CD	Controlled Drug
COCP	Combined Oral Contraceptive Pill
CSII	Continuous Subcutaneous Insulin Infusion

DMARD	Disease Modifying Anti-Rheumatic Drug
H_2RA	Histamine$_2$-Receptor Antagonist
HBIG	Hepatitis B Immune Globulin
IVIG	Intravenous Immunoglobulin
LMWH	Low Molecular Weight Heparin
MAOI	Monoamine Oxidase Inhibitor
NSAID	Non-steroidal Anti-inflammatory Drug
OTC	Over-the-Counter (drug)
POM	Prescription Only Medicine
POP	Progesterone Only (contraceptive) Pill
PPI	Proton-Pump Inhibitor
PTU	Propylthiouracil
SSRI	Selective Serotonin Reuptake Inhibitor
TNF	Tumour Necrosis Factor (inhibitor)
VZIg	Varicella zoster Immunoglobulin

MIDWIFERY CARE AND MEDICAL DISORDERS

1

S. Elizabeth Robson

Pre-conception Care
Antenatal Care
Intrapartum Care
Postnatal Care
General Considerations
Emergency Management
Preventing Maternal Mortality

1 Midwifery Care and Medical Disorders

INTRODUCTION

This chapter will give an overview of pre-conception, antenatal, intrapartum and postnatal care that would be given to a woman with a medical condition that either pre-exists or presents in pregnancy. The information here will not be repeated in each subject section, which will focus on the aspects specific to that particular medical disorder.

PRE-CONCEPTION CARE

In an ideal world all women would receive state-funded pre-conception care, however, about 50% of pregnancies are unplanned[1], and most women seek medical or midwifery attention once pregnant. For certain groups such as recent immigrants this first contact may happen late in the pregnancy[2].

For a woman with an existing medical disorder the need for pre-conception care is more pronounced, and early booking once pregnant is of paramount importance, as the disorder can affect the pregnancy and conversely the pregnancy can affect the disorder[3]. A woman with a previously well-controlled condition can become unstable with a domino effect on the pregnancy. Hence, such women should be advised to seek pre-conception advice from 'mainstream' medical or midwifery care prior to ceasing use of contraception.

In British practice a woman contemplating pregnancy may consult her general practitioner, practice nurse or midwife. Practice policies vary considerably[4], but can be summarised as follows:

1) *Nurse/midwife taking a history[5] to ascertain:*

- Medical, surgical, psychological or infectious conditions that could complicate a future pregnancy, including any current medications or treatment
- Family history of disease and handicap, including genetic history
- Vaccination status
- Substance use, e.g. alcohol, cigarettes and street drugs
- Past obstetric and gynaecological history
- Present employment – to identify occupational hazards
- Current diet and nutritional history
- Lifestyle, including diet and exercise

2) *Nurse/midwife observations and medical examination for:*

- Weight and height measurement for calculation of the Body Mass Index (BMI) (see Appendix 13)
- Baseline pulse, blood pressure, urinalysis measurement
- Pelvic examination to include a cervical smear and screening for infection such as *Chlamydia*
- Respiratory and cardiac function
- Other function screening – if history indicates
- Karotyping – if indicated by family history

- Blood samples for full blood count (FBC), VDRL and rubella
- If indicated, additional screening for TB, hepatitis B, HIV, chickenpox, cytomegalovirus and toxoplasma
- Haemoglobinopathy screening for women originating from: Africa, West Indies, Indian subcontinent, Asia, Eastern Mediterranean countries and the Middle East. If affected, partner screening should be offered with genetic counselling[6]

3) *Interventions that are advocated:*

- Folic acid: advise 0.4 mg daily[1]
- Vaccination, such as rubella or BCG for TB, dependent upon aforementioned antibody titres
- Contraceptive cover while investigations and treatment are initiated

4) *In relation to medical disorders, the doctor will usually:*

- Act upon any anomalies detected in the baseline observations and order additional tests such as glucose tolerance test (GTT) and initiate treatment
- Refer the woman back to any specialist clinic and physician who has previously treated her; immigrant women may need referral for the first time.
- Review current drug therapy to identify those on drugs associated with teratogenic effects or contraindicated in pregnancy, and initiate change
- Increase the folic acid dosage for a history of neural tube defects, haemoglobinopathies, rheumatoid arthritis, coeliac disease, diabetes or epilepsy
- Prescribe suitable contraceptive cover whilst the above is addressed
- Initiate counselling about prognosis for both mother and prospective child

5) *Specific advice, from a nurse/midwife, in relation to:*

- Keeping a menstrual diary
- Pregnancy testing and need for early booking
- Perinatal diagnosis – practical aspects
- Smoking and alcohol cessation
- Street drug avoidance and cessation
- Over-the-counter medicines and therapies
- Domestic violence
- Stress avoidance
- Sport, exercise and general fitness
- Occupational hazards
- Animal contact and infection risk
- Food hygiene and hand washing
- Weight adjustment
- Health education initiatives and leaflets
- Patient organisations, e.g. *Foresight*, with additional options such as hair analysis for mineral deficiencies[7]

ANTENATAL CARE

Antenatal care on the British model has followed the same basis for much of the twentieth century[8]. A woman reports a positive pregnancy test to her general practitioner (GP) then has a 'booking history' conducted by a midwife. Options for place of care and delivery are discussed and the mother should be offered choice of birth at a consultant unit, low-risk birth centre or at home. Risk for childbearing will be taken into consideration to avoid inappropriate bookings which are associated with maternal death (see Appendices 1.1 and 1.2). The mother is referred to an obstetrician and may have one appointment at a consultant clinic. Responsibility for care is shared between GP and obstetrician, hence the term *shared care*. Most appointments occur in the community at the GP premises with the midwife actually conducting the majority of the antenatal care, referring to either GP or obstetrician if problems are identified. Specialist investigations, such as ultrasonography and amniocentesis are conducted at a consultant unit, often in conjunction with an antenatal or specialist clinic.

Variations on care exist, with Domino, case-holding midwifery, and team-midwifery schemes aiming for women-centred care with continuity of carer and a focus on normality. Women on such schemes should have normal, uncomplicated pregnancies and a significant medical condition precludes inclusion on such a low-risk scheme.

With few exceptions a mother with a medical condition will require pregnancy management and care with involvement of hospital consultants. Some mothers may need to have some of their antenatal appointments at a specialist antenatal clinic, or at other clinics that combine obstetric care with involvement from a physician. Examples of such *combined clinics* are for diabetes and renal problems.

Such mothers tend to fit into a risk category of variable or high risk. Here an assumption might be made, wrongly, that no midwifery involvement is necessary, and in recent times the numbers of midwives and student midwives at high-risk clinics appears to have reduced. Whilst it might seem cost effective to have an auxiliary nurse chaperoning at a clinic and performing manual tasks, the knowledge and skills of a midwife should not be denied to a mother because she has a medical disorder and has a stereotypical label of risk.

The mother requires midwifery care and should be given the opportunity to build a rapport with a midwife and to get continuity of care as she would on a midwife-led scheme. The care that the midwife gives should be complementary to that of the obstetricians and physicians, with the mother and fetus being the cherished focus of attention.

Booking

The midwife must take and document a detailed, accurate booking history[10] which should encompass:

- Personal details – including name, address, date of birth, occupation, marital status, religion, GP, and official numbers such as National Insurance. Race is ascertained for screening of racially-specific conditions.
- Social factors – late booking, asylum seeker, drug misuse, domestic violence, known to social services, and other risk factors (see Appendix 1.1) of consequence.
- Histories – family, medical, surgical, psychological, gynaecological and obstetric histories; cross-reference with GP case notes or hospital records if access is possible. Medical records from other geographical areas may have to be obtained.

- Identification of risk factors for mother and fetus, which should encompass bio-physical factors, especially pre-existing medical disorders and current medication.
- Ascertain any hospital clinics previously attended in relation to a medical disorder or surgical operation. Determine if the mother is still attending, and discuss with the GP if the mother needs to be re-referred.
- Ascertain any pre-conception advice and care given.
- Calculate the expected date of delivery (EDD) from the menstrual history.

Be aware that a mother might not be fully forthcoming about an existing medical condition, or prognosis, if the booking history takes place with her husband/partner or in-laws in attendance. Any language translation should be conducted by a trained interpreter rather than a friend or relative. A mother may want certain details omitted from her handheld records if her domestic situation entails that her records would be viewed by family members – necessitating full details in the hospital records as a 'duplicate'[11].

A physical examination will identify baseline observations:

- General appearance and wellbeing
- Pulse and blood pressure
- MSU and urinalysis
- Weight
- Abdominal examination – to determine if the uterus is palpable and equates to dates

The doctor may additionally examine to determine:

- cardiac function
- lung function

NB: Pelvic examinations are no longer performed unless there is a specific indication to do so[8].

The following serum investigations[6] will be offered to the mother after explanation and informed consent:

- Identification of blood group and Rhesus factor
- Full blood count (FBC)
- Antibodies for rubella, hepatitis B, syphilis, and HIV
- Haemoglobinopathy screening for at-risk ethnic groups

Additional screening may be discussed and offered for:

- Down's syndrome risk
- Ultrasound for gestational age assessment
- Ultrasound for fetal structural anomalies after 16 weeks

Careful consideration is given as to where the mother is booked for antenatal care and for delivery. Mothers with a medical condition may be referred for antenatal care wholly or partly at a specialist antenatal or combined clinic (Table 1.1). The midwife should share ideas with the mother on a specific model of care, and discuss and agree a realistic birth plan.

Issues specific to antenatal screening are discussed. Then further advice is given in relation to:

- Occupation hazards
- Animal contact and infection risk
- Healthy diet with vitamins (Appendix 1.3) and safe eating
- Handwashing and food hygiene
- Domestic violence
- Smoking, alcohol and street drug cessation
- Sport, exercise and stress avoidance
- Maternity benefits
- Attending antenatal education parent-craft classes
- Important telephone and contact details

Table 1.1 Referral guide for specialist clinics*

Maternal Medicine Clinic	Fetal Assessment Unit
Neurological disorders, especially:	Previous fetal abnormality (live birth or ToP)
Epilepsy	Family history of genetic conditions
Multiple sclerosis	Monochorionic twins
Myasthenia gravis	Positive rhesus antibodies
Myotonic dystrophy	Homeless women and travellers (with no GP)
Cardiac disease, especially:	
Cardiomyopathy	**General Obstetric Clinic**
Congenital heart disease	Grand multiparity of >5
Marfan's syndrome	Previous stillbirth
Rheumatic heart disease	Previous abruption
Prosthetic valves	Previous precipitate labour
Gastrointestinal disease, especially:	Previous shoulder dystocia
Coeliac disease	Previous rotational forceps
Ulcerative colitis	Previous 3rd or 4th degree tear or other perineal morbidity
Crohn's disease	Previous retained placenta
Rheumatological/auto-immune disease, especially:	Previous primary postpartum haemorrhage (PPH)
Rheumatoid arthritis	Previous difficult labour/vaginal delivery
Systemic lupus erythematosus	Previous gynaecological surgery, other than fertility treatment
Severe back problem – including kyphoscoliosis	Previous caesarean sections
Liver and pancreatic disease – especially cholestasis	
Malignancy (current or previous)	**Specialist Obstetric Clinic** (Prematurity Prevention)
Substance misuse	Last pregnancy a pre-term birth (≤34 weeks)
	Last pregnancy a mid-trimester miscarriage
Specialist Obstetric Clinic (Fetal Growth)	Known uterine malformation
Previous small baby <2.5 kg at term	First pregnancy after a cone biopsy
Maternal weight <45 kg	
>2 first trimester miscarriages	**Specialist Gynaecology/Obstetrics Clinic**
Previous unexplained stillbirth	Multiple pregnancy
	Tubal surgery
	In vitro fertilisation pregnancies
Diabetes and Endocrine Clinic	Previous myomectomy
Diabetes mellitus	
Diabetes insipidus	**Hypertension Clinic**
Thyroid disorders	Booking BP >138/85
Pituitary disorders	Primigravidae with a mother or sister who had pre-eclampsia
Adrenal disorders	Primigravidae with hypertension outside of pregnancy
	Past obstetric history of raised blood pressure requiring
Haematology Clinic	treatment
Immune thrombocytopenic purpura (ITP)	
Von Willebrand's disease	**Renal Clinic**
Carriers of haemophilia	Any pre-existing renal disease
Antiphospholipid (Hughes) syndrome	Renal transplantation or dialysis patients
Hereditary thrombophilia	History of reflux nephropathy
Family history of thrombosis	Recurrent urinary tract infection
Acute thrombosis in pregnancy	Persistent first trimester proteinuria
Refractory anaemia	
Sickle cell disease	**Specialist/Consultant Midwife Referral**
Thalassaemia	Age ≤16 years
Low platelet count (<100 × 10^9/l) or rapidly falling platelet count	Age 17–19 years with housing or social issues, or any concerns to specialist or consultant midwife for teenage pregnancy
	Substance misuse – to drug liaison midwife
Anaesthetic Clinic	Hypertension – hypertension specialist midwife
Previous adverse drug reaction	Diabetes – to diabetic specialist midwife
Previous regional or GA problems	
Secondary referral from other clinic	

* Referral guide used for University Hospitals of Leicester, adapted and used with permission

Subsequent Antenatal Appointments

The frequency of routine antenatal visits has come under recent scrutiny, emphasising that schemes of care should be based on evidence rather than ritual[12]. However, recent research finds women actually wanting more frequent antenatal appointments, ultrasonic scans and support from their midwives[13].

Current UK recommendations[9] for routine antenatal care advocate visits at the following weeks of gestation. The regimen will vary between areas, but approximates to:

Week 8–12

- Initial booking with confirmation of pregnancy, identification of risk factors, and investigations as per previous page

Week 16

- BP and urinalysis
- AFP/serum screening for Down's risk
- Possibly ultrasound scan for fetal anomalies
- Discuss results from the booking blood tests

Week 18–20

- Discuss results from AFP or Down's risk
- Ultrasound scans for fetal anomalies, if not already done

Week 24–25

- Full antenatal examination to ascertain maternal well-being and to include BP, urinalysis, oedema, abdominal examination with symphysis pubis height measurement, fetal movements asked about and the fetal heart auscultated

Week 28

- Full antenatal examination as above
- FBC and antibody screen
- First dose of anti-D for rhesus negative women

Week 31–32

- Full antenatal examination as above

Week 34

- Full antenatal examination as above
- FBC and antibody screen
- Second dose of anti-D for rhesus negative women

Week 36

- Full antenatal examination as above, with emphasis on fetal position and presentation
- FBC

Week 38 (repeat at 40 weeks for nulliparae)

- Full antenatal examination as above

Week 41

- Full antenatal examination as above
- Assessment for induction of labour or increased fetal surveillance

A mother with a medical condition will require the same obstetric and midwifery care as a mother with a low-risk pregnancy on the above schedule, but with *additional* management and care from the specialists and the multidisciplinary team. Therefore midwives should consider:

- Arranging clinic appointments for both specialist clinics and antenatal clinics so that there is even spacing between them. These appointments should be made at a frequency suitable for the complexity of the medical condition and any additional fetal screening required
- If handheld notes are used the mother should be advised to keep these with her at all times
- Ensure the woman understands her condition, and the additional impact that pregnancy can have on the condition and vice versa. Further education may be necessary on a one-to-one basis
- Provide written information or leaflets to reinforce the advice given, seeking leaflets translated into other languages where necessary
- Ensure the woman understands signs and symptoms that may indicate the condition worsening, and give information on whom to contact, and what to do
- Accept that many women are fully informed about their medical condition and will be the first person to recognise an alteration in the condition
- Take the concerns of the woman and her husband/partner seriously
- Advise relatives, with the mother's consent, of acute situations that may arise, such as thrombo-embolism or an epileptic seizure, in which the mother may need emergency assistance, and give directions on first aid and whom to contact
- Be aware of, and report, any signs, symptoms and complications of a medical condition
- Carry out any treatment prescribed by the doctor, reinforcing any medical advice given. Be aware that many medical conditions have periods of remission and some mothers might be tempted to cease taking prescribed treatment if they feel their condition is stable or 'cured'. Always seek medical advice before acquiescing with any maternal decisions in relation to altering prescribed treatment
- Effective inter-disciplinary teamwork is of paramount importance for maximum feto-maternal benefit, so effective care pathways need to be established
- Normality is still possible for many aspects of the antenatal periods and labour and it is the midwife's duty to determine how best to empower the mother to achieve maximum fulfilment from her pregnancy and to make the process as natural as possible under the circumstances

INTRAPARTUM CARE

The medical condition may necessitate an elective caesarean section for many mothers. Some mothers may require induction of labour at, or before, term, dependent upon the condition and feto-maternal wellbeing during the antenatal period. Others may be able to labour normally. In these cases intrapartum care for labouring women with any other than a low-risk categorisation of a medical disorder should encompass:

- Delivery to be planned for a consultant unit with emergency facilities for both mother and baby
- The mother should have one-to-one care from a midwife, with adequate relief for breaks
- Care should be competent, compassionate and caring, with astute observation and vigilance in determining any deviations from anticipated progress
- Accurate history taking on admission to delivery suite to determine the onset and nature of the labour as well as feto-maternal wellbeing
- Baseline observations on admission of maternal temperature, pulse, blood pressure, urinalysis, oedema, and general wellbeing
- Full antenatal examination to include abdominal palpation and auscultation of the fetal heart
- Review of maternal case notes to ascertain the birth plan and care pathways for the medical and midwifery management of the medical condition in labour
- The mother would be seen by a member of the obstetric team as a matter of course, but also ascertain if a physician, paediatrician, anaesthetist or the neonatal unit needs to be informed that this mother is in labour
- Any specified treatment regimen should be implemented with full knowledge of the obstetric team on duty
- Seek medical advice before empowering the mother to eat during labour, as many such women have a high chance of operative delivery; often the mother may be on water *only* by mouth regimen
- Keep the mother well hydrated with water orally, or an iv infusion in line with medical guidance
- Prophylactic treatment to reduce acid content of the stomach, e.g. ranitidine 150 mg orally qds
- Assessment of first stage progress by abdominal palpation to assess descent, and vaginal examination at least four hourly, with results plotted on a partogram
- Abnormal progress of any of the three stages of labour must be reported to the obstetric team
- Suitable pain relief that is compatible with the planned treatment regimen
- Apt mobilisation of the mother whenever possible, or passive leg exercises if the mother has an epidural *in situ,* or is otherwise immobile
- Position should be changed regularly, and wedges placed under the mattress to prevent the mother's lying *flat on her back* resulting in pressure on the inferior vena cava leading to reduced uterine blood flow
- Some mothers may require TED stockings, especially if she is obese or has a history of thrombo-embolism
- Assistance to walk to the toilet, or bedpans, should be offered every two hours, with the urine measured and tested on every occasion
- Regular (hourly) observations of pulse and blood pressure, with temperature recorded at least four hourly

- Additional observations may be required in relation to the specific medical condition
- Monitoring of fetal wellbeing will, in most cases, necessitate continuous fetal heart monitoring throughout the first stage of labour
- Basic hygiene and comfort should be attended to regularly; if the mother is not mobile enough to use the shower, then a bowl and towel should be brought and the mother assisted to wash
- Water immersion in labour is discouraged because the mother does not meet the low-risk criteria[14]
- A normal vertex delivery can be managed by the midwife unless additional complications result
- The cord is usually clamped twice and cut, the baby dried and given to parents for a 'cuddle', if the condition permits
- The baby should have Apgar scores calculated at one and five minutes of life, and a low score should necessitate resuscitative measures and a paediatrician being called urgently
- The baby should be weighed and examined by a midwife to determine if there are any apparent abnormalities, and if the baby is making adequate adaptation to extra-uterine life
- Identification bracelets should be applied, having first been checked with the parents
- Third stage of labour often entails *active management* as this is not a low-risk labour and the midwife should check that the drugs used are compatible with the condition, e.g. Syntometrine is contraindicated with a number of conditions because of vaso-spasm[15], and Syntocinon may be prescribed instead
- The placenta and membranes should be examined for completeness and for signs of abnormality[15]; if there is any doubt the placenta should be retained for examination by a member of the obstetric team
- Be aware that after delivery specific blood samples might be required from the placenta, and advice should be sought if in doubt
- Post-delivery umbilical cord blood pH is usually measured in high-risk pregnancy and emergencies
- Occasionally the placenta may be sent to the laboratory for histological investigation
- Ascertain if any specific care is needed for the baby at, or shortly after, delivery
- Vitamin K is given to the baby, with maternal consent, to prevent haemorrhagic disease[16]
- Perineal trauma is assessed and sutured promptly
- The midwife must report any deviations from the anticipated progress of either the labour, or the medical condition, to the obstetric team
- Measures must be taken to prevent cross-infection in the delivery suite, with especial emphasis on hand washing and meticulous aseptic techniques
- All procedures should be performed with full explanation to the mother, and with informed consent
- There must be accurate and contemporaneous record keeping throughout labour[17]
- Whilst acknowledging the necessary medical management, the midwife should still be able to give woman-centred midwifery care, and many such women should still be able to have a normal vaginal birth under midwifery practice

POSTNATAL CARE

Postnatal care commences shortly after the birth and usually commences in hospital[18]. Within six hours of delivery the blood pressure should be recorded and the first urine void obtained and documented[19]. Gentle mobilisation is encouraged and opportunity given to talk about the birth. The midwife should be alert to life-threatening conditions in this period[19].

British midwives conduct home visits once the mother has been discharged home. These visits occur on a selective basis until the tenth postnatal day; however the midwife can extend these visits up to or beyond the 28th day[20]. After this, care is transferred to a specialist public health nurse (health visitor), who continues child health surveillance until the child is five years of age, when the child commences school[18].

A physical examination of the mother is conducted by the midwife to ascertain if her body is returning to the pre-pregnant state. The examination is repeated at home, and on a selective basis, and should determine:

- General wellbeing of mother and child
- Mother's emotional state
- Observations of pulse and blood pressure
- Presence of signs of infection
- Record temperature[19]
- Breast examination to ascertain initiation of lactation and sore/cracked nipples in breastfeeding mothers, as well as other problems such as breast engorgement
- Uterine involution
- Determine type of lochia, and if there are any anomalies such as heavy bleeding or passing of blood clots, or offensive odour which could indicate infection
- Perineum, with especial attention to wound healing, bruising and swelling
- Other wound inspection, especially if the mother delivered by caesarean section; a dry dressing may be re-applied to protect the wound from friction
- Legs to see if both calves are of equal size and temperature and if there is any pain (an abnormality of which could indicate a DVT)
- Fingers, pre-tibial area and ankles to ascertain if oedema exists, and if excessive
- Specific educational needs can be addressed on a one-to-one basis, such as making up infant feeds

The findings of the above examination should be recorded, and preferably plotted, to determine if there is a graphic pattern of the body returning towards the pre-pregnant state.

A postnatal visit often coincides with the newborn screening (Guthrie) test at 5–7 days of milk feeding.

The following additional considerations should be given to the mother with a medical condition:

- Some mothers need to remain in hospital for a longer period postpartum
- Follow-up appointments for mother and baby may need to be made before the mother is discharged home
- Physical observations may need to be conducted more frequently than customary home 'selective visiting'
- Drug treatment may need prompt alteration
- Some conditions can destabilise rapidly postpartum

GENERAL CONSIDERATIONS

Local Protocols

Management of routine midwifery care can alter and medical management of medical conditions may need to be changed promptly, especially in light of adverse event reporting. A midwife is obliged to follow local policies and protocols[21], as this is usually part of the employment contract. It is therefore important that midwives, doctors and other health care professionals regularly review:

- **Local guidelines**, which many health authorities now put on their own intranet
- **Unit protocols** – these may be in paper or intranet form and are usually specific to a specific area or ward
- **National guidelines** – in the UK the organisations of especial relevance are the National Institute for Clinical Excellence (NICE), the Royal College of Obstetricians and Gynaecologists (RCOG), the Royal College of Midwives (RCM) and the Nursing and Midwifery Council (NMC)

Complementary Therapies

By the nature of a chronic disease many women may already have tried complementary and alternative medications (CAM), perhaps feeling that conventional medicine has failed them. A woman may be self-administering CAM when she first consults the midwife, in the mistaken belief that because they are natural they are safe[22]. Whilst some interventions have some effectiveness, others require research before they can be recommended[23].

In a tactful way the midwife needs to explain that many complementary, homeopathic and herbal medicines have not been subject to research with adequate scientific rigour to ascertain if they are safe to use in pregnancy and therefore their continued use cannot be recommended[19,24]. If the mother is firmly adherent to her beliefs in a product, then the midwife should seek additional advice from a pharmacist or doctor.

Over-the-Counter Medication

Many medicines can be purchased over the counter (OTC) at a pharmacy or shop. The midwife may be the first health professional a pregnant woman sees to seek advice about these drugs for minor ailments[25] or to alleviate symptoms of their medical condition. There is a theoretical risk of a mother choosing OTC drugs in preference to those prescribed by a doctor, as she might mistakenly believe them to be 'safer'. Therefore the midwife should advise:

- To continue taking prescribed drugs until she has sought advice from her GP or specialist clinic
- To consider OTC drugs only if absolutely necessary
- Always to ask the advice of the pharmacist before making a purchase, making it clear that she is pregnant

Some drugs can be advised by the midwife, and common examples are bowel care medications, nutritional supplements and anti-fungal preparations[25], however the midwife should develop adequate knowledge about the products before advising about their use within the scope of midwifery practice[24,25].

Prescribed Medication

With many medical conditions the woman is likely to be receiving prescribed drugs, some of which might be contraindicated in pregnancy as their effect upon the fetus is unknown[26]. Some drugs are known to be teratogenic in animal studies, and therefore contraindicated for use in human pregnancy[26]. A few are already known to have caused human congenital anomalies and their use is strongly contraindicated unless in emergency situations[26]. Hence, the woman should have a review of her medication conducted by a doctor experienced in pregnancy prescribing, and safer alternative drugs selected.

A mother may panic about potential effects upon the fetus and cease taking her prescribed medication. In some cases sudden withdrawal of drugs can precipitate a medical crisis, such as an epileptic fit or lupus flare, with catastrophic effect on the pregnancy and fetal loss. For this reason a midwife should advise a woman to continue with her treatment until a medical practitioner with expertise in pregnancy prescribing has been consulted. The midwife may need to arrange an emergency appointment for the mother.

The NMC states[24] *'A practising midwife shall only supply and administer those medicines in respect of which she has received the appropriate training as to use, dosage and methods of administration.'* Therefore, a midwife may have to seek instruction or guidance in specific drugs to be able to meet the needs of certain mothers with medical conditions. She can seek recent information from reputable websites, in particular the British National Formulary or texts that specialise in prescribing in pregnancy (see reading list).

Nicotine, Alcohol and Illegal Drugs

Cigarette smoking, alcohol consumption and use of illegal drugs are of concern in pregnancy or puerperium. Smoking cessation should always be promoted by the midwife. Drinking should be discouraged, or, failing this, measures taken to reduce it to a minimum. Illegal drugs are strongly contraindicated. Alcohol and illegal drugs are addressed more fully in Chapter 16.

Termination of Pregnancy

Some medical conditions can exacerbate and tragically necessitate a mother facing the emotional dilemma of having to have a termination of a wanted pregnancy. This might be for congenital anomalies or to save the mother's own life. The gynaecological terminology is 'therapeutic abortion' but when speaking to the parents 'termination' should be used in preference to 'abortion'. CEMACH recommendations are for *termination of pregnancy services to be readily available for women with medical conditions precluding safe pregnancy*, and *an appointment should take no longer than three weeks*[27].

In the UK a midwife can be a conscientious objector to termination of pregnancy, however she cannot refuse to care for a mother if the termination is to save the life of the mother[28]. Confidentiality is also of paramount importance. The ethical, legal and emotional dilemmas cannot be addressed here, and it is strongly recommended that midwives read the RCM Position Statement No. 17 (see Essential Reading, this chapter).

Pre-term Birth

A maternal medical condition may result in pre-term induction of labour, caesarean section or a spontaneous pre-term delivery. If the presentation is cephalic the latter might be conducted by the midwife. The nature of the condition might also have caused growth restriction, and the baby may have a double set of problems. If time, surfactant prophylaxis is usually given to the mother (e.g. 12 mg betamethasone, two doses 24 hrs apart) to assist maturation of the fetal lungs.

The midwife should prepare for a pre-term delivery by: Notifying the neonatal unit and calling an experienced paediatrician to be present at delivery[29], then:

- Preparing neonatal resuscitation equipment in advance
- Avoiding use of narcotics which suppress infant breathing[29]
- Having a warm delivery room, and calm environment
- Have bonnet and plastic bag to prevent neonatal heat loss
- Preparing detailed records; duplicates may be needed to accompany the baby to the neonatal unit (NNU)
- Preparing identity bracelets in advance, and checking these with the parents
- Giving support and clear explanations to the parents

At delivery the midwife should:

- Leave adequate length of umbilical cord below the cord clamp to allow for catheter insertion on NNU
- Quickly dry the baby[29] and hand to the paediatrician
- Ask an assistant to apply the identity bracelets and, if the paediatrician permits, weigh the baby and pass to mother for a quick cuddle before the baby is taken to NNU
- Neonatal vitamin K (Konakion) should be given in the delivery room or on the neonatal unit

Care of the Mother of a Baby on the Neonatal Unit

If the baby has been admitted to a specialist unit for intensive care, the mother can feel bereft on the postnatal ward[29] or at home, and will benefit from psychological support and encouragement from the midwife. Postnatal care may have to be adapted if the mother is spending a lot of time in a paediatric hospital environment. In some cases the baby may be 'out of area' and arrangements must be made for a midwife to care for the mother in a different location. Accurate communication is needed, especially in relation to specific requirements of the medical condition.

Mother–infant attachment should be fostered by allowing a 'cuddle' with the baby whenever possible[29]. A photograph of the baby should be taken and given to her, and arrangements for visits made. The whole family are encouraged to visit the baby with due liaison with the neonatal unit. The staff there should give the parents regular explanations as to the progress and prognosis of the baby[29]. The midwife may need to reinforce some of the explanation as tired, anxious parents might find it difficult to assimilate information of this nature.

Mothers experience tiredness with frequent visits to a neonatal unit, and might be called throughout the night. A quiet, calm environment on the ward might assist relaxation and sleeping. As there is a chance of meals and drug rounds being missed, alternative arrangements should be made. Assistance should be given with breast pump use, and arrangements made for the storage of expressed milk.

Breast-feeding

In most cases, the midwife should promote and support breast-feeding even if concern may arise over drugs passing to the baby in breast milk. Here the midwife should confer with the physician, paediatrician and pharmacist as to the best course of action. In some cases the mother may need to express and dispose of breast milk until certain drugs have 'cleared' and she is able to breast-feed as normal. Alternatively she may have to continue with her 'pregnancy drugs' and delay a return to the former treatment regimen until breast-feeding has ceased.

The midwife should address practical aspects, such as equipment for expressing breast milk, cleaning and sterilisation of that equipment and storage of the milk, which will require refrigeration and labelling to comply with food handling requirements of the individual institution. Arrangements should be made to take the milk over to the neonatal unit if the mother is unable to go in person. Personal issues must not be forgotten, such as privacy when expressing breast milk, positive encouragement and relief of discomfort when expressing milk or breast-feeding the baby in either the postnatal ward or neonatal unit.

Some infectious conditions, of which Human Immune Deficiency Virus (HIV) is the most notable, could be passed on to the baby through breast-feeding, and this is expanded upon in Chapter 12.2. In these cases the midwife may have to educate the mother about formula feeding methods and sterilisation of feeding utensils. Non-pharmacological measures to suppress lactation should be taken.

Women Who Decline Blood Products or Blood Transfusion

Some mothers may decline the use of blood products or blood transfusion in pregnancy, or at any time. This may be for fear of infection, lack of understanding, religious conviction, or other reasons.

The religious group most usually associated with declining the use of blood products is the Jehovah's Witnesses. Followers accept most medical treatments, surgical and anaesthetic procedures, devices and techniques, as well as haemostatic and therapeutic agents that do not contain blood. They accept non-blood volume expanders and drugs to control haemorrhage and stimulate the production of red blood cells. However, they will *not* accept transfusions of whole blood, packed red cells, white cells, plasma and platelets. Neither are they likely to accept pre-operative autologous blood collection for later re-infusion. However, they *might* accept, on a basis of personal choice, cell salvage, haemodialysis, coagulation factors and immunoglobulins[30].

Closed loop intra-operative cell salvage may also be acceptable. Other women may consider cell salvage and autologous transfusion but need an individual care plan to be negotiated and documented.

It is important that two aspects of planning are addressed. First, as well as documenting refusal of blood products, there also must be a plan for minimisation of blood loss and for resuscitation as required. Second, women with additional risk factors for bleeding, e.g. multiple pregnancy, immune thrombocytopenic purpura (ITP) and those on anticoagulation therapy, must be delivered in a unit with experience of dealing with patients who decline blood products and expertise in alternative methods of treatment and resuscitation.

Declining blood products can pose certain challenges when caring for pregnant women with pre-existing medical conditions, because some conditions would normally require treatment with blood products. Furthermore, some conditions may predispose a mother to haemorrhagic situations, when blood products might be required in labour or emergencies. A Jehovah's Witness, is likely to produce a printed care plan (Appendix 14.2) at an antenatal visit and also when admitted to delivery suite and ask for a copy to be kept in the obstetric notes. This care plan *must* be discussed with the most senior clinician on duty.

Whatever the mother's religion or reason for declining blood products, the midwife should establish effective two-way communication and ensure that a supportive and non-judgemental attitude is displayed throughout. It is important that the midwife *listens* to the mother and understands the rationale underpinning any stated intention to decline blood products. Informed choice is an important issue here. The midwife may have to use her educational skills to explain why some products are advisable so that the mother fully understands the choices open to her. In some cases, a clearly put explanation may result in some mothers deciding to accept the treatment. In other cases the mother and her next of kin may have thought through the issues well in advance and be aware of the potential problems, including death, and be able to make a fully informed decision. The ethical and legal dilemmas that arise cannot be addressed within the scope of this book. If a mother continues to state she wishes to decline blood products the midwife should ensure that the mother is seen by a senior doctor with due experience in haematology or obstetrics, so that the issues can be discussed to a greater extent and appropriate plans made for care. Accurate records should be kept, especially of advice given and of decisions made.

It is important that all members of the multi-disciplinary team refer to their own institution's policies and guidelines for direction. Not only will the clinical aspects need to be addressed, but there are legal aspects of considerable importance requiring the mother and next of kin to sign a declaration with appropriate witnesses.

Conflict of Interest

Some women with a medical or addictive disorder may be high risk but are insistent upon a midwifery-led scheme of care. This places the midwife in a difficult position. The midwife has a role as the mother's advocate, but the level of risk creates a conflict of interest, especially when the fetus is taken into account.

A midwife cannot refuse to care for a mother, and should work in partnership with the woman and her family[21]. Negotiating skills should be used to coax the mother to attend an appropriate specialist clinic (Table 1.1). If the mother is adamant about rejecting high-risk care the midwife should consult her named supervisor of midwives in order that a plan of action is developed to support the midwife and colleagues, to care for the mother and fetus more effectively[27].

EMERGENCY MANAGEMENT

Midwives should have the skills to identify a deviation from normality and refer appropriately[31]. They must be able to initiate emergency measures in the doctor's absence, then assist the latter where appropriate[32]. Midwives should receive regular training on the signs and symptoms of critical illness including basic life support, with emergency 'drills' for maternal resuscitation practised regularly[27].

Pregnancy poses challenges for resuscitation of mothers, and there are some differences compared with standard adult resuscitation. Table 1.2 outlines considerations that should be taken into account when resuscitating a pregnant woman.

The midwife may be the first health professional to note a serious deterioration in a pregnant woman's condition and have to initiate emergency measures having called for medical aid. A scheme for midwifery management of sudden maternal collapse is given in Table 1.3.

It is not within the scope of this book to address advanced life support, and a number of authoritative texts already exist within the nursing/midwifery press that give this important subject detailed attention.

PREVENTING MATERNAL MORTALITY

The latest CEMACH report, **Saving Mothers' Lives**, devotes a chapter to issues for midwives[33], which all midwives should be encouraged to read (see Essential Reading, this chapter). Of particular relevance to medical disorders is the emphasis upon referral in order that timely interventions are implemented to prevent maternal death. Key physical signs that necessitate a midwife referring the mother to an appropriate doctor are:

- Heart rate of over 100 beats per minute
- Systolic blood pressure of over 160 mmHg
- Systolic blood pressure of *under* 90 mmHg
- Diastolic blood pressure of over 80 mmHg
- Body temperature of over 38°C
- Respiratory rate of over 21 breaths per minute; respiratory rate is often overlooked but rates over 30 per minute indicate a serious problem

The same report emphasises individual responsibility and states that if a midwife is unhappy with a medical opinion then s/he should consult a more senior doctor and seek support from a supervisor of midwives[33].

Table 1.2 Basic and advanced life support – considerations in pregnancy

Life Support Principles

These are similar as for non-pregnant individuals, but important additions are:

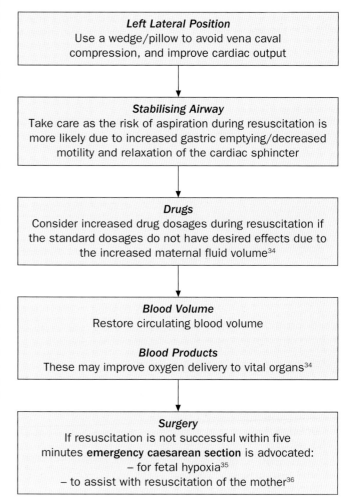

Left Lateral Position
Use a wedge/pillow to avoid vena caval compression, and improve cardiac output

↓

Stabilising Airway
Take care as the risk of aspiration during resuscitation is more likely due to increased gastric emptying/decreased motility and relaxation of the cardiac sphincter

↓

Drugs
Consider increased drug dosages during resuscitation if the standard dosages do not have desired effects due to the increased maternal fluid volume[34]

↓

Blood Volume
Restore circulating blood volume

Blood Products
These may improve oxygen delivery to vital organs[34]

↓

Surgery
If resuscitation is not successful within five minutes **emergency caesarean section** is advocated:
– for fetal hypoxia[35]
– to assist with resuscitation of the mother[36]

Table 1.3 Midwife management of sudden collapse in pregnancy

Prevention is paramount: recognise signs of maternal circulatory compromise, e.g. rapid, *thready* pulse, low BP, pale sweaty skin, altered consciousness levels/seek help immediately/treat any cause, e.g. haemorrhage/replace fluids /give oxygen/monitor condition[37]

Assess maternal condition: **D** (danger to self and woman)
R (response – level of consciousness – AVPU scale)
A (airway – is it open?)
B (breathing – is it normal?)
C (circulation – is the heart beating/is the circulation intact?)

↓

Shout/go for help: in the UK: hospitals – dial 2222/at home – dial 999

↓

If conscious:
Reassure, if pregnant tilt to left side, give oxygen via non-rebreathing mask, closely observe vital signs, seek obstetric referral, involve multi-disciplinary team and treat cause[37]

↓

If unconscious, but breathing normally and circulation adequate:
Tilt to left side, give oxygen via non-rebreathing mask, closely observe vital signs, seek obstetric referral, involve multidisciplinary team and treat cause[37]

↓

If breathing is absent or abnormal* and carotid pulse is absent[38]:
- Ensure help is on its way (see above)
- If no equipment immediately available commence continuous chest compressions
- Ask for/collect equipment/resuscitation trolley
- Treat where found, unless in immediate danger
- If pregnant, tilt to left side to reduce aortal–caval compression
- Once equipment/help is available, give 30 chest compressions to a depth of 1/3 of the chest at a rate of 100 times a minute
- Open airway using head tilt/chin lift manoeuvre and using a pocket mask or bag-valve-mask give 2 breaths
- Give oxygen at 15 l/min with the pocket mask (60% O_2 concentration) or via a reservoir bag on the bag-valve-mask system (100% O_2 concentration)
- Consider use of oropharyngeal/nasopharyngeal airways and suction to maintain airway[39]
- Continue at a rate of 30:2 until help arrives

*less than 10 times a minute/gasping

↓

Once help arrives:
Handover to medical team, including recent and relevant medical/obstetric history
Support medical team with ALS algorithms i.e.:
- Gaining iv access/administer iv drugs, i.e. *adrenaline, atropine* and *amiodarone*
- Assist with intubation
- Attaching ECG leads/analysing the cardiac rhythm and using the defibrillator, if rhythm dictates
If pregnant, the woman's condition will usually be stabilised before considering operative delivery, although emergency LSCS might improve maternal survival by increasing maternal cardiac output[37]

↓

After the event:
Ensure records are comprehensive and complete/provide support to relatives/liaise with other departments and professionals, e.g. ICU, as appropriate/complete risk management report

1 Midwifery Care and Medical Disorders

PATIENT ORGANISATIONS

Association for the Promotion of Preconceptual Care – Foresight.
178 Hawthorn Road
West Bognor
West Sussex PO21 2UY
www.foresight-preconception.org.uk

Association for Improvements in the Maternity Services (AIMS)
5 Ann's Court
Grove Road
Surbiton
Surrey KT6 4BE
www.aims.org.uk

Antenatal Results and Choices (ARC)
73–75 Charlotte Street
London W1T 4PN
www.arc-uk.org

Centre for Pregnancy Nutrition
University of Sheffield
Jessop Wing
Hallamshire Hospital
Tree Root Walk
Sheffield S10 2SF
www.shef.ac.uk/pregnancy_nutrition

La Leche League
PO Box 29
West Bridgford
Nottingham NG2 7NP
www.laleche.org.uk

Maternity Alliance
3rd Floor West
2–6 Northburgh Street
London EC1V 0AY
www.maternityalliance.org.uk

National Childbirth Trust (NCT)
Alexandra House
Oldham Terrace
London W3 6NH
www.nct.org.uk

Tommy's – The Baby Charity
Nicholas House
3 Laurence Pountney Hill
London EC4R 0BB
www.tommys.org

ESSENTIAL READING

Billington, M. and Stevenson, M. (2006) **Critical Care in Childbearing for Midwives**. Oxford, Blackwell.

BMJ books – Blackwell Scientific. **ABC series:**
ABC of Antenatal Care, ABC of Labour Care, ABC of Alcohol, ABC of Hypertension, ABC of Smoking Cessation, ABC of Sexual Health, ABC of Nutrition.

Briggs, G.G., Freeman, R.K. and Yaffe, S.J. (2005) **Drugs in Pregnancy and Lactation,** 7th Edn. USA, Lippincott.

British National Formulary www.bnf.org

Chan, K.L. and Kean, L.H. (2004) Routine antenatal management in later pregnancy. In: **Current Obstetrics and Gynaecology** 14:86–91.

Enkin, M., Keirse, M.J.N.C., Neilson, J., *et al.* (2000) **A Guide to Effective Care in Pregnancy and Childbirth**. Oxford, Oxford University Press.

Glenville, M. (2007) **Health Professional's Guide to Pre-Conception Care** (booklet). www.foresight-preconception.org.uk/booklet_healthproguide.htm

Henderson, C. and Mcdonald, S. (Eds) **Mayes Midwifery: A Textbook for Midwives**, 13th Edn. London, Elsevier.

Lewis, G. (Ed.) (2007) **Saving Mothers' Lives: Reviewing Maternal Deaths to Make Motherhood Safer**. 7th CEMACH Report. London, CEMACH.

National Institute for Clinical Excellence (NICE)
http://www.nice.org.uk/guidance/CG/guidelines.asp
Clinical guidelines: **CG46 Antenatal Care, CG45 Antenatal and Postnatal Mental Health, CG13 Caesarean Section, CG37 Routine Postnatal Care of Women and Babies**.

Redshaw, M. (2006) **Recorded Delivery: Women's perception of maternity care from a national survey**.
National Perinatal Epidemiology Unit.
www.npeu.ox.ac.uk/maternitysurveys/maternity-surveys_downloads/maternity_survey_report.pdf

RCM (1997) **Position Paper No.17 Conscientious Objection**.
London, Royal College of Midwives.
http://www.rcm.org.uk

Royal College of Obstetricians and Gynaecologists (RCOG)
http://www.rcog.org.uk
Green Top Clinical Guidelines: 40 listed.

SKIN DISORDERS

2

Catherine Gittins and Marian Parrish

2.1 Eczema

Incidence	Risk for Childbearing
Atopic eczema affects 9–20% of school children born after 1970 and 2–10% of adults[1]	None

EXPLANATION OF CONDITION

Eczema is a dry, itchy skin condition. It can occur anywhere on the body but typically it involves the flexures.

Acute eczema is hot, red, excoriated and scaly, sometimes with oozing, weeping and crusting.

Chronic eczema can result in fissuring, scaling and thickening (lichenification) of the skin.

Dermatitis means inflammation of the skin, a broader term than eczema. Most dermatologists now use the terms eczema and dermatitis interchangeably.

All skin conditions can cause a lowered quality of life and the psychosocial impact of eczema must also be considered.

COMPLICATIONS

Infection

- Bacterial infections: These are due to *Staphylococcus* and *Streptococcus*. Skin swabs which are positive for *Staphylococcus* are a major problem in atopic eczema. *Staphylococcus aureus* only needs treating if there is evidence of infection, e.g. crusting, weeping or deterioration in the eczema. Less commonly group A *Streptococcus* infection occurs and this always needs treating with antibiotics
- Viral: Herpes simplex can cause extensive generalised secondary infection which can occasionally be fatal

NON-PREGNANCY TREATMENT AND CARE

General Advice

- Explanation and education regarding the avoidance of irritants and furred or feathered animals
- Keep nails short

Topical Treatment (First-line Therapy)

- Emollient for the bath: daily lukewarm baths with 10–20 ml of bath oil (e.g. Oilatum or Diprobath bath emollients)
- No soap or shower gel; soap substitutes, e.g. aqueous cream or Epaderm, can be used
- Apply topical emollient after getting out of the bath while skin is warm and moist; apply emollient frequently during the day
- Topical steroids: a doctor will prescribe the weakest that works; low-potency steroids will not harm the skin if used long term (e.g. 1% hydrocortisone bd). Do not use anything stronger than this on the face
- Antihistamines do not stop the itching of eczema but sedative antihistamines will help adults with eczema sleep through the night if the itching is keeping them awake

- Secondary bacterial infection of eczema is treated with systemic antibiotics, e.g. flucloxacillin or erythromycin

Second-line Therapy

- Topical immune-modulators: tacrolimus and pimecrolimus are not recommended as first-line treatment of eczema
- Severe eczema is treated with oral prednisolone, azathioprine or ciclosporin, or PUVA (Psoralen with long-wave UVA light treatment)

PRE-CONCEPTION ISSUES AND CARE

The two main issues for eczema sufferers are counselling regarding disease progression in pregnancy and pharmacotherapy.

Atopic eczema is more likely to worsen than improve in pregnancy, although remission has been reported in up to 24% of cases[2].

Emollients, topical steroids, antihistamines and oral steroids are all safe to use.

Topical immune-modulators are contraindicated in pregnancy and should therefore be stopped.

There is no evidence that azathioprine is teratogenic, however there have been reports of premature labour/birth, low birth-weight babies and spontaneous abortion. There has been less experience with ciclosporine. it is thought to be no more harmful than azathioprine[4] therefore the midwife should advise the mother to seek medical advice in the peri-conception period, as their use is often supervised by specialist clinics (see Appendix 11).

Pregnancy Issues
- Eczema is the most common skin disorder in pregnancy (36% of total cases)[2]
- There have been no reports of adverse effects on fetal outcome
- It has been reported that infantile eczema may occur in up to 19% of babies born to mothers with eczema

Medical Management and Care
- Emollients, bath oils and soap substitutes are all safe and effective for eczema in pregnancy
- Use low- to moderate-potency topical steroids on any inflamed eczema
- If the eczema is severe then a short course of oral steroids can be used quite safely[4]
- For bacterial infection use flucloxacillin or erythromycin
- UVB light treatment is safe and occasionally used for eczema in pregnancy

Midwifery Management and Care
- After appropriate pre-conception counselling if a woman is not taking immune-modulating drugs she can be booked for low-risk care
- Encourage compliance with above treatment and reassurance of safety of treatments
- General advice (as for non-pregnant management, e.g. cotton clothing) applies when pregnant

Labour Issues
- Atopic eczema is not a contraindication to siting an epidural unless secondary infection is present

Medical Management and Care
- Continue topical treatment as above

Midwifery Management and Care
- Cotton clothing next to the skin and a cool environment will make eczema more comfortable in labour
- Midwifery care in labour can follow low-risk guidelines and protocols

Postpartum Issues
There is no conclusive evidence that breast-feeding will prevent atopic eczema. However, the overall evidence suggests that exclusive breast-feeding for at least four months may protect against atopic eczema in infants[3].

Hand dermatitis and nipple eczema may be a problem postpartum.

Medical Management and Care
- Encourage and support breast-feeding
- Hand dermatitis and nipple eczema can be treated with emollients, steroid creams and avoidance of irritants (see non-pregnancy treatment and care)
- Secondary infection with *Staphylococcus* is often a problem with nipple eczema and should be treated with appropriate antibiotics
- Tacrolimus, pimecrolimus, azathioprine and ciclosporin should all be avoided in breast-feeding unless under medical supervision[4]

Midwifery Management and Care
- Reinforce above advice, and support as necessary

2.2 Psoriasis

Incidence	Risk for Childbearing
2–3% of the UK population[1]	Low Risk
No gender differentiation	
Usual onset is in early adulthood[3]	

INTRODUCTION

Psoriasis is a common skin disease characterised by lesions which are bright red, raised, with well-defined edges and a silvery scale.

These lesions occur symmetrically, commonly involving the scalp, elbows, knees, sacral area and lower legs. However any part of the body can be affected including the flexures, hands, feet and nails.

There is a genetic susceptibility to psoriasis and it can be precipitated by infection (streptococcal sore throat), stress, trauma and hormonal changes.

All skin conditions can cause a lowered quality of life and the psychosocial impact of psoriasis must also be considered.

COMPLICATIONS

A small number of psoriasis patients will have joint involvement (**psoriatic arthropathy**).

Very occasionally a severe flare of psoriasis occurs. If this involves >90% of the body surface (a condition called **erythroderma**) then immediate admission to hospital is required for treatment and monitoring.

Generalised pustular psoriasis occurs rarely; this condition is often precipitated by oral or topical steroids, and also requires urgent admission for treatment.

NON-PREGNANCY TREATMENT AND CARE

General Advice

- Daily baths with emollients
- Avoid smoking and reduce alcohol intake
- Keep nails short
- There is no evidence that psoriasis is due to a dietary deficiency or food allergy

Topical Treatments (First-line Therapy)

- Emollients
- Salicylic acid ointments
- Vitamin D_3 analogues
- Dithranol
- Tar preparations
- Topical steroids
- Topical retinoids

Second-line Therapy

- Narrow band phototherapy; ultraviolet B (UVB) light treatment
- Bath PUVA (photosensitising medication in the bath with long-wave ultraviolet light treatment)

Systemic Treatments

- Psoralen + UVA light treatment, methotrexate, acitretin, ciclosporin, azathioprine and hydroxyurea
- When taking systemic treatment a reliable method of contraception needs to be used

PRE-CONCEPTION ISSUES AND CARE

The genetic susceptibility to psoriasis is controlled by several genes, so the familial tendency is variable. If one parent is affected then there is approximately a 10% chance of the child developing psoriasis[2].

Whilst trying to conceive, vitamin D_3 analogues, retinoid creams and PUVA should be avoided. Acitretin should be stopped two years before conception, and all other systemic treatment discontinued, if possible, at least three months before conception (see Section 2.1 Eczema).

If a woman's partner is being treated with methotrexate, this should be stopped three months prior to conception[4].

Pregnancy Issues
- Excessive weight gain can cause the skin to stretch and crack
- Women may have difficulty applying topical treatments to some areas as pregnancy progresses

Medical Management and Care
- Regular review of the condition and effectiveness of treatments
- Emollients, tar preparations, topical steroids, dithranol and UVB light therapy are all safe to use during pregnancy[6]

Midwifery Management and Care
The general principles of the pre-pregnant state management should be reinforced plus:
- Reassurance that vulval psoriasis does not preclude vaginal delivery
- Advise that the skin is kept well moisturised with emollients

It is important that the midwife demonstrates a willingness to touch and palpate the abdomen of a woman who has psoriasis in the usual way, and be sensitive to the need for privacy during examination if affected areas of the body are to be exposed.

Labour Issues
- A prolonged period of time in a warm, dry environment can irritate dry, scaly skin
- If fetal monitoring is required, the belts to secure transducers may cause discomfort
- Epidural analgesia is not contraindicated even if psoriatic plaques are present

Medical Management and Care
- Continue topical treatment as above

Midwifery Management and Care
- Ensure humidification of a warm, dry environment (a small bowl of water on a radiator will suffice)
- Careful placement of monitoring belts on abdomen; avoid unnecessary monitoring
- Assist with application of emollients
- Encourage the use of cool, loose cotton clothing

Postpartum Issues
- Psoriasis commonly deteriorates within four months post delivery, as does psoriatic arthropathy[5]

Medical Management and Care
- Treatment may need review
- PUVA, retinoids, methotrexate, ciclosporin and acitretin should all be avoided if breast-feeding
- Emollients, topical steroids, vitamin D analogues, tar preparations, dithranol and UVB light therapy are all safe to use whilst breast-feeding[4]

Midwifery Management and Care
- Explain that psoriasis may deteriorate postpartum
- Encourage and support the woman to establish successful breast-feeding

2 Skin Disorders

PATIENT ORGANISATIONS

National Eczema Society
Hill House
Highgate Hill
London N19 5NA
Tel: 0870 2413604 (Helpline)
Tel: 0207 2813553
Fax: 0207 816395
www.eczema.org

The Psoriasis Association
Milton House
7 Milton Street
Northampton NN2 7JG
Tel: 0845 6760076
www.psoriasis-association.org.uk

Psoriatic Arthropathy Alliance
PO Box 111
St. Albans
Herts. AL2 3JQ
Tel: 0870 703212
www.paalliance.org

British Association of Dermatologists
BAD House
19 Fitzroy Square
London W1P 5HQ
Tel: 0171 383 0266
www.bad.org.uk

The Skin Care Campaign
www.skincarecampaign.org

British Dermatology Nurses Group
4 Fitzroy Square
London W1T 5HQ
www.bdng.org.uk

Changing Faces
The Squire Centre
33–37 University Street
London WC1E 6JN
www.changingfaces.org.uk

ESSENTIAL READING

Ashton, R. and Leppard, B. (2005) **Differential Diagnosis in Dermatology**, 3rd Edn. Oxford; Radcliffe Publishing Ltd.

Berth-Jones, J., Tan, E. and Mailbach, H. (2004) **Fast Facts: Eczema and contact dermatitis**. Oxford; Health Press Ltd.

Mitchell, T. and Kennedy, C. (2006) **Your Questions Answered: Common Skin Disorders.** London; Elsevier.

NHS Skin Disorders Library
http://www.library.nhs.uk/skin/Default.aspx?pagename=HOME

Smith, C., Barker, S. and Munter, A. (2004) **Fast Facts: Psoriasis.** Oxford; Health Press Ltd.

HYPERTENSIVE DISORDERS

3

Trudy Boyce, Claire Dodd and Jason Waugh

3.1 Chronic (Essential) Hypertension

Incidence	Risk for Childbearing
2% of pregnancies	High Risk

INTRODUCTION

Hypertension in pregnancy is defined as a systolic blood pressure of ≥140 mmHg and/or a diastolic blood pressure of ≥90 mmHg. The significance of any blood pressure measurement is related to the gestation of the pregnancy and, in general terms, the earlier in pregnancy hypertension occurs the more likely it is to be chronic hypertension.

Chronic hypertension (CHT) describes all hypertension that exists pre-pregnancy. The majority of women in this group have essential hypertension, though many will be diagnosed for the first time in pregnancy.

Renal hypertension can complicate renal disease of any underlying pathology. Its presence increases maternal and perinatal morbidity and mortality though its management is as for other causes. The increased morbidity is usually related to the underlying renal pathology and it is concern for the maternal kidneys that usually precipitates delivery if problems arise.

Other causes of hypertension in pregnancy are:

- **Phaeochromocytoma**: rare but maternal mortality is ≥50%
- **Coarctation of the aorta**: high maternal mortality
- **Cushing's syndrome**: can be difficult to diagnose as features can be mimicked by normal pregnancy; associated with a high fetal loss
- **Conn's syndrome**: hypertension is associated with hypokalaemia

Chronic Hypertension *versus* Pregnancy Induced Hypertension (PIH)

In the first trimester of pregnancy the marked vasodilatation and drop in vascular resistance sees blood pressure fall in both normotensive and hypertensive women, (the drop being greater in the CHT group)[1]. As such hypertension may not be seen until the third or late in the second trimester. CHT can therefore only be diagnosed with reference to non-pregnant BP readings and this requires either prenatal BPs or more commonly detailed postnatal follow-up. Pharmacological management of CHT and PIH is identical and as a general rule if hypertension is present before 20 weeks CHT is more likely.

Women with CHT tend to be older, heavier and of higher parity.

COMPLICATIONS

Superimposed Pre-eclampsia

CHT is a major risk factor for pre-eclampsia[2]. The signs of superimposed pre-eclampsia are similar in this group but blood pressures (BP) will be higher or the BP picture will be difficult to interpret, due to CHT treatment with antihypertensives. In women with CHT the development of proteinuria is diagnostic of pre-eclampsia and is almost universally associated with fetal growth restriction. Another very predictive feature of pre-eclampsia in CHT is a high urate (uric acid).

If pre-eclampsia does not develop then women with CHT can expect a relatively uncomplicated pregnancy and outcome.

Fetal Growth Restriction

Even in the absence of other features of pre-eclampsia fetal growth restriction is more common in women with CHT. The underlying aetiology is usually poor placentation. Routine assessment of fetal growth with ultrasound scan (USS) from 28 weeks is commonplace.

Placental Abruption

Placental abruption is a rare but serious complication affecting 1% of CHT pregnancies[3]. It is unlikely that antihypertensive treatment would reduce this risk, but women should be advised of the risk and encouraged to stop smoking.

Severe Hypertension

Episodes of acute hypertension can occur in this group of women, who may stop medication when they conceive despite medical advice. The acute management is as for hypertension associated with severe pre-eclampsia and then oral therapy can be recommenced.

NON-PREGNANCY TREATMENT AND CARE

Excellent guidelines have been produced for management of hypertension[4]. Because the aetiology of the hypertension can be varied, different care pathways will exist and they are beyond the scope of this section. The majority of women with proven essential hypertension will be on one or more antihypertensive drugs as well as possibly other medications, and those with additional medical problems such as diabetes will have lower blood pressure targets.

All women should have been advised on lifestyle factors and their importance.

Initial therapy will be with either an angiotensin-converting enzyme inhibitor or angiotensin-receptor blocker or a beta-blocker and either a calcium channel blocker or a diuretic. For those with an interest the authors recommend the British Hypertension Society (BHS) guidelines for further reading.

Low-dose aspirin will be prescribed for the prevention of ischaemic cardiovascular disease in those who are more at risk (ten-year cardiovascular disease risk of >20%). This is rare in women under 50 years of age.

Statins are recommended for women either who already have evidence of cardiovascular disease and hypertension or who have a ten-year risk of cardiovascular disease of >20%.

PRE-CONCEPTION ISSUES AND CARE

- See Section 3.2 Pre-eclampsia for additional risk factor identification
- Antihypertensive medication changed to methyldopa
- Women should be encouraged to stop smoking and, where time permits, to lose weight if BMI >30

Pregnancy Issues

- Risk assessment and pre-eclampsia pro-phylaxis (see Section 3.2 Pre-eclampsia)
- Treatment of hypertension (for intra-partum treatment see Section 3.3 Eclampsia)
- Screening for pre-eclampsia (see Section 3.2 Pre-eclampsia)
- Screening for intrauterine growth restriction (IUGR)
- Timing of delivery

Medical Management and Care

All women with chronic hypertension should be referred for specialist input in the first trimester. This will include risk assessment, treatment review and pre-eclampsia prophylaxis[5] (see Section 3.2 Pre-eclampsia).

Blood pressure[6] – Blood pressure medication is commonly reduced or stopped in the first 20 weeks of pregnancy and is then required in increasing doses towards term.

- **Methyldopa**: this is the drug of choice for women pre-conceptually; very well documented safety profile for the fetus and newborn up to age 7 years; can be associated with sedation (which usually resolves within a week), depression and liver-function test changes
- **Labetalol**: combined alpha- and beta-blocker; some concern that prolonged use has been associated with fetal growth impairment and so its use should be limited to the third trimester; can be used in a parenteral form for acute BP control
- **Beta-blockers**: similar concerns to labetalol; contraindicated in asthma patients
- **Nifedipine**: increasingly common to prescribe in slow release form to supplement either methyldopa or labetalol
- **Hydralazine**: oral preparations can be used in refractory hypertension and parenteral preparations are used for acute hypertensive control
- **Third-line treatment**: diuretics can be used if necessary as can pra-zosin (an alpha-blocker); patients on this level of therapy will usually be in-patients
- **Angiotensin converting enzyme (ACE) inhibitors**: contraindicated in pregnancy

Midwifery Management and Care

- Regular antenatal assessments; blood pressure may be a poor sign of pre-eclampsia as it is either already raised or treated
- Dipstick testing of urine and clinical assessment of fetal growth are equally important

Labour Issues

- In the presence of significant hypertension induction of labour at term (39–40 weeks) is common
- Mode of delivery will depend on complications and other obstetric issues but vaginal delivery is not contraindicated
- Syntometrine/ergometrine should be avoided in the third stage of labour

Medical Management and Care

- NICE/RCOG recommend continual fetal monitoring for labour[7]
- An epidural in labour is not essential but may help control blood pressure

Midwifery Management and Care

- Regular blood pressure measurements in labour
- Blood pressure can often be managed by continuing oral antenatal medication
- Does not require a short second stage, can push as normal
- Oxytocin for active management of the third stage

Postpartum Issues[7]

- BP rise in the first four days postpartum and medication should be continued
- BP treatment should be modified to be supportive of breast-feeding and methyl-dopa should be stopped
- When possible, antihypertensive medication can be returned to pre-pregnancy regimes

If chronic hypertension is suspected but not confirmed then it is necessary for blood pressure to be further assessed in the postpartum period. It may take up to six months for blood pressure to return to non-pregnant levels but it is usually much quicker.

Medical Management and Care

- Nifedipine and labetalol are compatible with breast-feeding and can be continued postnatally
- Contraceptive advice may be dependent on blood pressure control

Midwifery Management and Care

- Check blood pressure regularly and liaise with specialist/GP for medication modifications and to change back to pre-pregnancy medications if required[4]
- Encourage continued antihypertensive drug use
- Support breast-feeding
- Advise on contraception (but consider referring to family planning clinic or GP) and for pre-pregnancy counselling next time

3.2 Pre-eclampsia

Incidence 2–7% of all pregnancies[1]	**Risk for Childbearing** High Risk

EXPLANATION OF CONDITION

Pre-eclampsia, or pre-eclamptic toxaemia (PET), is a major cause of maternal and fetal mortality and morbidity. It is a syndrome characterised by the development of new hypertension and proteinuria in the second half of pregnancy which will always resolve postnatally[1].

Pregnancy Induced Hypertension (PIH) or **Gestational Hypertension** (GH) are terms used to describe new onset hypertension occurring in the second half of pregnancy which resolves postnatally (similarly for gestational proteinuria).

Defining pre-eclampsia has always been controversial, but it is now recognised that for clinical purposes an appreciation of the other features of the syndrome, such as liver involvement (presenting as nausea and right upper quadrant pain), coagulation failure (thrombocytopaenia and clotting derangements), neurological involvement (headaches and visual disturbance) and fetal growth restriction are important in identifying women with the disease.

The exact aetiology of the condition is still not clear. We know that the origins of the disease are in the first and second trimesters of pregnancy with placentation problems and that the maternal endothelium is the target cell which leads to the clinical manifestations of the disease. However, the mechanisms which lead to endothelial cell dysfunction and their relationship to the placenta remain unclear.

Pre-eclampsia once established will always progress as long as the pregnancy continues. Symptoms for the woman are rare and progression can be gradual (2–4 weeks) or fulminant (24 hours).

Pre-eclampsia can begin antenatally, intrapartum or postnatally. Approximately 10% of all women will have PIH during their pregnancy. Within this group 3–4% will have pre-eclampsia, 5% PIH and 1–2% will have chronic hypertension.

COMPLICATIONS

The complications of pre-eclampsia are numerous and include placental abruption, intrauterine growth restriction, HELLP syndrome (**H**aemolysis, **E**levated **L**iver enzymes, **L**ow **P**latelet count), disseminated intravascular coagulation (DIC), renal failure, pre-term delivery, multi-organ failure, eclampsia (grand mal seizures in the presence of pre-eclampsia) and even death.

NON-PREGNANCY TREATMENT AND CARE

Pre-eclampsia is a disease unique to human pregnancy. Important issues for women who have had pre-eclampsia are:

- Has the condition resolved postnatally, or is there an element of chronic hypertension or renal disease on which the pre-eclampsia was superimposed?

- Does a history of pre-eclampsia predispose you to other cardiovascular disease in later life? This is currently the subject of considerable research and women should be advised at present regarding other cardiovascular risk factors such as weight loss, smoking cessation and exercise.

PRE-CONCEPTION ISSUES AND CARE

There are many risk factors that predispose to pre-eclampsia. These are listed with the approximate risk increase[2].

Antiphospholipid syndrome	9-fold increase
Previous pre-eclampsia	7-fold increase
Pre-existing diabetes	3.5-fold increase
Multiple pregnancy	3-fold increase
Nulliparity	3-fold increase
Family history	3-fold increase
Raised BMI pre-pregnancy	2.5-fold increase
Raised BMI at booking	1.5-fold increase
Age over 40	2-fold increase
Raised diastolic BP (>80 mmHg)	1.5-fold increase

The above risk factors can usually be sought through history and examination. It is clear that genetic, metabolic and environmental factors may all have a part to play, and the interaction of these risk factors is not fully understood. However it is likely that having more risk factors is generally worse and a history of pre-existing disease or previous early onset pre-eclampsia will increase the risk to approximately 20%.

Women often want to know whether pre-eclampsia can be prevented, and several agents have been investigated. Low-dose aspirin has been shown to reduce the risk of developing pre-eclampsia by 19% (additional benefits include 16% reduction in fetal death and a 7% reduction in pre-term delivery). It is estimated that 69 women will require treatment to prevent one case of pre-eclampsia. Aspirin prophylaxis is usually commenced at the end of the first trimester[3]. Women may also benefit from calcium supplementation with trials of 1 g/day suggesting a reduction in pre-eclampsia particularly in high-risk women. Calcium is however poorly tolerated in pregnancy as it causes gastrointestinal upset[4].

Pregnancy Issues

- Following an assessment of risk factors as for pre-pregnancy counselling a decision is made regarding pre-eclampsia prophylaxis
- The main feature of antenatal care is the careful surveillance of the woman, early diagnosis with appropriate intervention and timely delivery
- In the absence of risk factors for pre-eclampsia the NICE low-risk antenatal care guidelines can be applied
- Community guidelines to screen for pre-eclampsia have been published and the next level of care when pre-eclampsia is suspected is the obstetric day unit, which is present in most hospitals[5]

Medical Management and Care

Surveillance is a major component of ante-/intrapartum care and the reader is directed to more detailed accounts in Essential Reading.

- Women identified as *at increased risk* should be referred for specialist input; may involve investigation of underlying medical problems (urea and electrolytes [U&E], renal USS, thrombophilia screen)
- Assessment for aspirin/calcium prophylaxis
- Uterine artery Doppler screening at 20–24 weeks gestation; can be a useful additional test in high-risk women as it has a very high negative predictive value
- If pre-eclampsia is diagnosed then the balance between disease severity and fetal maturity will determine the timing of delivery

Midwifery Management and Care

- If low risk for pre-eclampsia: NICE Antenatal guidelines advocate BP and proteinuria assessments at 16, 28, 34, 36, 38 and 41 weeks in parous women, with additional visits at 25 and 31 weeks for nulliparae[5]
- Blood pressure measurement: When measuring blood pressure in pregnancy it is essential to use Korotkof sound 1 – sound appears (for systolic blood pressure) and 5 – sound disappears (for diastolic blood pressure). Accurate blood pressure measurement is essential for correct diagnosis. There are many new automated devices for blood pressure measurement and most are not accurate in pregnancy. Appendices 3.1 and 3.2 address device accuracy[6]
- Proteinuria measurement: Urine dipsticks remain the preferred method of choice for proteinuria assessment. These are also prone to observer error and the use of automated dipstick readers has been shown to improve accuracy[7]
- If signs of pre-eclampsia develop the midwife MUST refer the mother to an obstetrician promptly, and support any medical treatment
- Psychological support and advice regarding the condition should be given (see Section 3.1); any reassurance should be realistic

Labour Issues[8]

- Obstetric units/regions should all have guidelines for the management of severe pre-eclampsia
- Fulminating pre-eclampsia is an obstetric emergency requiring multi-disciplinary teamwork
- Delivery should be timed, performed in an appropriate unit and, if pre-term or urgent, will often require caesarean section
- Intensive observation (HDU/ITU care) is often required for up to 48 hours after delivery

Medical Management and Care[8] (see also Section 3.3 Eclampsia)

- **Blood pressure**: intravenous therapy may be required (see Section 3.3 Eclampsia)
- **Fluid balance**: strict fluid balance is employed often requiring invasive monitoring of central venous pressure
- **Eclampsia prophylaxis**: magnesium sulphate may be used peripartum

Midwifery Management and Care

- With severe pre-eclampsia, peripartum monitoring is intensified
- An HDU/ITU environment on delivery suite is used, incorporating:
  - non-invasive or arterial blood pressure measurement
  - fluid balance or central venous pressure monitoring
  - respiratory observations: pulse oximetry; respiratory rate if on magnesium sulphate
  - neurological observations: reflexes tested if on magnesium sulphate
  - haematological and biochemical tests every six hours
- Midwife may have to prepare for a pre-term delivery (see Chapter 1)

Postpartum Issues

Hypertension and proteinuria can take up to three months to resolve. Hence, the midwife may need to extend the period of postnatal visiting up to or beyond ten days, and should not delegate observations or care to those who are inappropriately qualified.

Medical Management and Care[8]

- Blood pressure medication is continued until hypertension resolves
- Postnatal review and pre-conception planning are recommended

Midwifery Care

- Documentation of resolved hypertension and proteinuria is essential to exclude CHT and renal disease

3.3 Severe Pre-eclampsia/HELLP/Eclampsia

Incidence	Risk for Childbearing
Eclampsia 5:10,000 pregnancies	High Risk
Severe pre-eclampsia 5:1000 pregnancies[1]	

INTRODUCTION

Eclampsia is the occurrence of one or more convulsions superimposed on pre-eclampsia. In eclampsia a case fatality rate of 1.8% has been reported and up to 35% of women suffer a major complication[1].

Severe pre-eclampsia should appropriately be considered alongside eclampsia. Severe pre-eclampsia is more difficult to define but blood pressures of systolic >170 mmHg or diastolic >110 mmHg with >1 g/l proteinuria is an accepted definition[1].

HELLP syndrome (**H**aemolysis, **E**levated **L**iver enzymes and **L**ow **P**latelet count) is an important variant of severe pre-eclampsia and will usually but not always also be associated with hypertension and proteinuria, though these may not be dominant features[1].

Clinical features of severe pre-eclampsia include:

* Severe headache
* Visual disturbances
* Epigastric pain
* Vomiting
* Liver tenderness
* Clonus/hyperreflexia
* Low platelets
* Papilloedema
* Abnormal liver function (ALT or AST >70 iu/l)

Severe pre-eclampsia and eclampsia can occur in pregnancy or the postpartum period. Up to 44% of cases of eclampsia have been described postnatally (up to four weeks). Up to 13% of women with pre-eclampsia will have underlying chronic or essential hypertension.

Strategy

Recent guidance from the Royal College of Obstetricians and Gynaecologists (RCOG) has suggested:

* Local and/or regional guidelines should be developed for the management of severe pre-eclampsia and eclampsia
* Careful assessment of blood pressure and proteinuria is required with consideration of the potential for the involvement of other organs including the feto-placental unit (for BP and proteinuria measurement see CHT section)
* Intensive monitoring of blood pressure and fluid balance is required, as well as regular blood tests for HELLP changes
* Delivery is dependent upon the woman being stable
* Delivery issues have been discussed in the pre-eclampsia section and eclamptic convulsions do not necessitate immediate delivery

* Severe early onset pre-eclampsia can be managed conservatively to prolong pregnancy for fetal maturation. This requires in-patient care in a unit with adequate neonatal facilities for pre-term infants. Evidence suggests that 7–15 days of extra gestation can be obtained and that this reduces neonatal respiratory morbidity

COMPLICATIONS

HELLP syndrome can present as a fulminant condition antepartum or postpartum. Recovery will take up to two weeks and there have been reports of hypercoagulability following cases of HELLP, so practitioners must be aware of the possibility of thrombo-embolic disease, which can be fatal.

Further complications in severe cases may result in bleeding under the liver capsule which can lead to rupture of the capsule, haemoperitoneum and, not infrequently, death.

NON-PREGNANCY TREATMENT AND CARE

Pre-eclampsia and eclampsia are conditions unique to human pregnancy. The important issues for women who have had pre-eclampsia or eclampsia are:

* Has the condition resolved postnatally or is there an element of chronic hypertension or renal disease on which the pre-eclampsia was superimposed?
* Does a history of pre-eclampsia predispose you to other cardiovascular disease in later life?

The latter is currently the subject of considerable research, and women should be advised regarding other cardiovascular risk factors and their avoidance by, e.g., weight loss, smoking cessation and exercise.

Treatment and care for pregnancy are given on the next page.

PRE-CONCEPTION ISSUES AND CARE

The RCOG recommends that women are seen for follow-up to determine that hypertension and proteinuria have resolved, and also to discuss the events of their pregnancy (de-briefing). This may include pre-conception counselling and preventative strategies for the future.

Pre-conception counselling and care are as for pre-eclampsia (see Section 3.2 Pre-eclampsia).

Pregnancy and Labour Issues[1]

1) Blood pressure control
(See Section 3.2 Pre-eclampsia for oral regimes)

Medical Management and Care[1]

- It can be possible to manage hypertension at immediate presentation with oral agents (labetalol or nifedipine); it is no longer recommended that sublingual nifedipine be used
- Parenteral administration of labetalol or hydralazine is common in units across the UK. These are usually given as an initial bolus and then as infusions, though exact protocols will vary. What is apparent from the most recent CEMACH report is that inadequate control of hypertension is responsible for most deaths in pregnancy. Blood pressures of >170/110 mmHg require urgent intervention

2) Fluid management
(See Section 3.2 Pre-eclampsia)

- It is not uncommon for units to pre-load women with severe pre-eclampsia with a bolus of fluid (usually 250 ml colloid solution) prior to treatment to reduce the incidence of CTG abnormalities seen when antihypertensive agents lower blood pressure
- Fluid restriction is advised to reduce the risk of fluid overload intrapartum or postpartum
- Usual regimes are 1 ml/kg/hr or 80–85 ml/hr
- Such regimes have seen a dramatic reduction in pulmonary oedema and death from this complication of pre-eclampsia; restriction is usually maintained until there is evidence of a postpartum diuresis
- This situation is further complicated if haemorrhage occurs, when fluid replacement is better guided by central venous pressure monitoring

3) Prevention of seizures

- Magnesium sulphate should be considered for women with severe pre-eclampsia, as it reduces the risk of an eclamptic seizure by about 58%. If severe, then 63 women will be treated to prevent one eclamptic fit, whereas if less severe women are treated then 109 will be treated to prevent one fit
- If a conservative management plan is proposed it is reasonable to defer magnesium until delivery is planned; should be continued for either 24 hours post-delivery or 24 hours post-seizure

4) Control of seizures

- Magnesium sulphate is the first-line treatment: 4 g by slow iv infusion (over 5–10 minutes) followed by an infusion of 1 g/hr for 24 hours
- If seizures are recurrent, either give a further bolus of 2 g or increase the infusion rate to 1.5–2 g/hr
- Magnesium toxicity can be detected by loss of deep tendon reflexes
- If seizures persist, then other agents in single doses (diazepam, thiopentone) can be used. These agents often necessitate intubation to protect the mother's airway and a period of ventilation on intensive care is the usual outcome
- If urine output drops to less than 20 ml/hr magnesium therapy should be stopped and it may be necessary to measure serum magnesium levels to monitor toxicity

Team Approach

- Teamwork is required, and this can be rehearsed in different clinical environments
- Basic principles of ABC (Airway, Breathing, Circulation) should be followed

Midwifery Management and Care

- Frequent observations, HDU/ITU monitoring and documentation as well as six-hourly review of blood tests
- Management of fluid balance and IV fluid pumps
- Administration of IV drugs as bolus and infusions

Labour Issues

- It is imperative to remember that general midwifery care, observations and support are essential

Medical Management and Care

- Delivery options as per Section 3.2 Pre-eclampsia

Midwifery Management and Care

- Continue with above high dependency care in labour
- Prepare for a potentially pre-term birth and/or compromised infant
- Pre- and post-operative care – depending upon mode of delivery

Postpartum Issues

- Postpartum eclampsia can occur

Medical Management and Care – see Section 3.2 Pre-eclampsia

Midwifery Management and Care – see Section 3.2 Pre-eclampsia

Maintain observations until stable. Usually women will remain as in-patients for four days, and the baby may be on NNU with the mother requiring supportive assistance. Breast-feeding is to be encouraged.

3 Hypertensive Disorders

PATIENT ORGANISATIONS

British Hypertension Society
BHS Administrative Officer
Clinical Sciences Building Level 5
PO Box 65
Leicester Royal Infirmary
Leicester LE2 7LX
www.bhsoc.org

Action on Pre-eclampsia – APEC
84–88 Pinner Road
Harrow
Middlesex HA1 4HZ
www.apec.org.uk

The Pre-eclampsia Society – PETS
Rhianfa
Carmel LL54 7RL
www.pre-eclampsia-society.org.uk

Blood Pressure Association
60 Cranmer Terrace
London SW17 0QS
www.bpassoc.org.uk

Australian Action on Pre-eclampsia
P.O. Box 29 Carlton South
Vic. 3053
Australia
www.aapec.org.au

New Zealand Action on Pre-eclampsia
34 Ridge Rd
Howick
Auckland
New Zealand
info@nzapec.com

The Pre-eclampsia Foundation
5353 Wayzata Blvd.
Suite 207
Minneapolis, MN 55416
United States of America
www.preeclampsia.org

The HELLP Syndrome Society
P.O. Box 44
Bethany
West Virginia 26032
United States of America
www.hellpsyndrome.org

ESSENTIAL READING

Billington, M. and Stevenson, M. (2006) Hypertensive disorders and the critically ill woman. In: **Critical Care in Childbearing for Midwives**. Oxford; Blackwell/Wiley.

Gilbert, E.S. (2007) Hypertensive disorders. In: **Manual of High Risk Pregnancy and Delivery**, 4th Edn. St. Louis, MO; Moseby/Elsevier.

Henderson, C. and Macdonald, S. (2004) Hypertensive disorders of pregnancy. In: **Mayes Midwifery: A textbook for Midwives**, 13th Edn. Ballière Tindall.

Johnson, R. and Taylor, W. (2006) Assessment of maternal and neonatal vital signs – blood pressure measurement. In: **Skills for Midwifery Practice**, 2nd Edn. Elsevier Churchill Livingstone.

Lip, G., Beevers, Y.H., O'Brien, G., Beevers, E. and Gareth, D. (2007) **ABC of Hypertension**, 5th Edn. Oxford; BMJ books/Blackwell.

RCOG (2006) **Clinical Guideline No. 10a: The management of severe pre-eclampsia/eclampsia**. London; Royal College of Obstetricians and Gynaecologists. On line as: www.rcog.org.uk/resources/Public/pdf/management_pre_eclampsia_mar06.pdf

Sibai, B., Dekker, G. and Kupferminc, M. (2005) Pre-eclampsia. **Lancet, 365**(9461):785–799.

HEART DISEASE

4

Moira McLean, Frances Bu'Lock and S. Elizabeth Robson

4.1 Mild Structural Heart Disease

Incidence:	**Risk for Childbearing**
Affects 1% of live births[1] 2500 adults present with congenital heart disease a year[2] 0.8% pregnant women have congenital heart disease[3]	Variable Risk (dependent upon repair and condition)

EXPLANATION OF CONDITIONS

Appendix 4.1 outlines cardiac terminology for the midwife, and cardiac abbreviations are in the glossary at the beginning of this book.

Of children born with congenital heart disease, 85% now survive to adulthood[1,4]. There are a wide range of lesions. Isolated valve lesions are dealt with separately. Other cardiac abnormalities are associated with shunts, missing chambers +/− abnormal connections. Mild conditions are outlined below, moderate and complex conditions in the next sections. Some conditions, especially atrial septal defect, may present or be detected for the first time in pregnancy. Most have previously been repaired but all require consideration and some require further management. Recurrence risks must also be addressed.

Shunts

A shunt is passage of blood through a channel that is not its normal one[5]. Severity is determined not only by the size of the shunt but also the complexity and repairability of associated lesions.

Atrial Septal Defect (ASD)

This is an incomplete closure of the wall between the upper chambers of the heart (left and right atria). It is commoner in women and may be associated with valve problems. It is generally repaired in childhood; transcatheter umbrella closure is now common.

Ventricular Septal Defect (VSD)

Ventricular septal defect is one or more openings in the wall separating the right and left ventricles. It is one of the most common congenital heart defects. About 60% of these close spontaneously or are too small to need surgery; the remaining 40% require open heart surgery, usually in infancy.

Patent Ductus Arteriosus (PDA)

This is the persistence of a normal fetal structure between the left pulmonary artery and the descending aorta. Persistence of this fetal structure beyond ten days of life is considered abnormal. It is commoner in pre-term infants and is generally closed either surgically or with a transcatheter umbrella-type device.

Tetralogy of Fallot

Tetralogy of Fallot has four components:

1. Ventricular septal defect (VSD)
2. Aorta dextroposition, which overrides a VSD
3. Right ventricular outflow tract obstruction
4. Right ventricular hypertrophy

Tetralogy of Fallot is the most common cyanotic heart defect, representing 5–7% of congenital heart defects. It can be associated with chromosome 22 deletion[6], and is generally repaired in infancy or early childhood.

COMPLICATIONS

Atrial Septal Defect

- Atrial fibrillation
- Heart failure
- Stroke

Ventricular Septal Defect

- Congestive heart failure and failure to thrive in infancy and early childhood
- Damage to the heart's electrical conduction system during surgery (requiring pacemaker or causing late arrhythmias)
- Infective endocarditis
- Aortic insufficiency (leaking of the valve that separates the left ventricle from the aorta)
- Pulmonary hypertension (high blood pressure in the lungs) leading to failure of the right side of the heart[7,8] (see Section 4.9 Pulmonary Hypertension)

Patent Ductus Arteriosus

Closure is usually completely successful, but there is an increased recurrence risk for the fetus.

Tetralogy of Fallot

- Post-repair, residual lesions are frequent
- Pulmonary regurgitation is common +/− stenosis, and the valve may need replacement
- Regular cardiological follow-up is essential
- Late arrhythmias also occur
- 22q deletion may not have been recognised previously and has 50% recurrence risk[9]

NON-PREGNANCY TREATMENT AND CARE

See above

PRE-CONCEPTION ISSUES AND CARE

- Seek expert congenital heart disease specialist advice as to whether further assessment required, e.g. PDA/ASD device closure relatively new
- Assess the requirement for endocarditis prophylaxis (only fully-closed defects are low risk)
- Consideration of pre-pregnancy interventions to optimise maternal and fetal wellbeing in pregnancy for ongoing/residual haemodynamic problems
- Clinical genetics referral for recurrence risk and need for fetal surveillance
- PDA and secundum ASD are **normal** in utero, hence fetal screening is not prognostic and postnatal echocardiography is recommended
- Other types of ASD (such as partial AVSD), VSD and Tetralogy of Fallot can be detected in utero; mild forms cannot be completely excluded

Pregnancy Issues

- Low risk if closed or repaired with surgery
- Increased recurrence risk in the baby, so specialised cardiac ultrasound screening may be indicated at specialist centres (see pre-pregnancy counselling)
- Fetal nuchal translucency screening may also be helpful[10]

Atrial septal defect
- May be newly diagnosed in pregnancy; if repaired, problems are unlikely[11]
- Open ASD increases risks of arrhythmia, thrombo-embolic stroke and right heart failure

Ventricular septal defect
- Previously closed defects very low risk; occasional arrhythmia issues
- Small defects near valves have increased endocarditis risks
- Large untreated defects are high risk (see Section 4.9 Eisenmenger's Syndrome)

Patent ductus arteriosus
- Previously closed/asymptomatic small shunts behave normally
- Large shunts' ducts can lead to pulmonary hypertension (see Section 4.9 Eisenmenger's Syndrome)
- 4% recurrence risk postnatally[12]

Tetralogy of Fallot
- If repaired, pregnancy generally tolerated well but needs cardiological supervision and antibiotic cover
- For unrepaired defects, see Section 4.3, Severe Structural Heart Disease

Medical Management and Care

Atrial septal defect
- Routine care if previously successfully closed, otherwise consider aspirin thrombo-prophylaxis

Ventricular septal defect
- Routine care if previously successfully closed (consider endocarditis prophylaxis for patch closures)
- Small shunts treated as normal, plus endocarditis prophylaxis
- Larger shunts need cardiological supervision
- Co-existing pulmonary hypertension: counselling for ToP etc. (see Section 4.9 Eisenmenger's Syndrome)
- Arrhythmias may occur
- Endocarditis is a risk with uncorrected or residual defect

Patent ductus arteriosus
- Closed – treat as normal
- Open/newly diagnosed – endocarditis prophylaxis and follow cardiological advice

Tetralogy of Fallot
- Assess for right outflow obstruction/pulmonary regurgitation, right ventricular function and other residual lesions
- Arrhythmia monitoring and treatment may be required
- Diuretics may be helpful but bed-rest is rarely necessary[17]
- In the absence of problems a normal vaginal birth is anticipated[13]

Midwifery Management and Care
All will require:
- Early booking with immediate referral to specialist
- Accurate booking history and baseline observations
- Advice on diet and iron supplements to maintain a normal Hb level
- Advice about antibiotic treatment for any dental or other procedures
- Observation for worsening tiredness and breathlessness
- If right ventricular failure develops prepare for a pre-term delivery

Labour issues
Symptomatic patients and those with open ASD have a higher risk of thrombo-embolic disease, are likely to require compression stockings[13] and anticoagulation considered if immobile[11].

Patients with active problems will require:
- Anaesthetic review prior to labour
- Plan of care drawn up, to include a strategy for oxytocic drugs[14] – generally as normal
- Antibiotic prophylaxis for rupture of membranes/active labour

Medical Management and Care

Atrial septal defect
- If unoperated, consider antibiotics to prevent endocarditis[13]

VSD/repaired tetralogy of Fallot
- Epidural may be preferable for pain relief
- Prescribe antibiotic prophylaxis[15]

Midwifery Management and Care
- Find, read and follow the care plan thoroughly
- Ascertain if antibiotics are to be given, and administer promptly
- TED stockings from onset of labour if to be used
- Careful monitoring of pulse, blood pressure and fetal wellbeing
- Assess progress in labour, with prompt referral if concerned
- Oxytocin is usually the drug of choice for third-stage management

Postpartum issues
The neonate is at risk of cardiac disease and requires screening according to cardiological advice[15].

Standard contraceptive advice is appropriate unless open ASD/concerns re pulmonary hypertension (see Section 4.9 Eisenmenger's Syndrome). Combined oral contraceptives are commonly used. Intrauterine devices may be appropriate but consider if endocarditis prophylaxis is warranted[16].

Medical Management and Care
- ASD – routine care if no complications
- VSD/corrected ToF – monitor fluid balance if potential for CCF
- Discuss contraceptive options
- Consider multi-disciplinary follow-up for six weeks after delivery[18]

Midwifery Management and Care
- Encourage ambulation to reduce risk of thrombo-embolic disease
- Ascertain if maintenance of fluid balance is to be continued
- Reinforce contraceptive advice as above
- Be alert for signs of cardiac disease in the neonate, which might initially present as lethargy or as a feeding problem
- The neonatal examination prior to discharge home is best performed by a paediatrician, not a midwife, due to the risk of cardiac disease

4.2 Moderate Structural Heart Disease

Incidence	Risk for Childbearing
Specified as per individual condition, see below	Variable and High Risk (dependent upon repair and condition)

EXPLANATION OF CONDITIONS

Coarctation of the Aorta

- 5–8% of CHD[1]
- Congenital narrowing of the aorta, generally at the site of ductal insertion, resulting in upper body hypertension and lower body hypoperfusion
- Aortic wall is often more diffusely abnormal; even with complete and timely repair there is a life-long risk of aneurysm formation and aortic dissection[2]
- Up to 50% have other heart defects, e.g. VSD, aortic or mitral valve disease (including bicuspid aortic valve)
- Up to 10% of older patients may have cerebral aneurysms at presentation[2]
- Most coarctations are detected and repaired in infancy or childhood; however diagnosis in adulthood and even during pregnancy is not uncommon

After coarctation repair many children were considered 'cured' and were discharged from follow-up, but there is an increasing appreciation of their premature morbidity and mortality[3,4] and the need for long-term cardiological supervision.

Transposition of the Great Vessels

This is uncommon (<1% CHD) but, like Tetralogy of Fallot, it has been successfully treated for more than thirty years, so there are significant numbers of women with it now entering reproductive life. The right ventricle gives rise to the aorta and the left ventricle the pulmonary artery[5]. Initial long-term survivors have generally undergone *Senning* or *Mustard* repairs[6] in which the venous blood is rerouted within the atrial chambers. Current techniques switch the great arteries, and coronary arteries to the correct chambers.

Valvular Heart Disease (see Section 4.4)

Cardiac Transplant Recipients

These patients are managed with their transplant unit for monitoring of anti-rejection drugs and cardiac status to assess for transplant rejection (see also renal transplant management in Section 6.4) Genetic issues for the pre-transplant condition should also be considered.

COMPLICATIONS

Coarctation of the Aorta

- Residual/re-coarctation after repair
- Associated aortic/mitral valve disease
- Hypertension
- Impaired LV function and CCF[7]
- Thoracic aortic aneurysm/dissection (higher risk in pregnancy)
- Cerebral aneurysm rupture (higher risk in pregnancy)
- Reduced life expectancy[3,7]
- Infective endocarditis[8,9]

Transposition of the Great Vessels

Of patients with atrial diversion operations, 30–50% have a degree of systemic ventricular dysfunction and systemic atrio-ventricular valve regurgitation, because the morphologic right ventricle and tricuspid valve are in the systemic circulation[10]. They are prone to atrial arrhythmias; both tachycardias and sinus node disease can be life threatening and need drugs or pacemaker. *Baffle obstruction* can occur, and can exacerbate problems from arrhythmias. Following the arterial switch operation there is a potential for coronary artery ostial stenosis and early coronary artery disease. Many patients have branch pulmonary artery stenosis and some have required pulmonary or aortic valve replacement.

NON-PREGNANCY TREATMENT AND CARE

Coarctation of the Aorta

Generally, infants/children treated surgically, with primary balloon dilatation or stenting used for older children or young adults, as is residual coarctation. Surgery in adulthood entails higher risk, often requiring conduit bypass of the narrowed segment. Hypertension requires aggressive treatment. Aneurysms are increasingly recognised, being managed with surgery or covered stents.

Transposition of the Great Vessels

Post-Mustard or Senning repair, many patients will be on ACE inhibitors +/− diuretics for ventricular dysfunction and systemic A-V valve regurgitation. Stenting for baffle obstruction, the use of atrial pacemakers and antiarrhythmic medication are common. Residual intracardiac shunts, and also pulmonary hypertension, need to be detected and managed.

PRE-CONCEPTION ISSUES AND CARE

Appropriate counselling regarding pregnancy should:

- Start in adolescence
- Give accurate, individual advice correcting misinformation about both contraception and pregnancy
- Identify potential effects of the defect on pregnancy in terms of maternal and fetal risks
- Discuss the effects of cardiac disease including risks of long-term deterioration, and even dying, and whether these will change with time or treatment

Coarctation of the Aorta

- MRI scan prior to pregnancy to exclude aneurysm[11] or significant obstruction, which should be dealt with if present
- Consider a genetic referral for underlying abnormalities such as 22q deletion
- Recurrence risk is around 4%, and fetal cardiac surveillance is recommended

Transposition of the Great Vessels

- MRI scan and echocardiogram to assess baffles and systemic ventricle or valve function
- Stent baffles if narrowed
- Holter monitoring for rhythm, and drugs/pacemaker initiated if required
- Cease ACE inhibitors

Pregnancy Issues

Coarctation of the Aorta

Most women reach childbearing age. Untreated coarctation carries a 3–8% increased fetomaternal risk[1]. Hypertension occurs in 30%, with additional risk of pre-eclampsia[12]. Uncorrected coarctation carries a risk of **aortic dissection** and cerebral haemorrhage in pregnancy, as well as fetal hypoperfusion. Only patients with evidence of dissection should undergo surgical repair during pregnancy[12]. However, most adult coarctation is now treated with percutaneous dilatation and stenting. This can be performed in pregnancy with a much lower risk to mother and fetus than surgery, particularly in the second trimester if there are problems with blood pressure control or concerns re fetal compromise. There is at least a 4% risk of recurrence.

Transposition of the Great Vessels

Well tolerated if good systemic ventricular function and competent valves[13]. May require diuretics, anti-arrhythmics +/− pacemaker. Pregnancy may exacerbate or unmask systemic ventricular dysfunction, baffle obstruction or arrhythmia. Recurrence risk for the fetus is probably low.

Medical Management and Care

Coarctation of the Aorta
- Control BP with beta-blockers and avoid ACE inhibitors[12]
- Consider elective caesarean section before term in case of aortic aneurysm formation or uncontrollable hypertension[14]
- Avoid balloon angioplasty in pregnancy[12], but stenting is probably safe

Transposition of the Great Vessels
- Monitor for signs of heart failure and arrhythmia[15]
- Diuretics for oedema
- Beta-blockers for tachycardias but may then need pacing
- Systemic venous baffle obstruction may need stenting

Midwifery Management and Care
- Early booking with immediate referral to a maternal medicine clinic and re-referral to the cardiologist
- Accurate booking history with baseline observations, especially pulse
- Check blood pressure in correct (usually right) arm as the left subclavian artery is often involved in coarctation repair
- Monitor blood pressure regularly for prompt identification of hypertensive disease, especially with coarctation of the aorta
- Maintain Hb levels, so give advice on diet and iron supplementation
- Advise on antibiotic treatment for any dental or other procedures
- Prepare the mother for the possibility of a pre-term delivery

Labour Issues

Labour is a risk period for acute cardiac decompensation or pulmonary oedema, and also for increased aortic wall stress. However, this may still be managed successfully in the majority of these women.
- Epidural analgesia may be useful as tachycardia secondary to pain increases cardiac work. Care with blood pressure and cardiac rhythm management is important
- Pushing increases vagal tone and may worsen bradycardia

Medical Management and Care
- Antibiotic prophylaxis
- Antihypertensive drugs may be needed to treat hypertension
- Prophylactic (even temporary) pacemaker may be considered for some TGA patients
- If normal birth anticipated consider shortening the second stage
- If there is evidence of aneurysm formation, caesarean section is preferable for delivery[13]
- Epidural use is recommended

Midwifery Management and Care
- The midwife *might* be able to conduct a normal delivery in uncomplicated cases, with an emphasis on a short second stage, which could require an episiotomy
- Alternatively the role might be to assist with an operative delivery, which may well be pre-term
- Otherwise the care is as in Section 4.1

Postpartum Issues
- As with mild structural defects (see Section 4.1) the neonate risks heart disease and requires screening
- The mother with transposition of the great vessels may be at increased risk of venous thrombo-embolism, but for most the risk is normal
- The same contraceptive issues arise as in Section 4.1

Medical Management and Care
- Review medications prior to discharge: some beta-blockers are excreted less in breast milk
- Blood pressure often settles rapidly
- Systemic ventricular dysfunction may continue or worsen postpartum so careful review pre-discharge is required
- ACE inhibitors may be restarted
- Cardiac follow-up 4–6 weeks post-delivery for problematic patients

Midwifery Management and Care
- This mother is not for discharge until reviewed by the medical team
- Basic post-operative care is required if post-caesarean section
- Basic observations might need to be continued for longer than usual, with an emphasis on blood pressure and fluid balance
- Advise and support specific to the needs of a mother with a baby on a neonatal unit if the delivery was pre-term (see Chapter 1)
- The basic care is the same as in Section 4.1

4.3 Severe Structural Heart Disease

Incidence	Risk for Childbearing
Varies as per individual condition	High Risk: life threatening; ≥5% maternal mortality[1]

EXPLANATION OF CONDITIONS

These are conditions in which pregnancy carries a significant risk (≥2–5%) for mother and/or fetus; i.e. pregnancy is either high/very high risk or contraindicated. Inevitably, despite counselling, some women will become/wish to remain pregnant. These women require intensive supervision, with which some will achieve an acceptable outcome. This includes women with:

- Unoperated/palliated cyanotic or complex congenital heart disease, including single ventricle conditions
- Women with poor systemic ventricular function (see Section 4.6 Cardiomyopathy)
- Women with Eisenmenger's syndrome (see Section 4.9)
- Women with Marfan's syndrome (Section 4.5)

Unoperated Cyanotic Heart Disease

Many women will be recent immigrants but, rarely, cyanotic heart disease may not be diagnosed until adulthood, even in the UK. Some conditions are balanced and may have been managed conservatively deliberately. Lesions include uncorrected Tetralogy of Fallot, pulmonary stenosis/atresia with ventricular septal defect, functionally univentricular heart conditions (e.g. tricuspid atresia) and Ebstein's anomaly with ASD.

Palliated Complex Heart Disease

Increasing numbers of children with complex cardiac abnormalities, including both single ventricle conditions and non-septatable VSD, +/− transposition, are surviving to adulthood with a Fontan circulation. This is a 'final common pathway' of surgeries for conditions in which the heart pumps blood solely around the systemic circulation, with the systemic venous return passing to the pulmonary arteries without being pumped by a ventricle. It permits separation of the arterial and venous sides of the circulation (hence most are 'pink'), and also offloads the heart, but pulmonary blood flow is dependent on the venous pump (from the calf muscles), respiratory 'suction' and gravity as well as a low-resistance circuit. Many of these patients are anticoagulated to reduce the possibility of thrombosis of rather sluggish pulmonary arterial circulation and increasing numbers are taking diuretics +/− ACE inhibitors. Atrial arrhythmias are common and some will have pacemakers +/− anti-arrhythmic drugs. Some may have had palliative shunt operations or intermediate/partial Fontan surgery, and hence remain hypoxic to some degree.

COMPLICATIONS

During pregnancy the fall in systemic vascular resistance and rise in cardiac output exacerbates any right-to-left shunting, worsening pre-existing cyanosis and hypoxia. The required increase in cardiac rate and output may also worsen the effects of valvular lesions and ventricular dysfunction.

Maternal complications depend mainly on functional classification of the mother (NYHA classification is in Appendix 4.2). NYHA classes I–II have a maternal mortality rate of <1%, whilst NYHA classes III–IV have a maternal mortality rate of 7% or greater[2]. This is largely determined by the degree of cyanosis, ventricular dysfunction and prior cardiac events, such as pulmonary oedema, arrhythmia, stroke, etc.[3] Complications include heart failure, arrhythmia, pulmonary/paradoxical embolism and haemorrhage. The effects on the fetus are marked, with a high incidence of spontaneous abortion, a 30–50% risk of premature delivery and low birth weight. The degree of maternal hypoxaemia is the most important predictor of neonatal outcome; oxygen saturations <85% give only 12% chance of livebirth[4]. NYHA class IV mothers also have a fetal mortality rate of around 30%. Recurrence risks are generally around 4% but may be up to 50% for patients with 22q deletion, which may not have been recognised previously.

NON-PREGNANCY TREATMENT AND CARE

These women should be under regular, careful supervision of cardiologists in tertiary centres specialising in the care of adults with congenital heart disease. They are monitored:

- Clinically, including oxygen saturation, and Hb estimation
- Functionally, with cardio-pulmonary exercise testing etc.
- Echocardiographically, plus CT or MRI as required
- Regular Holter monitoring for occult arrhythmia

Many will require trans-catheter or surgical interventions and indeed may benefit from new technology as time progresses.

PRE-CONCEPTION ISSUES AND CARE

Ideally, all women should be able to make an informed choice about pregnancy based on both maternal and fetal risks, long term prognosis and alternative options such as contraception, termination of pregnancy, adoption, surrogacy and IVF. Encourage realistic expectations, and advocate active preparation for pregnancy. This includes:

- Ensuring easy access to multi-disciplinary care
- Genetic counselling
- Pre-pregnancy surgery or intervention: e.g. change of valve type; consider risk of surgery versus reduction in pregnancy risk; catheter interventions; ablation of arrhythmia; and optimisation of cardiac function
- Optimal timing of pregnancy (pregnancy at a younger age is lower risk for some complex conditions)
- Avoidance of teratogens (medication may need to be changed prior to pregnancy, e.g. anticoagulants, ACEI, anti-arrhythmics) (see Cardiac Drugs in Appendix 4.3)
- Prompt initiation of iron supplementation
- General measures: smoking cessation and folic acid supplementation

Pregnancy Issues

Each woman will need management according to individual anatomical and functional status. Close liaison between cardiologists and obstetricians is essential.

- Admission for bed-rest +/− oxygen therapy may be required
- Anaemia should be avoided
- Fetal echocardiography is required as well as regular fetal wellbeing and growth monitoring
- Appropriate timing for delivery is crucial to balance maternal and neonatal morbidity and mortality
- A clear plan of management for labour and delivery should be established in advance, clearly documented and widely available

Medical Management and Care

- Iron deficiency – monitor red cell indices plus Hb, because cyanotic patients can be functionally anaemic even with a 'normal' Hb
- Warfarin may not be essential especially for Fontan patients; change to aspirin, or low-molecular-weight heparin
- Stop ACE inhibitors if not done pre-conceptually
- Regular outpatient review, echocardiography +/− Holter monitoring
- Beta-blockers for arrhythmia +/− pacemaker if indicated
- Diuretics for heart failure/breathlessness[5]
- Oxygen therapy may help severely cyanosed patients, especially if they have a reduced respiratory capacity

Midwifery Management and Care

- Early booking, with thorough history taking, and immediate referral to a maternal medicine clinic, then liaison with tertiary cardiologist
- Baseline observations, including oxygen saturation
- Maintain Hb levels as above, with additional dietary advice[5]
- Advise on antibiotic treatment for any dental or other procedures
- Teach the mother to keep a fetal movement chart after 24 weeks
- Prepare parents for potential pre-term/IUGR baby or fetal loss

Labour Issues

Labour requires careful monitoring of both mother and fetus. Pre-load and blood pressure should be monitored carefully and blood loss minimised. Antibiotic prophylaxis should be given during labour and delivery.

In general, vaginal delivery with low dose epidural is the mode of choice. Forceps or ventouse delivery may be used to shorten maternal expulsive effort in the second stage. Cardiac indications for caesarean section include aortic dilatation >40 mm, warfarin treatment and important systemic ventricular dysfunction.

Bolus doses of Syntocinon should be avoided in the third stage, as they can cause severe hypotension. Low dose oxytocin infusions are safer. Ergometrine is best avoided in most cases as it can cause acute hypertension. Uterine compression sutures are the most effective treatment in the management of uterine atony at caesarean section. The safety of misoprostol is yet to be determined.

Medical Management and Care

- Prophylactic (even temporary) pacemaker is considered for some women as pushing is vagotonic
- If normal birth is anticipated consider shortening the second stage
- If there is evidence of aneurysm formation, or major ventricular dysfunction, caesarean section is preferable[6]
- Epidural use is recommended
- Avoid supine position, especially for Fontan patients, because caval compression restricts pulmonary blood flow
- Invasive arterial +/− venous pressure monitoring may be helpful even for vaginal delivery
- Cyanotic patients may require intravenous hydration, especially if very nauseated
- Prescribe antibiotic prophylaxis

Midwifery Management and Care

- Intensive care setting is likely[5]; experienced staff required
- Administer the antibiotics and any other prescribed drugs as above
- Keep the mother in left lateral position throughout the first stage[7]
- The midwife may well be required to conduct a normal delivery under close medical supervision, with an emphasis on a short second stage, which could require an episiotomy
- Alternatively the role might be to assist with an instrumental/operative delivery, which may well be pre-term
- Otherwise the care is as in Section 4.1

Postpartum Issues

Following delivery, the return of the uterine blood flow into the systemic circulation results in an increase of cardiac output. Stroke volume, heart rate and cardiac output remain high for 24 hours post-delivery with rapid intravascular volume shifts in the first two weeks postpartum, thus the later stages of labour and early postpartum period are times of high risk for pulmonary oedema[1].

- The neonate may require intensive care in addition to heart screening
- Contraceptive issues are similar to the previous section
- Most require progesterone-only methods

Medical Management and Care

- Close medical supervision is still required after delivery with monitoring for at least 48 hours
- Review medications prior to discharge: restart ACE inhibitors and warfarin; some beta-blockers are excreted less in breast milk
- Systemic ventricular dysfunction may continue or worsen postpartum so careful review pre-discharge is required
- Cardiac follow-up 4−6 weeks post-delivery for almost all patients

Midwifery Management and Care

- This mother is not for discharge until reviewed by the medical team
- Basic post-operative care is required if post-caesarean section
- Basic observations may need continuation for longer than usual with emphasis on oxygen saturation, blood pressure and fluid balance
- Advise and support specific to the needs of a mother with a baby on a neonatal unit if delivery was pre-term (see Chapter 1)
- Bereavement care if a stillbirth occurred
- The basic care is as in Section 4.1

4.4 Valvular Heart Disease

Incidence	Risk for Childbearing
Prevalence varies as to the individual condition	Moderate to High Risk

EXPLANATION OF CONDITIONS

Stenosis is the narrowing of a valve restricting forward flow, commonly affecting the mitral, aortic and pulmonary valves. The latter is rarely problematic. Stenosis may be congenital or acquired as with rheumatic fever or SLE[1].

Regurgitation/insufficiency/incompetence results from incomplete valve closure that allows regurgitation of blood back to the preceding chamber. It can be congenital or acquired, e.g. rheumatic fever, or Marfan's or Ehlers-Danlos syndromes.

Rheumatic heart disease is a complication of rheumatic fever in which cardiac valve damage arises from immunologic injury in group A haemolytic streptococcal infection. Incidence remains high in developing countries and the UK immigrant population, hence it is re-emerging as a cause of maternal death[2].

Prosthetic heart valves are replacements for diseased heart valves. These can be *bioprostheses* (donor/animal tissue) or *mechanical*. They are mainly used on the left side and need lifelong anticoagulation; this complicates pregnancy.

COMPLICATIONS

Mitral valve disease: atrial fibrillation, heart failure, endocarditis or thrombosis may develop. Risk of stroke is increased and increased left atrial pressure may cause pulmonary oedema. Mitral regurgitation causes LV volume overload which may impair function.

Aortic valve disease: stenosis restricts the cardiac output increase required in pregnancy and may cause effort restriction, angina or syncope. Symptoms must be taken very seriously as they indicate a high risk of sudden death. Regurgitation is better tolerated but also leads to LV volume overload, myocardial failure and arrhythmia.

Pulmonary valve problems: isolated mild stenosis is common and of little consequence but more severe stenosis may be revealed during pregnancy by increased cardiac output. Pulmonary regurgitation is mainly post-intervention. Residual stenosis and regurgitation are common as part of more complex congenital heart disease.

Ebstein's anomaly: the tricuspid valve leaflets are displaced into the right ventricle. The valve is regurgitant and malformed. It is associated with other structural cardiac abnormalities. Incidence of arrhythmia is high[1].

Mixed disease is common (multiple valves +/− stenosis and regurgitation) complicating care and worsening prognosis.

Infective endocarditis: rare and potentially fatal for mother or fetus. Cardiac structural abnormality is a predisposition. Bacterial infection, especially in pregnancy, of heart valves/structures can initiate systemic or pulmonary embolism, so antibiotic prophylaxis is given within 2–3 hours of unexpected exposure and for predictable bacteraemia.

Antibiotic prophylaxis is advisable for:

- Previous bacterial endocarditis
- Prosthetic heart valves, conduits, other foreign material
- Complex cyanotic congenital heart diseases
- Valvular heart disease and cardiac shunts
- Hypertrophic cardiomyopathy
- Obstetric procedures in the presence of infection
- At the onset of labour, ARM/SRM or caesarean section
- Insertion of cervical cerclage and urinary catheterisation

Antibiotics are not required for:

- Physiological heart murmurs
- Isolated secundum/ASD, surgically-repaired ASD or PDA
- Cardiac pacemakers
- Certain procedures:
  - choriovillous sampling
  - amniocentesis
  - vaginal examination
  - transvaginal ultrasound scanning and insertion of regional analgesia[2,3,4]

NON-PREGNANCY TREATMENT AND CARE

- **Medication** might ease symptoms
- **Balloon dilatation** of valves may be performed safely for non-calcified valves (preferably after first trimester)
- **Surgical** repair or replacement requires cardiopulmonary bypass, and is high risk in pregnancy, (especially for the fetus) but can be life-saving
- **Metal prosthetic heart valves** – patients require long-term anticoagulation and antibiotic prophylaxis as above

PRE-CONCEPTION ISSUES AND CARE

- Expert clinical and echocardiographic assessment of:
  - functional status
  - previous cardiac events
  - ventricular and valvular function
  - pulmonary artery pressure
  - current medication[5]
- Discussion of risks associated with pregnancy
- Discuss risks and benefits of anticoagulant therapy
- Pre-pregnancy interventions, with contraceptive cover, to plan and optimise wellbeing for pregnancy[6]
- Identify if pregnancy is contraindicated, with either pulmonary hypertension or >2 risk factors below:
  - reduced LV systolic function (ejection fraction <40%)
  - left heart obstruction: aortic or mitral stenosis with valve areas of <1.5 cm^2 or <2.0 cm^2, respectively
  - past cardiovascular events (heart failure, TIA, stroke)
  - reduced functional capacity with a disease score of NYHA class II or higher[7] (Appendix 4.2) as the maternal death rate is 30–60%[8]

Pregnancy Issues

With unplanned pregnancies, consider risk of pregnancy continuation versus termination. Most valvular heart disease is manageable with expert input.

Mitral stenosis may cause pulmonary oedema or atrial arrhythmias during pregnancy or soon after delivery[9]. It may present for the first time in pregnancy, being poorly tolerated as the tachycardia and increased stroke volume of pregnancy cannot be supported through the narrowed valve. Left atrial pressure rises, causing pulmonary oedema[7,10]. Risk factors relate to severity:

- Decompensation (third trimester risk)[11]
- Death increases with left heart obstruction or NYHA class II disease[12] (Appendix 4.2)

Complications of pre-term delivery and IUGR.

Aortic stenosis becomes more significant during pregnancy if the valve area is severely compromised, as above. However, symptoms appear late due to left atrial capacitance. Pulmonary oedema, angina from reduced coronary flow and effort syncope are all ominous signs and urgent intervention is required.

Mitral and aortic regurgitation are usually well tolerated due to reduced systemic vascular resistance[13], but peripheral/pulmonary oedema benefits from diuretics.

Prosthetic heart valves are managed individually dependent on type and position of valve and cardiac function[9].

Medical Management and Care

- Regular appointments at a combined obstetric/cardiology clinic
- Baseline ECG, echocardiography, ultrasound and electrolytes, +/− chest X-ray
- Diuretics and beta-blockers may be helpful, +/− bed-rest[9]
- Risk of systemic emboli from atrial fibrillation, so anticoagulation is required, usually with low-molecular-weight heparin
- Heart rate control with digoxin, beta-blocker, calcium channel blocker or a combination of these[14]
- Pulmonary oedema – treat with oxygen and diuretics
- If deterioration, or severe symptoms, balloon mitral valve or aortic valvoplasty may be of benefit[11], preferably after the first trimester
- If surgery is required, careful monitoring of fetal wellbeing is necessary throughout; cardiopulmonary bypass with increased flow, if needed, to respond to fetal distress
- Anaesthetic agents used during surgery may have teratogenic effects[7]

Metal Prosthetic Valves and Anticoagulation

- Conception to week 12: consider the use of monitored and dose adjusted heparin if on >5 mg/day of warfarin; discuss drug teratogenicity versus the risk of valve thrombosis[9]
- Weeks 12–36: generally warfarin therapy is used
- Week 36+: discontinue warfarin; change to heparin titrated to a therapeutic activated partial-thromboplastin time, or anti-factor Xa level[15]
- Valve thrombosis: thrombolytic treatment first line as risks of embolism, bleeding or placental abruption are less than surgery risk

Midwifery Management and Care

- Newly arrived immigrants require a full examination by their GPs and referral if physical signs of cardiovascular disease are found[8]
- At/before booking, refer for combined obstetric/cardiology care
- Re-refer promptly if palpitations or breathlessness are reported, because it is difficult to differentiate cardiac decompensation from the physiological symptoms of pregnancy[5,8,16]
- Social support, and interpreters can improve outcomes
- Hospital admission for bed-rest, oxygen therapy, saturation monitoring and fluid balance estimation

Labour Issues

Labour is a risk period for acute decompensation/pulmonary oedema.

Epidural analgesia may be useful, because tachycardia secondary to pain increases cardiac work, predisposing to pulmonary oedema. However, excessive vasodilatation reduces coronary perfusion in aortic stenosis and must be prevented (e.g. with adrenaline/epinephrine).

Unexpected urgent delivery: If anticoagulated, reverse warfarin with fresh frozen plasma/vitamin K. Protamine sulphate reverses heparin[9].

Medical Management and Care

- Vaginal delivery anticipated and clear plan of care documented
- Heparin is discontinued for labour and delivery
- Antibiotic cover is essential for delivery
- ECG, IVI plus invasive monitoring for moderate or severe disease
- Avoid fluid overload

Midwifery Management and Care

- High dependency care and observations, fluid balance, EFM, oxygen and saturation monitoring, TED stockings[7]
- Avoid supine and lithotomy positions
- Avoid active directed pushing, as the consequent increase in heart rate might not be tolerated[9]
- Use a Syntocinon infusion rather than Syntometrine, and use uterine massage to reduce blood loss[7]

Postpartum Issues

The early puerperium is associated with increased venous return to the heart which can lead to heart failure[12], hence continued haemodynamic monitoring is required.

Breast-feeding is not contraindicated when using warfarin, as its high protein binding in the maternal circulation leads to very small amounts secreted into breast milk.

Medical Management and Care

- Resume warfarin therapy the night after delivery, providing no bleeding complications arise[15]
- Haemodynamic monitoring >24 hr
- Contraception counselling, with emphasis on progesterone implants

Midwifery Management and Care

- Gentle mobilisation and assistance with baby care
- Encourage neonatal vitamin K administration, and advise to empty the breasts when feeding as hind milk has a higher vitamin K level[17]
- Liaison with the multi-disciplinary team in readiness for discharge
- Supportive care to inspire confidence with parenting

4.5 Marfan's Syndrome

Incidence	Risk for Childbearing
Prevalence of 5 per 100,000 of population[1]	High Risk
5000 UK cases per annum, 10% being severely affected[2]	

EXPLANATION OF CONDITION

Marfan's syndrome was first described in Paris by Bernard Marfan in 1896[3]. It is an autosomal dominant condition on chromosome 15[3]. It is inherited in 50–75% of cases, and also occurs as a spontaneous mutation. Fibrillin (a fine fibre found in connective tissue) production is affected[3,4,5]. This connective tissue disorder presents in various body systems: musculoskeletal, ocular, cardiovascular, respiratory and integumentary[6].

Typically, there is a disproportionate length of long bones and little subcutaneous fat, presenting as a tall, thin physique with long fingers and toes and hyperflexibility of joints. Further signs of the condition vary considerably between individuals, who may have one or more of:

- Narrow 'pigeon' chest[3]
- Scoliosis[3] (curvature of the spine)
- Flat feet[3]
- Myopia (short-sighted)[2] and lens problems[3]
- High arched dental palate with overcrowding of teeth

Although the condition affects men and women equally[3,7] this appearance may be more exaggerated in men, with some women being undiagnosed[8].

The valve between the left chambers of the heart is defective and may be large and floppy, resulting in an abnormal valve motion when the heart beats. In some cases, the valve may leak, creating a heart murmur. Small leaks may not cause any symptoms, but larger ones can result in shortness of breath, fatigue, and palpitations.

Due to faulty connective tissue, the wall of the aorta is weakened and stretches causing **aortic dilatation**. This increases the risk that the aorta will tear (**aortic dissection**), or rupture. The rupture causes serious complications of mitral-valve prolapse, aortic-root dilatation or sometimes sudden death[5].

COMPLICATIONS

General Complications

- Joint pain and dislocations, due to joint laxity[3,7]
- Scoliosis (curvature) of the spine and consequent back pain and mobility restrictions[2,3,7]
- Spontaneous pneumothorax in >10%[3]
- Bronchiectasis, asthma and emphysema[3]
- Hernias[3,7]
- Fatigue[3]

Cardiac Complications

- Aortic dissection – accounting for 20% of maternal cardiac fatalities[8]
- Aortic aneurysm formation

- Mitral valve regurgitation – resulting in medical emergency or death
- Heart valve prolapse and leak
- Increased heart workload causing symptoms of shortness of breath, over-tiredness or palpitations
- Heart murmurs may present
- Cardiomyopathy may develop
- Dilatation of the aortic root can cause the aortic valve to become stretched and leak
- Arrhythmia may occur

NON-PREGNANCY TREATMENT AND CARE

General Treatment

Early diagnosis, meticulous echocardiographic follow-up and multi-disciplinary assessment are essential[9]. Restrictive lifestyle advice and drugs may have to be prescribed, but should be counterbalanced with the need of a child to develop and mature as normally as possible[9]. Exercise and a healthy, vitamin-rich diet is encouraged, and smoking strongly discouraged as it destroys elastin[3].

Cardiac Treatment

Beta-blockers might be used[9] to reduce aortic root dilatation[7]. If the aortic root is greater than 45 mm, root replacement may be considered, especially if pregnancy is contemplated[10].

PRE-CONCEPTION ISSUES AND CARE

- Start advice in adolescence, reinforced by effective contraception
- Genetic counselling as there is a 50% chance the prospective child could inherit the gene[3]
  - The implications for reproductive choices and relationships should be sensitively discussed alongside genetic counselling[11]
  - Feelings of guilt about passing on the condition to children, or of being a family member who has been found not to have the condition, have been reported[11]
- There should be access to expert pre-pregnancy care and implications for pregnancy should be discussed
- Echocardiography is essential
- If aortic root >40 mm advise about increased risk of adverse outcome; if the aortic root is <40 mm reassure about the lesser risk
- Beta-blockers should be used and continued throughout pregnancy[12,13]
- Discussion of pregnancy care and possible need for hospitalisation[14]

Pregnancy Issues

Pregnancy in women with Marfan's syndrome carries a lethal risk of acute aortic dissection[15]. All Marfan's pregnancies are therefore high risk throughout and multidisciplinary team management is needed at a specialist centre caring for high cardiac risk pregnancy.

If no pre-pregnancy assessment took place, it should be undertaken at first booking. Here counselling is vital. Antenatal staff should be made aware that the pregnancy is high risk, and management guidelines and emergency contact numbers should be clearly recorded.

There is a 50% chance of the woman having an affected child[15]. Prenatal diagnoses may be offered, in particular a detailed ultrasound at 20–24 weeks including echocardiography and careful limb measurement. Molecular diagnosis is only available if the family mutation is known.

- Premature labour and ruptured membranes are common[8,16]
- Pelvic instability and backache increase

Medical Management and Care

- Care plan devised and updated as delivery may occur at short notice[8]
- Aortic root diameter should be monitored throughout pregnancy with serial echocardiograms[15]
- Those with an aortic root diameter of less than 40 mm historically tolerate pregnancy well[5,17,18]
- Hypertension should be treated aggressively[8]
- Beta-blockers should be continued throughout pregnancy[8,18]
- A pre-delivery anaesthetic assessment is advised[8]
- MRI of the pelvis (to detect dural ectasia) may be useful to guide epidural catheter placement[8]
- Steroids if delivery likely <34 weeks, but this risks fluid retention and cardiac failure, hence diuretics should also be considered[19]
- Anticoagulants need reviewing
- Aortic-root dilatation may be a risk predictor, but aortic dissection may occur without a clinically significant dilatation[5]
- Surgery in pregnancy is possible if root dilatation presents[17]
- Gestational hypertension and pre-eclampsia may increase the risk of aortic rupture[20]

Midwifery Management and Care

- Astute booking history, refer promptly to obstetric cardiology clinic
- Monitor pulse and respiration alongside normal antenatal observation at each antenatal appointment
- Encourage iron and vitamins to reduce anaemia
- Prepare woman/family for possibility of third trimester bed-rest[21]
- Provide pelvic support girdle and teach techniques for safe movement, because of pelvic pain and laxity (see Section 9.2)
- Prepare woman for early labour and/or small baby

Labour Issues

If there are no cardiac complications and no obstetric risk factors, vaginal delivery is possible[17], with an assisted second stage. However, most specialist units recommend caesarean section for higher-risk women. Elective caesarean section if the aortic root exceeds 40 mm.

Epidural anaesthesia is recommended, however this should only be performed after the possibilities of dural ectasia or an arachnoid cyst have been excluded, as these can result in dilution of anaesthetic.

There is a higher risk of postpartum haemorrhage and inversion of the uterus[17].

Medical Management and Care

- Prostaglandins should be used with caution
- Prophylactic antibiotics for operative delivery if valvular involvement
- Instrumental delivery and active pushing
- Syntocinon via slow IVI for active management of third stage
- Ergometrine should be avoided if possible[19]
- Avoid carboprost and misoprostol and consider bimanual compression, uterine sutures or intrauterine balloons to reduce bleeding rather than pharmacological agents; careful risk–benefit assessment is required[19]
- Cardiac and invasive monitoring with an arterial line[8,22], but beware risks of endocarditis and emboli

Midwifery Management and Care

- Intensive care and support are needed, with rigorous monitoring of maternal and fetal condition and fluid balance
- TED stockings
- Left lateral/supported sitting position to assist placental oxygenation
- EFM as the fetus is dependent on maternal oxygenation when the mother is haemodynamically unstable; hypoxaemic reduced variability of FH may be an initial sign prior to maternal signs[23]
- Effective communication and adept interpersonal skills are necessary to maintain a positive atmosphere

Postpartum Issues

- The maternal risk continues
- Contraception is essential, as further pregnancy poses further risk to the mother
- Fetal and neonatal mortality[16] is 7%, therefore the neonatal examination and investigations should be performed by a paediatrician, with parental consent, for early diagnosis

Medical Management and Care

- Arrange cardiac assessment whilst still in hospital
- Surveillance should continue until eight weeks postpartum
- Review suitability for contraceptive pill, or IUS as an alternative, especially if there is hypertension or a risk of thrombo-embolism[24]
- Sterilisation is an option but carries anaesthetic risk[25]

Midwifery Management and Care

- Continue with blood pressure monitoring until otherwise directed
- Reinforce the need for contraception
- Note that this mother is not for early discharge from hospital

4.6 Functional Heart Disease: Cardiomyopathy

Incidence	**Risk for Childbearing**
1:5,000[1]	Variable and High Risk
Peripartum cardiomyopathy 1:10,000[2]; 1:3000–4000 live births[3]	

EXPLANATION OF CONDITIONS

The term 'cardiomyopathy' is derived from the Latin, meaning *disease of the heart muscle*. Characterised by ventricular dysfunction and eventual development of cardiac failure, this rare and potentially lethal condition has five manifestations.

Dilated Cardiomyopathy (DCM)

Progressive loss or damage of cardiac myocytes leads to chamber dilatation, cardiac enlargement and reduced systolic function. This leads to venous stasis in the lungs, pulmonary oedema, breathlessness, and eventually reduced cardiac output becoming **left heart failure. Right heart failure** can also follow, with fluid accumulation in the soft tissues, ankle/leg oedema, liver enlargement and ascites (abdominal fluid). The cause can be genetic in 25–30% of cases, with both autosomal dominant and recessive types. It can follow viral myocarditis, and be associated with other muscle diseases, collagen disorders, metabolic disorders, chemotherapy[4], autoimmune disease (Chapter 11), haemoglobinopathies, hypothyroidism and hyperthyroidism[2].

Hypertrophic Cardiomyopathy (HCM)

There is enlargement and abnormal fibre orientation of the cardiac myocytes. Impaired diastolic relaxation results, the heart does not fill properly and there may be left ventricular outflow obstruction. It can present in childhood but may manifest at any age. There may be no symptoms, or there may be:

* Chest pain (angina) due to increased cardiac muscle oxygen requirements and reduced coronary blood flow
* Dyspnoea (breathlessness)
* Syncope (fainting due to fall in blood pressure)
* Atrial or ventricular arrhythmias
* Heart failure[5]
* Sudden death

At least 70% of cases have a genetic basis[2]. Inheritance is generally autosomal dominant and it affects 0.2–0.5% of the population[6,7].

Restrictive Cardiomyopathy (RCM)

The ventricular walls are still and filling is markedly impaired. Pressure in both atria then rises, the atria dilate to compensate and fibrillation results[8]. Symptoms occur late and include: heart failure, arrhythmias, syncope and sudden death. Prognosis is very poor.

Arrhythmogenic Right Ventricular Cardiomyopathy (ARVC)

Right (and eventually left) ventricular muscle is replaced by fatty and fibrous tissue. Early symptoms are mainly palpitations/sudden death; heart failure develops late. The condition may present in pregnancy with arrhythmias, and the ECG is characteristic. Inheritance is frequently autosomal dominant.

Peripartum Cardiomyopathy (PPCM)

This refers to the onset of cardiac failure between the last month of pregnancy and five months postpartum, in the absence of a prior cause[2]. Although rare, it is frequently fatal[9], accounting for around 25% of maternal cardiac deaths[10,11].

Of uncertain aetiology[12], it is associated with higher maternal age, parity or gestation, as well as black race[13].

Presenting features include:

* Paroxysmal nocturnal dyspnoea and nocturnal cough
* Chest pain
* New regurgitant murmurs, and pulmonary crackles
* Raised jugular venous pressure
* Third trimester or postnatal, signs of heart failure[2]

Differentiation from normal pregnancy-associated dyspnoea, ankle oedema and tiredness can be difficult initially[3].

Sudden Collapse may occur in fluid overload situations, e.g. multiple pregnancy, Syntocinon infusion and epidural. Chest X-ray may reveal an enlarged heart, pulmonary oedema and pleural effusion

COMPLICATIONS

* Dilated cardiomyopathy – heart failure, sudden death[5]
* Hypertrophic cardiomyopathy – angina, sudden death
* Restrictive cardiomyopathy – arrhythmias, sudden death
* ARVC – palpitations, sudden death
* Peripartum cardiomyopathy – heart failure, sudden death[3]

NON-PREGNANCY TREATMENT AND CARE

* Drug therapy:
    – diuretics
    – ACE inhibitors
    – beta-blockers
    – anti-arrhythmics
    – warfarin and aspirin
* Cardioversion to stabilise heart rhythm
* Pacemakers/implantable defibrillators
* Heart transplant for severe cases

PRE-CONCEPTION ISSUES AND CARE

* History taking to identify a significant family history
* Genetic counselling
* Refer to cardiologist with experience of cardiomyopathy
* Echocardiogram
* Stop or change drugs, e.g. ACE inhibitors, warfarin
* Explain the physiological impact of pregnancy upon the heart with risk of sudden death
* The woman may be advised against pregnancy as it can result in cardiac failure and death
* Increased risk of recurrent PPCM in future pregnancies, for survivors of PPCM
* Termination of pregnancy may be advised

Pregnancy Issues

Cardiomyopathy symptoms are often seen in uncomplicated pregnancies. The significance may only be recognised late, when cardiomyopathy presents in an advanced state and treatment is difficult.

Puerperal cardiomyopathy manifests in the third trimester, the fetus is relatively mature and can be delivered reasonably safely prior to, or at, commencement of treatment.

Medical Management and Care

- Referral and collaboration with cardiologist, obstetric, anaesthetic and paediatric teams for combined care
- Clear care pathways to be documented and agreed antenatally
- Acute care may need to be in critical care unit

Midwifery Management and Care

- If this condition was previously diagnosed, or when symptoms present in pregnancy, refer immediately to maternal medicine clinic
- Sensitivity – this is a major, life threatening illness

Labour Issues

First Stage

- Invasive monitoring, guided by individual case details, is generally recommended
- Pain relief may relieve cardiac stress

Second Stage

- Aim to minimise cardiovascular stresses whilst maintaining adequate analgesia
- Vaginal delivery safe in most women[14]; advantages of reduced blood loss, greater haemodynamic stability, avoidance of surgical stress, less chance of post-operative infection and pulmonary complications
- Short second stage by instrumental delivery can minimise cardiovascular compromise

Third stage

- Intravenous oxytocin produces a small reduction in arterial BP followed by an increase in cardiac output[10,15]
- Oxytocin is associated with decreased cardiac contractility and heart rate[16], so ergometrine should be avoided[17]
- Carboprost and misoprostol are also contraindicated; use only if benefit outweighs risk
- Consider compression and intrauterine balloons for PPH rather than pharmacological solutions[16]

Medical Management and Care

- Plan the timing of induction of labour/delivery with extreme caution[16]
- Regional analgesia, with careful monitoring, unless anticoagulated
- Stabilisation of condition by multi-disciplinary team
- Monitoring for cardiac failure
- Avoid fluid overload
- Avoid hypotension
- Consider pulmonary arterial catheterisation
- ECG monitoring for cardiac arrhythmias
- Consider elective, instrumental, vaginal delivery
- Prophylactic antibiotics for labour and puerperium are recommended
- Once delivered, if condition unstable, transfer to the Intensive Care Unit

Midwifery Management and Care

- Labour may need to be induced; administration of oxytocin should be finely titrated and administered in low dosage to avoid hypotension[16]
- Care of the IVI throughout labour and maintain a strict fluid balance
- Vigilant monitoring and documentation of: BP, pulse, respiratory rate, ECG, oxygen therapy and oxygen saturation monitoring
- Continuous EFM
- Maintain adequate pain relief having conferred with anaesthetist
- Monitor progress of labour, and refer slow progress promptly
- Left lateral position for labour, with passive leg exercises if immobile
- The midwife might be able to conduct a normal vaginal delivery if second stage progress is brisk, alternatively, the midwife should assist an operative delivery and support the mother
- Physiological third stage may be most appropriate if labour has been spontaneous with no further risk factors (thrombo-prophylaxis)
- Avoid ergometrine and Syntometrine in the third stage[17]
- Care of the (pre-term) baby at birth and possible transfer to NNU

Postpartum Issues

- Major changes in cardiac output and plasma volumes continue >2 weeks postpartum, so ongoing cardiological surveillance required[18]
- Maternal condition usually returns to baseline by six months postpartum
- Cardiac function returns to normal in 50% women with PPCM but there is a risk of reoccurrence[19,20]
- Increased risks of pulmonary oedema, thrombo-embolism and rhythm disturbances
- Treatment with ACEI, beta-blockers and full anticoagulation is appropriate[10]
- Prognosis for PPCM is dependent on recovery of left-sided ventricular function; if left ventricular dysfunction is on-going, mortality rates are 85% over five years

If myocardial dysfunction is severe, a cardiac transplant may be required[18].

Medical Management and Care

- Multi-disciplinary care plan, prior to discharge, addressing dynamic disease change with treatment modification and recovery potential[12]
- Life-long treatment may be required if condition does not recede, so enlist the cardiologist's support and promote outpatient attendance
- Advise on need for pre-conception care, and prescribe contraception

Midwifery Management and Care

- Continue observation of vital signs, reporting any anomalies
- Baby on NNU – facilitate maternal interaction and establish lactation
- Plan care and counsel the mother in caring for infant and own health – seek assistance from family, friends, and social services for household and other support
- Advice in avoiding stress and anxiety and adequate rest
- Avoidance of extreme exertion – advise the family on adjustments to the baby's room and movement of equipment, to minimise exertion
- Extensive education regarding medications and their side effects
- Advice to mother/family of heart failure signs (weight gain, dyspnoea, cough, pallor, chest pain, arrhythmias) and reporting thereof
- Promote a healthy, low sodium, iron-rich diet

4.7 Functional Heart Disease: Arrhythmias

Incidence	Risk for Childbearing
2–4% simple arrhythmias in school girls and women >40yr[1]	Variable Risk
Incidence of each type of arrhythmia in pregnancy unknown[1]	

EXPLANATION OF CONDITIONS

Cardiac arrhythmia is any variation from the normal regular rhythm of the heart beat.[2] It is more common when pre-existing structural, functional or ischaemic heart disease interferes with the mechanisms controlling heart rhythm.[1] Arrhythmia can manifest as: tachycardia, palpitations (heart rate >100 beats per minute (bpm) or bradycardia (heart rate <60 beats per minute).

Tachycardia

This is a commoner problem during pregnancy. Pregnancy itself causes a physiological increase in heart rate, predisposes to atrial arrhythmias and exacerbates pre-existing arrhythmic tendencies.[3] If the rate is very high or the arrhythmia is sustained then chest pain (angina), dizziness (pre-syncope) or fainting (syncope) may occur.

Supraventricular Tachycardia (SVT)

This is a rapid heart rate emanating from the atria (upper chambers) of the heart.

Atrial Ectopy

Extra beats may be perceived as missed beats/chest thumping. The condition is benign requiring no treatment above reassurance.

Atrio-Ventricular Re-Entrant Tachycardias: Wolff-Parkinson-White Syndrome (WPW) and Atrioventricular Nodal Re-entrant Tachycardia (AVNRT)

There is a congenital deficiency in the 'electrical insulation' between the atria and ventricles which allows short-circuiting of the normal conduction pathway. Atrial ectopy can allow initiation of an atrio-ventricular electrical re-entry circuit producing a rapid heart rate. If atrial fibrillation occurs this can be life threatening. Many people have a predisposition to pre-excitation which may be unmasked during pregnancy.

Non-pregnancy treatment:

- Vagal stimulation – induced by **swallowing ice, the Valsalva manoeuvre, eyeball pressure or carotid sinus massage**[4,5] may terminate tachycardia but often iv adenosine is required
- DC cardioversion is rarely needed[5]
- Catheter ablation of re-entry pathway now treatment of choice, ideally before pregnancy[6]
- Risk of heart block from AVNRT ablation may mean medical therapy is preferred
- Maintenance drugs: beta-blockers, flecainide, amiodarone[5]

Atrial Flutter

- Associated with significant heart disease
- Atrial rates 240–400 bpm
- Generally ventricular rate about half atrial rate
- Can impede cardiac output, allow atrial thrombus formation and risks systemic embolisation[7]

Non-pregnancy treatment:

- Catheter ablation if possible

- Anticoagulation and rate control with digoxin or beta-blocker for chronic flutter
- Amiodarone for cardioversion and prevention[6,8]

ATRIAL FIBRILLATION

Rapid, chaotic depolarisation of the atria (300–500 bpm) with variable atrio-ventricular conduction.

- May be idiopathic or related to underlying cardiac disease
- Increased risk of thrombo-embolism[1]
- May be asymptomatic with low-ventricular-rate response

Treatment is as per atrial flutter.

Ventricular Tachycardia (VT)

Rapid rhythm emanating directly from the ventricles.

- More common in women with structural/ischaemic heart disease or long QT syndrome[3]
- Rarely asymptomatic
- Palpitations, dyspnoea and syncope
- Increased risk of sudden death[1]
- Long QT syndrome hereditable

Non-pregnancy treatment:

- Treatment of underlying disease
- Catheter ablation if possible
- Anti-arrhythmic medication tailored to cause
- Implantable pacemaker or defibrillator

Treatment in pregnancy is as for pre-pregnancy, but avoid amiodarone and excessive radiation exposure if possible.

Bradycardia

- May be sinus bradycardia
- Present in otherwise normal individuals
- Common in well-trained athletes and during deep sleep[9]
- Rarely, it may be related to myocardial disease
- Can be vagally induced[5]

Non-pregnancy treatment: ignore if asymptomatic, otherwise it generally responds to atropine or adrenaline[9] and rarely needs a pacemaker[5].

Treatment in pregnancy generally consists of pacemaker insertion.

PRE-CONCEPTION ISSUES AND CARE

- Many conditions now amenable to catheter ablation which should be performed pre pregnancy if possible[10]
- Avoid amiodarone if possible due to fetal thyroid disease and its long half-life[11,12]
- Discuss hereditable conditions, e.g. long QT syndrome
- Beta-blockers may cause slight reduction in fetal weight
- Discuss risks/benefits of warfarin individually
- Optimise treatment of underlying heart disease but avoid ACE inhibitors
- Balance between symptoms and fetal risk
- General health promotion: smoking cessation, weight loss, healthy diet, BP measurements, cholesterol level, encourage exercise and avoiding stress

Pregnancy Issues
- New onset arrhythmias are common in pregnancy[13]
- Pre-existing arrhythmias increase
- Low incidence of serious arrhythmia[14]

Supraventricular tachycardia
- Premature atrial beats are present in 50% pregnant women, being generally well tolerated[14]
- WPW, AVNRT may worsen with catheter ablation required for uncontrollable, or life-threatening, symptoms
- Digoxin, adenosine and beta-blockers are generally safe, but amiodarone best avoided due to fetal thyroid toxicity

Ventricular arrhythmia, atrial fibrillation/flutter
- Frequently indicates underlying heart disease needing to be excluded or treated, e.g. hypertrophic cardiomyopathy, ischaemic heart disease; these are high risk indicators for sudden death[15]
- Long QT syndrome and Brugada syndrome are also life threatening and need accurate diagnosis and treatment[3,16]

Atrial flutter/fibrillation is commoner in patients with atrial septal defects and atrial scars from surgical repair. Catheter ablation for this is possible, but complex, with prolonged X-ray exposure. Therefore, it is generally managed medically with rate control and anticoagulation during pregnancy.

Automatic implantable cardio-defibrillators:
- Limited literature but no device or therapy complications are reported
- Implantation is possible during pregnancy if indicated, such as ARVD

Bradycardia
Pathological bradycardia is rare in pregnancy. It is usually benign, but heart block may require pacemaker insertion.[17]

Medical Management and Care
For new onset arrhythmias:
- ECG – note that arrhythmia might have subsided by time ECG done!
- Symptom diary and 24-hour Holter monitor
- Serum investigations in order to exclude metabolic abnormalities, particularly hyperkalaemia, acidosis and hypoxaemia
- Try simple measures first, such as vagal stimulation for tachycardia
- Asymptomatic arrhythmia should not be treated unless life threatening
- Recurrence of arrhythmias has adverse fetal or neonatal effects[14]
- Digoxin or beta-blockers for first line management[10,18]. Although beta-blockers cross the placenta and can potentially result in fetal bradycardia, hypoglycaemia, premature labour, low birth weight and metabolic abnormalities, they are usually well tolerated during pregnancy and are widely used[19]
- Adenosine is safe in second and third trimesters[20] but needs to be given by experienced practitioner in a monitored area with equipment ready for resuscitation; continual electronic fetal monitoring (EFM) to observe for fetal bradycardia[14,15]
- DC cardioversion if haemodynamically unstable[5]
- EFM throughout due to the small risk of fetal arrhythmia
- If catheter ablation required, safest period is third trimester[1]
- Exclude hyperthyroidism
- Be alert to risk of thrombo-embolism especially with atrial fibrillation or flutter[21]

Midwifery Management and Care
- Recognise signs and symptoms (breathlessness, chest pain, pre-syncope)
- Take accurate history of onset, frequency and duration to differentiate from physiological symptoms of advancing pregnancy
- Rule out pre-existing anaemia
- Give advice about avoiding stimulants such as caffeine, cigarettes and alcohol and illicit drug use
- Remember may be more symptomatic in third trimester and refer
- Women with severe arrhythmia and who are unstable should be on coronary care unit where more familiar with drugs and treatments
- Assist with vagal manoeuvres – educate woman that the Valsalva manoeuvre, or cold drink, may terminate the episode
- Assess fetal growth if woman on beta-blockers

Labour Issues
- **Tachycardia** – manage according to symptoms and haemodynamics
- **Bradycardia** – usually transient and due to vagal stimulation; atropine/adrenaline useful

Medical Management and Care
- Monitor with ECG, only treat if symptomatic[13]
- Blood samples for U&E and cardiac enzymes

Midwifery Management and Care
- Avoid Valsalva manoeuvre as this can worsen bradycardia
- Care with epidural
- PO$_2$ monitoring
- Continual pulse and blood pressure monitoring
- Continual EFM for fetal bradycardia secondary to beta-blockers

Postpartum Issues
- If occurrence was for first time in pregnancy, postnatal follow-up is required

Medical Management and Care
- If condition persists, or worsens, initiate ongoing ECG monitoring
- Referral for investigation

Midwifery Management and Care
- Neonatal care – monitor carefully for metabolic abnormalities especially hypoglycaemia and thyroid function[12,22]

4.8 Ischaemic Heart Disease: Angina and Myocardial Infarction

Incidence	**Risk for Childbearing**
1:10,000–1:30,000; incidence is increasing four-fold according to the 2003–2005 CEMACH report[1,2]	High Risk – maternal mortality rate of 37% 33% maternal cardiac disease deaths are ischaemic[2,7]

EXPLANATION OF CONDITION

Ischaemic heart disease is due to inadequate myocardial blood flow related to coronary arterial narrowing. This may be temporary, **angina pectoris** (angina), or permanent, **myocardial infarction** (MI). It manifests as chest pain or discomfort, and may radiate to the left arm or jaw. It is accompanied by feelings of constriction/suffocation. Angina is generally precipitated by exertion or stress, but more severe cases may present at rest. The pain of myocardial infarction is generally more severe and may be accompanied by sweating, nausea and a feeling of impending death or collapse.

Coronary artery disease is due to gradual and incomplete occlusion of the coronary vessels by fatty deposits, (atheromatous plaques) accumulating in the endothelial cells lining the arterial walls. Symptoms occur when myocardial oxygen demands exceed possible supply.

Complete occlusion of a diseased coronary artery may occur suddenly due to clot formation within the narrowing (**coronary thrombosis**). It may also arise from coronary artery spasm, or dissection of coronary arteries[2]. The supplied myocardium will infarct (die) unless the obstruction is relieved rapidly.

Risk Factors for Ischaemic Heart Disease in Women

- Age >35 yr – but 10% women with MI are under 35[1]
- Cigarette smoking – and cardiac effects are more pronounced in pregnancy[3]
- Obesity, diabetes or cocaine abuse
- Family history of cardiovascular disease[4]
- Hypertension
- Ethnicity – Black and Asian women have higher risk[3]
- In pregnancy, risk is increased by:
  - pre-eclampsia and eclampsia
  - phaeochromocytoma
  - sickle cell and collagen vascular disease[3,5]
  - infection and postpartum haemorrhage (PPH)[6]

Presentation in Pregnancy

- Can be confusing as chest discomfort, nausea and breathlessness are common in pregnancy and may be confused with gastro-oesophageal reflux (heartburn)
- Typical presentation – ischaemic chest pain with an abnormal ECG and elevated cardiac enzymes (MI)
- Symptoms may be masked/unclear during labour or delivery
- ECG and cardiac enzymes can be insensitive
- Cardiac specific troponin I greater than 0.15 ng/ml is a more specific indicator of myocardial infarction than creatinine kinase muscle–bone (CK–MB) levels, which increase during normal labour[6,7]
- Differential diagnosis of ischaemic chest pain includes haemorrhage, sickle crisis, pre-eclampsia, acute pulmonary embolism and aortic dissection – be aware of systolic hypertension[2]
- There may be no symptoms at all (especially in diabetics) with the presentation as for cardiomyopathy

COMPLICATIONS

Associated with exacerbation of angina in pregnancy or progression to *de novo* myocardial infarction are:

- **Arrhythmias**
  - ventricular tachycardia/fibrillation
  - heart block
- **Haemodynamic problems**
  - pericarditis
  - tamponade
  - LVF
  - cardiogenic shock
  - acute mitral regurgitation
- **Mortality** is 37–50% in pregnancy, with greatest risk if:
  - the infarct occurs late in pregnancy
  - the woman is *under* 35 years of age
  - pulmonary/amniotic fluid embolism, haemorrhage, placental abruption, eclampsia, or drug toxicity arise

Sudden severe chest pain in a previously fit pregnant woman may be caused by dissection of the aorta +/– coronary arterial dissection. If suspected, withhold thrombolytics and immediate CT/coronary angiography.

- The indication for coronary intervention depends on the site and apparent size of the evolving infarct
- Acute aortic dissection itself requires urgent surgery

NON-PREGNANCY TREATMENT AND CARE

- Reduction of obesity, smoking cessation and statins
- Glyceryl trinitrate (GTN) spray or tablets – administered under the tongue
- Early recognition and treatment of MI by history taking, ECG results and raised cardiac enzymes
- Drug therapy includes aspirin, beta-blockers, ACEI, calcium channel blockers and statins
- Treat pain, nausea and vomiting
- Early thrombolysis/intervention improves outcome in MI
- Basic and advanced life support
- Angioplasty[2]

PRE-CONCEPTION ISSUES AND CARE

- Previous coronary bypass surgery does not of itself contraindicate pregnancy
- Impaired LVF is one of the main determinants of maternal and neonatal outcome[1]
- Seek expert cardiological input:
  - echocardiography to evaluate left ventricular ejection fraction and exclude structural anomalies
  - coronary angiography to ascertain disease severity +/– angioplasty/stenting
  - echocardiography and exercise testing three months prior to stopping contraception is helpful
- Optimise medication prior to cessation of contraception:
  - ACE inhibitors contraindicated
  - aspirin[9], beta-blockers and GTN to be encouraged as directed
- Promote smoking cessation
- Encourage daily exercise and weight reduction/control
- Advocate diet low in fat, salt and cholesterol
- Advise on stress avoidance, including control measures e.g. deep breathing, muscle relaxation and imagery

Pregnancy Issues

IHD has a rising incidence[1,2], with midwives increasingly likely to see women with angina or myocardial infarction. Smoking, obesity, diabetes mellitus, increasing maternal age and familial lipid disorders are responsible.

Recent myocardial infarction:

- Low dose aspirin advised[9]
- Risk of complications high: cardiac arrhythmias (PVC), ventricular tachycardia or fibrillation, bradycardia, pericarditis, tamponade, LVF, mitral regurgitation, ventricular septal defect, free wall rupture, systemic or pulmonary embolism and cardiogenic shock[10]
- Some women may develop symptoms *during pregnancy* and need investigation and treatment to maintain sufficient coronary flow reserve to survive the pregnancy; timely and expert cardiological input are crucial
- Severe chest pain requiring opiate analgesia must be investigated by CT chest/ MRI/echocardiogram[2]
- Diabetic women require attention as they may have 'silent' myocardial ischaemia
- Discuss genetic consequences of having a child with a hereditary genetic predisposition to premature ischaemic heart disease

Medical Management and Care

- Close cardiological supervision is essential
- Beta-blockers, aspirin/heparin, nitrates and calcium antagonists are reasonably safe[1] as needed (Appendix 4.3)
- If acute MI suspected, diagnosis based on ECG and troponin I levels (as CK–MB unreliable peripartum)
- Echocardiography helpful to assess LV function, regional wall motion and valvar abnormalities and guide management
- Coronary angiography/angioplasty/stenting may be needed[7]
- Thrombolytic therapy for life-threatening massive, acute MI has been used to favourable effect, but risks haemorrhagic complications[1,7]

Midwifery Management and Care

- Careful booking history, noting drug regime and symptoms
- Book at a consultant unit
- Refer to maternal medicine clinic, and re-refer to the cardiologist those with known disease or risk factors and ischaemic-sounding chest pain
- Advise limited physical activity +/− salt and fluid intake; self-weigh
- Monitor BP, pulse, oedema etc. for pre-eclampsia/CCF
- Remember angina can present for the first time in pregnancy, hence significant chest discomfort should not be dismissed as 'heartburn'
- Counselling and support re challenges of motherhood with an underlying cardiac condition, and any potential interventions
- Effective communication with the multi-disciplinary team
- Support smoking cessation programmes
- Clinical assessment of fetal growth and wellbeing supplemented by ultrasound growth, liquor volume and Doppler to exclude IUGR
- If the mother reports angina symptoms associated with driving, report to the medical team and advise the mother that she should cease driving until the cardiologist has reviewed her condition[16]

Labour Issues

- Vaginal delivery avoids surgical stress, reduces blood loss and risk of infection and permits early ambulation
- Use of instrument delivery and regional analgesia reduce the second stage and some elements of unpredictability
- Recent MI – if possible delay delivery until the infarct has time to heal, as mortality is higher within two weeks of event[11,12]
- Ergometrine is best avoided as it can cause coronary artery spasm[13]
- Caesarean section with an epidural may be more appropriate if the infarct is recent[14]

Medical Management and Care

- Agree care plan between mother and all team members
- Carefully document in records: delivery options, drug, fluid and monitoring regimes and methods
- Anticoagulants discontinued 12–24 hrs prior to regional anaesthesia
- Plan a strategy for potential primary or secondary haemorrhage

Midwifery Management and Care

- Feto-maternal monitoring by: EFM, ECG, BP, pulse, respirations
- IV access, strict fluid balance
- Supplementary oxygen and saturation monitoring if indicated
- Left or right lateral position advised
- Use compression (TED) stockings
- Monitoring of analgesia requirement and effectiveness
- Careful use of oxytocic drugs, **avoid** ergometrine (coronary spasm)
- Resuscitation skills and equipment to hand
- Avoid active closed glottis 'pushing'; passive descent is beneficial
- Assist with operative delivery and support the mother

Postpartum Issues

- Spontaneous coronary artery dissection most common cause of MI in postnatal period[15]
- Avoid ergometrine, as it can cause coronary artery spasm[13]
- Thrombolysis is generally contraindicated with acute MI, as it increases the risk of haemorrhage
- Oestrogen-based contraception is contraindicated due to risk of venous thrombo-embolism (VTE)

Medical Management and Care

- Observe for exacerbation of the underlying condition and arrhythmia
- Consider drug regimes and breast-feeding (Appendix 4)
- Advise on future pregnancy options, and contraception choice

Midwifery Management and Care

- Continue vital signs observations 1/4-hourly post birth until stable
- Continue with fluid volume assessment and watch for bleeding
- Avoid ergometrine for PPH, unless life threatening
- TED stockings, and administer prescribed anticoagulants
- Encourage rest and avoiding exertion
- Diet – well balanced, high iron and fibre content (avoid constipation)
- Consider social support issues
- Reinforce contraceptive advice, explaining use of POP or IUCD
- Encourage rest and gentle mobilisation

4.9 Pulmonary Hypertension and Eisenmenger's Syndrome

Incidence	Risk for Childbearing
1:20,000 of which approximately 6% appears to be familial[1,2]	High Risk – maternal mortality ≥56%[9]

EXPLANATION OF CONDITION

Pulmonary hypertension (PH) is progressive elevation of pulmonary artery pressure leading to right ventricular failure and death. It is due to increased pulmonary vascular resistance impeding blood flow through the lungs. It is defined as an elevated mean pulmonary artery pressure of 25 mmHg or greater at rest or 30 mmHg with exercise. This is commoner in women, aged 30–40, with a ratio of female to male of 1.7–3.5:1[3].

Classification[4]
- Pulmonary arterial hypertension (PAH)
- PH with left heart disease
- PH with lung disease and hypoxaemia
- PH due to thrombotic/embolic disease
- Miscellaneous

Pulmonary Arterial Hypertension

Pulmonary arterial hypertension is due mainly to changes in the pulmonary arterioles. It may be **idiopathic** (IPAH) or **familial** (FPAH), often with autosomal dominant inheritance, and there may be worsening of the disease in subsequent generations[5]. PAH is often **associated** (APAH) with one or more triggering factors (+/− a genetic pre-disposition), resulting in endothelial injury, vasoconstriction and vascular remodelling. The main triggers are:

- Connective tissue diseases such as scleroderma, CREST, rheumatoid arthritis, and SLE
- Congenital systemic to pulmonary shunts (mainly cardiac)
- Portal hypertension[6,7]
- Viral infection – especially HIV
- Drugs and toxins, especially appetite suppressants
- Pulmonary veno-occlusive disease
- Persistent pulmonary hypertension of the newborn
- Miscellaneous triggers, e.g. autoimmune and storage diseases

Signs and Symptoms

The signs and symptoms are usually insidious, with advanced presentation, with several years elapsing prior to diagnosis.

- Dyspnoea main symptom until late in the disease
- Pre-syncope or syncope
- Chest pain and palpitations
- Cyanosis if atrial shunting present
- Raised jugular venous pressure, right-ventricular heave, loud pulmonary component of the second heart sound, tricuspid or pulmonary regurgitant murmurs and right heart failure (see above) occurs late[8]

Eisenmenger's Syndrome

Eisenmenger's syndrome is the end-stage reaction of the pulmonary vasculature to the increased pulmonary blood flow (and pressure) from systemic to pulmonary shunting in congenital heart disease. There is usually severe cyanosis and restricted effort tolerance.

COMPLICATIONS

- Mortality from PAH is high, with <3 year from diagnosis to death, mainly from RV failure or sudden death; some treatments now available which may improve this
- Patients with Eisenmenger's syndrome generally survive longer due to preserved RV function
- Pregnancy is very poorly tolerated, irrespective of cause of PAH, with mortality >50%[10]

NON-PREGNANCY TREATMENT AND CARE

Screening, with ECG and echocardiography, should be offered to women with a family history of PAH, as well as those with HIV, scleroderma or other known triggers.

Drug Treatment

- Pulmonary vasodilator therapy – nifedipine of benefit in a small group with reactive pulmonary vasculature; iv or inhaled prostenoids may also be of long term benefit but are very expensive and have major lifestyle implications
- Anticoagulants – warfarin reduces risk of pulmonary thrombosis and may be life prolonging[11]
- Phosphodiesterase 5 inhibitors, such as sildenafil (Viagra®), and endothelin receptor antagonists, such as bosentan (Tracleer®), are more recent therapies (Appendix 4.3)
- Diuretic therapy reduces breathlessness and oedema
- Oxygen therapy may be required, often overnight

Interventions

- Atrial septostomy may be life saving when there is severe PAH: enlargement of the *foramen ovale* (between the atria) permits right-to-left shunting which augments cardiac output, albeit at the expense of cyanosis
- Heart–lung or double lung transplant, once drugs and therapy become ineffective

PRE-CONCEPTION ISSUES AND CARE

- Advise strongly **against** pregnancy[12]
- Contraceptive advice – sterilisation, progesterone only oral contraceptive pill, Mirena (progestogen eluting) coil
- Genetic counselling
- Management of underlying diseases

If Pregnancy Occurs

- Prompt liaison with specialist PAH unit (most patients are already under their care but denial can be a problem)
- Termination of pregnancy – rapid referral with specialist anaesthesia if instrumentation required
- Supportive treatment with nebulised iloprost, oxygen therapy, anticoagulation, etc. is possible but carries a very high risk to mother and fetus (Appendix 4.3)
- Bosentan is contraindicated as it is teratogenic

Pregnancy Issues

Consider termination of pregnancy:
- Risk of heart failure
- Ensure women have made informed choice if they plan to continue
- Prior treatment with pulmonary vascular therapy for over a year with improved right ventricular function slightly improves outcome but there is still considerable risk
- Limited experiences of newer therapies with pregnant women especially first trimester (some cases teratogenic in animal studies)[8]
- Low cardiac output state means women cope poorly with physiological changes of pregnancy
- Fetal morbidity and mortality are considerable, with premature delivery and restricted fetal growth occurring in 50% of cases
- Only 15–25% pregnancies reach term

Medical Management and Care

- Contact and refer to the national designated specialist centre
- Drug therapies: prostaglandin therapy, e.g. iv or nebulised iloprost
- Newer treatments may be teratogenic, but calcium channel blockers, e.g. nifedipine, may be helpful
- Monthly specialist appointments; as pregnancy progresses more frequent – exercise capacity, oxygen saturation, 'echo', etc.
- Multi-disciplinary team approach
- Early hospital admission may be appropriate
- Fetal growth and development – clinical assessment and ultrasound and Doppler studies
- Anticoagulant therapy

Midwifery Management and Care

- **Urgent** referral to consultant unit and cardiologist team; should be referred to **specialist referral centre** or own team contacted
- Support of family and woman
- Consider legal issues, especially guardians for the baby if the parents are unmarried and there is an adverse outcome
- Support if needed for additional appointments, especially if travelling to regional centres
- Preparation for hospital admission and prolonged stay
- Recognition of signs and symptoms of heart failure
- Promote a healthy and nutritious diet
- Preparation for a growth restricted and pre-term baby

Labour Issues

- **One of the times most at risk**
- **Cardiac intensive care** setting – if on delivery unit skilled professionals at hand, close team work essential
- Pulmonary artery pressure monitoring may be useful during delivery and several days afterwards
- Prepare resuscitation equipment, plus ventilation with inhaled nitric oxide
- **Dangers:**
  - post-operative or delivery fluid shifts
  - **high-risk time** for sudden death
- *Spontaneous labour is preferred*, but induction is safe using prostaglandins[13]
- Operative delivery may be indicated
- Regional analgesia advantageous, but not single spinal analgesia (hypotension risk – right ventricle inadequate response)[8]

Medical Management and Care

- Labour birth plan made early in collaboration with the combined team and woman/family, documented clearly in the case notes and *adhered to*; an ITU bed must be booked
- Pre-term birth is likely for worsening maternal condition
- Planned lower section caesarean section (LSCS) in many cases with team all available[8]
- LSCS may be in general/cardiac theatres; closer to ITU if needed
- Invasive monitoring arterial line CVP
- Stop anticoagulants pre-delivery/regional anaesthesia

Midwifery Management and Care

- Intensive monitoring of ECG, CVP, BP, pulse, respirations and oxygen therapy with saturation monitoring and arterial blood gases
- Foley catheter hourly readings; accurate fluid balance, avoid overload and early recognition of reduced urine output
- Continual EFM, risks of IUGR and/or pre-term birth
- Vaginal birth may be possible but elective LSCS is more usual as early induction of labour is often not possible
- Lateral tilt for labour, compression stockings, passive exercises
- Second stage – avoid 'bearing down'; forceps/ventouse electively
- Third stage – avoid or minimise oxytocic drugs; either physiological third stage or carefully titrated oxytocin with careful monitoring[10] to minimise blood loss

Postpartum Issues

- **Mortality high in the postnatal period**
- Care in intensive care for at least a week
- Risk of pulmonary oedema
- **Sudden death** risk due to right heart failure
- Follow-up with cardiology team is essential to assess heart function
- Providing information to family members frequently, concisely and honestly[14]
- Counselling re risks of another pregnancy
- Contraception – advise about sterilisation (but risks with surgery): intrauterine system or subdermal implant are as effective[12]

Medical Management and Care

- Oxygen therapy, thrombo-embolism prophylaxis, fluid balance, and observations remain vital
- Inhaled nitric acid and/or iv prostacyclin is continued or initiated[8]

Midwifery Management and Care

Immediate – close monitoring continues, plus:
- Regular visits from the midwifery team if the mother is on ITU
- Advice re maternal–infant interaction, photos/video of baby (may be in SCBU or NICU dependent on gestation)
- Lactation – advice with support re breast-feeding/pumping/timing related to drug therapy

Longer term:
- Support with recovery and the practical aspects of baby care

4 Heart Disease

PATIENT ORGANISATIONS

Antenatal Results and Choices
73–75 Charlotte Street
London W1T 4PN
www.ARC-UK.org

Birth Defects Foundation
BDF Centre
Hemlock Way
Cannock
Staffs. WS11 2GF
www.BDFcharity.co.uk

British Heart Foundation
14 Fitzhardinge Street
London W1H 6DH
www.bhf.org.uk/default.aspx

Children's Heart Federation
Level One
2–4 Great Eastern Street
London EC2A 3NW
www.childrens-heart-fed.org.uk/

Arrhythmia Alliance
PO Box 3697
Stratford upon Avon
Warwickshire CV37 8YL
www.arrhythmiaalliance.org.uk

Cardiomyopathy Association
40 The Metro Centre
Tolpits Lane
Watford WD18 9SB
www.cardiomyopathy.org

Echo UK
www.echocharity.org.uk

Grown Up Congenital Heart Patients Association
http://www.guch.org.uk

Marfan Association UK
Rochester House
5 Aldershot Road
Fleet
Hampshire GU51 3NG
http://marfan.org.uk

Max Appeal
Supporting families affected by DiGeorge syndrome VCFS
and 22q11.2 deletion
http://www.maxappeal.org.uk

ESSENTIAL READING

Billington, M. and Stevenson, M. (Eds) (2007) **Critical Care in Childbearing for Midwives.** Oxford; Blackwell.

De Swiet, M. (Ed.) (2002) Heart disease in pregnancy. In: **Medical Disorders in Obstetric Practice**, 4th Edn, pp. 125–158. Oxford; Blackwell.

Edwards, G. (2004) **Adverse Outcomes in Maternity Care – Implications for Practice, Applying the Recommendations of the Confidential Enquiries**. London; BFM/Elsevier.

Gilbert, E.S. (2007) Cardiac disease. In: **High Risk Pregnancy and Delivery**, 4th Edn. London; Mosby/Elsevier.

James, D.K., Steer, P.J., Weiner, C.P. and Gonik, B. (2006a) Cardiac disease. In: **High Risk Pregnancy**, 3rd Edn, pp. 798–827. London; Elsevier.

James, D.K., Steer, P.J., Weiner, C.P. and Gonik, B. (2006b) Critical care of the obstetric patient. In: **High Risk Pregnancy**, 3rd Edn, pp. 1624–1640. London; Elsevier.

Nelson-Piercy, C. (2005) Heart disease. In: **Handbook of Obstetric Medicine**, 2nd Edn. London; Martin Dunitz.

RCOG (2002) **Maternal Morbidity and Mortality** Study Group Statement. www.rcog.org.uk/index.asp?PageID=1738

Steer, P.J., Gatzoulis, M.A. and Baker, P. (Eds) (2006) **Heart Disease and Pregnancy**. London; RCOG Press.

Thorne, S., Nelson-Piercy, C., MacGregor, A. *et al.* (2006) Pregnancy and contraception in heart disease and pulmonary arterial hypertension. **Journal of Family Planning and Reproductive Health Care**, **32**(2):75–81.

RESPIRATORY DISORDERS

5

Michelle Goldie, Jane Scullion and Christopher Brightling

5.1 The Breathless Pregnant Woman

Incidence/prevalence 60–70% pregnant women, either as a normal physiological response or due to underlying pathology	**Risk for Childbearing** Low Risk – physiological causes Variable Risk – pathological causes

EXPLANATION OF CONDITION

Breathlessness is the sensation of feeling *out-of-breath* or unable to *catch your breath*. The normal respiratory rate is 12–20 breaths/minute at rest. A persistent respiratory rate at rest >24 breaths/minute is abnormal[1].

Breathlessness in pregnancy is extremely common and may reflect the normal anatomical and physiological changes that occur in pregnancy or may be a consequence of an underlying pathology.

The normal changes of pregnancy that may influence the respiratory rate, perception of breathlessness and decreased exercise capacity comprise:

- Increase in weight
- Elevation of the diaphragm by up to 4 cm, although its excursion is not impaired
- Capillary enlargement throughout the respiratory tract with increased mucosal oedema and hyperaemia
- Increased transverse and antero-posterior diameter leading to an increase in the sub-costal angle and up to 7 cm increase in chest circumference
- 20% increase in oxygen consumption
- 15% increase in maternal metabolic rate
- Increased tidal volume but normal respiratory rate
- Increased progesterone leading to hyperventilation
- Increased free cortisol

Pathological Causes of Breathlessness

- Respiratory disease:
  - asthma
  - chest infection and/or pneumonia
  - thrombo-embolic disease
  - interstitial lung disease, e.g. sarcoid or secondary to a connective tissue disorder
  - pneumothorax
  - amniotic fluid embolism
- Cardiac disease:
  - arrhythmias
  - ischaemic heart disease
  - cardiomyopathy
- Endocrine disease:
  - diabetes mellitus leading to hyperventilation in the setting of acute ketoacidosis
  - acute thyrotoxicosis
- Haematological:
  - chronic anaemia
  - acute haemorrhage
- Renal disease:
  - hyperventilation to compensate for metabolic acidosis secondary to acute renal failure

This list is not exhaustive and further details on all of these conditions are outlined in the relevant chapters.

COMPLICATIONS

Breathlessness is experienced by 60–70% of women during pregnancy, especially in the second and third trimesters. Physiological breathlessness does not cause complications.

Breathlessness due to a pathological cause can result in complications and these are detailed in the chapters relating to specific conditions.

NON-PREGNANCY TREATMENT AND CARE

Breathlessness is a normal physiological response to exercise. However, breathlessness at rest and breathlessness in response to minimal exercise out of proportion to an individual's normal level of fitness needs to be investigated. When a pathological cause of breathlessness is suspected, a detailed history and examination need to be taken.

First line investigations should include:

- Full blood count
- Renal function
- Glucose
- Simple lung function tests
- Urine dipstick
- Chest radiograph

Additional tests may include:

- D-dimers
- ECG
- Full lung function tests
- Thyroid function tests
- Computed tomography of the chest, with or without pulmonary angiography
- Echocardiogram
- Detailed cardiopulmonary exercise testing

Treatment should be directed at the specific cause. In the setting of hyperventilation, physiotherapy to instruct patients in breathing control techniques may be of benefit.

PRE-CONCEPTION ISSUES AND CARE

Whether the cause of breathlessness has pre-conception implications is dependent upon the cause of the breathlessness, and the reader needs to refer to the individual chapters on the management of specific conditions that can cause breathlessness.

Strongly encourage smoking cessation.

Pregnancy Issues

In most cases breathlessness in pregnancy is due to a normal physiological response[2]. Pathological causes need to be considered when there is a clinical suspicion.

The risk–benefit ratio of investigations for breathlessness needs to be evaluated. Most radiological investigations expose the woman and baby to radiation, which needs to be minimised, but chest radiography is generally regarded as safe.

In extreme circumstances, in the setting of respiratory failure, whether the woman and baby are sufficiently oxygenated needs to be considered.

Medical Management and Care

- If a pathological cause is suspected the woman needs to be investigated[2] and, in particular, conditions that are more common in pregnancy, e.g. pulmonary emboli, need to be considered
- Treatment needs to be specific for the cause of breathlessness but the potential risks of treatment need to be considered, e.g. antibiotic choice for pneumonia
- Details of the management of specific conditions are outlined in the other relevant chapters

Midwifery Management and Care

- The midwifery care needs to be tailored to the woman's needs. This should be focused on education through antenatal care and support for physiological breathlessness. With pathological breathlessness this will involve referral to a consultant obstetrician to assess the woman's case and need for further investigations
- Regular antenatal appointments with the community midwife to ensure that the baby is not compromised and to ensure the woman's health does not deteriorate
- At all stages of pregnancy, whether at the booking visit or midtrimester the midwife must recognise any complications and give full explanations of these and potential consequences to the mother. This is important in order for her to make informed decisions about where she may want to give birth. If she had intended to give birth at home or in a midwifery-led unit this may not be the most appropriate place

Labour Issues

Breathlessness is very common in labour, but breathlessness in early labour that is not associated with contractions is unusual. This, together with other symptoms or abnormal vital signs should alert the carer to potential pathological causes of breathlessness.

Early referral to a doctor is indicated in the setting of pathological breathlessness because delivery options need review.

Medical Management and Care

- In the setting of pathological breathlessness, augmented labour or early caesarean section may need to be considered

Midwifery Management and Care

- On admission to delivery suite the midwife needs to make an initial assessment of her immediate condition and needs
- This should involve basic observations – recording of maternal pulse, blood pressure, temperature and respiratory rate
- Take a detailed history taking into account any investigations which may recently have been carried out
- Carry out abdominal palpation and auscultation of the fetal heart. If maternal or fetal observations are outside of normal parameters then the midwife should refer to a doctor for further advice. This is also true if the woman has been admitted to a midwifery-led unit or is labouring at home
- If pathological breathlessness is suspected then the baby needs to be continuously monitored with maternal vital signs recorded at more frequent intervals

Postpartum Issues

Breathlessness in the postpartum period is unusual and is likely to reflect a pathological cause such as pulmonary emboli or haemorrhage.

Breathlessness in combination with changes in vital signs is suggestive of a serious complication. The move towards early discharge after delivery places even more importance on the postnatal examination by the midwife in the community.

Medical Management and Care

- Postpartum breathlessness should be taken seriously
- It is important to be mindful of the potential pathological causes of postpartum breathlessness, e.g. pulmonary emboli or anaemia
- A low threshold for seeking further medical advice is required

Midwifery Management and Care

- The midwife needs to be mindful of the potential seriousness of a woman with postpartum breathlessness
- A mother with signs of breathlessness should not be discharged from hospital without having first had a medical review
- Once home, thorough postnatal examinations with astute observation of the physical condition should be conducted. Where necessary instigate appropriate investigations and refer to the primary care physician, or as an emergency to hospital, as warranted

5.2 Asthma

Incidence	Risk for Childbearing
10–15% of UK children and 5–10% of UK adults[1] 3–12% of pregnant women[2]	Variable Risk

EXPLANATION OF CONDITION

Asthma is a common condition in western societies, affecting up to 15% and its prevalence and incidence are increasing.

Asthma is a chronic inflammatory disease of the airways, which is characterised by intermittent episodes of wheeze, shortness of breath, chest tightness and cough. It is a variable disease in which, in response to certain stimuli, or triggers, inflammation and structural changes occur in the lungs. This causes airway hyper-responsiveness and variable airflow obstruction leading to the symptoms described. Symptoms of asthma tend to be variable, intermittent and worse at night.

Patients suffer from *flare-ups* or exacerbations of their disease either in response to an acute infection, which is usually viral in origin, or due to poor control of their airway inflammation.

Triggers for Asthma

- Smoking
- Allergens, e.g. house dust mite, pollen, etc.
- Exercise
- Occupational exposure
- Pollution
- Drugs, e.g. aspirin, beta-blockers, including eye drops and as part of an anaphylactic response to other drugs
- Food and drinks such as dairy produce, alcohol, peanuts and orange juice
- Additives such as monosodium glutamate and tartrazine
- Medical conditions, e.g. rhinitis and gastric reflux
- Hormonal, e.g. pre-menstrual conditions and pregnancy

There is a strong link between asthma and atopy (the tendency to become sensitised to allergens and to develop allergic disease).

COMPLICATIONS

Asthma is a major burden not only on the patient, but also for health care provision and on society, causing time off work.

There are currently around 1500 asthma deaths per year. Many factors are believed to be responsible for these, including:

- A long history of asthma
- Marked peak flow variability
- Non-adherence to medication, especially inhaled corticosteroids
- Psychosocial problems
- Previous admissions with asthma, particularly if ventilated or if life-threatening features were present

The majority of asthma deaths occur in patients who present late for treatment, often despite having symptoms. Poor patient education, an underestimation of the severity of the asthma by both the patient and the health care professional and inappropriate treatments have also been implicated in asthma deaths. On occasion, fatal attacks occur rapidly with little time for intervention, but this is uncommon[3,4].

NON-PREGNANCY TREATMENT AND CARE

British Thoracic Society (BTS) guidelines for the management of asthma have been in existence since the 1990s. These are now living guidelines and can be accessed through the BTS website (www.brit-thoracic.org.uk).

Aims of Asthma Management

- Control of symptoms
- Prevention of exacerbation
- Achievement of the best pulmonary function for the patient with minimal side effects

Good Asthma Care[5]

- Correct diagnosis: a history consistent with a diagnosis of asthma, supported by objective tests and after consideration of possible differential diagnoses
- Control of symptoms
- Pharmacological management – in a stepwise manner
- Non-pharmacological management: avoidance of triggers[6]
- Smoking cessation advice: to avoid fixed airway obstruction in later life[6]
- Self-management: essential for any chronic disease[6]

In a third of patients symptoms will get better, in a third symptoms will worsen and in a third they will stay the same.

PRE-CONCEPTION ISSUES AND CARE

It is important that women with asthma are optimally managed in the pre-conception period. The treatment may require review, and the woman might need to be re-referred to a specialist clinic. The Royal College of Physicians suggests three questions[3], which can be incorporated as part of the woman's assessment:

- Have you had difficulty sleeping because of your asthma symptoms, including a cough?
- Have you had your usual asthma symptoms during the day, such as a cough, wheeze, chest tightness or breathlessness?
- Has your asthma interfered with your usual activities, e.g. housework, work, school, etc.?

Pregnancy Issues
- Poorly-controlled asthma confers an increased risk to the mother and fetus[2,7]
- Asthmatic women are more at risk of low birth weight neonates, pre-term delivery and complications such as pre-eclampsia, especially in the absence of actively managed asthma treated with inhaled corticosteroids[2]
- There is no contraindication to most first-line treatments for asthma when used in pregnancy
- Smoking cessation is an important part of general obstetric advice, but is important in asthma to reduce symptoms and the efficacy of inhaled corticosteroids is reduced in asthmatics who smoke

Medical Management and Care
Details about the management of asthma are available in the BTS/SIGN guidelines (see Essential Reading this chapter).
- It is important to optimise the control of the woman's asthma, as this will reduce the potential of asthma-related morbidity during pregnancy. This includes addressing issues related to trigger factors and adherence to medication
- Inhaled corticosteroids alone or in combination with long-acting bronchodilators are safe in pregnancy
- Leukotriene antagonists are relatively contraindicated in pregnancy due to the lack of information about possible teratogenic effects. These medications are rarely a critical part of asthma care and therefore should not be initiated in pregnancy. Alternative therapy should be considered
- Oral corticosteroids should be used for acute severe exacerbations
- Maintenance systemic corticosteroids should be reserved for women with severe refractory asthma and need to be reviewed by respiratory and obstetric specialists

Midwifery Management and Care
- Pregnancy does not appear to have a consistent effect on asthma control, which can either worsen or improve, hence, it should be stressed to the woman that well-controlled asthma is *better for baby* and pregnancy outcomes
- Explain that asthma medication is generally safe in pregnancy
- Education about good control and adherence to medication is an essential part of early antenatal care
- In unstable asthma, shared care with obstetrician, midwife and GP is advisable
- Advise women who smoke about the dangers and give appropriate advice about smoking cessation
- Encourage attendance at parent-craft and relaxation classes
- Reinforce health education advice with appropriate leaflets (see Appendix 5 for an example)

Labour Issues
- Acute, severe or life-threatening exacerbations of asthma during labour are extremely rare
- Women who have been on regular oral steroids may require hydrocortisone during labour
- Ergometrine[7], Syntometrine and prostaglandin may cause bronchoconstriction and should be used with caution

Medical Management and care
- In the absence of acute asthma, caesarean section should only be carried out when indicated
- If anaesthesia is required then an epidural is preferential to a general anaesthetic[7]

Midwifery Management and Care
- Advise women that acute asthma is rare in labour
- Women should continue their usual asthma medications in labour
- A mother who has well-controlled asthma should be able to have low risk care, with labour managed normally by the midwife
- Normal pain relief can be given and Entonox is considered safe[7]
- Syntocinon is the preferable drug for active third stage management

Postpartum Issues
Primary care physicians (GPs) can manage most women with asthma, but women with severe disease, particularly if systemic corticosteroids are considered, need to be managed by respiratory physicians.

WHO recommends women should exclusively breast-feed for at least six months[8]. Whether breast-fed children have a reduced risk of developing allergic disease including asthma is contentious, but this does not detract from the overwhelming benefit of breast-feeding.

Medical Management and Care
- Women need to continue on their regular medication
- It is unusual for asthma to become uncontrolled in the immediate postpartum period
- Generally there are no changes in therapy requirements

Midwifery Management and Care
- Breast-feeding should be discussed in the antenatal period for the mother to gain greater awareness of the long-term health benefits of breast-feeding and feel more confident to try breast-feeding
- Advise the mother that food allergy appears less likely if foods are introduced at a later stage
- As outlined for medical care above standard asthma therapy can be used as normal during breast-feeding[7]

5.3 Pneumonia and Chest Infections

Incidence	Risk for Childbearing
4:1000 per year – higher in older people	Variable Risk – except in the rare circumstances of severe pneumonia or unusual complications

EXPLANATION OF CONDITION

Pneumonia is an acute infection within the lower respiratory tract occurring twice as often in the winter months as in the summer.

COMPLICATIONS

Most cases of pneumonia are not severe and can be easily managed at home with appropriate rest and, if necessary, antibiotics. Complications are unusual but include:

- Severe respiratory failure requiring ventilatory support and admission to intensive care
- Parapneumonic pleural effusion and empyema which may require pleural intubation and drainage and sometimes surgery for decortication
- Abscess formation and embolic abscesses
- Generalised septicaemia

NON-PREGNANCY TREATMENT AND CARE

British Thoracic Society guidelines for the management of community-acquired pneumonia[1] have been in existence since the 1990s. These are now living guidelines and can be accessed through the BTS website (www.brit-thoracic.org.uk).

The treatment of pneumonia is guided by an assessment of the severity of the pneumonia and knowledge of the likely causative pathogens[1]. This is often influenced by host factors, epidemiological or circumstantial factors and geographical variations.

In adults, 70% of community-acquired pneumonia cases are caused by bacteria; atypical bacteria cause 20% of cases, and 10% of cases are viral. *Streptococcus pneumoniae* is the commonest pathogen found in around half of identified cases. Other pathogens will vary in importance in relation to host or environmental factors.

Hospital-acquired pneumonia is unusual in pregnancy and mostly affects the elderly in hospital with multiple medical problems. Hospital-acquired pneumonia is often due to the aspiration of bacteria which then colonises the upper respiratory tract, often in association with impaired immunological and mechanical host defences[2].

Assessment

Severity of pneumonia is assessed by scoring one point for each of these factors that are present[1]:

- Confusion
- Urea >7 mmol/l
- Respiratory rate ≥30/min
- Blood pressure (systolic <90 mmHg or diastolic ≤60 mmHg)
- Age ≥65 years

Interpretation of score:

- 0–1: likely suitable for home treatment
- 2: consider supervised hospital treatment
  - short stay in-patient
  - hospital supervised out-patient
- >3: manage in hospital as severe pneumonia
- 4–5: assess for intensive care unit admission

Treatment

Treatment includes supportive care such as bed-rest, analgesia, anti-pyretics, fluids and oxygen if required. In addition, antibiotics are usually given empirically, guided by the severity of the pneumonia, but if there is microbiological confirmation of the causative organism and sensitivities the antibiotic therapy needs to be adjusted accordingly.

The empirical antibiotics of choice, based on severity, are as outlined below[1]:

- **Home-treated, not severe**: Oral amoxicillin or, if penicillin allergic, oral erythromycin or clarithromycin
- **Hospital-treated, not severe** (admitted for non-clinical reasons or previously untreated in the community): as for Home-treated, not severe
- **Hospital-treated, not severe**:
  - **either** oral amoxicillin plus erythromycin or clarithromycin 500 mg bd
  - **or**, if intravenous therapy is needed, use ampicillin plus erythromycin/clarithromycin
  - in cases of penicillin allergy, or where penicillin has already been given, treat with either levofloxacin or moxifloxacin
- **Hospital-treated, severe**: intravenous co-amoxiclav or cefuroxime plus erythromycin or clarithromycin
  - in cases of penicillin allergy use levofloxacin

PRE-CONCEPTION ISSUES AND CARE

Pneumonia is an acute infection and not a chronic condition and therefore does not have significant pre-conception effects. However, antibiotics do reduce the efficacy of the oral contraceptive pill and women need to be advised about alternative contraception whilst treated with antibiotics.

Pregnancy Issues

Pneumonia is no more common in pregnancy than at other times, but requires prompt attention and, if severe, may have serious complications compromising the woman and baby[3].

The selection of antibiotics needs to be made while remaining cognisant of potential teratogenic effects.

Medical Management and Care

- The management of pneumonia in pregnancy is essentially the same as for the non-pregnant woman
- Care needs to be taken in the selection of antibiotics:
  - penicillin, cephalosporin and macrolides safe in pregnancy
  - quinolones, tetracycline and trimethoprim contraindicated
- Careful consideration required to consider the benefit to the woman with severe pneumonia of using contraindicated antibiotics against the risk to the fetus

Midwifery Management and Care

- If the midwife suspects that the woman may have a chest infection, initiate a plan of care:
  - send a sputum sample
  - make an urgent referral to a doctor
- If the woman is being managed at home, antenatal home visits need to be increased to monitor progress, and adherence to medication should be encouraged
- A further referral may need to be made if, after a course of treatment, symptoms have not improved
- Once the infection has cleared and the woman is back to her usual state of good health she can be transferred back into low risk care

Labour Issues

Sufficient oxygenation of the woman and baby need to be maintained.

Unless maternal oxygen saturations are low, the woman should not need additional oxygen therapy.

There is a risk of pre-term labour, possibly related to pyrexia[2].

Medical Management and Care

- Severe pneumonia in late pregnancy is unusual and in the setting of acute respiratory failure caesarean section and respiratory support may need to be considered

Midwifery Management and Care

- Support and monitoring of baby and woman need to be increased, including continuous EFM
- The woman should have regular blood pressure, temperature, pulse, respiratory rate and oxygen saturations measured and documented appropriately
- With any findings outside normal parameters refer on to appropriate medical staff
- In certain cases the midwife may need to prepare for a pre-term delivery

Postpartum Issues

Potential complications of antibiotic therapy need to be considered.

Medical Management and Care

- Pneumonia in the postpartum period needs to be managed as for pregnancy
- Quinolones, tetracycline and trimethoprim are contraindicated for a breast-feeding woman

Midwifery Management and Care

- In the case of severe pneumonia the woman needs to be adequately monitored in hospital
- If treated at home adherence to medication needs to be encouraged and advice given about potential antibiotic-related side effects, such as diarrhoea, vomiting and reduced feeding, in the breast-feeding child
- With good support from community midwives and other agencies (for example breast-feeding support groups) there should be no reason why the women should not be successful in breast-feeding
- Reassurance should be given that any side effects will be temporary and that the benefit of long-term feeding outweighs the short-term inconvenience

5.4 Tuberculosis

Incidence	Risk for Childbearing
1.7 billion affected and 3 million deaths worldwide per annum 6000 cases in England and Wales per annum, TB being prevalent in cities with a high ethnic minority population	High Risk

EXPLANATION OF CONDITION

Tuberculosis (TB) is a bacterial infection, caused by *Mycobacterium tuberculosis*, which is spread by direct contact with an infected individual.

Initial infection with TB often occurs without symptoms, although a positive tuberculin test may show that it has occurred. Only 10–15% of those infected will develop clinical disease over their lifetime, with the highest risk being in the first year after infection. Tuberculosis can affect most parts of the body, but most commonly presents as pulmonary TB[1].

COMPLICATIONS

- TB is associated with significant morbidity and mortality worldwide but in the UK due to careful management and access to appropriate treatment death due to TB is unusual.
- The symptoms, signs and complications of TB relate to the sites in the body that are affected. Importantly, TB medication may cause considerable morbidity and in rare cases death so carers need to be mindful of potential complications of treatment as outlined in the section below.
- 85% of post-primary TB affects the lungs and sufferers may present with respiratory symptoms such as cough, haemoptysis and breathlessness together with constitutional symptoms like fever, night sweats and weight loss.
- Other sites of infection include:
  - peripheral lymph nodes – usually presents with constitutional symptoms alone
  - bones and joints – may present in any joint but most importantly can affect the spine and may lead to cord compression
  - pericardium – may cause a large pericardial effusion, which may compromise the function of the heart and require drainage
  - meninges – TB meningitis is rare in the UK but is associated with significant mortality
  - miliary TB – TB may become generally disseminated, particularly in immunocompromised subjects, and lead to miliary TB, which has a significant mortality

NON-PREGNANCY TREATMENT AND CARE

British Thoracic Society guidelines for the management of TB have been in existence for many years[2]. These are now living guidelines and can be accessed through the BTS website (www.brit-thoracic.org.uk). Current NICE guidance can be accessed through the same website. Due to the potential complications associated with treatment for TB, it is important that the diagnosis should only be made in the presence of a strong clinical suspicion together, where possible, with microbiological confirmation of TB, histological evidence of TB in tissue samples and a positive interferon-gamma test.

Patients diagnosed with active TB should be referred to an appropriate physician trained in treating patients with TB.

The standard treatment regimen for TB is:

- Six months of isoniazid and rifampicin initially, plus pyrazinamide and ethambutol for the first two months
- This regimen is appropriate for all types of TB except CNS infection, when treatment is for 12 months in combination with corticosteroid therapy
- Multi-drug-resistant TB and atypical mycobacterial infections particularly associated with an immunocompromised host (e.g. a mother with HIV/AIDS), remain unusual in the UK but pose a considerable challenge to management and require close supervision by appropriate specialists

Side effects from TB treatment are common, although serious complications are rare.

Common side effects include:

- mild nausea
- rashes
- pruritus
- arthralgia
- orange discoloration of urine
- sweat (due to rifampacin)

Serious Side Effects

All of the first-line drugs except ethambutol can cause liver toxicity. This is idiosyncratic and not dose-related. Therefore, liver function is monitored with tests before and throughout the treatment period.

Ethambutol can cause retro-bulbar neuritis, and acuity needs to be tested before treatment. Patients and carers need to be mindful of potential problems with vision and consider stopping treatment and referring to an eye specialist should problems arise.

Isoniazid can cause a neuropathy due to its effect on vitamin B_6 metabolism. Therefore, in patients where dietary intake of this vitamin is a concern, vitamin supplementation with pyridoxine should be given.

PRE-CONCEPTION ISSUES AND CARE

Due to the pressing need to treat TB, the medication is not contraindicated during pregnancy. However, women are advised not to consider pregnancy when undergoing treatment.

TB medication reduces the efficacy of the oral contraceptive pill and therefore women need to be advised about the use of alternative contraception.

Pregnancy Issues

It is well recognised that treatment for pulmonary TB is safe in pregnancy.

There is better neonatal and perinatal survival if treatment is adhered to[3,4].

Even in multi-drug-resistant TB the benefits of treatment outweigh the risks. Of the small number of studies there seem to be few if any teratogenic effects on newborns.

Transmission of pulmonary TB from mother to baby is rare; there has only been a single case report of a mother with endometrial TB who transmitted TB to her unborn baby.

Medical Management and Care

Medical management in pregnancy is the same as for a non-pregnant patient[3,4]:

- Six months of isoniazid and rifampicin initially, plus pyrazinamide and ethambutol for the first two months

Midwifery Management and Care

- It is now recommended that all new UK entrant pregnant women and children under 11 have a Mantoux test; midwife should ascertain at the booking visit that this has been done
- A pregnant woman with TB should have shared care with a TB specialist, obstetrician (preferably in a joint clinic), midwife and GP
- Ensure adherence to treatment through regular antenatal visits
- If admitted to antenatal ward will need to be in a single room
- If multi-drug-resistant TB then should be in a specialist centre offering a negative pressure room

Labour Issues

Issues in labour relate to the site and severity of infection.

Epidural anaesthesia will be contraindicated.

Medical Management and Care

- Women established on anti-TB therapy are likely to have an uncomplicated labour
- If the woman has multi-drug-resistant TB or has a new diagnosis and has not been established on TB treatment for at least two days then she should be managed in a negative pressure room and precautions taken to prevent infection
- General anaesthetic may be required for operative delivery, so the anaesthetist should review this mother early in the labour

Midwifery Management and Care

- Most women can have a normal labour with delivery conducted by the midwife
- Particular care is required if the woman has a new diagnosis of TB or has multi-drug-resistant TB as the woman will need a negative pressure room
- Women with extra-pulmonary TB may require specific management e.g. women with spinal TB will need to be assessed as to their suitability for normal delivery and may require particular attention during labour
- Discuss options for pain relief

Postpartum Issues

Treatment needs to be continued.

Breast-feeding is *not* contraindicated.

Medical Management and Care

- Women should be maintained on their current therapy

Midwifery Management and Care

- Encourage continued adherence to anti-TB treatment
- Reassure the woman that there are no contraindications for breast-feeding on standard TB therapy
- Ensure newborn has BCG vaccination[3]
- Baby should have isoniazid or isoniazid and rifampicin combination chemoprophylaxis as per NICE guidelines (www.brit-thoracic.org.uk)
- Paediatric review prior to discharge
- Liaison with community midwife and health visitor for further childhood and family surveillance

5.5 Cystic Fibrosis

Incidence	Risk for Childbearing
1:2500 UK live births	High Risk – maternal mortality ≥12%, related to the risk of maternal hypoxia and pulmonary hypertension[2]

EXPLANATION OF CONDITION

Cystic fibrosis (CF) is the most common life-threatening genetic disorder in Caucasian people. It is an autosomal recessive disorder and the carrier frequency is 1 in 25[1].

The CF gene sits on the long arm of chromosome 7 and encodes for a protein known as the CF transmembrane conducting regulator (CFTR). This protein acts as a chloride channel and also services regulatory functions over membrane chloride channels. Essentially, CF is a disorder in which there are abnormalities in the sodium chloride concentrations in the secretory epithelia occurring throughout the body. This may affect:

- Respiratory tract
- Male reproductive system
- Pancreas
- Hepato-biliary system
- Gastrointestinal tract

Cystic fibrosis often presents in early childhood with cough, loose stools and failure to thrive. Other symptoms include meconium ileus, prolonged neonatal jaundice and rectal prolapse. Heel prick (Guthrie) tests are routinely made in the newborn and additional neonatal screening can be made at 6–9 weeks where a screening policy exists.

COMPLICATIONS

Symptoms and morbidity in general relate to the effects of CF on the respiratory system. However due to the multisystemic effects of the disease other symptoms and complications can occur:

Complications include[1]:

- Nasal polyps
- Recurrent sinusitis
- Bronchiectasis
- Haemoptysis
- Allergic bronchopulmonary aspergillosis
- Recurrent pneumothoraces
- Intestinal obstruction
- Pancreatic insufficiency
- Malnutrition
- Portal hypertension
- Cirrhosis
- Gallstones
- Male infertility
- Insulin-dependent diabetes
- Osteoporosis
- Vitamin and salt deficiency
- Delayed puberty
- CF associated arthritis

The median survival age of CF sufferers is currently the mid-thirties, but this has increased from a median age of survival of ten years old some 30 years ago. Therefore it is only recently that women with CF have been able to conceive.

NON-PREGNANCY TREATMENT AND CARE

Diagnosis is critical and is usually made in early childhood, although late presentations have been reported.

Goals of management are to:

- maintain lung function
- maintain quality of life

There is a need to ensure treatment regimens are negotiated with patients, so that adherence to therapy is achieved and longer-term effects are minimised.

The patient should undertake daily physiotherapy to clear the lungs, but this, combined with the many medication regimens that patients have to undertake, can be problematic. Hence, it is important to assess compliance with treatment.

Regular assessment, with measurement of lung function, is important, as is early aggressive management of infection. Pulmonary exacerbations, in particular colonisation of the respiratory tract with *Pseudomonas aeruginosa, Staphylococcus aureus, Stenotrophomonas maltophilia* and particularly *Burkholderia cepacia*, need prompt and aggressive treatment. *Burkholderia cepacia*, in particular, causes rapid decline in patients. Often intravenous antibiotics to which the particular organism is sensitive are the treatments of choice and care and management may include teaching patients to manage their own intravenous regimens.

Dietary supplementation is important and patients are often prescribed treatments such as Creon to allow them to absorb their food.

Patients appear to do better under specialised centres and this should always be an option. Often, secondary centres are attached to tertiary centres but care is shared due to the logistical problems of travel. Clearly multi-disciplinary input helps address the many problems these patients have.

PRE-CONCEPTION ISSUES AND CARE

There is significant maternal morbidity and mortality, and most women with CF are unlikely to live to see their children reach adulthood. Therefore pre-conception advice and counselling needs to be offered to women with CF and management of the disease optimised.

- Management of women with CF requires specialist multi-disciplinary care and needs to be individualised[2]
- Women should be screened for diabetes and advised that a prospective child will be a carrier of cystic fibrosis[3]

Pregnancy Issues

The issues in pregnancy are the same as in the non-pregnant woman, but are more exaggerated.
- Adequate dietary supplementation
- Recurrent infections
- Respiratory failure
- Pulmonary hypertension

Prenatal diagnosis, with careful consideration of termination of pregnancy, becomes an issue.

Medical Management and Care
- The most serious complications are related to the further compromise of a woman with respiratory failure and pulmonary hypertension. It is important to remember that this can lead to maternal mortality
- Antibiotic therapy may be complicated in CF, and in some circumstances antibiotics that are not recommended in pregnancy (such as quinolones) may need to be given after careful consideration of the benefits versus risks
- Growth scans for prompt identification of IUGR[3]

Midwifery Management and Care
- The management of women with CF is complex and requires a multidisciplinary approach from midwives, physiotherapists, dieticians and clinicians
- Booking at a consultant-led unit
- Role of midwife is to support the woman during pregnancy, to reinforce adherence to treatment and ensure engagement with other health care professionals
- Promote a healthy lifestyle with emphasis on a nutritious diet
- CF does not only affect the respiratory system and pancreatic insufficiency occurs; dietary supplementation is standard treatment
- Monitor closely noting any signs such as increasing breathlessness which will assist in the early recognition of complications; these should be reported promptly to the relevant doctor

Labour Issues

Respiratory failure may compromise the oxygenation of the woman and baby.
  Delivery may well be pre-term[3].

Medical Management and Care
- Most women with CF can have a normal labour, but in those with respiratory failure and/or pulmonary hypertension an elective caesarean section needs to be considered
- General anaesthesia may be contraindicated[3], so early review by the anaesthetist is recommended

Midwifery Management and Care
- The midwife needs to be particularly mindful of the potential risk to the woman and baby with respect to respiratory failure and monitoring requirements
- Ensure that oxygen is available in the delivery room, and maternal oxygen saturations should be measured at intervals
- Continuous electronic fetal monitoring[3]
- Avoid prolonged pushing and the Valsalva manoeuvre[3]
- If necessary, prepare for a pre-term delivery and make the paediatricians aware that the mother is in labour

Postpartum Issues

Respiratory infections are common, and whether antibiotics are contraindicated in the breast-feeding woman needs to be considered.

Medical Management and Care
- With most women the postpartum period is uncomplicated, but again be mindful of all of the potential complications of CF

Midwifery Management and Care
- It is important that the woman continues her regular management regimen and additional support may be required in the immediate postpartum period
- Be alert for signs of respiratory infection
- Infant feeding may be an issue if the woman is prescribed quinolones (see Section 5.3 Pneumonia and Chest Infections); apart from this promote breast-feeding
- Nutritional supplements are still required, especially if breast-feeding
- If paternal genetic screening was negative for the CF gene there should be no neonatal issues for disease inheritance

5.6 Sarcoidosis

Incidence	**Risk for Childbearing**
Sarcoidosis is rare. The prevalence of active disease is approximately 0.2% and the incidence is 0.1%	Variable Risk – most patients High Risk – small minority of patients with significant disease

EXPLANATION OF CONDITION

Sarcoidosis is a systemic granulomatous condition of unknown cause characterised by frequent pulmonary involvement, although any part of the body may be affected.

There are no specific tests to diagnose sarcoidosis. The diagnosis is made by the presence of typical radiological features together with supporting evidence of raised serum levels of angiotensin converting enzyme (ACE), immunoglobulin and calcium.

Sarcoidosis is a rare condition and is unlikely to complicate pregnancy.

COMPLICATIONS

Pulmonary sarcoidosis is radiologically staged:

- **Stage I:** bilateral hilar lymphadenopathy
- **Stage II:** as for stage I plus interstitial infiltrates
- **Stage III:** infiltrates without hilar lymphadenopathy
- **Stage IV:** dense fibrosis

Most patients present incidentally with hilar lymphadenopathy, identified when a chest radiograph is performed for another reason. Therefore, in most subjects, the condition is asymptomatic. Even in those with pulmonary involvement the disease is usually self-limiting within two years, although the changes in lung function and lung damage are permanent. It is unusual for the disease to become active again after a period of quiescence.

A minority of patients develop progressive lung disease, with increasing symptoms of breathlessness and lethargy, together with respiratory failure. In extreme circumstances sarcoidosis may cause death due to respiratory failure.

The other organs affected by sarcoidosis include:

- Skin
  - non-specific maculopapular rash
  - erythema nodosum
  - lupus pernio
- Heart – may cause heart block
- Eyes
  - scleritis
  - iritis
  - uveitis
- Joints and muscles
  - arthritis
  - myopathy
- Nervous system
  - peripheral neuropathy
  - spinal sarcoid
  - psychiatric symptoms
- Kidneys
  - renal failure secondary to interstitial nephritis
  - glomerulonephritis
  - IgA nephropathy
  - nephrocalcinosis and nephrolithiasis secondary to hypercalcaemia

NON-PREGNANCY TREATMENT AND CARE

In the presence of symptomatic progressive lung disease and/or significant hypercalcaemia patients should be treated with oral corticosteroids. Vitamin D supplementation can exacerbate the hypercalcaemia and should be avoided in those with active disease. This treatment improves symptoms, reduces progression of disease and hastens resolution. The dose of corticosteroids is high for the first few months and then can be reduced to low dose maintenance therapy.

Treatment for involvement of other organs is also systemic corticosteroids (topical for skin disease), occasionally in combination with corticosteroid-sparing agents.

A respiratory specialist usually manages sarcoidosis, but the management of other organs involved will require specialist care with each relevant organ-based specialist.

In addition to the complications of the condition noted above treatment with oral corticosteroids is also associated with significant side effects. These include corticosteroid-induced myopathy, osteoporosis, diabetes mellitus and hypertension. This list is not exhaustive and highlights the potential issues of systemic corticosteroid therapy.

PRE-CONCEPTION ISSUES AND CARE

Sarcoidosis is not usually a contraindication to pregnancy[3]. In the vast majority of women with sarcoidosis there are no pre-conception issues. Women with significant active disease need to be managed in a specialist clinic.

Particular care is needed with patients treated with systemic corticosteroids due to the increased risk of diabetes mellitus and hypertension. In the rare circumstance of patients with significant respiratory failure women should be advised against pregnancy.

Pregnancy Issues

In most cases there are no pregnancy issues. Rarely respiratory failure and other severe complications may need to be considered.

Medical Management and Care
- The medical management of sarcoidosis is the same in the pregnant and non-pregnant woman
- In most women there are no specific issues, except for those with significant disease and on systemic corticosteroids where particular care is required with respect to complications secondary to the disease and treatment

Midwifery Management and Care
- This is a rare condition in pregnancy and severe sarcoidosis in pregnant women is very unusual[3]
- The woman should be booked in a joint specialist clinic with obstetrician and respiratory consultant care
- Acute breathlessness in a pregnant woman with sarcoidosis is more likely to be due to an alternative cause, e.g. chest infection or PE
- In rare circumstances a woman with sarcoidosis may develop respiratory failure; presents as progressive decline in exercise capacity and development of excessive breathlessness and requires prompt review by a respiratory specialist
- In those women requiring drug therapy the midwife needs to encourage adherence to treatment, but needs to be aware of the potential problems related to corticosteroid therapy
- Advise the mother not to take vitamin D supplements, which may precipitate hypercalcaemia[4]

Labour Issues

Labour is rarely complicated by sarcoidosis except in severe disease.

Medical Management and Care
- Women treated with corticosteroids will require corticosteroid cover during labour[4]
- In the rare circumstance of a woman with significant respiratory failure an elective caesarean section may be required

Midwifery Management and Care
- Only in the exceptional circumstance of respiratory failure does sarcoidosis require any additional midwifery management
- In this setting, as with any woman with respiratory failure, increased monitoring is required to assess whether the woman and baby are adequately oxygenated
- Continuous electronic fetal monitoring

Postpartum Issues

There are no specific postpartum issues with sarcoidosis.

Medical Management and Care
- The woman needs to continue with current therapy and have follow-up arrangements made as appropriate

Midwifery Management and care
- Breast-feeding is not contraindicated and should be encouraged and supported
- Follow-up with a respiratory specialist is indicated for women with sarcoidosis diagnosed in pregnancy or for those women already under review

5 Respiratory Disorders

PATIENT ORGANISATIONS

British Lung Foundation
73–75 Goswell Road
London
EC1V 7ER
www.lunguk.org

Asthma UK
Summit House
70 Wilson Street
London
EC2A 2DB
Email: info@asthma.org.uk
www.asthma.org.uk

TB Alert
22 Tiverton Road
London
NW10 3HL
United Kingdom
www.tbalert.org

Cystic Fibrosis Trust
11 London Road
Bromley
Kent
BR1 1BY
www.cftrust.org.uk

Sarcoidosis and Interstitial Lung Association
www.sarcoidosis.org.uk
info@sarcoidosis.org.uk

ESSENTIAL READING

BTS/SIGN British Guideline on the Management of Asthma (2003) **Thorax**, 58 (Supplement I), 2004 Update.
www.brit-thoracic.org.uk

Diffuse Parenchymal Lung Disease Group of the British Thoracic Society (1999) **Thorax**, 54 (Supplement I).

Dilworth, J.P. and Baldwin, D.R. (2002) **Respiratory Medicine Specialist Handbook**. London; Martin Dunitz.

Guidelines for the Management of Community Acquired Pneumonia in Adults (2001) **Thorax**, 56 (Supplement IV), 2004 Update.
www.brit-thoracic.org.uk

NICE (2006) **Clinical Diagnosis And Management Of Tuberculosis, And Measures For Its Prevention And Control**. Guideline **CG033.**
www.nice.org.uk

Price, D., Foster, J., Scullion, J. and Freeman, D. (2004) **Asthma and COPD**. London; Churchill Livingstone.

Sarcoidosis European Respiratory Monograph (2005) **32:**1–339.

Scullion, J.E. (2007) **Fundamental Aspects of Nursing Respiratory Disorders**. London; Quay Books.

RENAL DISORDERS

6

Nigel J. Brunskill and Andrea Goodlife

6.1　Urinary Tract Infections

Incidence	Risk for Childbearing
1–3% of pregnancies are complicated by urinary tract infection, 2–10% by asymptomatic bacteriuria[1]	Moderate Risk

EXPLANATION OF CONDITION

Urinary tract infection (UTI) is caused by bacteria in the urinary tract. Bacteria usually originate from the bowel and the most common causative organism is *Escherichia coli*, which accounts for 80–90% of all acute UTI. In pregnancy UTI may be manifest as the urethral syndrome, acute cystitis (2% of all pregnancies) or acute pyelonephritis (1–3% of pregnancies).

Features of the **urethral syndrome** are frequency and dysuria, whereas those of **acute cystitis** include frequency, urgency and dysuria, offensive smelling urine, haematuria and suprapubic discomfort. Urethral syndrome may be caused by sexually transmitted genital infections such as *Chlamydia trachomatis*. **Acute pyelonephritis** may present with pyrexia, rigors, abdominal/flank pain, nausea and vomiting[1,2,3,4].

The presence of $>10^5$/ml of the same bacterial species in a midstream specimen of urine (MSU) in the absence of symptoms is called *asymptomatic bacteriuria* (ABU). This is of greatest significance in pregnancy, and in non-pregnant individuals with structurally abnormal urinary tracts, renal stones or diabetes mellitus[2,5,6].

COMPLICATIONS

- **Acute symptomatic urinary tract infection**
  - developed by ≥30% of women with asymptomatic bacteriuria
  - can lead to pyelonephritis
  - untreated infection may cause kidney damage[2,5,6]
- **Acute cystitis**
  - not usually dangerous but may cause significant discomfort and inconvenience
  - usually an isolated event but can be recurrent and may follow sexual intercourse
  - if untreated may progress to acute pyelonephritis
- **Pre-term labour**
  - in many non-pregnant women uncomplicated asymptomatic bacteriuria resolves spontaneously
  - in pregnancy ABU is associated with premature delivery and low birth weight and is therefore treated with antibiotics
  - ABU occurs in 2–10% of all pregnancies[1]
- **Acute pyelonephritis**
  - a more serious infection
  - if very severe, or inadequately treated, septicaemia may result in acute renal failure, multiple organ failure and death
  - repeated episodes of acute pyelonephritis may be associated with the development of renal scars[4]

NON-PREGNANCY TREATMENT AND CARE

- Identify causative organism by testing an MSU, and treat with appropriate antibiotics
- On completion of antibiotic therapy, an MSU is retested to ensure that the urine is now free of infection
- Treatment is not required in non-pregnant women with uncomplicated asymptomatic bacteriuria
- Affected individuals should be warned to be alert for symptoms suggestive of active urinary infection

Advise on ways to reduce the risk of recurrent UTI:

- Drink 2 l of fluid daily, with frequent voiding of urine
- Wipe from 'front to back' after passing urine
- Void to empty the bladder after intercourse
- Drinking cranberry juice may reduce the risk; the dosage is unclear, but approximately 200–300 ml (or by capsule), daily appears to be potentially effective[7,8,9]
- Consider prophylactic antibiotics if recurrent UTI

If UTI is recurrent, consider investigation of underlying cause, such as renal stones or ureteric reflux, with:

- Renal ultrasound
- Abdominal X-ray
- Cystoscopy

Acute pyelonephritis may require:

- Hospitalisation
- Intravenous hydration, monitor fluid balance
- Intravenous antibiotics, changing to oral antibiotics when infection is controlled
- Monitor U&E, urine and blood cultures
- Four-hourly observation of temperature

PRE-CONCEPTION ISSUES AND CARE

- Investigate renal function, and possible underlying causes, prior to pregnancy if recurrent infections have occurred
- Treat and eliminate infections
- Women at risk should be counselled regarding the need for regular urine culture, and the possible requirement for antibiotic therapy during pregnancy
- Advise that there is an increased risk of UTI in pregnancy. This is as a result of relaxation and dilation of the ureters due to hormonal changes and compression at the pelvic brim by the enlarging uterus and ovarian vein[2]. As the pregnancy advances, upward displacement of the bladder into the abdomen results in elongation of the urethra. Under these circumstances, incomplete bladder emptying allows urinary stasis, which in turn encourages infection. If this is accompanied by vesicoureteral reflux ascending bacterial migration and infection is facilitated[2]

Pregnancy Issues

All pregnant women should be offered routine screening for asymptomatic bacteriuria by an MSU culture in early pregnancy, followed by prompt treatment. UTI in pregnancy has been shown to be associated with pre-term birth and low birth weight, although this is controversial[1,3,4].

Generally, if adequately treated, there are no significant effects on the fetus. If the mother has reflux nephropathy as a predisposing cause for UTI there is an increased risk that the baby may also suffer from this condition.

If the organism responsible for the UTI is Group B *Streptococcus* (GBS), this will need to be treated with antibiotics at the time of diagnosis. Intrapartum antibiotics will also be advised. GBS bacteriuria is associated with an increased risk of early onset neonatal sepsis; although the risk is increased, it is not quantified[10].

Medical Management and Care

- Treat confirmed UTI including asymptomatic bacteriuria, promptly[11]
- Ensure antibiotic chosen is safe in pregnancy
- Avoid trimethoprim in the first trimester, as it is a folate antagonist[12]
- Augmentin increases the risk of neonatal necrotising enterocolitis if taken around the time of a premature delivery[13]
- Consider prophylactic antibiotics to prevent recurrent UTI
- In the case of acute pyelonephritis, hospitalise, commence iv antibiotics, converting to oral when tolerated, iv hydration and adequate analgesia
- Monitor renal function and consider renal ultrasound

Midwifery Management and Care

Monthly MSU – more frequently if clinically indicated by:

- Dysuria
- Increased frequency of micturition
- Urine dipstick positive for haematuria/proteinuria or nitrates
- Lower abdominal pain or renal tenderness
- Pyrexia

Always do a *test of cure* MSU after any treatment of UTI and encourage compliance with prescribed antibiotic regime.

Advise:

- Drinking 2 l of fluid daily
- Empty bladder after intercourse
- Always wipe from front to back after urinating
- Drinking 200–300 ml cranberry juice (or capsule) daily may reduce the risk of recurrent UTI[7,8,9]

If GBS is the causative organism, inform the woman, placing an alert note on the case notes for antibiotic cover in labour[10].

Pyelonephritis:

- Refer to hospital if acute pyelonephritis suspected
- Administer analgesia and antibiotics as prescribed
- Observations: hourly temperature, BP, pulse
- Record fluid balance accurately

Labour Issues

If the mother has a UTI in labour, and is pyrexic and tachycardic, this may result in fetal tachycardia. In this case electronic monitoring of the fetal heart rate in labour is indicated.

Urinary catheterisation increases the risk of UTI, so avoid if possible, but if this is required utilise a strict aseptic technique.

Medical Management and Care

- Commence antibiotics and monitor fetal wellbeing especially if the mother is pyrexic in labour. Otherwise manage as normal.

Midwifery Management and Care

- Encourage regular emptying of the bladder
- Avoid urinary catheterisation as this increases the risk of UTI
- Administer any prescribed treatment
- Ensure adequate hydration, if pyrexic iv fluid may be required

Postpartum Issues

If mother has recurrent UTI due to reflux nephropathy, then there is a risk that the baby could also have this condition.

Early detection and prompt treatment of urinary infections in the newborn can help prevent renal scarring and chronic kidney disease later in life.

Medical Management and Care

- Liaise with the GP if there have been recurrent UTIs in pregnancy
- If UTI persists postpartum further investigation is warranted
- A renal ultrasound scan, for reflux nephropathy, should be arranged for the baby

Midwifery Management and Care

- Postnatal care can usually be managed from a normal perspective by the midwife
- The mother may need reassurance that antibiotics are safe to be taken when breast-feeding

6.2 Chronic Kidney Disease

Incidence	Risk for Childbearing
11% of UK adult population may have CKD[1]	High Risk

EXPLANATION OF CONDITION

Chronic kidney disease (CKD) implies longstanding kidney problems often, but not always, associated with loss of excretory function. CKD is classified according to estimated glomerular filtration rate (eGFR). Five stages are recognised:

1. **Normal:** GFR >90 ml/min/1.73 m^2 with other evidence of chronic kidney damage*
2. **Mild impairment:** GFR 60–89 ml/min/1.73 m^2 with other evidence of chronic kidney damage*
3. **Moderate impairment:** GFR 30–59 ml/min/1.73 m^2
4. **Severe impairment:** GFR 15–29 ml/min/1.73 m^2
5. **Established renal failure**: GFR <15 ml/min/1.73 m^2 or on dialysis

   other evidence may be urinary dipstick abnormalities or structural abnormalities detected by ultrasound scanning

Estimated GFR is automatically reported by chemical pathology laboratories using a formulaic calculation based on serum creatinine[2], but it is not validated in pregnancy.

Proteinuria in the first trimester of pregnancy may be the first indication of CKD, as this is often the first time a woman's urine has been tested.

COMPLICATIONS

- **Hypertension** – common with CKD
- **Fluid retention** – may cause ankle oedema and contribute to hypertension
- **Anaemia** – increased risk as the kidney produces erythropoietin which stimulates the bone marrow to produce red blood cells; erythropoietin is often deficient
- **Heavy proteinuria** – in the nephrotic range (>3 g per 24 hours); can cause hypoalbuminaemia and oedema
- **Metabolic acidosis** – can develop
- **Renal bone disease** – may occur
- **UTI** – increased risk of infection
- **Impaired renal function** – this may relentlessly and predictably deteriorate over time
- Patients may be given dietary restrictions to help control blood pressure and potassium levels within safe limits

NON-PREGNANCY TREATMENT AND CARE

- Investigations into the cause of CKD may include renal ultrasound scanning or occasionally renal biopsy
- Some causes of CKD may require specific treatments, such as immunosuppression with steroids
- Regular monitoring of renal function in nephrology clinic or primary care
- Antihypertensive medication
- Diuretics to treat fluid retention

- Subcutaneous erythropoietin for anaemia
- Referral to a dietician if dietary restrictions are required to maintain safe blood chemistry levels
- Patient education about disease and treatment
- Dialysis or transplantation is required for stage 5 CKD

PRE-CONCEPTION ISSUES AND CARE

- Referral to a renal/obstetric or maternal medicine clinic for personalised specialised advice and counselling
- The predicted outcome of a pregnancy depends on, and is directly proportional to:
  - how well controlled the blood pressure is at booking
  - the level of renal impairment
  - magnitude of proteinuria
  - the underlying disorder responsible for CKD[3,4,5,6]
- Ascertain cause of CKD; if actively under investigation it is prudent to await results before conception
- Always consider previous obstetric history and underlying medical conditions, e.g. patients with lupus nephritis could also have antiphospholipid syndrome[7]
- With progressively worsening CKD decreasing fertility and need for early conception is balanced against the risk of deteriorating renal function in a pregnancy
- Optimal BP control is essential, and alteration to medications may be required
  - ACE inhibitors are commonly used for patients in CRF because of their protective effect on the kidneys, but they are contraindicated in pregnancy as they cause fetal anuria and subsequent oligohydramnios[8]
- Heavily proteinuric patients are at increased risk of thrombo-embolism in pregnancy
  - prophylactic daily injections of low-molecular-weight heparin might be considered if they become pregnant; must be balanced against the increased risk of bleeding[9]
- Some individuals have familial renal disease and may require referral to clinical genetics for counselling
- Pre-eclampsia risk increases with CKD, being difficult to differentiate from deterioration of underlying CKD
- Increased risk of UTI, so regular MSU testing required with early treatment of symptoms
- If there is significant proteinuria, it may be difficult to accurately measure the alpha-feta protein (AFP) level
  - meaningful interpretation of Down's syndrome screening blood test, usually offered around the 15th week of pregnancy, may not be possible
  - if the kidney is leaking protein AFP may also, theoretically, be lost in the urine
- Once pregnant, the woman will need to have regular hospital appointments, at a specialised centre

Pregnancy Issues

If the woman did not receive pre-conceptual counselling she should be made fully aware of the effect and risks of pregnancy upon herself, her renal function and her fetus.

The woman should be managed at a maternal medicine or renal/obstetric clinic.

In pregnancy, CKD is associated with:

- IUGR
- Pre-eclampsia
- Premature delivery
- Fetal loss
- UTI
- Deteriorating renal function[3,4,5,6]

The predicted outcome of the pregnancy is directly proportional to blood pressure control at booking, the degree of hypertension, the level of renal impairment, magnitude of proteinuria and the underlying disorder responsible for CKD[3,4,5,6].

Close supervision of renal function, blood pressure and proteinuria are required.

Although eGFR is now reported as a measure of renal function with all requests for serum creatinine, eGFR is not validated as an accurate measure of renal function in pregnancy[2].

Medical Management and Care

- Specific treatment for underlying renal disease should continue
- Monitoring renal function necessitates regular blood testing
- Careful blood pressure monitoring is required (see Chapter 3.1)
- Current medications should be reviewed; some agents may need to be omitted or changed to those which are safe for pregnancy
- Administration of erythropoietin may be required to treat anaemia
- Monitor urine for increasing protein excretion
- If heavily proteinuric and/or there is a low serum albumin, it may be necessary for the mother to commence anticoagulant therapy[9]
- Monitor renal function carefully by serum creatinine
- Declining renal function may occasionally necessitate institution of dialysis during pregnancy
- Regular fetal growth scans

Midwifery Management and Care

- Early referral to a renal/obstetric or maternal medicine clinic
- Baseline U&E and LFT with booking blood tests
- Advise about alternative screening methods for Down's syndrome if the serum test was unreliable due to heavy proteinuria; an alternative is nuchal translucency scanning
- Monthly MSU
- Advise the woman about the signs and symptoms of pre-eclampsia
- Encourage compliance with prescribed medications and reassure regarding the safety of the drugs for the fetus, and whilst breast-feeding
- Refer to the pharmacist if further information is required
- Teach administration of anticoagulant injections, if prescribed, and give information about the symptoms of DVT and PE; reinforce with general advice about reducing the risk of thrombosis[9]

Labour Issues

There is no reason why the patient should not have a normal vaginal delivery. However the woman will be at increased risk of an emergency LSCS, or induction of labour for either maternal or fetal complications.

The ergometrine component of Syntometrine is associated with hypertensive episodes.

Medical Management and Care

- Monitor renal function and BP carefully
- Strict fluid balance
- Monitor fetal wellbeing, being vigilant for fetal distress

Midwifery Management and Care

- If the fetus is premature or growth restricted then continuous fetal monitoring will be indicated
- If the woman is hypertensive, oxytocin will be required for active third-stage management instead of Syntometrine

Postpartum Issues

There is still potential in the immediate postnatal period for instability in the maternal renal function and blood pressure control.

The baby will require a renal ultrasound if the mother has ureteric reflux, because of the familial nature of these conditions.

If the woman suffers from uncontrolled hypertension, or is breast-feeding, the combined oestrogen and progesterone oral contraceptive will be contraindicated.

Medical Management and Care

- Monitor renal function carefully in immediate postpartum period
- Blood pressure should be well controlled
- Recommence and change to pre-pregnancy medication if required (avoiding nephrotoxic medications), however this may be delayed if the mother wishes to breast-feed, dependent upon any contraindications
- Ensure adequate hydration
- Send notification to the woman's lead nephrologist and GP detailing care and pregnancy outcome
- Arrange a renal ultrasound for the baby if required

Midwifery Management and Care

- Follow-up appointment should be arranged in the mother's routine nephrology department
- If alterations are made to hypertensive treatment, more frequent BP monitoring should be arranged
- The woman will not be suitable for an early discharge
- Discuss the alternative methods of contraception available

6.3 Dialysis in Pregnancy

Incidence
Uncommon – less than 1% of women of childbearing age on dialysis become pregnant each year.

Risk for Childbearing
High Risk

EXPLANATION OF CONDITION

Dialysis is a means of removing waste products and water from the body of patients whose kidneys have failed and have lost their ability to excrete water and dissolved waste products as urine. These patients would otherwise die.

Two types of dialysis are available.

Haemodialysis

In haemodialysis (HD) blood is circulated through a machine where it is purified before being returned to the patient. This type of dialysis is usually performed on three occasions per week in hospital. HD patients require access to their circulation, usually in the form of an arteriovenous fistula or a semipermanent plastic catheter inserted into a large vein.

Peritoneal Dialysis

In peritoneal dialysis (PD) the patient has a soft tube inserted into the peritoneal cavity. This is used to drain up to 2.5 l of fluid *in and out* of the peritoneal cavity, typically four times a day, by patients in their own home.

Each patient has an individual dialysis prescription and a target 'dry' weight to ensure that the correct amounts of waste products and fluid are removed by their dialysis.

Women of childbearing age receiving dialysis either have reduced fertility or are infertile.

COMPLICATIONS

- Dialysis is an imperfect substitute for normally functioning kidneys and dialysis patients have a reduced life expectancy
- Nearly all dialysis patients are hypertensive and anaemic due to the failure of damaged kidneys to produce erythropoietin
- Dialysis patients suffer from secondary hyperparathyroidism and renal osteodystrophy
- Dialysis patients have greatly increased morbidity and mortality, predominantly as a result of infection and especially cardiovascular disease, including heart disease, cerebrovascular disease and peripheral vascular disease
- Arteriovenous fistulae can clot off and become blocked, and permcaths can become blocked or infected; an urgent alternative has to be arranged
- Patients receiving peritoneal dialysis can develop peritonitis as a result of bacteria entering the peritoneal cavity through the dialysis tube; treatable with antibiotics but a potentially very serious complication

NON-PREGNANCY TREATMENT AND CARE

The patient needs close supervision and care from a multidisciplinary team including doctors, nurses, dieticians, pharmacists and dialysis technicians.

Treatment

- Dialysis – to be performed regularly
- Nearly all patients need antihypertensive medication and erythropoietin injections to prevent severe anaemia
- Strict dietary restrictions to limit intake of fluid, potassium and phosphate
- Regular review clinics are required to assess adequacy of dialysis treatment and to prevent dialysis complications

PRE-CONCEPTION ISSUES AND CARE

Because of the low likelihood of pregnancy occurring in women receiving dialysis, very few actually seek preconceptual advice. However, conception is possible and those of childbearing age should take appropriate contraception precautions to avoid an unwanted pregnancy.

Psychosexual problems are common in dialysis patients and may limit the ability to conceive.

Refer to a joint renal/obstetric or maternal medicine clinic, where they can be seen jointly by a consultant nephrologist and obstetrician and specialised midwife. In some cases this may involve considerable travelling to the appropriate unit.

Advise that pregnancy is at high risk of problems such as:

- Anaemia
- Hypertension
- Pre-eclampsia
- IUGR
- Polyhydramnios
- Premature labour

- **Haemodialysis** – HD requirements will increase, and to help stabilise the blood values dialysis would be performed approximately six days a week (compared with three occasions per week as described above)
- **Peritoneal dialysis** – As the pregnancy advances, then smaller, more frequent fluid exchanges may need to be performed; changing to haemodialysis may have to be considered
- If renal transplantation is imminent it may be sensible to wait until after transplantation before trying for a pregnancy
- Down's screening tests will not be interpretable in dialysis patients; nuchal translucency screening or diagnostic tests would have to be considered if requested
- The underlying renal disorder may have an impact on the pregnancy, and this will need to be considered
- Current medications will need review, and probable alteration, by the renal team

Pregnancy Issues

A high-risk pregnancy[1,2,3,4] with the risk of:

- IUGR and pre-term labour
- Severe pre-eclampsia (difficult to diagnose in renal patients)
- Polyhydramnios – as the fetus is exposed to high urea levels which increase the diuresis
- Peritonitis with continuous ambulatory peritoneal dialysis
- Dietary restrictions will require modification to accommodate any change in the dialysis prescription
- Anaemia, because the kidney is responsible for erythropoietin which stimulates red cell production

The aim is to minimise the effect of the uraemic maternal environment on fetal development and to prevent large fluctuations in maternal blood chemistry, fluid status and blood pressure.

Target weights need frequent re-assessment as weight increases throughout pregnancy. Excellent teamwork and communication between the different members of multi-disciplinary team will be essential.

Peritoneal Dialysis (PD)

- More frequent smaller exchanges as the pregnancy advances
- Good exchange technique to avoid peritonitis

Haemodialysis (HD)

- Increase dialysis frequency to six days per week
- Avoid hypotensive episodes as dialysis can reduce placental blood flow

Medical Management and Care

- Ensure the woman *understands* risks of proceeding with a pregnancy
- Aim to deliver in a unit with both obstetric and nephrology support
- Consider if the underlying disease has any impact on the pregnancy
- Assess current medications for their compatibility with pregnancy
- Increase the frequency and duration of dialysis through pregnancy
- Frequent monitoring of:
  - serum biochemistry
  - haemoglobin
  - bacteriuria
  - fluid balance
  - maternal weight
- Close input from specialised renal dietician
- Regular ultrasound scans for fetal growth
- Conventional Down's syndrome screening investigations will be difficult to interpret as a result of the dialysis so discuss alternatives such as nuchal translucency screening or amniocentesis
- Aim to maintain haemoglobin >10 g/dl, which may require increasing erythropoietin, iron supplementation, or having a blood transfusion

Midwifery Management and Care

- Refer to renal/obstetric or maternal medicine clinic
- No phlebotomy or taking of BP on the arm if there is an arteriovenous fistula as this increases the risk of damaging the access for dialysis
- Monthly MSU
- Advice on prevention of urinary tract infection
- Educate about the symptoms of pre-eclampsia; ensure the mother has appropriate contact numbers if there is concern
- Plan regular antenatal appointments
- Encourage compliance with dietary advice, medication and treatment
- Liaise closely with the renal unit, coordinate care and try to avoid repetition of blood tests which could be taken whilst on haemodialysis
- Due to increasing hospitalisation and visits, consider referral to social services or support group to offer financial or practical support, such as assistance with transport problems
- If a pre-term delivery is likely arrange a tour of the relevant neonatal unit for the mother and significant others

Labour Issues

The dialysis mother could in principle have a normal delivery, but there is an increased likelihood that they will need to be delivered early because of pre-eclampsia, concerns about IUGR or for maternal reasons. Hence, the majority of pregnant dialysis women will be delivered by caesarean section.

Medical Management and Care

- Dialysis prior to elective delivery with close monitoring of blood biochemistry
- Strict blood pressure control and fluid balance
- If caesarean section performed PD should be discontinued, and all PD fluid drained out pre-operatively; PD can be restarted immediately post-delivery if there are no complications

Midwifery Management and Care

- Continuous electronic fetal monitoring, being alert for fetal distress
- Strict control of any iv fluids and record fluid balance
- Liaise with renal team/nurses regarding prescribed dialysis
- Clearly document and report up-to-date blood results

Postpartum Issues

The mother can now return to pre-pregnancy medications (if not breast-feeding) and dialysis prescription.

Caesarean section should not preclude continuation of PD, however if unable to do PD following abdominal surgery, temporary HD may be required until wounds healed.

Medical Management and Care

- Review medications and dialysis prescriptions
- The Mirena intrauterine system (IUS) would be the contraceptive of choice; reduces menstrual blood loss, therefore reduces anaemia, and is very effective in preventing unplanned pregnancies

Midwifery Management and Care

- Ensure specific dietary requirements are met whilst an in-patient
- Liaise with renal unit regarding dialysis requirements
- Breast-feeding is possible, although awkward whilst actually on HD

6.4 Renal Transplantation

Incidence	Risk for Childbearing
Over 14,000 pregnancies have been documented in renal transplant recipients	High Risk

EXPLANATION OF CONDITION

The patient will have developed end-stage renal failure as a consequence of either acute or chronic kidney disease. At this stage renal replacement therapy is required. The options are haemodialysis, peritoneal dialysis or renal transplantation. Most patients spend some time receiving dialysis before receiving a kidney transplant. Kidneys for transplantation may be obtained from a cadaver donor or be donated by a living relative. Although non-functional, the patient's own kidneys do not cause a significant problem and are not removed.

The transplanted kidney is placed superficially in the lower part of the abdomen in the left or right iliac fossa. To avoid rejection the patient requires lifelong immunosuppressive therapy.

The success of the transplant may vary. Most transplanted kidneys function well for many years, whereas others function less well or not at all. Commonly however, kidney transplants work well initially, but their function declines slowly over time.

COMPLICATIONS

- Risk of rejection and loss of renal function
- Immunosuppressive treatment increases the risk of infection and malignancy
- The patient may experience side effects from the immunosuppressive medications
- Transplant patients are commonly hypertensive, and are at particular risk of cardiovascular disease
- Progressive decline in transplant kidney function may occur, until the transplant fails and dialysis is needed

NON-PREGNANCY TREATMENT AND CARE

Regular hospital appointments are needed to address:

- Blood and urine analysis to monitor kidney function and immunosuppressive treatment
- Annual review for long-term stable transplant patients
- Ensure well-controlled blood pressure
- Advice on general good healthy lifestyle, no smoking, good weight control, dietary intake and good hygiene
- Importance of seeking prompt treatment if unwell or if infection is suspected

For women of childbearing age, transplantation improves libido, and restores fertility[1], therefore discussions need to take place around family planning, and contraceptive advice.

PRE-CONCEPTION ISSUES AND CARE

- If the underlying disease is an inherited condition, the patient may require a clinical genetics referral to discuss potential implications for the fetus, and the possibility of prenatal testing
- Referral to renal/obstetric or maternal medicine clinic for specific individual advice and counselling is very important
- Prospective mothers with transplanted kidneys, and their partners, should be informed that pregnancy in renal transplant recipients is associated with an increased risk of pre-eclampsia, intrauterine growth retardation, premature delivery and fetal loss
- Risks increase as kidney transplant function declines or if blood pressure is poorly controlled[2]
- Regardless of the level of transplant function all patients should be regarded as having renal insufficiency
- Advise the woman to wait for at least one year after transplant, with no evidence of rejection in past year, before attempting pregnancy[3]
- Aim for stable and adequate kidney function
- Achieve good blood pressure control
- The woman should be taking maintenance doses of immunosuppressive drugs at stable dosages. Some newer immunosuppressive drugs are not safe for the fetus in pregnancy (see Appendix 11) and will require changing before conception; this process is associated with an increased risk of rejection
- Women may be taking other medications that are not safe in pregnancy, e.g. ACE inhibitors or statins, which need to be changed for safer drugs, or discontinued pre-conception[2]
- Outcome of pregnancy may be influenced by other co-existing morbidity:
  - diabetes
  - cardiovascular status
  - level of transplant function
  - hypertension
  - aetiology of the original kidney disease
- Generally, pregnancy outcomes in kidney transplant recipients are good

Pregnancy Issues

It is essential that the pregnancy is managed jointly by nephrologists, obstetricians and midwives who are experienced in renal disease and pregnancy[1,2,3,4].

Pregnancy outcome is highly dependent on stable transplant with good function, well-controlled blood pressure and minimal co-morbidity. If these factors are optimised then this will improve the outcome of the pregnancy[1,2,3,4].

The woman is at risk of pre-eclampsia, hence she requires careful blood pressure monitoring.

Kidney transplant rejection can occur in pregnancy and may require transplant biopsy.

Signs of infection may be less obvious or unusual with immunosuppressant therapy and must not be overlooked.

Medical Management and Care

- Review medications, and change or omit drugs which are contraindicated in pregnancy
- Regular renal function checks with serum investigations, and urinalysis for proteinuria
- Monitor immunosuppressive drug levels, altering dosages as required
- Regular MSU to check for urinary infection
- Regular fetal growth scans
- Be alert for pre-eclampsia
- Remain aware that transplant rejection may occur, or that underlying renal disease may have an impact on transplant function during the pregnancy[3,4]
- Maintain a good haemoglobin level

Midwifery Management and Care

- Refer early to a specific joint renal/obstetric or maternal medicine clinic for high-risk care
- Regular antenatal appointments and prompt referral if there are any concerns, ensuring the midwifery team and the mother have appropriate contact telephone numbers
- If the mother has an arteriovenous fistula used for previous dialysis, avoid that arm for phlebotomy or blood pressure measurement
- Minimise risk of UTI (see Section 6.1)
- Reassure the woman that the baby will not 'squash' the new kidney, and the baby will have room to grow
- Ensure compliance with medications and emphasise their importance in optimising pregnancy outcome
- Be alert for signs of infection, referring if problems are suspected
- Breast-feeding may not be contraindicated, dependent on the drugs used; refer to a pharmacist for specialised advice if required

Labour Issues

A normal vaginal delivery is not contraindicated because of the presence of a transplanted kidney. Caesarean section is reserved for standard obstetric indications.

If the labour is protracted or complicated by pre-eclampsia, there must be good fluid balance control, particular avoidance of dehydration and hypotensive episodes, which would reduce renal blood flow and increase the risk of acute renal failure.

Medical Management and Care

- Increase steroid cover during labour
- Monitor blood pressure regularly in labour
- Strict input/output fluid balance
- Prompt fluid replacement if there is significant haemorrhage
- Inform and involve the renal team of the woman's admission, updating them if there are any medical concerns in labour

Midwifery Management and Care

- Administer any prescribed (including regular) medications
- Maintain an accurate fluid balance record
- Encourage regular micturition, but avoid bladder catheterisation
- Report any hyper- or hypotensive episodes

Postpartum Issues

Ensure renal function is stable, and blood pressure well controlled (therefore the mother is not suitable for early discharge).

The baby will require a renal ultrasound if the mother has scarring nephropathy or ureteric reflux, due to the familial nature of these conditions.

For non-rubella immune mothers, the live rubella vaccine should be avoided as it is contraindicated with immunosuppressants[1].

If the woman has uncontrolled hypertension the combined oral contraceptive will not be advised.

Medical Management and Care

- Monitor renal function and immunosuppressive drug levels in the immediate postpartum period
- Aim for well-controlled blood pressure
- Re-commencement of pre-pregnancy drugs may be required, but ensure there are no contraindications if the patient is breast-feeding
- Arrange a renal ultrasound of the baby if required
- Arrange an appointment at the routine transplant clinic

Midwifery Management and Care

- Good hygiene, being alert for early signs of sepsis, as the woman is immunosuppressed, with prompt medical referral if concerned
- Administer medications as prescribed
- Regular blood pressure monitoring, reporting hypo- or hypertensive episodes
- Advise on contraception available to the woman

6.5 Nephrotic Syndrome

Incidence	Risk for Childbearing
Uncommon	High Risk

EXPLANATION OF CONDITION

Nephrotic syndrome is a classical clinical syndrome of renal disease compromising a triad of features:

1. Proteinuria (usually >3.5 g/24 hours)
2. Low plasma albumin
3. Oedema

Most patients also have high cholesterol and high triglyceride levels. The loss of protein into the urine results in a fall in plasma albumin concentration, but other circulating proteins are also lost. Falling plasma oncotic pressure encourages fluid to leave the circulation, and this results in oedema.

The development of nephrotic syndrome indicates that the patient has renal disease affecting the glomerulus, i.e. glomerulonephritis. Many different types of glomerular disease may cause nephrotic syndrome (e.g. membranous nephropathy, diabetic nephropathy) and a renal biopsy is usually required to make a precise histological diagnosis.

COMPLICATIONS

- Oedema
- Hypertension
- Infection
- Hyperlipidaemia – may result in atherosclerosis over time
- Thrombo-embolism – loss of protein in the urine results in an imbalance in blood clotting systems with increased risk of thrombo-embolic disease
- Kidney failure – for some patients with nephrotic syndrome

NON-PREGNANCY TREATMENT AND CARE

- Fluid retention and oedema are treated with diuretics, often in high dosages, and dietary restriction of salt
- Hypertension may require treatment; ACE inhibitors and angiotensin receptor blockers (ARB) are the agents of first choice
- Even if nephrotic patients are normotensive, they will receive either an ACE inhibitor or an ARB since these agents reduce protein leakage into the urine and protect kidney function
- Some patients may receive a statin
- Some patients may be anticoagulated
- Some patients may receive treatment aimed specifically at the cause of the nephrotic syndrome, usually some form of immunosuppression

PRE-CONCEPTION ISSUES AND CARE

The woman requires referral to a renal/obstetric or maternal medicine clinic for specialised advice. This encompasses:

- Ascertain the underlying cause of nephrotic syndrome by renal biopsy prior to pregnancy if possible
- Determine the level of renal functional impairment if present
- Ensure hypertension is controlled prior to conception
- The combination of pregnancy (a hypercoagulable state), and nephrotic syndrome, will put the woman at a markedly increased risk of thrombo-embolism[1]; prospective mothers should be advised to:
  - reduce their weight if obese
  - stop smoking
  - wait, if possible, until the protein loss is minimal and stable
- Be aware that during pregnancy daily sc injections of low-molecular-weight heparin may be prescribed; this is balanced against the risk of causing bleeding problems
- Consider cessation of ACE inhibitors and angiotensin receptor blockers as they are contraindicated in pregnancy; if used as an antihypertensive they can be changed to methyldopa[2]
- Consider cessation of other drugs (e.g. diuretics, statins)
- The Down's screening test may not be reliable in pregnancy (as yet unproven), but if serum protein is lower because of increased excretion, then serum levels of alpha-feta protein could also be lower; nuchal translucency scanning or diagnostic tests (amniocentesis) are to be considered if required
- Advise the prospective mother that pregnancy entails increased risk of:
  - Pre-eclampsia, although this is difficult to distinguish from deteriorating renal function, therefore regular monitoring and frequent blood and urine testing would be required
  - IUGR
  - Premature delivery

Pregnancy Issues

There is increased risk of:
- Pre-eclampsia
- IUGR
- Deteriorating renal function
- Thrombo-embolism

Because of the high risk and complex nature of nephrotic syndrome in pregnancy[3], the woman will need to be referred to a specialist renal/obstetric or maternal medicine clinic.

The woman must be made aware that pregnancy itself is a hypercoagulable state, and she will be at an increased risk of thrombosis if the pregnancy continues.

There is no clear evidence as to what level of proteinuria, and/or lowered serum albumin requires commencement of prophylactic anticoagulation. This is usually given as daily sc injection of low-molecular-weight heparin. A careful balance of the risk of thrombosis versus the concern about haemorrhage must be made in discussion with the mother.

Developing pre-eclampsia may be difficult to distinguish from deterioration of the underlying renal condition. Regular assessment of all signs and symptoms of pre-eclampsia must be evaluated carefully.

Although there is heavy urine protein loss, increasing dietary intake of protein is not indicated as this simply results in increased urinary protein leakage.

Urinary tract infection is more common.

Medical Management and Care

- Aim to deliver in a unit with obstetric and nephrology support
- Outline risks of thrombosis with continuing pregnancy
- Monitor: U&E and LFT (specifically plasma albumin levels), urine protein, creatinine ratios and 24-hour urinary protein excretion
- Consider investigation of underlying cause of nephrotic syndrome by renal biopsy, if not already identified
- Assessment of thrombosis risk factors:
  - overweight
  - limited mobility
  - previous thrombotic episodes
  - low plasma albumin <30 g/l
  - 24-hour urinary protein loss > 3 g/24 hours
  - smoking
- Consider prescribing low-molecular-weight heparin anticoagulant therapy, by daily sc injection[1]
- Consider referral to haemostasis clinic for monitoring of heparin assay levels if low-molecular-weight heparin is prescribed (see Chapter 15)
- Careful monitoring and good control of BP
- Down's risk screening test will be difficult to interpret; consider nuchal translucency screening or diagnostic tests (amniocentesis) if required
- Fetal growth surveillance by regular ultrasound scans
- Monthly MSU

Midwifery Management and Care

- Refer to a renal/obstetric or maternal medicine clinic
- Investigations for U&E and LFT simultaneous with 'booking bloods'
- Teach self-administration of low-molecular-weight heparin injections
- To reduce the risk of thrombosis, advise the mother:
  - do not sit with legs crossed
  - at rest, raise legs on footstool, make circle movements with feet
  - wear support stockings, evenly applied (no creases)
- Advise on the signs and symptoms of thrombosis or embolism (and to seek immediate help if occur) (see Chapter 15)
  - acutely painful swollen calf
  - pleuritic pain, cough or breathlessness
- Weigh regularly (helps to monitor for fluid retention)
- Be alert for signs and symptoms of pre-eclampsia
- Fortnightly antenatal appointments

Labour Issues

Whilst there is an increased risk of labour being induced if the pregnancy is complicated, there are no reasons for the woman not to have a normal delivery.

In order to reduce the risk of postpartum haemorrhage, low-molecular-weight heparin is omitted on the day of delivery.

Medical Management and Care

- Omit low-molecular-weight heparin on the day of delivery
- If receiving steroids an increase in 'cover' will be required for labour

Midwifery Management and Care

- Mobilise the mother as much as possible throughout the labour
- Strict fluid balance
- If Fragmin has been given, be aware of the increased risk of PPH
- Apart from the above, labour can usually be managed normally by the midwife

Postpartum Issues

The increased risk of thrombosis continues into the postpartum period. Six weeks appears to be the acceptable time frame to continue with anticoagulant therapy[4].

Serum albumin and total protein urine excretion will need to be assessed along with the patient's risk factors for thrombosis, in order to individualise care.

Avoid the combined oral contraceptive pill, because of the increased risk of DVT.

Medical Management and Care

- Continue with anticoagulants for approximately six weeks, dependent upon serum albumin and proteinuria levels[1]
- Monitor for signs of infection
- Arrange follow-up appointment in a general nephrology clinic

Midwifery Management and Care

- TED stockings to be worn whilst in hospital
- Reassurance that it is safe to breast-feed whilst on anticoagulants
- Give advice on alternative contraception

6 Renal Disorders

PATIENT ORGANISATIONS

National Kidney Federation
6 Stanley Street
Worksop
Nottinghamshire S81 7HX
www.kidney.org.uk/main/nkf_work.html

British Kidney Patient Association
Bordon
Hants. GU35 9JZ
www.britishkidney-pa.co.uk

Kidney Alliance
26 Oriental Road
Woking
Surrey GU22 7AW
www.kidneyalliance.org.uk

Kidney Research UK
Kings Chambers
Priestgate
Peterborough PE1 1FG
www.kidneyresearchuk.org

Kidney Patient Guide
www.kidneypatientguide.org.uk

American Association of Kidney Patients
www.aakp.org

Edinburgh Royal Infirmary Patient Information
www.renux.dmed.ed.ac.uk/edren/EdRenINFOhome.html

Group B Strep Support
P O Box 203
Haywards Heath
West Sussex RH16 1GF
www.gbss.org.uk

Action on Pre-eclampsia – APEC
84–88 Pinner Road
Harrow
Middlesex HA1 4HZ
www.apec.org.uk

ESSENTIAL READING

Barcelo, P., Lopez-Lilo, J., Cabero, L. and Del Rio, G. (1986) Successful pregnancy in primary glomerular disease. **Kidney International**, 30:914–919.

Davison, J.M. (2001) Renal disorders in pregnancy. **Current Opinion in Obstetrics and Gynaecology**, 13:109–114.

Hou, S. (1999) Pregnancy in chronic renal insufficiency and end stage renal disease. **American Journal of Kidney Disease**, 33:235–52.

James, D.K., Steer, P.J., Weiner, C.P. and Gonik, B. (Eds) (2006) Thromboembolic disorders, pp. 938–48; Autoimmune disease, pp. 949–85; Renal disorders, pp 1098–1124; Pregnancy after renal transplantation, pp. 1174–1186. In: **High Risk Pregnancy: Management Options**. W.B. Saunders, Philadelphia.

Jepson, R.G., Milhaljevic, L. and Craig, J. (2004) Cranberries for preventing urinary tract infections. **The Cochrane Database of Systematic Reviews**, Issue 2.Art.No.CD001321. DOI:10.1002/14651858.CD001321.

McKay, D.B. and Josephson, M.A. (2006) Pregnancy in recipients of solid organs – effects on mother and child. **New England Journal of Medicine**, 354:1281–1293.

Queenan, J.T. (Ed) (1999) Renal disease. In: **Management of High Risk Pregnancy**, pp. 236–245. Blackwell Science, Oxford.

RCOG (2003) Prevention of early onset neonatal group B streptococcal disease. **Guideline No 36**, p. 6.

Smaill, F. (2002) Antibiotics for asymptomatic bacteriuria in pregnancy. **The Cochrane Database of Systematic Reviews**, Issue 2. Art. No.: CD000490. DOI: 10.1002/14651858. CD000490.

Thorsen, M.S. and Poole, J.H. (2002) Renal disease in pregnancy. **Journal of Perinatal Neonatal Nursing**, 15:13–26.

Williams, D.J. (2001) Renal disease and fluid balance in pregnancy. **Current Obstetrics and Gynaecology**, 11:146–152.

7 ENDOCRINE DISORDERS

Rob Gregory, Diane Todd and Mairie Halliday

7.1 Hypothyroidism

Incidence	Risk for Childbearing
0.3–0.7% Hypothyroidism	Variable Risk
2.2–2.5% Subclinical hypothyroidism	

EXPLANATION OF CONDITION

Hypothyroidism comprises a lack of thyroid hormones, thyroxine (T4) and tri-iodothyronine (T3). This may be primary (impaired functioning of thyroid tissue) or central (due to pituitary or hypothalamic disease).

Causes

The commonest causes encountered in pregnancy are autoimmune thyroiditis, with or without goitre (Hashimoto's or atrophic thyroiditis), and a history of thyroidectomy or radioiodine treatment.

Autoimmune thyroid disease occurs in families; sometimes in association with other organ-specific autoimmune diseases, e.g. type 1 diabetes, reflecting a genetic predisposition to organ-specific autoimmunity. Auto-antibodies to thyroid peroxidase (TPO) are usually present in serum.

Symptoms

The symptoms are independent of the cause and may affect multiple systems. They include:

- Weight gain
- Constipation
- Cold intolerance
- Alopecia
- Dry skin
- Hoarseness
- Lethargy
- Ataxia
- Cognitive impairment
- Normochromic normocytic anaemia
- Menorrhagia
- Bradycardia[1]

However, the majority of cases have few or no symptoms at diagnosis.

Signs

Slow-relaxing ankle reflexes, coarse skin, cool skin, periorbital puffiness.

Subclinical hypothyroidism is defined biochemically as a raised TSH concentration with normal free T4 (fT4) and free T3 (fT3) concentrations[2]. This condition can resolve spontaneously, but 2.6% of antibody negative and 4.3% of antibody positive subjects become hypothyroid per year.

Investigations

Investigation consists of the measurement of circulating thyroid hormones with thyroid function tests. In primary hypothyroidism thyroid stimulating hormone (TSH) will be raised, free thyroxine (fT4) will be reduced, as will fT3, although this is not always measured. In central hypothyroidism the TSH will also be low.

TPO antibodies are usually positive in autoimmune thyroiditis. Up to 5% of women have positive antibodies in early pregnancy.

COMPLICATIONS

Myxoedema coma is a rare complication that occurs in undiagnosed or chronically untreated hypothyroidism. There is loss of consciousness with hypothermia, hypoventilation and bradycardia.

There are pregnancy associated complications:

- To mother:
  - Reduced fertility
  - Pregnancy induced hypertension
- To baby:
  - Low birth weight
  - Psychomotor retardation

NON-PREGNANCY TREATMENT AND CARE

The standard treatment is thyroid hormone replacement with oral L-thyroxine at a dose sufficient to restore TSH to the normal range – usually 50–150 micrograms once daily.

In central hypothyroidism the dose is adjusted to keep the fT4 in the normal range.

PRE-CONCEPTION ISSUES AND CARE

Women with hypothyroidism may have anovulation and may present with infertility.

Pre-conception care is especially important, as the prospective mother and future child are at risk of:

- **Pregnancy induced hypertension** – this is 2–3 times as common in overt or subclinical hypothyroidism
- **Low birth weight** – but there is no excess of congenital malformations
- **Reduced psychomotor development** – associated with hypothyroidism in early pregnancy
- **Lower IQ in children at age eight years** – associated with untreated maternal hypothyroidism; fetal thyroid starts to produce hormones at 10–12 weeks and early fetal brain development depends on small amounts of maternal thyroid hormone that cross the placenta[3]

Women who are known to have hypothyroidism should be informed of the above issues, but can be reassured that adequate treatment with thyroxine will reduce the risks to a minimum. They should be reminded to take their thyroxine regularly throughout the pregnancy.

A measurement of fT4 and TSH should be taken as baseline and the dose of thyroxine adjusted if necessary to ensure the woman is euthyroid at the time of conception.

Women with recently-diagnosed hypothyroidism should be advised to delay conceiving until their TSH is restored to a normal level.

Women with subclinical hypothyroidism, who are contemplating pregnancy, should be treated with thyroxine to correct the TSH concentration.

As weight gain and lethargy are common problems, the BMI should be estimated (see Appendix 13) and if overweight a reducing diet advised and an exercise plan recommended.

Pregnancy Issues

Women may be diagnosed with hypothyroidism at any stage of pregnancy and should be treated promptly.

In pregnancies complicated by hypothyroidism the TSH rises, indicating a rising demand for thyroxine. The usual increase in dose is 25–50%.

Medical Management and Care

- Check fT4 and TSH at booking and 4–6 weekly throughout the pregnancy
- Adjust the dose of thyroxine to maintain TSH in the lower half of the reference range[2]
- Encourage compliance with thyroxine supplementation
- If previous intrauterine growth restriction associated with hypothyroidism has occurred, then serial fetal growth scans are indicated

Midwifery Management and Care

- Mother is suitable for routine, shared antenatal care, unless there are any other medical or obstetric issues
- Any concerns regarding restricted fetal growth, refer immediately to the obstetric unit
- Ensure that regular fT4 and TSH blood tests are performed and acted upon
- Be alert for pregnancy-induced hypertension

Labour Issues

As for normal pregnancy.

Medical Management and Care

- No specific medical issues

Midwifery Management and Care

- As for low-risk pregnancy – unless there are any other underlying medical or obstetric issues
- At examination of the placenta take a 10 ml sample of umbilical cord blood (standard clotted sample) for neonatal screening[5]

Postpartum Issues

- Reduced demand for thyroxine to pre-pregnancy level
- Neonatal screening is of paramount importance
- The parents are likely to be anxious that the baby could have inherited the maternal condition

Medical Management and Care

- Reduce dose of thyroxine to pre-pregnancy dose (assuming the woman was euthyroid then) in order to avoid overtreatment postpartum
- Check fT4 and TSH six weeks after delivery

Midwifery Management and Care

- Routine care for type of delivery
- Breast-feeding should be encouraged
- Arrange paediatric review of baby[6]
- Emphasise to the mother the importance of attending any outpatient appointments arranged, especially for the baby
- It is important that the neonatal screening blood test (Guthrie test) is performed promptly and well, and mention made of the maternal condition on the request form[6]
- Support and reassure the mother who may have been alarmed over indiscreet mention of 'cretinism' and fearful for long-term prospects of the baby

7.2 Thyrotoxicosis

Incidence	**Risk for Childbearing**
Graves' disease approximately 1:1000 Other causes are rare	High Risk

EXPLANATION OF CONDITION

Thyrotoxicosis is the clinical syndrome caused by high serum concentrations of thyroid hormones. Symptoms and signs include:

- Heat intolerance
- Weight loss (despite good appetite)
- Insomnia
- Agitation
- Tremor
- Retraction of the upper eyelid
- Sweating
- Tachycardia and bounding pulse
- Diarrhoea
- Oligo- or amenorrhoea

Since several of these features occur in normal pregnancy, the clinical diagnosis of thyrotoxicosis can be difficult to make in this context. The combination of raised serum free thyroxine (fT4), and low thyroid stimulating hormone (TSH) confirms the diagnosis. Occasionally the fT4 is in the normal range, but if the fT3 is raised T3 toxicosis occurs[1].

Causes

Graves' disease: Most women with primary hyperthyroidism in pregnancy will have Graves' disease (GD), an autoimmune condition in which thyrotoxicosis is caused by auto-antibodies to the thyroid stimulating hormone receptor (TSHR). These thyroid stimulating immunoglobulins (TSIg) mimic the effects of TSH on its receptor, but in an unregulated way. Endogenous TSH falls in response to high levels of fT3 and fT4, but production and release of these hormones continues to be stimulated by TSIgs. A smooth, symmetrical goitre (enlarged thyroid gland) is often present, over which a *bruit* may be heard. In some cases Graves' disease is associated with other organ-specific autoimmune conditions, e.g. type 1 diabetes and pernicious anaemia.

Excess thyroid hormone ingestion: This may be iatrogenic (overtreatment of hypothyroidism) or factitious (taking thyroid hormone surreptitiously, perhaps to aid weight loss).

HCG-dependent hyperthyroidism: Human chorionic gonadotrophin (HCG) shows a degree of homology with TSH, and can act as a weak TSHR agonist. Conditions characterised by raised concentrations of HCG may cause hyperthyroidism. The commonest is hyperemesis gravidarum which results in transient hyperthyroidism in one third of cases. Trophoblastic tumours such as hydatidiform mole may rarely cause thyrotoxicosis[1].

COMPLICATIONS

- **Graves' ophthalmopathy** (GO) describes the range of eye symptoms and signs seen in up to 50% of patients with GD. These range from a stare due to retraction of the upper eyelid to exophthalmos of one or both eyes that may result in diplopia and even blindness due to optic nerve compression. Corneal damage can occur when the patient cannot close her eyes properly. Smoking is a risk factor for GO. The disease is thought to be due to an immune response directed against orbital antigens resembling TSHR[2].

- **Graves' dermopathy** is an uncommon feature characterised by localised, usually pre-tibial, myxoedema.
- **Thyrotoxic storm** is severe life-threatening thyrotoxicosis, usually precipitated by the withdrawal of antithyroid drug treatment or intercurrent illness. Features include high fever, tachycardia, drowsiness and coma[3].

NON-PREGNANCY TREATMENT AND CARE

Antithyroid Drugs

Carbimazole (CBZ) (methimazole in the US) and propylthiouracil (PTU) block the organification of iodine – an essential step in the manufacture of thyroid hormones. They are also weakly immunosuppressive and may induce long-term remission of GD.

Treatment is usually started at a high dose, which reduces fT4 and fT3 to normal in approximately four weeks. Propranolol, a non-selective beta-blocker, may be prescribed to relieve symptoms during this phase, but is not required long term. In order to avoid iatrogenic hypothyroidism it is necessary either to reduce the dose of CBZ or PTU to that required to keep the concentration of fT4 in the normal range (*dose titration*) or to continue with high dose CBZ or PTU in combination with L-thyroxine (*block and replace*). After treatment for 12–18 months with dose titration, or 6–12 months with block and replace, medication is stopped.

Remission is induced in 60% of cases. Some who relapse opt for long-term CBZ or PTU (titrated dose), others choose radioiodine treatment or surgery. Side effects include urticaria and arthralgia. Agranulocytosis (incidence 0.2–0.5%) is potentially life threatening and patients must be counselled when starting treatment[1].

Radioiodine (^{131}I)

The thyroid gland in GD is avid for iodine and will take up ^{131}I given orally. This radioactive isotope causes a thyroiditis that eventually destroys sufficient thyroid tissue to lower thyroid hormone levels to normal, or subnormal. Women are counselled not to conceive for six months following ^{131}I treatment.

Thyroidectomy

Subtotal thyroidectomy is usually reserved for cases of GD uncontrolled by large doses of antithyroid drugs, or where there is a large goitre.

PRE-CONCEPTION ISSUES AND CARE

The woman is at risk of oligo-/amenorrhoea and consequently reduced fertility.

There are additional risks of fetal and neonatal transfer of the thyroid antibodies causing neonatal thyroid dysfunction.

Women on block and replace treatment are switched to a titrated dose of CBZ or PTU. The woman should be euthyroid by fT4 before conception. If uncontrolled by drug therapy, surgery is considered prior to cessation of contraception.[2] Women on radioiodine should continue with contraception for six months following ^{131}I treatment.

Aplasia cutis is a rare defect of the skin of the scalp. It has only been reported in babies born to mothers who took CBZ and not PTU in pregnancy. Some endocrinologists recommend using PTU rather than CBZ in pregnancy[4].

Pregnancy Issues

Thyrotoxicosis increases the risk of miscarriage. Diagnosis of thyrotoxicosis may be difficult because some of the symptoms and signs are mimicked by normal pregnancy. Serum investigations are necessary.

Graves' disease (GD) tends to improve in pregnancy, and may remit completely during the second half of pregnancy.

Fetal or neonatal thyrotoxicosis affects 2–10% of Graves' disease pregnancies. This can cause a *small for dates* baby, premature labour and intrauterine death or neonatal death. It is also associated with craniostenosis.

Overtreatment of maternal thyrotoxicosis will cause fetal hypothyroidism and goitre.

If ultrasound scans show a fetal goitre the differential diagnosis is fetal hypothyroidism or fetal thyrotoxicosis. This is an indication for cordocentesis to measure fetal TSH and fT4[2].

Medical Management and Care
- The aim of treatment is to achieve maternal euthyroidism (normal thyroid function) and maintain this for the entire pregnancy
- fT4 should ideally be in the upper half of the reference range
- Block and replace regimens are contraindicated in pregnancy because, while CBZ and PTU cross the placenta, relatively little thyroxine does and this would cause fetal hypothyroidism
- The lowest dose of CBZ or PTU that achieves target fT4 levels is used
- Serial measurements of fT4 and TSH every four weeks will usually allow withdrawal of antithyroid drugs in the third trimester
- If large doses of CBZ or PTU appear to be required to treat maternal thyrotoxicosis, it is worth considering referral for subtotal thyroidectomy after the first trimester to avoid fetal hypothyroidism
- The risk of fetal/neonatal thyrotoxicosis is highest in women with uncontrolled thyrotoxicosis in later pregnancy, those who have had this complication before, and those who have had radioiodine or surgical treatment
- Measurement of TSIg in the third trimester in such cases may help those at highest risk, but this assay is not readily available in the UK and many centres rely on careful obstetric monitoring of fetal thyroid status

Midwifery Management and Care
- Accurate booking history and early referral to specialist obstetric unit
- Ensure regular fT4 and TSH tests are performed and acted upon
- Serial ultrasound growth scans should be organised
- Regular assessment of fetal heart rate to detect fetal tachycardia (>160/min is suggestive) is essential

Labour Issues

Detection of previously undiagnosed fetal thyrotoxicosis.

Medical Management and Care
- To manage as high risk[2]

Midwifery Management and Care
- Manage as high-risk labour
- Continuous fetal monitoring to detect fetal tachycardia
- Alert the paediatrician when labour is established

Postpartum Issues

Management of neonatal thyrotoxicosis
Neonatal thyrotoxicosis, caused by placental transfer of maternal TSIgs, is self-limiting, but gets worse transiently when the maternally-transferred antithyroid drugs disappear.

Relapse
Graves' disease can 'flare' postpartum.

Antithyroid drugs and breast-feeding
PTU is preferred to carbimazole if the mother wishes to breast-feed, as it is transferred to breast milk less readily. However carbimazole in low dose (<15 mg daily) does not affect infant thyroid function.

Medical Management and Care
- The baby may require temporary treatment with antithyroid drugs and propranolol
- Maternal thyroid hormone levels must be checked six weeks postpartum to identify relapse of GD and treatment reintroduced or increased as necessary[5]

Midwifery Management and Care
- Extend the period of postnatal observations, with emphasis on pulse
- Promote breast-feeding and reassure the mother that low dose carbimazole does not affect infant thyroid function
- When examining the baby, be vigilant for signs of goitre (swollen neck) and if suspected report this immediately
- Be alert for signs of neonatal thyrotoxicosis, which may be delayed for a week[6], and include: weight loss, jitteriness, tachycardia, irritability and poor feeding
- The baby may be transferred to a neonatal unit, in which case the mother requires support and measures to promote infant 'bonding'

7.3 Type 1 Diabetes Mellitus

Incidence	Risk for Childbearing
2–4:1000 pregnancies	High Risk

EXPLANATION OF CONDITION

Type 1 diabetes mellitus (T1DM) accounts for 15–20% of all diabetes mellitus. Since it usually presents in childhood or early adulthood, it accounts for the majority of cases of pregestational diabetes. It is caused by autoimmune destruction of the insulin-producing β-cells of the pancreatic islets leading to insulin dependency, and there is a genetic pre-disposition to the condition.

The symptoms are of hyperglycaemia and include thirst, polydipsia, weight loss, fatigue and blurred vision. If not diagnosed at this stage, diabetic ketoacidosis may develop – a medical emergency, characterised by dehydration, and metabolic acidosis, that can lead to coma and death. Diagnostic criteria are included in Appendix 7. Most patients with T1DM would have had symptoms at presentation and a raised fasting or random venous plasma glucose.

COMPLICATIONS[3]

Microvascular Complications

These are caused by chronic hyperglycaemia and are preventable if patients can achieve near normal blood glucose concentrations for much of the time.

Retinopathy

The early stages are asymptomatic, so annual photographic screening is essential. The stages progress from background (requiring no specific treatment) through pre-proliferative to proliferative retinopathy in which retinal ischaemia has stimulated new vessel formation on the optic disc or in the periphery of the retina. New vessels are prone to tear leading to vitreous haemorrhage. The fibrous stalk carrying the new vessels can cause traction retinal detachment. Each scenario can cause blindness. Laser photocoagulation is an effective treatment for pre-proliferative and proliferative retinopathy.

Nephropathy

The earliest sign is microalbuminuria (albumin:creatinine ratio >3.5 mg/mmol). Angiotensin converting enzyme inhibitors (ACEI) are indicated at this stage to reduce the risk of progression. The next stage is overt proteinuria (Albustix® positive). Renal function deteriorates and blood pressure increases. Renal failure progresses to chronic kidney disease (CKD). Some may require dialysis or transplantation.

Neuropathy

The commonest presentation is with a symmetrical sensory polyneuropathy of the feet and legs; this confers a risk of foot ulceration. Less commonly there may be diabetic mononeuropathies and autonomic neuropathy that can cause postural hypotension, gastroparesis, diarrhoea and bladder dysfunction.

Cataract Formation

3–4 times more likely in those under the age of 60 years.

NON-PREGNANCY TREATMENT AND CARE

The aims of treatment are to prevent symptomatic hyper- and hypoglycaemia, and the development of complications. Treatment is with subcutaneous insulin injections. Although insulin preparations are of standard strength, they differ considerably in the rate of onset and duration of action. Patients may take 2–5 injections per day. Injections are given with disposable syringes and needles or with pen-injectors. Some patients use a continuous subcutaneous insulin infusion (CSII) (insulin pump).

The diabetic diet is designed to achieve and maintain a healthy weight. It is high in unrefined carbohydrate (60%) and low in fat (<30%).

Patients are encouraged to monitor their own capillary glucose concentrations to help them to achieve target values. Carbohydrate counting and appropriate adjustment of the insulin dose is the cornerstone of modern diabetes management. However, not all patients achieve ideal control. Routine care includes assessment of diabetic control by measuring HbA1c, physical examination for complications, retinal photography, screening urine for microalbumin and measurement of serum creatinine.

PRE-CONCEPTION ISSUES AND CARE

Pre-pregnancy counselling is essential because of the risks of miscarriage, congenital anomalies, IUGR, pre-eclampsia, macrosomia, polyhydramnios and IUFD. This should be part of routine diabetes care wherever this is provided, but women who are considering pregnancy should have access to a multi-disciplinary pregnancy preparation service.

The aim is a planned pregnancy with the woman taking high-dose folic acid (5 mg daily)[3] and having the best possible diabetic control at the time of conception[4]. Women with sub-optimal diabetic control (HbA1c >7%) should be encouraged to use contraception while efforts are made to improve control[1,2]. There should be a thorough assessment of complications, as retinopathy and nephropathy can deteriorate as a result of pregnancy, placing both mother and baby at risk.

Medication should be reviewed and where possible changed to agents that are safer in pregnancy. In particular ACEI should be stopped, and, where treatment for hypertension is required, methyldopa substituted. Insulin regimens may be intensified – twice daily injections with biphasic preparations are unlikely to allow sufficient flexibility of dose adjustment. Only *insulin aspart* (NovoRapid®) is licensed for use in pregnancy. Theoretical concerns about insulin glargine (Lantus®) and animal insulins mean that human isophane insulins or *insulin detemir* (Levemir®) are preferred as basal insulins[1] (though increasing evidence now supports insulin glargine use in pregnancy).

Pregnancy Issues

Booking:
- Dating/viability scan
- HbA1c
- Complication check and retinal examination
- Medication review
- Blood glucose monitoring strategy
- Dietetic review
- *Potential issues*
  - miscarriage*
  - hypoglycaemia
  - hyperemesis gravidarum
  - Down's risk assessment (nuchal thickness and amniocentesis)

Week 20:
- Detailed ultrasound scan
- *Potential issues*
  - congenital malformation*

Weeks 28, 32, 36:
- Growth scans
- *Potential issues*
  - IUGR*
  - macrosomia*
  - polyhydramnios*
  - premature labour
  - pre-eclampsia

Week 35 onwards:
- Plan mode and timing of delivery
- Plan insulin management during labour and postpartum
- *Potential issues*
  - unexplained fetal death*
  - *Outcomes influenced by diabetic control*

Medical Management and Care
- Planned pregnancy – check if pre-pregnancy actions were carried out
- Unplanned pregnancy – start folic acid 5 mg daily[3], review insulin regimen and alter if necessary, and undertake pre-pregnancy actions
- Arrange retinal screening and, if retinopathy detected, arrange regular ophthalmological monitoring
- Advise about risk of hypoglycaemia (especially if vomiting is a problem); ensure the woman and her partner are equipped to treat hypoglycaemia – glucose tablets or drinks (GlucoGel®) and glucagon injection (GlucaGen®)
- Advise and assist the woman to achieve target blood glucose levels (<5 mmol/l pre-meals and <7 mmol/l two hours after meals)
- From 20–36 weeks of gestation maternal insulin resistance increases due to placental production of counter regulatory hormones, especially human placental lactogen; insulin dose will need to be increased to deal with this
- Delivery should be at term unless there is any concern about fetal growth or wellbeing or if the diabetic control has been suboptimal, in which case earlier delivery may be recommended

Midwifery Management and Care
- Immediate referral to combined diabetes–obstetric antenatal clinic
- Maintain regular contact with specialist team either by clinic attendance or telephone every 1–2 weeks
- Ensure plan for delivery has been made in partnership with the woman and is clearly and accurately documented in the notes
- Advise woman to come to the unit if she becomes unwell or has concerns about fetal movements
- Offer parent-craft education including advice on the management of diabetes during delivery and postpartum

Labour Issues
- High-risk labour (not suitable for home delivery or birthing pool)
- Management of diabetes
- Monitoring fetal wellbeing – there is a risk of fetal distress
- Paediatricians should be available for delivery

Medical Management and Care
- Managed as per high-risk pregnancy
- Optimise blood glucose control at 4–7 mmol/l using intravenous insulin and D-glucose as per local guidelines (for suggested insulin regimen for labour see Appendix 7)
- Prevent maternal hyperglycaemia and neonatal hypoglycaemia
- Avoid maternal hypoglycaemia
- Prophylactic antibiotics for operative or instrumental delivery

Midwifery Management and Care
- Hourly measurement of maternal blood glucose
- Continuous EFM is indicated
- Anticipate shoulder dystopia (awareness of local obstetric protocols)
- Notify paediatricians once labour is established, and call for delivery

Postpartum Issues
- Neonatal hypoglycaemia
- Insulin regimen
- Breast-feeding
- Contraception advice

Medical Management and Care
- Insulin sensitivity increases promptly after delivery
- Stop insulin infusion once the woman has re-commenced eating
- Optimise maternal blood glucose levels, avoiding hypoglycaemia
- Adjust postpartum insulin doses according to blood glucose levels
- Breast-feeding typically reduces insulin requirements by 30%

Midwifery Management and Care
- Routine postnatal care appropriate for the type of delivery and observe for maternal hypoglycaemia
- Infants should be offered early feeding, observe baby closely for signs of hypoglycaemia (jitteriness)
- Neonatal blood glucose levels should be monitored as per local policy
- Breast-feeding should be actively encouraged[5]
- Not appropriate to have early six-hour discharge
- Information should be offered regarding future pregnancies, and pre-pregnancy care[5]
- A follow-up appointment should be made with the diabetes team

7.4 Type 2 Diabetes Mellitus

Incidence	Risk for Childbearing
Approximately 1:1000 pregnancies, but depends on ethnicity of the clinic population	High Risk

EXPLANATION OF CONDITION

Type 2 diabetes (T2DM) accounts for 80–85% of all diabetes mellitus. The prevalence of T2DM is rising worldwide, but the rate of rise is fastest in developing countries. It usually presents in middle age or later life, but along with the global epidemic there is a trend for earlier presentation, particularly in minority ethnic populations, so women with T2DM are becoming pregnant. Some of these women will have had gestational diabetes previously.

T2DM is characterised by two metabolic defects – insulin resistance and impaired insulin secretion. There is an inherited predisposition (polygenic) that can be unmasked by obesity and physical inactivity. Besides raised blood glucose, non-esterified fatty acid (NEFA) concentrations are raised. NEFA reduce the uptake of glucose by muscle, and stimulate gluconeogenesis in the liver.

Early in the disease patients respond to diet or oral hypoglycaemic agents, but many ultimately require insulin treatment. T2DM was commonly regarded as 'mild diabetes' because patients did not need to be treated with insulin to keep them alive, however the adjective is inappropriate because patients are at increased risk of cardiovascular mortality and morbidity.

COMPLICATIONS[4]

Microvascular Complications

Microvascular complications are caused by chronic hyperglycaemia and are preventable if patients can achieve near normal blood glucose concentrations for much of the time.

Macrovascular Disease

Macrovascular disease occurs because insulin resistance is part of the 'metabolic syndrome' (see Appendix 7), each component of which is a risk factor for cardiovascular disease. Consequently the management of T2DM is not just about controlling blood glucose concentrations: it encompasses the management of as many of these risk factors as possible.

Pregnancy Complications

- Miscarriage
- Congenital malformations
- IUGR
- Macrosomia
- Polyhydramnios
- IUFD

NON-PREGNANCY TREATMENT AND CARE

The aims of treatment are to prevent symptomatic hyper- and hypoglycaemia and the development of micro- and macrovascular complications.

Initially, lifestyle modification (increasing physical activity and reducing dietary energy consumption) that leads to weight reduction may improve glucose tolerance and control diabetes adequately.

With time it is often necessary to use oral antidiabetic agents. Metformin is the drug of choice for overweight patients and is increasingly used in polycystic ovarian syndrome (PCOS) to augment ovulation induction. Other agents include sulphonylureas (e.g. glibenclamide, gliclazide, glipizide) and thiazolidinediones (rosiglitazone and pioglitazone). If oral agents alone or in combination are ineffective then insulin injections are added or substituted, and management of this is as for T1DM.

Patients are often prescribed antihypertensives (especially ACEI), statins to lower cholesterol concentrations and aspirin as primary prophylaxis against cardiovascular events.

Routine care is as for T1DM (see Section 7.3).

PRE-CONCEPTION ISSUES AND CARE

Pre-pregnancy counselling is essential for all women of childbearing age with T2DM. This should be part of routine diabetes care wherever this is provided, but women who are considering pregnancy should have access to a multidisciplinary pregnancy preparation service. There is evidence to suggest that women with T2DM are more likely to be cared for in primary care and are less likely to receive pregnancy advice than women with T1DM. This is associated with worse outcomes[1,2].

The aim is the same as for women with T1DM.

Pre-pregnancy assessment is as for women with T1DM. Women with T2DM are likely to be overweight or obese and they should be actively encouraged to lose weight before conceiving if possible.

Pre-pregnancy medication review is very important. Women are likely to be taking potentially teratogenic drugs including statins and ACEI, which must be discontinued.

Oral antidiabetic/hypoglycaemic agents should be discontinued and treatment with insulin started as for T1DM. Increasing evidence indicates metformin is not teratogenic, and some clinicians advise women with PCOS who conceive whilst receiving it to continue to take it at ≥12 weeks.

Women with suboptimal diabetic control (HbA1c >7%) should be encouraged to use contraception while efforts are made to improve control[1,6].

Pregnancy Issues

Booking:
- Dating/viability scan
- HbA1c
- Complication check and retinal examination
- Medication review
- Blood glucose monitoring strategy
- Dietetic review
- *Potential issues*
  - miscarriage*
  - hypoglycaemia
  - hyperemesis gravidarum
  - Down's risk assessment (nuchal thickness and amniocentesis)

Week 20:
- Detailed ultrasound scan or fetal echocardiogram
- *Potential issues*
  - congenital malformation*

Weeks 28, 32, 36:
- Growth scans
- *Potential issues*
  - IUGR*, macrosomia*
  - polyhydramnios*
  - premature labour
  - pre-eclampsia[1,3]

Week 35 onwards:
- Plan mode and timing of delivery
- Plan insulin management during labour and postpartum
- *Potential issues*
  - unexplained fetal death*
  - * *Outcomes influenced by diabetic control*

Medical Management and Care

- Planned pregnancy – check if pre-pregnancy actions were carried out
- Unplanned pregnancy – start folic acid 5 mg daily[3], review insulin regimen and alter if necessary, and undertake pre-pregnancy actions
- Arrange retinal screening and, if retinopathy detected, arrange regular ophthalmological monitoring
- Advise about risk of hypoglycaemia (especially if vomiting is a problem); ensure the woman and her partner are equipped to treat hypoglycaemia – glucose tablets or drinks (Glucogel®) and glucagon injection (Glucagen®)
- Advise and assist the woman to achieve target blood glucose levels (<5 mmol/l pre-meals and <7 mmol/l two hours after meals)
- From 20–36 weeks gestation maternal insulin resistance increases due to placental production of counter-regulatory hormones, especially human placental lactogen; insulin may be required to compensate for this
- Delivery should be at term unless there is any concern about fetal growth or wellbeing or if the diabetic control has been suboptimal, in which case earlier delivery may be recommended

Midwifery Management and Care

- Immediate referral to combined diabetes–obstetric antenatal clinic
- Maintain regular contact with specialist team either by clinic attendance or telephone every 1–2 weeks
- Ensure plan for delivery has been made in partnership with the woman and is clearly and accurately documented in the notes
- Advise woman to come to the unit if she becomes unwell or has concerns about fetal movements
- Offer parent-craft education including advice on the management of diabetes during delivery and postpartum

Labour Issues
- High-risk labour (not suitable for home delivery or birthing pool)
- Management of diabetes
- Monitoring fetal wellbeing – there is a risk of fetal distress
- Paediatricians should be available for delivery

Medical Management and Care
- Managed as per high-risk pregnancy
- Optimise blood glucose control at 4–7 mmols/l using intravenous insulin and D-glucose as per local guidelines (for suggested insulin regimen for labour see Appendix 7)
- Prevent maternal hyperglycaemia and neonatal hypoglycaemia
- Avoid maternal hypoglycaemia
- Prophylactic antibiotics for operative or instrumental delivery

Midwifery Management and Care
- Hourly measurement of maternal blood glucose
- Continuous EFM is indicated
- Anticipate shoulder dystocia (awareness of local obstetric protocols)[4]
- Notify paediatricians once labour is established, and call for delivery

Postpartum Issues
- Neonatal hypoglycaemia
- Insulin regimen
- Breast-feeding
- Contraception advice

Medical Management and Care
- Insulin sensitivity increases promptly after delivery
- Stop insulin infusion once the woman has re-commenced eating
- Optimise maternal blood glucose levels, avoiding hypoglycaemia
- Adjust postpartum insulin doses according to blood glucose results
- Breast-feeding typically reduces insulin requirements by 30%

Midwifery Management and Care
- Routine care as appropriate for the type of delivery
- Observe baby closely for signs of hypoglycaemia (jitteriness)
- Monitor neonatal blood glucose levels as per local policy
- Breast-feeding should be actively encouraged[5]
- Oral antidiabetic agents should not be used until weaning
- Insulin treatment is preferred
- Information should be offered regarding contraception (suitable for oral contraceptives), future pregnancies and pre-pregnancy care[1]
- A follow-up appointment should be made with the diabetes team or local GP

7.5 Gestational Diabetes Mellitus

Incidence	Risk for Childbearing
2–3% of pregnancies (depending on definition used and on population studied)	High Risk

EXPLANATION OF CONDITION

Gestational diabetes (GDM) is glucose intolerance that is diagnosed during pregnancy. This may represent previously undiagnosed type 1 or type 2 diabetes, but the majority of cases are due to transient, pregnancy-induced glucose intolerance.

Pathophysiology

Glucose tolerance changes during normal pregnancy: fasting blood glucose concentration falls and postprandial glucose concentration rises up to 36 weeks gestation. From week 20 increasing levels of placental hormones, including human placental lactogen, are responsible for increasing maternal insulin resistance. If the woman has sufficient insulin secretory reserve, then the rise in plasma glucose is minor: if she has limited reserve, then glucose intolerance or diabetes may result.

Definition

There is no international agreement on the definition of GDM. In the US, the diagnostic test is a 100 g, three-hour oral glucose tolerance test (OGTT), whereas in Europe the 75 g, two-hour OGTT is used (see Appendix 7). The US definition relates to the risk of the woman developing diabetes after the index pregnancy – 50% within eight years.

The degree of glucose intolerance that is deemed to merit intervention is still being debated. Some would only treat biochemical diabetes, others impaired glucose tolerance and others somewhere in between, for example the Pregnancy Study Group of the European Association for the Study of Diabetes advocates intervening if the two-hour glucose >9 mmol/l.

The reason for the inconsistency is that although studies have shown that pregnancy outcomes in women with any degree of glucose intolerance are worse than in those with normal glucose tolerance[1], only one randomised controlled trial to date has demonstrated a beneficial effect of treatment[2]. A definitive answer is expected from the larger on-going international Hyperglycemia and Adverse Pregnancy Outcome (HAPO) trial funded by the National Institutes of Health.

Screening

Since nearly all women with GDM will be asymptomatic, it will be necessary to screen. The prevalence in the general maternity population is too low to justify universal screening. The National Institute for Clinical Excellence (NICE) Routine Antenatal Guidance 2003 states: 'The evidence does not support routine screening for gestational diabetes mellitus (GDM) and therefore it should not be offered.' However, it also states: *'Throughout the entire antenatal period, healthcare providers should remain alert to signs or symptoms of conditions which affect the health of the mother and fetus, such as . . . diabetes.'*

Selective screening of high-risk groups is justified[3]. Groups at high risk include women with:

- Previous gestational glucose intolerance
- Previous large baby (>4 kg)
- Previous unexplained stillbirth
- First degree relative with diabetes
- Maternal obesity >120% ideal body weight
- Polyhydramnios in current pregnancy

To these may be added non-white ethnic group and polycystic ovarian syndrome.

Glucosuria is a poor predictor of GDM and usually reflects hyperfiltration of pregnancy. However, glucosuria before 20 weeks is unusual and should not be ignored as it may indicate pre-existing undiagnosed diabetes.

A two-stage screening test is usual in the US. A 50 g oral glucose challenge is administered non-fasting at 24–28 weeks. If the venous plasma glucose measured after one hour is >7.8 mmol/l, an OGTT is performed. This reduces the number of GTT needed. Elsewhere, one-stage screening is with an OGTT alone.

COMPLICATIONS

Increased maternal glucose concentration leads to increased delivery of nutrients to the fetus, which stimulates fetal insulin production. The potential effects of diabetes on the fetus include:

- Polyhydramnios
- Macrosomia (risk of shoulder dystocia)
- Hepatomegaly
- Polycythaemia
- IUFD
- Hyaline membrane disease
- Neonatal hypoglycaemia

Since the onset of GDM is after 12 weeks, it does not confer an increased risk of congenital malformation or miscarriage.

TREATMENT AND CARE

Unless the woman has symptomatic hyperglycaemia it is usual to start by offering lifestyle advice and home blood glucose monitoring. Most women (80%) will be adequately controlled by diet and exercise. A dietetic assessment is essential. Women should be advised to eat regular meals, and to take 50% of their diet as unrefined carbohydrate. If they are overweight it is safe to aim for no further weight gain during the pregnancy, by modest energy restriction. Aerobic arm exercise has been shown to be an effective and safe adjunct.

The memory of the blood glucose meter should be interrogated at each clinic visit. Consistent failure to meet target blood glucose concentrations is an indication to start insulin treatment. Oral antidiabetic agents are not generally used, although glibenclamide (glyburide) has been claimed to be safe and effective.

Raised post-meal glucose values are best treated by short-acting analogues *insulin aspart* (NovoRapid®) or *insulin lispro* (Humalog®), while raised pre-meal values are treated with human isophane insulin or *insulin detemir* (Levemir®).

Pregnancy Issues

- Explanation of condition
- Dietetic advice
- Blood glucose monitoring instruction
- Dietetic review
- Review maternal blood glucose results: if consistently above target, commence insulin treatment and titrate dose until targets achieved

Weeks 28, 32, 36:
- Growth scans
- *Potential issues*
    - macrosomia*
    - polyhydramnios*
    - premature labour
    - pre-eclampsia
    - IUGR

Week 35 onwards:
- Plan mode and timing of delivery
- Plan insulin management during labour if necessary
- *Potential issues*
    - unexplained fetal death*
    Outcomes influenced by diabetic control

Medical Management and Care

- Advise and assist woman to achieve target blood glucose levels (<5 mmol/l before meals and <7 mmol/l two hours after meals)
- From 20–36 weeks gestation maternal insulin resistance increases, due to placental production of counter-regulatory hormones, especially human placental lactogen; insulin may be required to compensate for this
- Delivery should be at term unless there is any concern about fetal growth or wellbeing or if the diabetic control has been suboptimal, in which case earlier delivery may be recommended

Midwifery Management and Care

- Full explanation of GDM and the implications for pregnancy should be given
- Maintain regular contact with specialist team either by clinic attendance or telephone every 1–2 weeks to permit adjustment of treatment where necessary and to arrange regular ultrasound scans
- Ensure plan for delivery has been made in partnership with the woman and is clearly and accurately documented in the notes
- Advise the woman to come to the unit if she becomes unwell or has concerns about fetal movements
- Offer parent-craft education including advice on the management of diabetes during delivery and postpartum

Labour Issues

- High-risk labour (not suitable for home delivery or birthing pool)
- Management of diabetes
- Monitoring fetal wellbeing – there is a risk of fetal distress
- Paediatricians should be available for delivery

Medical Management and Care

- If insulin-treated, manage as per type 1 DM high-risk pregnancy
- Optimise blood glucose control using intravenous insulin and D-glucose as per local guidelines – as for type 1 and type 2 diabetes
- If on diet treatment alone, monitor blood glucose levels as per local guidance, no requirement for insulin therapy in labour if blood glucose levels are normal
- Prophylactic antibiotics for operative or instrumental delivery

Midwifery Management and Care

- In addition to routine labour care, take hourly measurements of maternal blood glucose, and adjust insulin as appropriate
- Continuous EFM is indicated
- Anticipate shoulder dystocia (consult local obstetric protocols)
- Notify paediatricians once labour is established, and call for delivery

Postpartum Issues

- Neonatal hypoglycaemia
- Assess glucose intolerance
- Encourage breast-feeding
- Lifestyle advice
- Contraceptive advice

Medical Management and Care

- Stop insulin immediately after delivery and monitor maternal blood glucose concentrations before meals for 24 hours
- If blood glucose >7 mmol/l seek advice from diabetes team
- Arrange repeat glucose tolerance test at six weeks postpartum
- Classify glucose tolerance according to result and manage accordingly

Midwifery Management and Care

- Observe baby closely for signs of hypoglycaemia (jitteriness)
- Neonatal blood glucose levels should be monitored as per local policy
- Breast-feeding should be actively encouraged
- Ensure understanding of increased risk of type 2 diabetes and advise about lifestyle modifications to minimise that risk. Educate about symptoms of diabetes and recommend an annual test of glucose tolerance
- Advise that the woman should have an oral GTT before she conceives again, and during every subsequent pregnancy to screen for type 2 diabetes mellitus

7.6 Addison's Disease (Adrenal Insufficiency)

Incidence	Risk for Childbearing
Rare <1:1000	High Risk

EXPLANATION OF CONDITION

Adrenal insufficiency is the deficiency of gluco- and mineralocorticosteroids produced by the cortex of the adrenal glands[1]. This may be primary (damage to the glands) or secondary, due to the lack of pituitary adrenocorticotrophic hormone (ACTH).

Addison's disease refers to primary adrenal insufficiency. Of all cases, 70–90% are due to autoimmune destruction of the adrenal cortex (either alone or associated with other organ-specific autoimmune conditions, e.g. type 1 diabetes, autoimmune thyroid disease). Of the remainder, most cases are due to tuberculosis. Autoantibodies to the enzyme 21-hydroxylase are often present in autoimmune Addison's disease.

Symptoms

Symptoms include:

- Anorexia
- Nausea
- Vomiting
- Weight loss
- Weakness
- Lassitude
- Syncope
- Hyperpigmentation (not in secondary adrenal insufficiency)
- The patient may be hypotensive or have postural hypotension

Diagnosis

Biochemical changes include:

- Low serum sodium
- Raised potassium
- Hypoglycaemia

but they may be absent. A low plasma cortisol concentration at 9 am supports the diagnosis.

A paired ACTH measurement is needed to differentiate primary (ACTH raised) from secondary (ACTH low) cases. If the morning plasma cortisol is borderline, the ability of the adrenal cortex to respond to synthetic ACTH (tetracosactrin) is tested by measuring plasma cortisol before and 30 minutes after an intramuscular injection of synthetic ACTH – the 'short Synacthen® test'. The incremental rise in plasma cortisol is subnormal in Addison's disease[1].

COMPLICATIONS

Acute Adrenal Crisis (Addisonian Crisis)

This is a medical emergency in which a patient with primary adrenal insufficiency suffers a stressful event such as an intercurrent infection or trauma. The normal physiological increase in corticosteroid secretion cannot occur. The patient presents in hypovolaemic shock with features of the precipitating event.

Pregnancy Complications

- IUGR – if undiagnosed
- Hypovolaemic shock – following labour

NON-PREGNANCY TREATMENT AND CARE

Patients are treated with oral corticosteroids for life. Typically glucocorticoid replacement is with hydrocortisone 20–30 mg daily, given as 2–3 doses. The adequacy of the dose is assessed by patient wellbeing, supplemented by measurement of 24-hour urinary free cortisol excretion (which should be in the reference range) and possibly plasma cortisol profiles measured as a day case. It is important to avoid chronic over replacement in order to avoid osteoporosis and other features of Cushing's syndrome. Patients should increase their dose to cover intercurrent illness, and carry medical alert information about their diagnosis and treatment. They should seek urgent medical help if vomiting and unable to absorb oral steroids.

The stress of elective or emergency surgery is covered by the administration of intramuscular hydrocortisone in high doses tapering to normal over several days.

Mineralocorticoid replacement is also required in patients with primary adrenal insufficiency: 9α-fluorohydrocortisone (fludrocortisone) is given at a dose of 50–200 micrograms once daily. This should abolish postural hypotension and correct electrolyte abnormalities. Excessive doses may cause hypertension and hypokalaemia.

PRE-CONCEPTION ISSUES AND CARE

There should be no adverse effects on pregnancy of treated adrenal insufficiency. It is important to check that the woman is adequately but not excessively replaced with steroids as above. She should be advised to carry a steroid card and medical alert bracelet or tag with her at all times.

Although there is no need to increase the steroid doses routinely in pregnancy, the woman should be aware that she should seek medical advice in the event of vomiting in early pregnancy that prevents her absorbing oral steroids[2]. She should also be counselled about the need *to cover* labour and the puerperium with higher doses of steroids[2].

Pregnancy Issues

No changes in regular treatment required

Special circumstances:
- Hyperemesis
- Intercurrent illness
- Risk of Addisonian crisis

Medical Management and Care
- Hyperemesis may result in insufficient oral steroid being absorbed by women with treated adrenal insufficiency
- Admission for parenteral steroid administration may be necessary
- Undiagnosed Addison's disease should be suspected in women with persistent nausea and vomiting beyond 20 weeks gestation, especially if this is associated with fatigue and weight loss

Midwifery Management and Care
- High-risk pregnancy – shared care with community and obstetric teams
- Women with intercurrent illness during pregnancy should be reminded to increase their corticosteroid dose exactly as they would do normally
- Promote correct administration of medication
- Immediate admission for signs of adrenal crisis, e.g. nausea and vomiting, profound epigastric pain or hypotension

Labour Issues
- Increased corticosteroid requirement for labour and delivery
- Intravenous fluids to prevent hypovolaemia

Medical Management and Care

Suggested labour regimen:
- Hydrocortisone: 100 mg 6-hourly im

Midwifery Management and Care
- This is a high-risk labour, managed by the obstetricians although the midwife should be able to deliver the baby if the labour itself progresses normally
- Continuous EFM is required
- Hourly blood pressure monitoring
- Care of the IVI and strict recording of fluid balance
- Send for immediate medical assistance for signs of adrenal crisis, e.g. nausea, vomiting, profound epigastric pain or hypotension
- Be aware that epidural anaesthesia may mask epigastric pain
- Promote correct administration of steroids
- Ensure that appropriate pharmacological therapy is available for an adrenal crisis[2]

Postpartum Issues
The physiological diuresis of the puerperium may cause significant hypotension.

Medical Management and Care
- Steroid dose should be tapered gradually over 6 days to cover the physiological diuresis in the puerperium
- *Suggested labour regimen:*
  - Day 1: Hydrocortisone 100 mg 6-hourly intramuscularly
  - Day 2: Hydrocortisone 50 mg 6-hourly intramuscularly
  - Day 3: Hydrocortisone 40 mg morning, 20 mg evening orally
  - Days 4 and 5: Hydrocortisone 30 mg morning, 15 mg evening orally
  - Day 6: Usual maintenance dose
- Ensure the woman is taking her maintenance dose of steroids on discharge

Midwifery Management and Care
- Routine care appropriate for type of delivery
- This mother is not suitable for early discharge from hospital
- Continue to monitor blood pressure and observe for signs of adrenal crisis
- Breast-feeding is considered safe and should be actively encouraged[2]

7.7 Prolactinoma

Incidence	**Risk for Childbearing**
Rare <1:1000	High Risk

EXPLANATION OF CONDITION

Prolactinomas are the commonest hormone-secreting pituitary adenomas and the only ones likely to be encountered in routine obstetric practice. They arise from the monoclonal proliferation of a lactotroph cell in the anterior pituitary gland. These cells synthesise and secrete prolactin (PRL), the hormone that promotes lactation. Of these adenomas, 90% are microadenomas (<10 mm diameter) and 10% are macroadenomas (≥10 mm). Microadenomas may regress spontaneously and do not usually grow significantly, with very few enlarging to become macroadenomas. Macroadenomas are more likely to expand[1].

The clinical features are due to hyperprolactinaemia and the space-occupying effects of the tumour. Hyperprolactinaemia causes secondary amenorrhoea and infertility; it inhibits pulsatile GnRH (gonadotropin releasing hormone) release which results in anovulation and low oestrogen levels. Raised PRL levels can also cause galactorrhoea.

Serum prolactin is always raised: in general higher levels are seen with macroprolactinomas. It is important to exclude other causes of hyperprolactinaemia (pregnancy, untreated hypothyroidism, antipsychotic and antiemetic drugs) before imaging the pituitary with MRI.

COMPLICATIONS

If the prolactinoma is large enough, it may compress the surrounding normal pituitary cells, causing partial or complete hypopituitarism, with deficiencies of growth hormone (GH), adrenocorticotrophic hormone (ACTH), leading to hypocortisolaemia, and thyroid stimulating hormone (TSH), leading to hypothyroidism.

Large macroadenomas may cause pressure symptoms with headache, and, if optic chiasmal compression occurs, visual field defects, usually bitemporal hemianopia. Further expansion beyond the pituitary fossa may cause diplopia due to involvement of cranial nerves III, IV and VI.

NON-PREGNANCY TREATMENT AND CARE

Microprolactinoma

Medical treatment with a dopamine (DA) agonist is almost always successful in restoring normal prolactin concentration and stopping galactorrhoea. Bromocriptine was the first drug to be used. Cabergoline and quinagolide are alternatives. Bromocriptine is cheapest, but has to be taken 2–3 times daily, is less well tolerated and marginally less effective than cabergoline. Cabergoline is taken once or twice a week.

All have side effects:

- Nausea
- Vomiting
- Constipation
- Postural hypotension
- Nasal congestion
- Raynaud's phenomenon

Women must be warned about these effects. Compliance is helped by starting with a low dose and slowly increasing. Long-term use has been associated with pulmonary, pericardial and retroperitoneal fibrosis.

Since 10–20% microprolactinomas remit after medical treatment, it is reasonable to withdraw medication every 2–3 years to see whether it is still required.

Trans-sphenoidal surgery to remove the adenoma is reserved for women who cannot tolerate, or who do not respond to, DA agonists. It is as effective as medical treatment, but carries greater risks, including a degree of hypopituitarism.

Macroprolactinoma

First-line treatment, even with the largest adenomas, is with DA agonists. These induce falls in prolactin concentrations within 24 hours and tumour shrinkage within weeks. These improvements continue with duration of treatment. The visual field defects usually recede, and PRL concentrations return to normal in 58% of cases. Rapid shrinkage may result in a leak of cerebrospinal fluid from the nose (CSF rhinorrhoea).

If tumours do not shrink as expected, trans-sphenoidal surgery to debulk the tumour mass in the sella followed by radiotherapy is recommended.

PRE-CONCEPTION ISSUES AND CARE

There is a risk of amenorrhoea and infertility.

Safety of DA Agonists

There is no evidence of increased rates of spontaneous abortion, ectopic pregnancy or teratogenicity with bromocriptine therapy. There is much less experience with cabergoline, which is therefore not first choice agent for women wishing to conceive. Women receiving DA agonists should be advised to use barrier methods of contraception for the first few menstrual cycles, which may be irregular, to facilitate accurate dating of pregnancy.

Risk of tumour expansion

As oestrogen levels rise in pregnancy they stimulate the growth of lactotrophs that, in normal women, cause the pituitary gradually to double its size: prolactinomas may also grow. The risk of clinically significant expansion of microprolactinomas is very low, compared with 20% of macroprolactinomas. Women with microprolactinomas should be advised to stop taking the DA agonist as soon as pregnancy is confirmed.

The management of macroprolactinoma depends on the size of the tumour. If it is confined to the sella, the DA agonist can be stopped after conception. In women with larger macroadenomas, options to be considered before making an individualised plan include:

- Trial withdrawal of DA agonist
- Continuing bromocriptine throughout pregnancy
- Pre-pregnancy trans-sphenoidal surgery to debulk the tumour

Pregnancy Issues
Monitor for symptoms and signs of tumour expansion.

Medical Management and Care
Since normal pregnancy is associated with increasing PRL concentrations, it is not possible to use PRL measurements to indicate prolactinoma enlargement.

Microprolactinomas
- Discontinue DA agonist
- Monitor clinically for symptoms and signs of tumour expansion
  - headache
  - visual symptoms
- Check visual fields clinically by direct confrontation

Macroprolactinomas
Decide whether to continue with DA agonist. Monitor clinically for symptoms and signs of tumour expansion as for microprolactinoma. In addition perform monthly visual perimetry to detect early signs of optic chiasmal compression. Serial MRI scanning is not recommended in view of a lack of proof of its safety in pregnancy.

If there is a suggestion of tumour expansion, this should be confirmed with an urgent MRI scan and bromocriptine started immediately. The subsequent management involves endocrinologist, obstetrician and neurosurgeon. Lack of response to bromocriptine is a neurosurgical emergency.

Early delivery may be indicated according to the gestational age.

Midwifery Management and Care
- Accurate booking history, noting any past treatments/surgery and current medication
- Care shared with community midwife and medical obstetric team
- Routinely ask about headaches and visual symptoms
- Refer to specialist unit if indicated

Labour Issues
No particular issues except if a woman is known to have an expanding macroprolactinoma.

Medical Management and Care
If the woman has an expanding tumour, she will need to be prepared for elective forceps delivery to avoid a rise in intracranial pressure during labour.

Midwifery Management and Care
- Routine shared care, unless expanding tumour as above or any other underlying obstetric or medical complications
- Be prepared for induction of labour before 38 weeks and prepare for a pre-term delivery

Postpartum Issues

Breast-feeding
Suckling has no effect on PRL concentrations and there is no evidence that it causes tumour expansion. DA agonists should not be given while breast-feeding.

Contraception
Oestrogens in combined oral contraceptives might stimulate growth of prolactinomas.

Restarting medical treatment
In most cases there should be no immediate need to restart DA agonist treatment after delivery. It is reasonable to wait and see whether the original symptoms return and to measure serum PRL if they do.

Medical Management and Care
- Advise the woman to report a recurrence of her original symptoms
- Confirm hyperprolactinaemia before restarting medical treatment
- Note that PRL concentrations return to normal by three weeks postpartum in normal women
- Women with macroprolactinomas should have an MRI scan postpartum to estimate tumour size

Midwifery Management and Care
- Routine postnatal care appropriate for type of delivery
- Encourage breast-feeding provided the woman does not need to restart DA agonists
- Discuss contraceptive options; theoretical risk of oestrogen-containing oral contraceptives should be discussed

7 Endocrine Disorders

PATIENT ORGANISATIONS

British Thyroid Foundation
PO Box 97
Clifford
Wetherby
West Yorkshire LS23 6XD
www.btf-thyroid.org

Diabetes UK
10 Parkway
London NW1 7AA
www.diabetes.org.uk

The Addison's Disease Self Help Group
21 George Road
Guildford
Surrey GU1 4NP
www.adshg.org.uk

The Pituitary Foundation
PO Box 1944
Bristol BS99 2UB
www.pituitary.org.uk

ESSENTIAL READING

Billington, M. and Stevenson, M. (2007) **Critical Care in Childbearing for Midwives**, pp. 55–62. Blackwell Science, Oxford.

Girling, J.C. (2006) Thyroid disorders in pregnancy. **Current Obstetrics and Gynaecology**, **16**:47–53.

Maresh, M. (2002) Diabetes. In: de Swiet M (ed.) **Medical Disorders in Obstetric Practice**, 4th Edn, pp. 386–414. Blackwell Science, Oxford.

Taylor, R. and Davison, J.M. (2007) Type 1 diabetes and pregnancy. **British Medical Journal**, **334**:742–745.

Turner, H.E. and Wass, J.A.H. (Eds) (2002a) **Oxford Handbook of Endocrinology and Diabetes**, **Part 1**, pp. 21–48 and 69–76. Oxford University Press, Oxford.

Turner, H.E. and Wass, J.A.H. (Eds) (2002b) **Oxford Handbook of Endocrinology and Diabetes, Part 1**, pp. 135–144 and 309–320. Oxford University Press, Oxford.

Wier, F.A. (2006) Clinical controversies in screening women for thyroid disease during pregnancy. **Journal of Midwifery and Women's Health**, **51**(3):152–158.

NEUROLOGICAL DISORDERS

8

Jo Matharu, Eleanor Burns-Kent and Edmund Howarth

8.1 Migraine and Headaches

Incidence	**Risk for Childbearing**
Most common neurological disease	Variable Risk – dependent on cause
Migraine affects 15% of females, 6% of males[1]	

EXPLANATION OF CONDITION

Headache is an extremely common neurological disorder, the most common type being 'tension' type headaches. These are thought to occur due to scalp muscle contraction resulting in a sensation of tightness in the head and pressure behind the eyes. Often related to stress, such headaches may be precipitated by noise, depression, fatigue and concentrated visual work. The diagnosis is made by reported symptoms with physical signs of tension in nuchal and scalp muscles.

Cluster Headaches

Cluster headaches usually appear rapidly, without an aura, and peak within ten minutes. Pain is usually non-pulsatile and unilateral and may be centred on one eye. Symptoms include lacrimation, oedema and rhinorrhoea with 60% of cases causing ptosis and miosis. Attacks usually last <1 hour and often occur in clusters of 1–3 every day.

Migraine

Migraine without aura (common migraine) is the typical type of migraine. There are usually no, or vague, prodromal visual symptoms, the headache is usually unilateral and pulsatile, lasting 6–24 hours and is often associated with nausea, vomiting, photophobia, phonophobia and malaise.

Migraines with aura (classical migraine) occur when patients undergo a prodromal phase of up to 48 hours. Symptoms include depression, irritability and yawning, difficulty concentrating, stiff neck and food craving. Other symptoms may include visual disturbances affecting one side of the visual field (scintillating scotoma, geometric patterns) and unilateral paraesthesia or numbness. Headache begins during the aura period or within an hour of the aura ceasing and manifests in the same way as migraine without aura.

Migraine headache is thought to be due to vasodilation of cerebral blood vessels and stimulation of cerebral nerves. The release of 5-hydroxytryptamine, a vasoactive substance, is known to rise at the onset of prodromal symptoms and fall during the headache.

Migraines may be induced in a minority of patients by:

- Stress
- Anxiety
- Head or neck trauma
- Dietary factors (particularly cheese, chocolate, alcohol and citrus fruits)
- Fatigue

Oral contraceptives and vasodilators may exacerbate migraines.

COMPLICATIONS

Migraine with aura is associated with a six-fold increase in the risk of stroke.

NON-PREGNANCY TREATMENT AND CARE

Headache

- Investigation to confirm the benign nature of the headaches
- Simple analgesia: paracetamol and/or an NSAID
- Avoid agents which may exacerbate headache, e.g. alcohol, nicotine
- Cluster headaches are primarily treated as migraine

Migraine

A detailed neurological examination should be performed to ensure accurate diagnosis. Hemiplegic, visual and hemisensory symptoms must be distinguished from thrombo-embolic transient ischaemic attacks (TIA). In addition:

- Patient to complete a diary to ascertain any triggers
- Discontinue oral contraceptives if appropriate
- Simple analgesia as a first-line treatment, with or without an anti-emetic
- Ergotamine tartrate (a vasoconstrictor) can be used during an attack. May be given po, pr or by subcutaneous injection
- Sumatriptan, a $5HT_1$ agonist is commonly used for acute attacks (oral, nasal spray or injection)
- Beta-blockers are used as prophylaxis
- Pizotifen, a serotonin agonist is used as prophylaxis
- Feverfew, a herbal remedy, may decrease the number of headaches experienced by a patient with a history of frequent migraines[2]

PRE-CONCEPTION ISSUES AND CARE

Women should be accurately counselled regarding the risks and benefits of continuing any medication prescribed or bought over the counter.

Pregnancy Issues

Migraine and headache account for 33% of neurological problems in pregnancy[2]. Headaches may occur due to eye strain, fatigue, emotional changes and sinusitis or be a continuing chronic problem[3]. Tension headaches do not usually improve in pregnancy[4].

Of women with pre-existing classical migraine, 50–90% will improve during pregnancy[3]. However some women will develop migraine for the first time in pregnancy[5].

Differential diagnosis includes:
- Sub-arachnoid haemorrhage
- Meningitis
- Encephalitis
- Cerebral vein thrombosis
- Benign intracranial hypertension
- Pre-eclampsia
- Intracranial mass lesions

Ergotamine[6] and feverfew (which contain ergot alkaloids) should be avoided throughout pregnancy.

NSAIDs have been associated with increased risk of first trimester miscarriage. In the third trimester they have been associated with increased risk of neonatal intracranial haemorrhage, an effect on fetal/neonatal renal function and the theoretical risk of premature closure of the ductus ateriosus[6]. As such they should only be used under specialist supervision.

Medical Management and Care
- Careful diagnosis, history taking and neurological examination
- Prolonged neurological signs and symptoms for >12 hours require further investigation
- Simple analgesia; avoid NSAIDs in the first and third trimesters
- Avoid ergotamine
- Consider prophylaxis if attacks are frequent or long lasting; aspirin 75 mg once daily is safe and effective[3]
- Consider beta-blockers; note that use of these in pregnancy has been associated with IUGR (see Appendix 4.3)
- If beta-blockers and aspirin are ineffective consider tricyclic anti-depressants (25–50 mg amitriptyline)
- Consider anti-emetics if presentation of nausea and vomiting; metoclopramide decreases gastric atony and increases absorption of other administered medications[7]

Midwifery Management and Care
- Advise about hydration – pregnant women should drink four litres of water per day
- Advise reduction in tea and coffee consumption and avoidance of any known triggers
- Encourage use of relaxation techniques
- Careful history taking with women presenting with symptoms
- Ensure physical observations noted to exclude other diagnosis
- Women who present with headaches in late second and third trimester should be screened for pre-eclampsia (blood pressure measurement and urinalysis) and referred for urgent medical assessment if necessary (see Section 3.2)

Labour Issues

Triggers such as stress, pain and starvation can induce headache or a migraine attack.

Medical Management and Care
- As above

Midwifery Management and Care
- Condition may cause anxiety about labour and analgesia; discuss and refer to anaesthetic team if necessary
- Encourage normal diet and adequate hydration
- Utilise relaxation techniques

Postpartum Issues
- Differential diagnosis – migraine and headache may be confused with post-dural puncture headache
- Migraine often recurs in the postpartum period[7]

Medical Management and Care
- Careful examination and history taking; post-dural headache will usually improve when the mother is lying prone
- Women with classical migraine should not take oestrogen-containing oral contraceptives
- Consider pre-pregnancy treatment, ensuring no contraindication if breast-feeding

Midwifery Management and Care
- Carefully history taking
- Referral to medical team if necessary
- Advise regarding rest, hydration and relaxation

8.2 Epilepsy

Incidence	Risk for Childbearing
General population 4–10:1000[1]	Variable Risk – depending on nature of epilepsy and seizure control
Affects 0.6–1% of pregnant women[2]	

EXPLANATION OF CONDITION

Epilepsy is a disorder of brain function characterised by sudden onset, recurrent seizures[3]. The temporary physiological brain dysfunction is caused by an abnormal electrical discharge of cortical neurons. During a seizure, groups of neurons are activated repeatedly and hypersynchronously. A failure of the inhibitory synaptic contact between the neurons causes high voltage spike and wave activity on an electroencephalogram (EEG).

Epilepsy can be broadly classified into two categories, partial and generalised seizures.

Partial Seizures

Partial seizures originate from either the frontal or temporal lobe of the brain. They may or may not be associated with loss of consciousness and may extend to become generalised seizures. Many patients with partial seizures experience a warning 'aura'[4].

Generalised Seizures

Generalised seizures involve both hemispheres of the cerebral cortex and are further classified:

- **Absence seizures** (*petit mal*) usually last <20 seconds and seizures are often a disorder of childhood, that manifest as brief episodes of impaired consciousness with no aura or post-ictal confusion
- **Myoclonic seizures** consist of brief, jerking, arrhythmic motor movements
- **Tonic–clonic seizures** (*grand mal*) typically follow a warning and consist of sudden, rigid, tonic extension or flexion of limbs, head and/or torso lasting up to a minute followed by convulsions consisting of rhythmic motor jerking movements, with or without impaired consciousness, lasting a few seconds to a few minutes
- **Atonic seizures** occur in epileptic patients with serious neurological abnormalities and consist of loss of tone and generalised *floppiness*

COMPLICATIONS

- **Status epilepticus** – a medical emergency that occurs when a patient experiences repeated seizures without any recovery of consciousness between them
- **Trauma** occurring at the time of the convulsion, including tongue biting, head trauma, hot water burns, etc.; patients with epilepsy should be counselled regarding precautions and how to minimise harm
- **Cardiorespiratory failure** arising from *status epilepticus* where treatment was delayed
- **Sudden adult death** – phenomenon whereby patient with epilepsy dies suddenly and no anatomic or toxicological cause of death is revealed[5]

NON-PREGNANCY TREATMENT AND CARE

The aim of treatment is to achieve optimum, seizure-free status without adverse effects. Anti-epileptic drugs (AEDs) are generally recommended for all patients having experienced more than one seizure.

As in pregnancy, monotherapy carries less risk than polytherapy and careful monitoring of patients is required to balance efficacy with long-term side effects of AED (see Appendix 8.1 for drug therapy).

PRE-CONCEPTION ISSUES AND CARE

- Women considering pregnancy should seek pre-conceptual advice from an appropriately experienced health care professional
- Women should be counselled regarding their current treatment, the risk of major malformations in the fetus and the use of folic acid[6]
- Women with epilepsy and particularly those taking AEDs are at increased risk of folate deficiency and neural tube defects[7,8], and should be prescribed folic acid 5 mg per day before conception and up to 12 weeks gestation[9]
- Pregnancy should be deferred until seizure control is optimal. Women who have been seizure free for a minimum of two years may consider withdrawing AEDs. This should be planned well before conception and implications for driving and risk of seizure recurrence should be explored
- Women who require AEDs to maintain seizure control should be treated with the lowest dose of the lowest number of drugs. Polytherapy increases the risk of major congenital malformations (MCMs)[1]
- Sodium valproate is associated with an increased risk of MCM and fetal valproate syndrome. Wherever possible, alternative AEDs should be utilised in order to maximise seizure control whilst minimising risks to the fetus and long-term sequelae for the neonate and child. Carbamazepine is associated with the lowest risk of MCM, when used as monotherapy[1] (see Appendix 8.1)
- Women must be fully informed and involved in the decision making process regarding the use/change of AEDs. An awareness of the side effects of AEDs for the patient, risk of abnormality in the fetus, importance and necessity of seizure control and the social and psychological impacts of balancing these issues should be paramount

Pregnancy Issues

- Of women with epilepsy, 25–30% will see an increase in the frequency of seizures in pregnancy; 54% will see no change[9]
- Seizures may increase as a result of:
  - poor or non-compliance with medication
  - decreased drug levels due to nausea and vomiting
  - decreased gastrointestinal absorption and increased hepatic and renal clearance resulting in insufficient drug levels
  - lack of sleep[10]
- The greater the frequency of seizures before pre-conception the more likely they are to increase in frequency in pregnancy
- Gestational epilepsy has been described[11], however its existence as a separate entity is not universally acknowledged
- Frequent *grand mal* seizures may result in fetal hypoxia and consequently IUGR; partial seizures do not have the same effect
- Epilepsy accounted for 8.4% of indirect deaths reported in the 2004 confidential enquiry into maternal deaths[12]
- All AEDs cross the placenta with varying rates of teratogenicity
- AEDs interfere with folate metabolism, which results in increased risk of neural tube defects (NTDs)
- Major congenital malformations (MCMs) occur in <5% of fetuses of women taking AEDs during pregnancy[1]
- Polytherapy regimes increase the risk of MCM therefore monotherapy is suggested wherever possible
- Sodium valproate is associated with an increased risk of MCM; carbamazepine is associated with the lowest risk[1]
- The effects of newer AEDs, such as lamotrigine, topiramate and others, remain the subject of investigation; current data does not suggest an increase in risk over the more traditional AEDs[13]
- 95% of mothers taking AEDs during pregnancy will deliver normal healthy babies[1]

Medical Management and Care

- Prescribe 5 mg per day folic acid early in first trimester if not commenced pre-conceptually
- Women taking sodium valproate should continue with 5 mg per day folic acid for the remainder of the pregnancy
- All women with epilepsy should have detailed fetal ultrasound performed at 18–22 weeks to screen for anomalies
- Women should be advised to have serum screening with AFP for neural tube defects
- Women taking enzyme inducing AEDs should receive vitamin K 10 mg per day from 36 weeks gestation until delivery or for four weeks prior to delivery[14]; these AEDs include:
  - carbamazepine
  - phenytoin
  - phenobarbitone
  - primidone
  - topiramate
  - oxcarbazepine
- Women taking AEDs should be treated with a single AED wherever possible. If this is inefficient at maintaining seizure control then consider alternative monotherapy. Polytherapy should only be considered when monotherapy has been unsuccessful (see Appendix 8.1 for review of AEDs).
- Encourage British women to register with UK Epilepsy and Pregnancy Register to contribute to greater understanding of epilepsy and AED use in pregnancy

Management of status epilepticus

- Senior obstetric and anaesthetic staff to be present
- Maintain airway
- Oxygen therapy
- Ensure safe environment to maintain safety of patient
- Prolonged seizures should be treated with iv lorazepam 4 mg
- Lorazepam has been shown to be less sedative and longer acting than diazepam[15]
- Investigations – FBC, U&E and consider AED levels
- Consider alternative causes
- Seek advice from neurologist if lorazepam is not effective
- Consider iv phenytoin with continuous EEG monitoring
- If phenytoin is not successful then paralyse and sedate the woman and ventilate mechanically
- Consider delivery of the fetus at this point

Midwifery Management and Care

- Take detailed booking history and refer for early assessment at a consultant-led unit
- Antenatal care should be provided by a multi-disciplinary team consisting of obstetrician, neurologist and midwife
- Advise against hot baths and steamy environments
- Ascertain expectations, and discourage from unrealistic schemes, such as water-birth
- Advise regarding importance of compliance with medication regimen
- Refer to medical staff if increase, or onset, of seizures occurs

Labour Issues

Risk of seizures increases around the time of delivery.

- Of pregnant women with epilepsy, 1–2% will have a seizure in labour
- Hyperventilation, exhaustion and dehydration can induce a seizure
- Prolonged or repeated seizures can cause fetal hypoxia
- *Status epilepticus* is a medical emergency (see above)
- Pethidine is metabolised to norpethidine and may induce a seizure; its use should be avoided in labour[16]

Medical Management and Care

- Continue normal AED regime[6]
- Serial or prolonged seizures should be treated with iv lorazepam 4 mg
- *Status epilepticus* necessitates input from obstetric and anaesthetic teams

Midwifery Management and Care

- All women with epilepsy should deliver in a consultant-led obstetric unit[9]
- Use of the birthing pool is contraindicated on safety grounds
- Ensure compliance and continuation of prescribed AEDs
- Limit stress due to pain and anxiety, consider appropriate pain relief and ensure adequate hydration
- Continuous EFM is not essential for women with epilepsy who are seizure-free during labour
- One-to-one care should be provided
- Women with epilepsy should not be left alone in labour
- Adhere to unit policy for the management of epilepsy

Postpartum Issues

- During the first 24 hours postpartum there is an additional 1–2% risk of *grand mal* seizures
- Physiological changes that occurred in pregnancy are reversed, which may lead to an increase in AED levels[17]
- AEDs have been shown to interfere with vitamin K metabolism in the newborn and may lead to haemorrhagic disease
- Sedation, poor feeding, hypotonia and respiratory distress are occasionally seen in the neonate with increased AED levels
- New onset seizures require investigation to rule out other causes (e.g. eclampsia, infection, intracerebral haemorrhage)

Medical Management and Care

- Review AED regime and levels; consider return to pre-pregnancy dosage if increased in pregnancy
- Ensure appropriate contraception prescribed; enzyme inducing AEDs decrease the efficacy of COCP and POP

Midwifery Management and Care

- All neonates should receive 1 mg vitamin K intramuscularly post delivery[13]
- Women should be encouraged to breast-feed. AEDs are secreted in breast milk but the dose received is less than the therapeutic level for neonates and less than that received *in utero*
- Women receiving lamotrigine should be advised of an association with a severe neonatal necrolysing skin rash and warned to discontinue breast-feeding if a reaction occurs[17]
- Advise women how to minimise risks when caring for the baby in case of seizure[18] (see Appendix 8.2)
- Observe neonate closely, report any concerns to paediatric staff promptly
- If the neonate is drowsy or needing to be roused for feeds consider feeding prior to the administration of AEDs[9]

8.3 Cerebrovascular Disease and Stroke

Incidence	Risk for Childbearing
Sub-arachnoid haemorrhage: 1–5:100,000 pregnancies[1] Cerebral vein thrombosis: 1:2500[2]–10:10,000 deliveries[3]	High Risk

EXPLANATION OF CONDITION

Cerebrovascular accidents (CVA), also known as **strokes**, are the result of cerebral infarction and are the most common brain disorder in the general population[4]. They occur when the flow of blood carrying essential oxygen to the brain is disrupted, causing brain cells to die[5].

Stroke is divided into 3 categories:

1. **Ischaemic:** from decreased blood flow as a result of vascular occlusion by embolism or atherosclerosis[4] within an artery
2. **Thrombotic:** a venous event
3. **Haemorrhagic** (sub-arachnoid haemorrhage [SAH]) due to a ruptured blood vessel in the brain

With CVA there can be an abrupt onset of neurological symptoms that vary in severity due to the location and extent of the damage caused. They range from mild strokes, where recovery occurs within 24 hours, to severe brain damage or death[5]. In the case of a small CVA the body has the ability for neurons near to the damaged area to sprout new dendrites, make new synaptic connections and take over some of the functions of the lost neurons[4], thereby reducing the patient's physical neurological symptoms.

Risk Factors

- **Ischaemic stroke:**
  - hypertension
  - hypercholesterolaemia
  - heart disease
  - previous transient ischaemic attacks
  - diabetes
  - smoking
  - obesity
  - excessive alcohol intake[4]
- **Thrombotic stroke:**
  - thrombophilias
  - dehydration
  - infection[6,7]
  - smoking
  - in pregnancy, operative delivery
- **Haemorrhagic stroke** may be associated with hypertension and the use of vasoactive drugs such as amphetamines and cocaine

Whilst history and risk factors may give guidance as to which type of CVA has occurred, there is considerable symptom overlap and appropriate imaging is essential. For example, cerebral vein thrombosis (CVT) may have an insidious symptom onset with headache followed by impairment of consciousness, and SAH classically presents with a 'bursting' headache, vomiting, hypertension and progressive loss of consciousness[1], but neither history is conclusive.

COMPLICATIONS

Ischaemia resulting from a CVA is a major cause of permanent disability and death[7]. Permanent neurological disability may be experienced as:

- Dizziness
- Weakness
- Numbness
- Paralysis in a limb or a side of the body
- Headache
- Slurred speech
- Difficulty understanding speech
- Partial loss of vision
- Nausea and vomiting[4]

NON-PREGNANCY TREATMENT AND CARE

If a SAH is left untreated, half of all patients will die[7]. The aim in treating CVAs is the prevention of neurological complications and death. Urgent investigation is appropriate.

Blood/urine toxicology would be beneficial to rule out substance misuse. Cerebrospinal fluid (CSF) examination is beneficial if an infection is suspected[6], and for the presence of blood if a SAH is suspected[7]. If cardiac origin is suspected, an ECG and echocardiogram should be performed.

Ultimately, the management is dependent upon the precise type of CVA. Brain imaging is essential either by CT or MRI to determine the type of CVA.

The presence of significant haemorrhage is a contraindication to anticoagulation[1], whereas therapeutic anticoagulation is essential to prevent further episodes if thrombotic stroke is diagnosed.

Surgery may be necessary to remove the blood clot, or to repair a ruptured aneurysm, if there is a SAH.

PRE-CONCEPTION ISSUES AND CARE

Women who have had a stroke are unlikely to have a recurrence in pregnancy unless there is an underlying risk factor[8]. Those women who have had six or more pregnancies have an increased risk of all types of stroke[9].

Women who have previously had an **ischaemic stroke** will be receiving anti-platelet medication, most commonly aspirin, dipyridamole or clopidrogel. If receiving either of the latter two, then conversion to aspirin 75–300 mg per day prior to pregnancy would be recommended. Discontinuation of all anti-platelet medication would be unwise.

Thrombotic stroke is seen throughout gestations but is most commonly identified 3–30 days postpartum[1].

Although the exact cause is unknown, it is thought the profound coagulation changes occurring during a pregnancy and the puerperium may be a factor. If a woman has had a thrombotic stroke previously and is taking warfarin, consideration should be given to changing this to subcutaneous heparin prior to attempting conception.

Pregnancy does not appear to increase the incidence of **sub-arachnoid haemorrhage**, although the physiological changes occurring during pregnancy such as increased blood volume, stroke volume and cardiac output, as well as increased oestrogen levels resulting in vasodilatation of an already abnormal vessel, can precipitate this[7].

Pregnancy Issues

- Previous CVA
- At risk of CVA due to underlying risk factor (i.e. poorly controlled hypertension, thrombophilia, vasculitis)
- Development of CVA during pregnancy

Medical Management and Care

- The nature of previous CVA, persisting neurological disability and current treatment dictate care during pregnancy
- If previous **ischaemic** stroke, then anti-platelet therapy in the form of aspirin 75–300 mg per day should be continued
- If previous **thrombotic** stroke, commence anticoagulation in the form of subcutaneous heparin as prophylaxis continued for at least six weeks postnatally
- If currently receiving warfarin, risk of warfarin embryopathy (6%) should be acknowledged, and request for termination of pregnancy respected
- If wishing to continue with pregnancy, subcutaneous heparin should be substituted for warfarin
- If no persisting vascular malformations, then pregnancy carries no specific care needs for women who have previously had a **sub-arachnoid haemorrhage**, although if this was in relation to substance misuse, then a urine toxicology screen to exclude persistent use of these recreational drugs should be considered
- The existence of pre-existing risk factors should alert clinicians to appropriate investigations should a woman present with relevant symptoms and signs
- Careful clinical assessment and documentation of neurological findings and relevant history and risk factors
  - early imaging is essential, and, where available MRI is the investigation of choice
  - CT scans may be performed providing appropriate abdominal shielding is used[1]
- Full anticoagulation is of benefit in the presence of cerebral vein thrombosis, but may cause bleeding into an ischaemic stroke and lead to its extension
- Once the acute treatment has been initiated, early physiotherapy and speech therapy are essential in maximising recovery

Midwifery Management and Care

- Appropriate referral for care is essential
- Women should be advised to continue their medications until medical review
- Persisting neurological disability should be recognised and appropriate arrangements for care should be in place and may include:
  - ensuring the availability of disabled parking at the maternity unit for appointments
  - advice regarding childcare
  - alerting the maternity unit to any special needs when admitted
- The existence of pre-existing risk factors should alert clinicians to appropriate investigations should a woman present with relevant symptoms and signs
- The risk of SAH with poorly controlled hypertension should be a particular concern
- Support, reassurance and basic nursing care are essential; these women may require help with toileting and pressure-area care
- Contribution to physiotherapy in the form of guided exercises under the direction of the physiotherapy services will aid recovery

Labour Issues	Medical Management and Care
1. Labour and delivery after SAH	1. Treatment of SAH by surgical or neuroradiological intervention should be undertaken initially; fetal outcome is dependent on maternal outcome[7]. After successful treatment, earlier authors recommended elective caesarean section; illogical in the absence of persisting arterial malformation, and labour and vaginal delivery pose no additional risk to mother and baby[10]
2. Labour and delivery after CVT	2. If receiving low-molecular-weight subcutaneous heparin prophylactically, then this should be discontinued on the day of delivery to permit use of regional anaesthesia if required. Prophylactic heparin does not contribute to excessive blood loss at delivery. Adequate hydration and mobilisation, along with TED stockings are important
3. Labour and delivery after ischaemic stroke	3. Should be treated as normal. If taking clopidrogel, then this needs to be discontinued at least a week before labour if regional anaesthesia is anticipated

Midwifery Management and Care

General DVT prevention is essential, therefore ensure:

- TED stockings are worn
- The mother is well hydrated and well mobilised
- Regular maternal observations are taken
- Supportive care related to any neurological disability is undertaken
- See also Section 15.1

Postpartum Issues	Medical Management and Care
- Thrombo-embolic risk - Persisting disability and childcare	- An assessment of risk should be made on all women undergoing LSCS and prophylaxis instituted as appropriate[11] - Women who have had a CVT and/or persisting limited mobility require anticoagulation for at least six weeks postpartum - Continued involvement with physiotherapy, occupational therapy and speech therapy services may be required to assist the woman in providing care for her baby

Midwifery Management and Care

- As per medical entry
- Women with persisting disability may require additional help in achieving breast-feeding
- Collaborative working with other services will help to ensure that the woman has a safe, supportive setting in which to care for her child as independently as possible

8.4 Other Neuropathies

Incidence	Risk for Childbearing
Bell's Palsy: 50:100,000 pregnancies[1]; 17: 100,000 general population[1] Carpal Tunnel Syndrome: 20–25% of pregnancies[2]	Low Risk

EXPLANATION OF CONDITION

Bell's Palsy

Bell's palsy results from inflammation or compression of the cranial nerve VII within the temporal bone, which causes unilateral facial weakness. It is often discovered in the morning. Sense of taste may be diminished over the anterior two thirds of the tongue as well as an inability to close the eye on the affected side, even during sleep. Hyperacusis is common as is pain in and around the ear. The underlying cause is not known, although occurrence in late pregnancy may be caused by oedema or be secondary to infection[3,4,5].

Carpal Tunnel Syndrome

Carpal tunnel syndrome results from compression of the median nerve as it passes from the forearm into the hand via the carpal tunnel at the wrist[6]. It results in pain, pins and needles, weakness and numbness of the thumb and fingers (forefinger, middle finger and half of the ring finger) supplied by the median nerve. In severe cases, wasting of the muscle at the base of the thumb (*thenar eminence*) can occur[6].

A decrease in the size of the carpal tunnel or an increase in the volume within the tunnel results in compression of the median nerve, as with trauma, oedema and repetitive flexion of the wrist[7] as occurs with long-term use of crutches and walking sticks. Symptoms are worse at night and often disrupt sleep. It tends to occur in the dominant hand but can be present simultaneously in both hands.

COMPLICATIONS

Bell's Palsy

Due to an inability to close the eyelid as well as a reduction in the production of tears, damage and infection to the eye can occur. For similar reasons, it is cosmetically disfiguring.

Pain is common in and around the ear. Frequently, a misdiagnosis of Ramsay Hunt syndrome (facial palsy due to *Herpes zoster* of the geniculate ganglion) is made.

Carpal Tunnel Syndrome

There is a loss of manual dexterity and weakness in grip resulting in dropping things. Injuries to numb fingers are common. Sleep is often disturbed by pain or the pins and needles sensation. If severe, it can be disabling and cause muscle wasting.

NON-PREGNANCY TREATMENT AND CARE

Bell's Palsy

- The diagnosis is made clinically
- An examination of the external auditory meatus and soft palate for herpetic vesicles is necessary to prevent being mistreated as Ramsay Hunt syndrome

- If the herpes virus is evident, treat with acyclovir
- Commencement on high-dose corticosteriods within 72 hours of onset may speed the recovery[5], although Bell's palsy will improve spontaneously if left untreated
- Eye care is essential to prevent morbidity and should include eye drops and the use of a patch or glasses
- Physiotherapy may be of some benefit
- The prognosis for a facial palsy is usually good and complete recovery often occurs within 3–6 weeks

Carpal Tunnel Syndrome

- The diagnosis is made clinically from the history given and if positive to Phalen's test and Tinel's sign[6]; electrophysiological tests will show a decreased conduction in the median nerve[3] but are rarely required
- Physiotherapy referral is a treatment option; splinting of the wrists into a neutral position opens the carpal tunnel and thus minimises pressure on the median nerve
- Anti-inflammatory analgesics to reduce pain and swelling are often necessary
- Diuretics to reduce fluid retention[8] are of uncertain benefit
- Injections of steroids (sometimes combined with a local anaesthetic[5]) into the carpal tunnel reduces the inflammation and can provide temporary relief[6,8] but in severe cases surgical decompression and release of the trapped nerve will be required

PRE-CONCEPTION ISSUES AND CARE

Bell's Palsy

- Pregnancy is not contraindicated if a woman is being treated for a Bell's palsy
- Acyclovir is safe in pregnancy[9]
- If a woman has experienced a Bell's palsy outside of pregnancy, it may recur during pregnancy, particularly during the third trimester and the postpartum period

Carpal Tunnel Syndrome

- Pregnancy is not contraindicated
- Women should be advised that the fluid retention brought about by hormonal changes of pregnancy can result in further swelling within the carpal tunnel, and the pregnancy hormone relaxin may result in further narrowing of the carpal tunnel thus increasing compression of the median nerve[6] and worsening the symptoms
- If a women has suffered with carpal tunnel syndrome in a prior pregnancy it may recur in subsequent pregnancies[10]
- If a woman requires walking aids, she may benefit from wrist splinting prior to developing symptoms
- Excessive weight gain is a predisposing factor[3] so ideal weight management should be emphasised

Pregnancy Issues

Bell's palsy
- Acute onset with an increased frequency during the third trimester and postpartum period[3,5]
- Pain
- Disfiguring

Carpal tunnel syndrome
- Usually presents in the second and third trimesters
- Pain
- Disturbed sleep
- Disabling

Medical Management and Care

Bell's palsy
- Prednisolone is safe during pregnancy[11]

Carpal tunnel syndrome
- Corticosteroid injection into the carpal tunnel may be indicated, and is safe during pregnancy[12]
- Nerve decompression under local anaesthesia is safe during pregnancy, but is best avoided since symptoms resolve or are significantly reduced soon after birth

Midwifery Management and Care

Bell's palsy
- At the onset of symptoms, referral to the appropriate medical practitioner for the exclusion of Ramsay Hunt syndrome and commencement of corticosteroids
- Reassurance of the short-term nature of Bell's palsy and that it does not affect the course of pregnancy[4]
- Referral to physiotherapy may be of benefit
- Paracetamol for analgesia if painful
- Ensure adequate eye care is given

Carpal tunnel syndrome
- Conservative management aimed at the relief of symptoms is preferred
  - referral to a physiotherapist for splinting may be of benefit
  - paracetamol for analgesia
- Give a thorough explanation of carpal tunnel syndrome and reassurance that it almost always settles after birth

Labour Issues

Bell's palsy
- If the mother had prolonged antenatal corticosteriod use, she will require hydrocortisone cover during labour

Carpal tunnel syndrome
- Digital numbness and weak wrists

Medical Management and Care

Bell's palsy
- Consider the necessity of hydrocortisone cover

Carpal tunnel syndrome
- Avoid cannulation in the affected hand or hands

Midwifery Management and Care

Bell's palsy
- IV access is required for steroids during labour

Carpal tunnel syndrome
- Avoidance of birthing positions that involve flexion of the wrists for prolonged periods, e.g. kneeling on all fours
- Hydrotherapy for labour and/or birth will allow ease of movement

Postpartum Issues

Bell's palsy
- As for antenatal issues

Carpal tunnel syndrome
- May present for the first time during the puerperium
- Loss of manual dexterity, making caring for baby difficult
- Difficulty positioning baby for breast-feeding
- Weakness of hands
- Risk of developing carpal tunnel syndrome in later life if experienced during pregnancy

Medical Management and Care

Bell's palsy
- Prednisolone is safe for breast-feeding

Carpal tunnel syndrome
- Surgical decompression if symptoms persist or are significantly troublesome

Midwifery Management and Care

Bell's palsy
- Provide reassurance of a good prognosis and swift recovery

Carpal tunnel syndrome
- Ensure help is available to assist the mother with the trickier tasks of changing and nursing a newborn
- Extra help and support whilst establishing breast-feeding
- Encourage feeding positions that result in little pressure on the wrists, e.g. using pillows for support
- If wrists are weak and gripping is an issue, advise the mother against holding the baby whilst standing and walking with the baby in her arms, until some strength has returned

8.5 Multiple Sclerosis

Incidence	Risk for Childbearing
100–120:100,000[1]	Variable Risk
Twice as many women as men have MS[2]	
Affects 2.5 m people worldwide[3]	

EXPLANATION OF CONDITION

Multiple Sclerosis (MS) is an unpredictable, progressive demyelinating disease that affects the central nervous system (CNS) at different levels and at varying times[4]. It is a chronic, disabling condition[5]. The white matter within the brain or spinal cord becomes inflamed then destroyed by the person's own immune system. The inflamed areas of myelin sheaths on neurons deteriorate and become scarred to become scleroses in multiple regions. This destruction of the myelin sheath slows and short-circuits the conduction of nerve impulses[5], resulting in neurological symptoms. Often there is an acute onset of symptoms, including:

- Diplopia
- Vertigo
- Bladder incontinence
- Loss of vision
- Fatigue
- Muscular weakness[6]

Multiple sclerosis has an unknown aetiology[7,9]. It typically presents during child-bearing years[8] and is more common in females (two out of three sufferers).[9]

There are several clinical types of MS, but the most common types are:

- *Relapsing–remitting*: Clearly defined disease relapses with good recovery between relapses. There are variations in severity and frequency of relapses[7]. 80% of patients have this form of MS at the onset[1]. Some are normal for years between attacks
- *Secondary progressive*: Initially relapsing–remitting course followed by progression with or without an occasional relapse. 50% of people with relapsing–remitting MS develop secondary progressive MS during the first ten years of their illness[1]
- *Primary progressive*: Disease progresses from its onset, with temporary minor improvements; 10–15% have this form from the onset[1]

COMPLICATIONS

- **Optic neuritis** (inflammation of the optic nerve): often acute in onset and painful, resulting in a reduction or loss of vision in an eye[1]
- **Transverse myelitis**: impairment of motor control, sensory function and control over bladder, bowel and sexual functions[1]

NON-PREGNANCY TREATMENT AND CARE

Diagnosis

There is no single test that can confirm an MS diagnosis. It is diagnosed clinically by accumulating evidence from history, examinations and investigations.

Common investigations are:

- Brain imaging to identify lesions
- CSF studies for the presence of oligoclonal bands

Treatment

In MS the majority of interventions are targeted at the symptoms rather than the disease itself. Pharmacological treatment for MS patients with relapsing–remitting disease or with secondary progressive MS may involve using interferon beta or glatiramer acetate[10].

Acute episodes are treated with a course of high-dose corticosteriods and should be started as soon as possible after onset of relapse.

Further pharmacological therapies are dependent on the severity of the relapse and the specific problem. They generally include antispasmodics, analgesics and medications for bladder urgency.

Referral to a specialist neurological rehabilitation service, which involves occupational therapists, speech therapists and physiotherapists, is essential for every person with MS.

PRE-CONCEPTION ISSUES AND CARE

- MS does not affect fertility, but sometimes MS sufferers experience difficulties with intercourse[2], from severe spasticity of the legs or the presence of indwelling catheters, and may require assisted conception
- It is ideal to plan a pregnancy during a remission period when the woman may be off medication
- The teratogenic effects of MS medication are uncertain, and many therapies are for symptomatic relief only. Review of medication prior to pregnancy and discontinuation where appropriate is important. Waiting for three months prior to conception is advocated[2]
- The woman contemplating pregnancy can be advised that MS has no apparent adverse effects on pregnancy, labour and delivery. There does not appear to be an increased risk of spontaneous abortion, congenital malformation or stillbirth
- Pregnancy does not affect the overall rate of disease progression[11]. There can be improvement of MS during the pregnancy with fewer relapses occurring[12]. There is a marked increase in relapses during the initial postpartum period with 20–40% of patients affected[11]. This is attributed to immune activation following delivery, and hormones returning to non-pregnant levels
- Children of MS mothers have a 1:50 risk of acquiring the disease, compared to a population risk of 1:800[13]

Pregnancy Issues

- Having MS has no effect on pregnancy, labour and birth
- Women with MS are no more likely to experience complications than other women[11]
- Half of all people with MS may have impaired ability to learn and remember[1]
- If there is urinary tract involvement, screen regularly for asymptomatic bacteriuria[6]
- Any physical therapy and stretching exercises required prior to pregnancy should be continued[6]
- Relapses during pregnancy tend to be mild and leave no or minimal residual deficits[11]

Medical Management and Care

- Mild relapses may only need supportive treatment
- Severe relapses are usually treated with high-dose corticosteriods[14]

Midwifery Management and Care

- Continuity of midwifery care would be beneficial
- The midwife should check the woman has understood all issues and provide written material where available
- Good communication between health care professionals is essential in the management of these women
- Refer to an obstetrician who has the knowledge of supporting women with disabilities
- Referral to anaesthetists so a plan of labour analgesia can be drawn up and documented[9]
- Refer to local services and support groups for mothers with disabilities
- Parent-craft groups are beneficial for the support element from other pregnant women

Labour Issues

- If the mother has had prolonged antenatal corticosteriod use, she will require hydrocortisone cover during labour[6]
- More likely to become exhausted quickly
- Many women suffer with urinary retention outside of pregnancy, and this can be a particular problem during labour
- Those mothers who are immobile are at an increased risk of pressure ulcers and DVT
- For those with restricted mobility, the use of a birthing pool may be beneficial
- Epidural analgesia is safe and does not increase the rate of relapse[8,11]
- Relapse may occur after a stressful event, such as delivery of a baby[9]

Medical Management and Care

- No need for continuous fetal monitoring in the absence of obstetric complications

Midwifery Management and Care

- Bladder care is essential
  - attention to urinary output and palpation for a bladder are necessary
  - catheterisation may be required
- For those who are immobile, use pressure-relieving procedures
- Inspect the skin areas at risk, and record a pressure-ulcer risk score; use of an appropriate specialist mattress may be needed
- DVT prevention (TED stockings, leg exercises and adequate hydration) is essential (see Section 15.1)
- Access to a birthing pool will provide analgesia as well as aiding mobility, however a hoist must be available
- Provide reassurance to those mothers who have epidural analgesia regarding the temporary loss of sensation
- Careful documentation of pre-existing neurological deficit in legs to avoid any postpartum exacerbation of MS being inappropriately attributed to a regional block[8]
- Adequate analgesia for the benefit of reducing stress in labour[9]

Postpartum Issues

- Exacerbation of MS is reported to increase 20–40% during first six months after delivery[11]
- Nearly all new mothers are fatigued; this can be exacerbated in MS sufferers, and therefore it is important that extra help and support is made available
- Longer maternity leave may be required to cover the period of highest risk of relapse[2]
- Breast-feeding should be encouraged, unless prescribed medication precludes it
- Infections have been associated with worsening of disability and can trigger a relapse[1]
- Since MS does not affect fertility, the usual decisions about contraception need to be made[2]

Medical Management and Care

- Re-starting therapy shortly after delivery may decrease the frequency of postpartum relapse[11]

Midwifery Management and Care

- If mobility is affected or if a severe relapse occurs following the birth, the mother may require thrombo-prophylaxis for the initial six weeks postpartum (see Section 15.1)
- Those with disability will require extra help with infant care[8]
- Breast-feeding does not have an adverse effect on the rate of relapse[2,8,11]
- If manual dexterity is reduced the mother will require extra help and support with feeding
- Be vigilant for the signs and symptoms of infections and act promptly
- The type of contraception will be dependent on the areas affected by the MS and the other medications that are being taken. If manual dexterity is reduced, barrier methods are impractical. If bladder problems are experienced, diaphragms may increase the likelihood of UTI. If mobility is an issue or if the mother is on medication and oral contraceptives are used, the mother may be susceptible to DVT or to reduced efficacy of the 'pill'
- There should be thorough discussion of contraception between the mother and an appropriate health professional

8.6 Myasthenia Gravis

Incidence	Risk for Childbearing
2–10:100,000[1]	High Risk – both maternal and fetal
Female to male ratio 2:1[2]	

EXPLANATION OF CONDITION

Myasthenia gravis (MG) is a chronic autoimmune disease. Its name literally translated from Latin means grave muscle weakness. First reported in 1672, MG is characterised by fatigue on exertion and skeletal muscle weakness[3]. This occurs as a result of breakdown in the communication between the nerve and muscle at the neuromuscular junction, due to the presence of autoantibodies which block the acetylcholine receptors.

It is suggested that an abnormal thymus gland induces the developing immune cells to produce autoantibodies. Of patients with MG, 50–60% exhibit lymphofollicular hyperplasia and 10–20% have a thymoma[4].

Patients with MG will present with erratic muscle weakness that worsens with sustained or repeated exertion and recovers with rest[5]. MG may affect any voluntary muscle although in many cases it is limited to the ocular muscles. The degree of muscle weakness may vary greatly, ranging from the localised ocular form to a generalised form affecting bulbar, limbic and respiratory muscles. Symptoms may include:

- Ptosis (drooping eyelid)
- Diplopia (double vision)
- Unstable gait
- Limb weakness
- Dysphagia (impaired swallowing)
- Dysarthria (impaired speech)
- Dyspnoea (impaired breathing)

COMPLICATIONS

- Respiratory arrest
- **Myasthenic crisis** as a result of exacerbation of MG characterised by acute bulbar or respiratory paralysis which may necessitate mechanical ventilation; death may occur as a result of severe respiratory muscle fatigue[1]
- **Cholinergic crisis** caused by overdosage of anticholinesterase drugs, resulting in:
  - severe muscle weakness
  - hypersalivation
  - constriction of pupils
  - sweating
  - vomiting
  - lacrimation
- Adverse drug response

NON-PREGNANCY TREATMENT AND CARE

MG is one of the most treatable neurological disorders[3], with several therapies available to improve muscle weakness.

- Therapeutic anticholinesterase agents used include neostigmine and pyridostigmine
- Pyridostigmine currently the most utilised long-acting medication for the treatment of MG: oral pyridostigmine 240–1500 mg per day[1]
- Immunosuppressive drugs include:
  - prednisone (60–80 mg per day)
  - ciclosporin
  - azathioprine
  - significant side effects may occur
  - use with caution (see Appendix 11)
- Plasmapheresis – plasma exchange involving the removal of abnormal antibodies from blood
- Intravenous immunoglobulin (IVIG), high dosages of which temporarily modify the immune system, providing the recipient with normal donated antibodies
- Thymectomy reduces symptoms in >70% of patients without thymoma; usually performed in patients under 45 years of age[6]

PRE-CONCEPTION ISSUES AND CARE

Onset of MG can occur at any age. Female incidence peaks in the third decade therefore during peak childbearing age. Evidence suggests there is a greater risk of death from MG during a pregnancy in the first year of the disease, with a marked decrease in risk after this time. It is suggested that pregnancy be postponed in women with newly-diagnosed MG. Therapeutic abortion is not advocated[7].

- Ensure medical advice is sought early to ensure maximum clinical improvement prior to conception
- Advise small increased risk of spontaneous abortion[7]
- Adjustment of medication to establish good control of symptoms, although generally the usual drug therapy may be maintained
- If disease severity is minimal consider discontinuing medication
- Educate women with regard to the need for close supervision, potential for increased fatigue and respiratory compromise and the risk of pre-term birth and neonatal myasthenia gravis

Pregnancy Issues

The effect of myasthenia gravis on pregnancy is variable and unpredictable:

- Disease may remain stable, result in partial or complete remission or deteriorate and may differ in each pregnancy
- Relapses or remissions tend to occur in the first trimester[7]
- Effect of nausea and vomiting on gastric emptying may influence medication levels
- Exacerbated by stress, physical exertion, minor infections and fatigue
- Exacerbation in pregnancy less likely if patient has undergone previous thymectomy
- Hypermagnesaemia inhibits release of acetylcholine
- Acetylcholinesterase receptor antibodies in the mother may cross to the fetus and cause arthrogryposis (limb contracture)

Medical Management and Care

- Specialist multi-disciplinary team approach; input required from neurology and anaesthetic teams, to ensure medications that may precipitate a crisis are avoided
- Assess extent of muscle weakness
- Continuous monitoring of disease and fetus (including regular USS)
- Discussion regarding mode of delivery, depending on severity of the disease
- Treat if necessary with acetylcholinesterase inhibitor therapy: drug of choice is pyridostigmine 240–1500 mg orally, in divided doses 3–8 hourly[1]
- Thymectomy is not recommended in pregnancy
- Magnesium sulphate for treatment of pre-eclampsia, should *not* be used in patients with MG, as it may precipitate a crisis

Midwifery Management and Care

- Encourage rest
- Ensure women are referred to appropriate medical staff
- Frequent antenatal appointments for maternal and fetal assessment
- Advise regarding fetal movement
- Advise to avoid stress, limit exercise and to ensure prompt treatment of infections
- Consider referral to anaesthetic team for discussion re labour

Labour Issues

- Increased risk of respiratory insufficiency and aspiration of gastric contents in severe disease[8]
- Expulsive efforts in second stage may be reduced
- Acetylcholinesterase inhibitor requirements may be difficult to estimate, due to reduced gastric absorption and worsening weakness
- Insufficient dosage may lead to severe weakness (myasthenic crisis); excessive dosage may induce a cholinergic crisis (muscle weakness, sweating and abdominal colic)

Medical Management and Care

- Prophylactic antacids in labour
- Consider the need for instrumental delivery
- Caesarean section is not warranted unless for obstetric reasons
- Consider need for medication to be administered parentally to avoid erratic absorption
- Avoid gentamicin, ritodrine, salbutamol and narcotics, which may exacerbate muscle fatigue[2]

Midwifery Management and Care

- Careful observation and monitoring of excessive fatigue
- Avoid stress and prolonged second stage of labour
- Regional analgesia may minimise stress of labour and prevent sedative effects of Entonox and opioids
- Women may have concerns about possible effects of regional analgesia on disease

Postpartum Issues

- Decreasing circulating volume post delivery may require rapid adjustment of medication
- Myasthenia gravis is exacerbated by stress and infection
- Acetylcholine receptor antibodies may enter fetal circulation via the placenta; 12% of babies born to mothers with MG may display transient muscle weakness (this usually resolves within eight weeks)

Medical Management and Care

- Close observation in short-term postnatal period in order to adjust drug therapy
- In the longer term it is necessary to re-establish pre-pregnancy treatment regime

Midwifery Management and Care

- Ensure support for women at home and advise regarding rest
- Assistance with baby care is needed following birth
- Advise and observe for signs of uterine and wound infection; refer for treatment promptly if appropriate
- Observe neonate for signs of muscle weakness, e.g. floppiness, feeble cry, poor feeding and respiratory distress
- Advise that pyridostigmine is not contraindicated if breast-feeding

8 Neurological Disorders

PATIENT ORGANISATIONS

Migraine Action Association
Unit 6 Oakley Hay Lodge Business Park
Great Folds Road
Great Oakley
Northants. NN18 9AS
www.migraine.org.uk

The Migraine Trust
2nd Floor
55–56 Russell Square
London WC1B 4HP
www.migrainetrust.org

Epilepsy Action (British Epilepsy Association)
New Anstey House
Gate Way Drive
Yeadon
Leeds LS19 7XY
www.epilepsy.org.uk

National Society for Epilepsy
Chesham Lane
Chalfont St Peter
Bucks. SL9 0RJ
www.epilepsynse.org.uk

Multiple Sclerosis Society
MS National Centre
372 Edgware Road
London NW2 6ND
www.mssociety.org.uk

Multiple Sclerosis International Federation
3rd Floor
Sky Line House
200 Union Street
London SE1 0LX
www.msif.org

Stroke Association
Stroke House
240 City Road
London EC1V 2PR
www.stroke.org.uk

Bell's Palsy Association
www.bellspalsy.org.uk

Myasthenia Gravis Association
First Floor
Southgate Business Centre
Normanton Road
Derby DE23 6UQ
www.mgauk.org

ESSENTIAL READING

Adab, N. and Chadwick, D. (2006) Management of women with epilepsy in pregnancy. **The Obstetrician and Gynaecologist**, **8**(1):20–25.

Billington, M. and Stevenson, M. (2007) **Critical Care in Childbearing for Midwives**. Oxford; Blackwell.

Briggs, G.G., Freeman, R.K. and Yaffe, S.J. (2005) **Drugs in Pregnancy and Lactation**, 7th Edn. Philadelphia, USA; Lippincott.

Epilepsy Action booklets:
– *Epilepsy for everyone*
– *Women*
– *Epilepsy and pregnancy*
From: www.epilepsy.org.uk

James, D., Steer, P., Weiner, C. and Gonik, B. (Eds) (2006) Neurologic disorders, 1067–1074; Autoimmune disease 949–85. In: **High Risk Pregnancy: Management Options**, 3rd Edn. London; Elsevier.

Lewis, G. and Drife, J. (2002) **CEMACH 6th report: Why Mothers Die 2000–2002** Confidential Enquiries into Maternal and Child Health. London; RCOG Press.
NB: 7th report pending publication Dec 2007

Lowe, S.A. and Sen, R. (2005) Neurological disease in pregnancy. **Current Obstetrics and Gynaecology**, **15**:166–173.

MS Essentials Booklet 15 – Multiple Sclerosis Society
From: www.mssociety.org.uk

NICE Clinical Guidelines:
20: *The Epilepsies – The diagnosis and management of the Epilepsies in adults and children in primary and secondary care settings.*
8: *Multiple sclerosis; Management of multiple sclerosis in primary and secondary care.*
From: www.nice.org.uk

Rozette, C. and Houghton-Clemmey, R. (2003) A review of carpal tunnel syndrome in pregnancy. **British Journal of Midwifery**, **11**(3):136–139.

MUSCULOSKELETAL DISORDERS

9

S. Elizabeth Robson, Javed Iqbal and Edmund Howarth

9.1 Back and Pelvic Pain

Incidence	Risk for Childbearing
Back pain – 33.3% of pregnant women[1] Sciatica – 1% of pregnant women[2]	Variable Risk

EXPLANATION OF CONDITION

Back pain is a common disorder, and a childbearing woman may have a past history of 'backache'. Alternatively, it may present for the first time in pregnancy. Lower back pain is so common in pregnancy that it is described as one of the minor disorders of pregnancy[3]. 'Backache' is a loose term. The common presentations of more significant back pain are:

- Low back pain
- Sacroiliac dysfunction
- Sciatica

Diagnosis is complex. Backache is often referred pain, in particular from the pelvic organs. This needs consideration prior to assuming that the pain is orthopaedic in nature.

COMPLICATIONS

- Worsening mobility
- Impaired driving ability
- Difficulty continuing with everyday tasks, work commitments, or caring for other children
- Insomnia leading to tiredness and irritability

NON-PREGNANCY TREATMENT AND CARE

Careful assessment and treatment are required for any back or pelvic joint dysfunction. This could include referral to a specialist physiotherapist. Treatment is specific to the cause.

Low Back Pain

Symptoms usually occur between 4–7 months of pregnancy[4]. Pain is usually low in the back, sometimes radiating into the buttocks and thighs, and occasionally down the legs as sciatica. There is also a great variation in the severity of symptoms between individuals. Some women have transitory stiffness or discomfort, whilst others are severely affected[4]. The pain is usually exacerbated by prolonged standing or sitting, forward bending and lifting. Some women also experience pain over the symphysis pubis or thoracic spine at the same time.

Associated factors include[5]:

- Increased parity
- Fetal position, especially malposition
- Back pain in a previous pregnancy
- Increased weight and tiredness
- Postural changes and adaptations
- Joint and ligamentous laxity

Treatment includes:

- Individual education can reduce symptoms[6] by empowering women to understand their condition[7]
- Back care and postural advice[4]

- Management of activities of daily living to keep pain level as low as possible[4]
- Women are encouraged to maintain the level of activity that they are comfortable with[8]
- Analgesia may be prescribed on a gradient, or 'pain ladder' (see Appendix 9) and adjusted accordingly[9]

Sacroiliac Dysfunction

Pregnancy can affect the sacroiliac joints in several ways:

- Joint laxity may allow enough repetitive new movement at one or both joints to cause pain (a hypermobile joint)
- Alternatively, the newly permitted movement could result in the uneven joint surfaces moving on one another and then becoming 'stuck' (a hypomobile joint)[10]

Treatment includes:

- Appropriate exercise and advice will be given by the obstetric physiotherapist
- It is sometimes appropriate for *gentle* manipulative or self-manipulative techniques to be tried[4]

Sciatica

This is pain in the distribution of the sciatic nerve[11], which may accompany backache and sacroiliac dysfunction and rarely occurs alone. The sciatic nerve runs immediately in front of the sacroiliac joint and could become involved in any dysfunction or inflammatory process that is occurring there. The most common cause is a prolapsed intervertebral disc[11]. An exaggerated lumbar curve could also affect the nerve, especially in lying and standing.
Treatment includes:

- Assessment by a physiotherapist or doctor to exclude other back problems and assess the sacroiliac joints[2]
- Pelvic support might be fitted to assist with a co-existing problem such as pelvic instability[2,8]
- Advise the woman to sleep on her side with a pillow between her knees[2]
- Advise the woman to roll over in bed keeping knees and shoulders in line to avoid twisting[2]

PRE-CONCEPTION ISSUES AND CARE

- Women who have had back problems in previous pregnancies are more susceptible in subsequent pregnancies, and may benefit from referral to an obstetric physiotherapist early in the pregnancy for advice and treatment
- Women with current back symptoms need a medical review of current drug treatments, especially for fetal risk, and substitutions made where indicated (see Appendices 9 and 11)
- A referral for stability exercises pre-conceptually may be appropriate for some women

Pregnancy Issues

Previous back pain can be exacerbated by the release of progesterone and relaxin, which relaxes the pelvic ligaments. Alternatively, there can be a respite from discomfort if the pain is ligamentous in origin.

Back pain can present for the first time in pregnancy, influenced by the above hormones and postural changes due to the gravid uterus altering the woman's centre of gravity. This condition gets progressively worse as the pregnancy continues.

Back pain can impede mobility, driving and child caring ability. Furthermore, the woman's employment may be affected, and if her job cannot be adapted she might have to take sick leave or take maternity leave sooner than anticipated.

Physiotherapy is effective in treating 75% of antenatal back pain, with most women reporting an improvement in their symptoms after one treatment episode[12].

Vitamin D deficiency/osteoporosis can present in pregnancy. Initial symptoms may be symmetrical lower back pain spreading to the pelvis and upper legs and ribs[13].

Medical Management and Care

- Physical examination
- Investigations of any neurological symptoms
- Analgesia with regular review, and augmentation dependent upon the severity of symptoms (see Appendix 9)
- Early maternity leave may be needed, and 'sick note' required

Midwifery and Physiotherapy Care

- Accurate booking history to identify any previous 'backache'
- Be aware that backache can be musculoskeletal or can be associated with other pelvic conditions such as infection
- Advise to wear low-heeled shoes and *bend at the knees* when lifting
- Monitor the progress of the backache to determine if the advice is helping, and if not then physiotherapy referral may be necessary
- The obstetric physiotherapist can advise the multidisciplinary team about the most suitable positions for labour and delivery
- Encourage parent-craft attendance where the woman and her birth supporter can be advised about labour and birth positions
- The care and advice of non-pregnancy (previous page) in relation to the specific type of back pain should be reinforced
- A planned exercise programme has been shown to reduce pain[17]
- Water exercise has reduced pain enabling women to remain at work[1]
- Acupuncture[1] and TENS[9] can be beneficial for chronic back pain
- Regular use of a pelvic belt decreases mobility of the sacroiliac joints[18] and reduces pain intensity whilst increasing mobility[19]
- Women of short stature have difficulty with fitting a belt effectively[19]
- Be aware that increasing lower back pain in dark-skinned or veiled women may indicate vitamin D deficiency requiring medical referral
- Maternal concerns should be taken seriously; a 'just accept it' attitude by staff should be replaced by assessment for therapy[19]

Labour Issues

- Some women are best remaining comfortably supported in labour rather than moving around, which could exacerbate symptoms[14]
- Epidurals are not harmful per se, but the relief they give allows positions to be adopted which may further exacerbate the pre-existing condition

Medical Management and Care

- Review analgesia options
- Avoid, or take care with lithotomy position which may cause nerve root compression from disc protrusion

Midwifery Management and Care

- Agree a birth plan which allows for flexibility with choice of mobility or rest during labour, and position for delivery
- If the mother wishes for water immersion in the first stage, discuss this with the obstetrician, ensuring that a hoist is available as there is a theoretical chance of difficulty in getting out of a bath/pool
- Suitable delivery positions may include side-lying, kneeling on all fours or semi-reclining with the legs well supported[14]
- If the woman requires assistance to move her legs, they must be moved together

Postpartum Issues

- The ligamentous changes that take place during pregnancy can take up to six months to reverse[8]
- Many women who have back pain during pregnancy find that it persists, or recurs, after the birth[12,15]
- Persistent postpartum backache requires accurate investigation and a diagnosis made before further pregnancies are planned, as the pain may result from an underlying condition such as osteoporosis, which could be exacerbated by subsequent childbearing[16]

Medical Management and Care

- As for antenatal care
- Women who continue to have poor postpartum mobility may require venous thrombo-embolism prophylaxis

Midwifery and Physiotherapy Care

- Re-refer to the obstetric physiotherapist if pain persists
- Arrange any necessary outpatient appointments
- Midwife and physiotherapist to give consistent advice on:
  - good posture when feeding, nappy changing, etc.
  - wearing flat-heeled shoes
  - appropriate postnatal exercises
  - the best time to resume pre-pregnancy exercise regimes
  - seeking advice and medical consultation if the back pain persists beyond the postnatal period

9.2 Diastasis Recti Abdominis

Incidence	**Risk for Childbearing**
66% of third trimester mothers[1]	Low Risk – unless there is a pendulous abdomen

EXPLANATION OF CONDITION

Diastasis of recti abdominis, also known as *divarication* of recti abdominis, is a separation of the recti abdominis muscles, often appearing in the second or third trimester, or as a result of bearing down during delivery[1].

The abdominal muscles are stretched and elongated during pregnancy, and can become separated along the linea alba, which has become softer and more elastic. The hormonal and mechanical stresses placed on the abdominal wall are believed to facilitate this separation[2].

The diastasis can vary from a small vertical gap 2–3 cm wide and 12–15 cm long, above or below the umbilicus, to a gap measuring 12–20 cm wide and extending almost the whole length of the recti muscles[3]. This weakens the abdominal support, which potentially could increase the vulnerability of the back to injury.

Women Most at Risk

- Multiple pregnancy
- Polyhydramnios
- Multiparae
- Women with a narrow pelvis and large baby
- Women with weak abdominal muscles pre-pregnancy

COMPLICATIONS

If left untreated, diastasis recti abdominis can lead to long-term problems, in particular:

- Abnormal posture
- Back pain
- Pendulous abdomen (with sequelae of fetal malpresentation and malposition in subsequent pregnancies)

NON-PREGNANCY TREATMENT AND CARE

All newly-delivered women with the condition should ideally be referred to an obstetric physiotherapist, who is likely to first check the width of the gap.

With the woman in crook lying, supported on one pillow, she raises her head to reach with her hands towards her feet. With the fingertips of one hand placed widthways across the abdomen in the midline, just below the umbilicus, the medial edges of the two recti muscles can be palpated as the woman raises her head. The degree of separation is measurable in fingertip widths[4].

The physiotherapist will then:

- Teach appropriate abdominal exercise[5]
- Advise regarding activities of daily living
- Encourage constant awareness of the abdomen, so that the woman retracts her abdominal muscles frequently[6]

- Encourage the woman to roll onto her side to get into and out of bed, reducing the amount of strain placed on the muscles and the back
- Determine if the woman would benefit from wearing an abdominal support such as Tubigrip, in the interim period, to provide some abdominal support
- Review the woman regularly until the diastasis has improved.

In extreme cases, where the condition persists after physiotherapy and abdominal musculature is severely impaired, corrective surgery by abdominoplasty may be considered. This entails suturing the rectus bellies together and removing the distended pendulous fat and skin[6].

PRE-CONCEPTION ISSUES AND CARE

It is thought that women who take regular exercise before pregnancy have a reduced risk of developing diastasis recti abdominis because their muscle tissue is healthier as a result[7]. Hence all women should be encouraged to exercise, and this especially applies to women with a past history of diastasis as well as women generally in the pre-conception period.

The woman with a past history of the condition should be encouraged to:

- Use effective contraception until the diastasis has improved, and effective muscle tone has been achieved
- Exercise regularly, especially swimming
- Have a well-balanced diet to reduce obesity
- Adopt a positive body image
- Avoid, or take care, with lifting – especially lifting her own children[5]

If a woman has had surgical treatment by abdominoplasty, further pregnancies are not usually recommended, as the repaired abdominal muscles may not stretch adequately in pregnancy. If a woman still wishes for a pregnancy she would benefit from advice and counselling, because she is likely to experience increasing discomfort as the pregnancy progresses.

Pregnancy Issues

- Healthy pregnant women should be encouraged to remain active. Mild to moderate exercise is beneficial, provided that overheating or exhaustion does not occur[4]
- Swimming provides a toning and strengthening activity which increases physical fitness as well as promoting a sense of wellbeing
- A mild diastasis, with inter-recti distance of two finger widths is considered normal, and should not prevent the mother from having low-risk midwifery care, unless further complications occur
- An inter-recti distance of four or more finger widths is considered abnormal
- Fetal parts are readily identifiable on abdominal palpation, and the fetus is theoretically more vulnerable to trauma under the diastasis gap. Skin over the gap may be inflamed or itchy
- There is a theoretical risk of pendulous abdomen developing in grand multiparae, which can pre-dispose to fetal malpresentation or malposition
- Women with previous abdominoplasty will experience significant pain and discomfort. It is difficult to palpate the abdomen, and it is misleading to measure fundal height against the umbilicus, necessitating ultrasonic scans

Medical Management and Care

- Examine the mother and monitor the condition if referred
- No specific medical interventions are proven
- Skin treatment may have to be prescribed if moisturisers have failed
- Refer to the obstetric physiotherapist for treatment as below

Midwifery and Physiotherapy Management and Care

- Be aware that a mother with a previous diastasis may have a recurrence in the current pregnancy, and that diastasis can also present for the first time in the second/third trimester[1]
- Take care when performing abdominal palpation, as a mother with diastasis may feel especially sensitive in the midline
- Advise the use of moisturiser cream for itchy/flaky abdominal skin
- If a pendulous abdomen develops refer to the obstetrician, and be alert for fetal malpresentation or malposition
- Ascertain if the mother has an occupational risk of contact pressure on her abdomen, which may necessitate adaptation of occupation
- Refer the mother to the obstetric physiotherapist if the diastasis presents (or re-occurs) with an inter-recti distance ≥4 finger widths
- The physiotherapist might fit a tubigrip abdominal support in late pregnancy or in readiness for labour[10]

Midwife and physiotherapist should advise the mother
- To roll onto her side to get in and out of bed, to reduce excessive strain on the abdominal muscles
- To avoid strenuous abdominal exercises (sit-ups) and contact sports
- To attend aquanatal classes, informing the instructor of her condition
- That labour is likely to be normal, unless other problems develop

Labour Issues

- A woman with a significant diastasis may benefit from wearing a piece of size 'L' Tubigrip (xiphisternum to symphysis pubis) during labour to help to support the abdomen, if tolerated

Medical Management and Care

- This is dictated by fetal malposition, otherwise labour can be managed normally by the midwife

Midwifery Management and Care

- Gentle, but accurate, abdominal examination in labour as it is important to identify fetal malposition or malpresentation
- Assist the mother with significant diastasis to put on the Tubigrip belt, and be aware that the mother may feel 'hot and sweaty' under the belt and require assistance with washing
- Labour should otherwise be managed normally

Postpartum Issues

- Whilst the inter-recti distance should reduce after delivery, some degree of diastasis may persist for 30–60% of postpartum women[1] and non-resolution postpartum is associated with chronic lower back pain[8]
- Advice and treatment in the puerperium remains the same as for non-pregnancy
- The inter-recti distance should reduce naturally, but some degree of the gap is likely to persist for up to 12 weeks postpartum[9]. The gap is larger when measured in a resting posture postpartum[9]

Medical Management and Care

- Be aware of the risk of bowel incarceration, which can result when muscle tone improves and the gap narrows

Midwifery Management and Care

- Assess the inter-recti distance as part of the routine postnatal examination, measuring in both active and resting positions[9]
- Re-refer the mother to the obstetric physiotherapist, who is likely to assess the width of the diastasis gap, and advise on abdominal exercise (see previous page)
- Reinforce the advice of the obstetric physiotherapist
- Give practical advice to the mother on posture and picking up her baby, and returning to pre-pregnancy fitness; in particular, to 'draw-in' her abdomen when walking and prior to picking up the baby
- Advise the mother that this condition could recur with future pregnancies, and she should wear abdominal support promptly[10]

9.3 Symphysis Pubis Dysfunction

Incidence	Risk for Childbearing
Symphysis pubis dysfunction (SPD)[1] 1:36 Diastasis of the symphysis pubis (DSP)[2] 1:569	Variable Risk

EXPLANATION OF CONDITION

Symphysis Pubis Dysfunction

Symphysis pubis dysfunction (SPD) encompasses symphysis pubis malfunction due to ligament relaxation giving rise to varying degrees of immobility or disability[3], of which the definitions vary[4]. The condition is also known as *pelvic girdle relaxation, pelvic relaxation syndrome, pelvic insufficiency* or *pubo-pelvic arthropathy*[5].

There are no definitive tests that prove or disprove the presence of symphysis pubis dysfunction[5], the diagnosis being made on the basis of symptoms alone.

Signs and symptoms of SPD include:

- Mild to severe pain in the symphysis pubis joint, hips, groin, lower abdomen, inner thighs and back
- Exacerbated by all weight-bearing activities, especially walking, stairs, sitting to standing, standing on one leg, abducting the legs (e.g. getting in and out of a car)
- Painful to roll over in bed
- Some women may be aware of clicking or grinding of the symphysis pubis
- Women often walk in a 'waddling' fashion

N.B. Palpation of the symphysis pubis should be performed cautiously as it can be extremely tender.

The pelvic girdle is responsible for the transference of large forces from the upper body onto the legs during walking. It is therefore essential that the three joints of the pelvis are strongly supported and stable.

Stability of the pelvic ring is provided by close fitting joint surfaces, strong pelvic ligaments and support from pelvic and trunk muscles. This means that any dysfunction (stiffness or hypermobility) at one joint could have an effect on the others. Women presenting with SPD often complain of low back pain and vice versa.

During pregnancy, pelvic stability can be compromised by ligamentous laxity that occurs as a result of hormonal changes. It is thought that progesterone and relaxin bring about collagen remodelling which allows for the baby to pass more easily through the pelvis at delivery[6]. The normal gap between the pubic bones in pregnancy varies from 4.5–9 mm. However, separation can exceed 10 mm. In some cases, severe dysfunction and pain can occur as a result of these changes.

Symphysiolysis

Symphysiolysis is the name given to pain in the symphysis pubis only. This group of patients tend to hormonally-mediated changes alone[7,8] (the other groups have additional biomechanical and articular changes) and the best outcome with full postpartum recovery[7].

Diastasis of the Symphysis Pubis (DSP)

Diastasis of the symphysis pubis (DSP) may develop from chronic SPD, or present acutely with the same symptoms.

Definitive diagnosis can, however, only be made radiologically. The definition is separation of the symphysis pubis of 10 mm or more, and a vertical shift of 5 mm or more[9]. It has been noted that there is often no association between the severity of symptoms and the degree of separation at the symphysis pubis[10]. Traumatic separation can occur as a result of:

- Precipitous delivery
- Cephalo-pelvic disproportion
- Excessive abduction of the thighs during delivery[3]
- Pelvic girdle pain in a previous pregnancy
- Previous pelvic damage

COMPLICATIONS

- Long-term morbidity can be experienced by some women, who may ultimately require internal fixation
- Long-term disability impacts on every aspect of daily life and relationships
- Some women experience postnatal depression because of the physical problems they have had
- Increased risk of recurrence in subsequent pregnancy

NON-PREGNANCY TREATMENT AND CARE

Symptoms may persist postpartum and women may require physiotherapy for several months with an emphasis on:

- Advice on adapting to daily living and employment
- Promoting good posture
- Teaching core stability exercises

Most cases resolve by six months postpartum[4]. In non-resolving cases orthopaedic referral may be necessary. In extreme cases orthopaedic surgery for internal fixation of the symphysis pubis may be necessary.

PRE-CONCEPTION ISSUES AND CARE

- If a woman had symphysis pubis dysfunction during a previous pregnancy it is likely, though not inevitable, that it will recur in subsequent pregnancies
- SPD often starts earlier in subsequent pregnancies, and symptoms can be more pronounced
- It is helpful for the woman to recover as well as possible from a previous pregnancy before embarking on another, hence effective contraception is required
- Good general fitness, a healthy diet and pre-conception pelvic stability exercises assist in the management of a subsequent pregnancy
- Once pregnant early referral to a physiotherapist is advisable for assessment and prompt symptom control

Pregnancy Issues

- SPD can present at any stage during pregnancy. The mother may experience a range of severity with symptoms and complications, which include:
  - pain
  - instability
  - immobility
  - inability or difficulty with weight-bearing
- The condition gets worse with multiple pregnancy[11]
- The disabling nature of the condition is under-recognised[6]
- Women experience practical difficulties caring for themselves and their children, and become increasingly dependent upon others[12]
- Disabling situations and pain can influence[12]:
  - domestic mobility
  - driving ability
  - employment situation
  - social isolation
  - psychological wellbeing
  - family relationships
  - sexual function
  - enthusiasm for the pregnancy

Medical Management and Care

- Analgesia should be prescribed and amended on a gradient as symptoms alter (see Appendix 9)
- Antenatal epidural has been described in extreme situations[14], necessitating hospital admission
- Women with limited mobility will require VTE prophylaxis

Midwifery and Physiotherapy Management and Care

- Midwife should liaise with an obstetric physiotherapist for assistance in managing the condition. This would include:
- Advice on back care and exercises
- Management of joint dysfunction
- Correction of muscle imbalance
- Assess effectiveness of a pelvic support belt if used, as there is conflicting evidence as to its effectiveness[15,16]
- Provision of elbow crutches
- Check pain-free range of hip abduction prior to labour and liaise management of labour with the named midwife
- Advise the mother to:
  - reduce non-essential weight-bearing activities, e.g. lifting, shopping
  - rest – in short doses, as long periods usually aggravate symptoms when starting to walk again
  - avoid straddle movements
  - sit to get dressed
  - wear flat-heeled shoes
- Referral to the multi-disciplinary team may be required as follows:
  - occupational therapist for appropriate aids and wheelchair
  - home assessment if symptoms are severe
  - medical social worker if assistance with benefits, home help or childcare assistance is required

Labour Issues

- If the woman 'pushes' with her feet on the midwife's hips, this can lead to SPD worsening to become diastasis
- This can be 'masked' if a mother has an epidural or spinal analgesia[12]
- Acute presentation of diastasis in the second stage, with audible 'popping' noise has been associated with McRoberts manoeuvre for shoulder dystocia[13]

Medical Management and Care

- Epidural can be used, but care is needed with lithotomy position
- Keep lithotomy position to the shortest time period possible, and legs should be moved into position at the same time

Midwifery Management and Care

- Enable woman to adopt the most comfortable position in all stages of labour, e.g. side lying, kneeling, but avoid squatting position[17]
- Keep hip abduction to a minimum[12]
- Vaginal examinations in the most comfortable position, often lateral
- The woman should **not** rest her feet on the attendant's hips
- Labour can be managed normally
- Water-birth is not encouraged due to handling risks[17]

Postpartum Issues

- The disability of the antenatal period is likely to continue into the puerperium, although some level of pain might abate[7]
- The mother with mobility problems is at risk of venous thrombo-embolism (VTE) and postnatal depression
- Whilst diastasis might have occurred acutely in labour, it might be recognised first in the puerperium, possibly after the mother has been discharged home, hence all cases of postpartum supra-pubic pain should be taken seriously

Medical Management and Care

- Analgesic/anti-inflammatory medication if possible
- Anticoagulants if bed-rest exceeds 24 hours
- If symptoms persist, imaging may be required (flamingo posture by standing on one leg) and an orthopaedic referral arranged[18]

Midwifery and Physiotherapy Management and Care

- Bed-rest until acute pain subsides, usually 24–48 hours
- TED stockings and leg exercises if on bed-rest[17]
- Basic nursing care of mother and baby while on bed-rest
- Wheelchair to toilet, and gradual mobilisation as pain allows
- Ascertain status of social services support
- Community midwife to extend period of postnatal visiting
- Innovative ways to promote maternal–infant attachment[19]
- Be alert for signs of depression
- Counselling – 68–85% risk of recurrence in future pregnancies[18]

9.4 Hypovitaminosis D and Osteomalacia

Hypovitaminosis D Incidence
Up to 90% of certain migrant women to North West Europe, 3% indigenous women in North West Europe

Risk for Childbearing
Variable Risk

EXPLANATION OF CONDITION

Vitamin D

Vitamin D is essential for calcium and phosphorus absorption for skeletal mineralisation[1]. Vitamin D has a variety of functions and deficiency has been associated with a range of conditions[2,3,4] and in the elderly the risk of falls and fractures[5,6].

Under sunlight, the skin synthesises the major source of vitamin D_3, cholecalciferol[7,8]. Smaller amounts of vitamin D (vitamin D_2), ergocalciferol, and some cholecalciferol are obtained in certain foods. The supply of vitamin D from standard European diets is inadequate[7,9]. In the UK fortification of food is not a policy[10].

Vitamin D_2/D_3 is transported to the liver to produce the main circulating form, 25(OH)VitD (calcidiol) which is further metabolised in the kidney to produce the active hormonal form of vitamin D, 1,25-dihydroxyvitamin D (1,25(OH)$_2$VitD) (calcitriol). Calcidiol measurement in blood reflects supply of vitamin D and in the UK shows seasonal variation, with high levels during late summer and early autumn and low levels in early spring[1,11]. The fetus is entirely dependent on vitamin D supply from the mother[12].

Hypovitaminosis D

Serum calcidiol level of <50 nM/l indicates vitamin D insufficiency; <25 nM/l indicates deficiency[13,14]. Other characteristic biochemical changes occur. Serum calcium and phosphorus may become low, but parathyroid hormone (PTH) and later the serum bone alkaline phosphatase rise[15,16] (see Appendix 9.2). These changes can be diagnostic in any age group. Although mild hypovitaminosis D seems to be prevalent in many populations worldwide, resurgence of severe vitamin D deficiency, first described in the 1960s in migrants from the Indian subcontinent to the UK[17], seems to be a continuing problem[18,19,20,21]. This has also been described in other recent migrants from the Middle East and the Afro-Caribbean regions[13,19,20,22]. As migration has occurred to other northwest European countries[23,24] and Australia[25,26] vitamin D deficiency has been reported to be particularly prevalent in women of child-bearing age.

Risk Factors for Hypovitaminosis D/Osteomalacia

- Migrant women from the Southeast Asian Indian subcontinent, Middle East, Afro-Caribbean countries coming to the UK and Europe or Australia
- Indigenous European women from poor backgrounds
- Those on anticonvulsant therapy

COMPLICATIONS

Osteomalacia

With severe vitamin D deficiency, calcium and phosphorus supply to bone are diminished and an excess of new collagen, osteoid, is formed. This is diagnostic of osteomalacia (bone softening) and is diagnosed on bone biopsy[27,28]. Clinically there may be:

- Bone pain
- Pseudofractures, partial linear stress lines in the cortex of bone, can progress to complete fractures of:
  - pelvis
  - upper femora
  - ribs
- With hypocalcaemia there is risk of paraesthesia and seizures
- Mild muscular pains, which are not uncommon, can progress to severe proximal myopathy with paresis[27,28]

Rickets

Bone softening results in bowing of the legs (typically at age 1–2 years when walking begins), knock knees in older children, swollen wrists, dental hypoplasia, frontal bossing and/or rickety rosaries (swollen costochondral joints)[29].

Cardiac Complications

Rare serious cardiac complications in adults and children have been described[30,31].

Pregnancy and Neonatal Seizures

Severe skeletal complications including fractures of the femur and pelvic deformity and fracture[32,33,34] have been described in pregnancy. As the fetus is entirely dependent on the mineral supply from the mother, intrauterine rickets may ensue[35,36]. Vitamin D deficiency is particularly common in breast-fed infants[37], and in those that have *not* been taking supplements[38,39].

Neonates of mothers with vitamin D deficiency, in the weeks and months following birth, are prone to hypocalcaemia[40], with seizures resulting, which can be difficult to treat[41].

NON-PREGNANCY TREATMENT AND CARE

- Women who follow Southeast Indian subcontinent culture and cover themselves are advised to take regular vitamin D supplements
- A treatment regime of im cholecalciferol (300,000 IU) twice monthly with an oral course of calcium (1000 mg) and cholecalciferol (20 micrograms daily) should resolve vitamin D deficiency within three months[42]
- 'Sensible sunlight' exposure should be encouraged

PRE-CONCEPTION ISSUES AND CARE

- Ideally all *at risk* prospective mothers should be routinely supplemented with vitamin D
- Those with severe deficiency should avoid pregnancy until this has been corrected
- Vitamin and mineral deficiencies may be precipitated by repeated pregnancies at short intervals – appropriate family spacing is a way of minimising this risk

Pregnancy Issues

Ideally, as the population most at risk from vitamin D deficiency is well defined, routine supplementation with vitamin D, 400 IU should be given daily. This should avoid any of the rare cases of advanced osteomalacia presenting in pregnancy with possible skeletal complications.

The Committee on Medical Aspects of Food and Nutritional Policy (COMA) has recommended vitamin D supplementation of 10 micrograms daily to all pregnant women, especially women with a cultural background predisposed to vitamin D deficiency, who should take supplements under medical supervision even if not pregnant.

Medical Management and Care

- Prescribe vitamin D 400 IU daily supplements to a*t risk* mothers from onset of pregnancy
- If vitamin D deficiency is encountered later in pregnancy other dosage schedules have been used: from the third trimester onwards 1000 IU of vitamin D daily[43] or a single dose of 100,000–200,000 IU of vitamin D in the sixth or seventh month of pregnancy[44] (the latter should only be used under specialist supervision)
- Generalised musculoskeletal symptoms may be difficult to evaluate and blood biochemistry is diagnostic: raised serum alkaline phosphatase of bone origin indicates more advanced vitamin D deficiency with possible skeletal complications and these women need careful monitoring

Midwifery Management and Care

- Report any musculoskeletal symptoms to the medical team
- Encourage mother to comply with nutritional doses of vitamin D supplements
- Advise women that if they use antacids heavily this could inhibit their vitamin D absorption[45,46]

Labour Issues

- In women with a contracted pelvis from childhood complications and osteomalacia, deformity will need to be carefully assessed

Medical Management and Care

- Careful assessment to see if caesarean section will be required

Midwifery Management and Care

- If pre-pregnancy treatment has been successful with no pelvic anomalies, then labour can be managed normally
- Careful observation of the progress of labour and relate to pelvic shape on vaginal examination
- Be aware that asynclitism can be an indication of a rachitic, contracted pelvis[46]

Postpartum Issues

Mother
- The mother should have been taking calcium and vitamin D supplements, and these should be continued postpartum

Neonate
- There may be some days before neonatal hypocalcaemia develops and mother and baby may already be discharged, so it is important to assess the biochemistry before discharge. Any jitteriness, muscular jerks or twitching should be taken seriously and appropriate treatment considered before full-blown grand mal seizures occur
- Infant biochemistry is diagnostic. Low 25(OH) vitamin D levels lead to low serum calcium and phosphate, raised serum alkaline phosphatase and parathyroid hormone levels (PTH). Some of these tests may take longer to obtain (25[OH] vitamin D and PTH)
- Treatment should be instigated in the infant on empirical grounds, but especially if there is hypocalcaemia and/or a raised alkaline phosphatase

Medical Management and Care

- Mothers will need assessment of their vitamin D status with appropriate biochemistry and consider bone densitometry
- Women with severe symptoms plus abnormal biochemistry may need pelvic and femoral X-rays after delivery to exclude pseudofractures
- Check the neonate's biochemistry (see Appendix 9.2) and give appropriate calcium and calciferol supplements
- If neonatal fits occur, paediatric assessment will be essential
- **Vitamin D deficiency in the mother**: if there has been any suspicion of this during pregnancy, especially during late pregnancy, then very careful assessment of the newborn will be required; close liaison should be kept with a neonatologist

Midwifery Management and Care

- If breast-feeding, women will require adequate vitamin D supplementation, and advice about avoidance of a further pregnancy until the condition is completely resolved
- Breast-feeding should not be prolonged in the presence of maternal hypovitaminosis D or osteomalacia
- Upon discharge the parents should be advised about signs of neonatal seizures and the need to seek urgent medical advice

9.5 Osteoporosis

Incidence	Risk for Childbearing
1:3 post-menopausal women[1]	Variable Risk
Rare in pregnancy	

EXPLANATION OF CONDITION[1,2]

Osteoporosis

Osteoporosis is a progressive, systemic skeletal disease characterised by low bone mass and micro-architectural deterioration of bone tissue with a consequent increase in bone fragility and susceptibility to bone fracture.

A more clinically relevant definition of osteoporosis is made on bone mineral density measurement (BMD). BMD is usually measured at the lumbar spine, hip and the radius. Results are expressed in grams per centimetres squared (g/cm^2) as an area density expressed as standard deviations related to the BMD of young adults (T-score). Results can be expressed as standard deviation related to age; this constitutes the Z-score. The WHO diagnostic classification is:

- T-score -1 or better: normal
- T-score between -1 and -2.5: osteopenia
- T-score below -2.5: osteoporosis
- T-score below -2.5 plus one or more osteoporotic fractures: clinical osteoporosis.

These criteria strictly apply to women, and at the sites of measurement of hip, spine and forearm.

Osteoporosis Associated with Pregnancy[2,3,4]

This is a rare condition in which women present with severe back pain and height loss due to vertebral collapse, usually in the third trimester of pregnancy. Often the diagnosis is not made until after delivery. Lateral spinal X-rays will show vertebral collapse. The aetiology is not clear but may be related to previous prolonged amenorrhoea, anorexia nervosa or mild forms of **osteogenesis imperfecta**. Osteogenesis imperfecta is an inherited bone disorder due to defective collagen known colloquially as 'brittle bone disease' that results in fractures of varying frequency and severity.

Pregnancy-related Osteoporosis of the Hip (transient)

This is a rare condition characterised by pain in the hip in the late second or third trimester of the pregnancy. There is no associated history of trauma or illness. Physical examination is essentially normal apart from pain in the hip on hip movement. This needs to be differentiated from joint infection or fracture and although X-rays are relatively contraindicated they need to be considered. This condition may be due to neurovascular ischaemia.

COMPLICATIONS[1,2]

Osteoporosis leads to bone fracture, especially lower radius, vertebral and hip fractures. There are estimated to be around 250,000 osteoporotic fractures each year in the UK.

Osteoporosis is common, with up to one in three women over the age of 50 years affected, especially very elderly women. In women of child-bearing age, osteopenia and osteoporosis are less common, but those with a family history of repeated fractures, prolonged amenorrhoea, and steroid use are at risk of worsening bone density during pregnancy and breast-feeding. This may increase chances of worsening post-menopausal bone health with risk of fractures in later life.

NON-PREGNANCY TREATMENT AND CARE

Women of child-bearing age who have osteopenia or osteoporosis will require appropriate medical attention either in primary and/or secondary care. Advice on diet and exercise are as below. Also see note below regarding bisphosphonate therapy.

PRE-CONCEPTION ISSUES AND CARE

Women with osteoporosis or osteogenesis imperfecta contemplating pregnancy should be encouraged to seek pre-conception care. This should be tailored to the physical condition and personal circumstances, to encompass:

- Re-referral to a physician if an existing treatment is associated with osteoporosis, in particular low-molecular-weight heparin (LMWH) and certain steroids
- Calculate the body mass index (see Appendix 13) to determine if weight needs to be gained, as with anorexia nervosa, or lost, as with obesity[4]
- Encourage a well-balanced diet, rich in calcium, vitamin D and other vitamins[4] (daily dietary requirements are to be found in Appendix 1.3)
- Some mothers may require vitamin supplementation
- Smoking and alcohol consumption should be strongly discouraged[4]
- Encourage regular, gentle exercise of which swimming is a good example[4]
- Specific relaxation techniques to help with pain, and exercises to develop muscle strength, are found in the National Osteoporosis Society's booklet (see Essential Reading)
- Advise that breast-feeding may not be possible for some
- Old fractures to femur, hip or spine can cause sexual difficulties, so advice on coital position may be needed[4]
- Women receiving bisphosphonate therapy should be made aware that the safety of these drugs is unproven in pregnancy and lactation[5] and are therefore contraindicated in pregnancy; bisphosphonates remain in bones for a long time, and will continue to be released into the woman's circulation ≥18 months[6]
- Women having had osteoporosis in a previous pregnancy need careful assessment and advice prior to planning a future pregnancy

Pregnancy Issues

Osteoporosis associated with pregnancy
Vertebral collapse presenting for the first time in pregnancy is rare and making the diagnosis is all important. Characteristically, vertebral collapse occurs in the third trimester but may occur any time until after delivery. Sudden, severe back pain in the thoracic and/or lumbar spinal region, persisting for some weeks or even months, are the main clinical features.

Pregnancy-related osteoporosis of the hip
For cases of sudden onset of pain in the hip, fracture, infection, tendonitis and muscle sprain osteoporosis will need to be considered.

Related issues
Some medications – steroids, prolonged heparin therapy – are associated with increased risk of osteoporosis.

Identification of fractures in pregnant women raises a possibility of domestic violence. Hence, there is a theoretical risk of misattribution of fractures to domestic violence with the possibility of osteoporosis being overlooked.

Medical Management and Care

Osteoporosis associated with pregnancy
- Lateral spinal X-rays showing vertebral collapse would be diagnostic, and careful judgement would be needed about the need to do these as there is a relative contraindication
- Other imaging modalities may be discussed with local radiology services
- Pain management (see Appendix 9.1)
- Apart from calcium and vitamin D preparations other specific treatment for osteoporosis can be deferred until after delivery

Pregnancy-related osteoporosis of the hip
- To exclude possible infection of the hip: pulse and temperature, together with FBC including WBC and CRP, will be needed
- To exclude hip fracture X-rays will need to be considered and this will require careful clinical judgement about the need to do this
- Reduced bone density on X-rays is characteristic of this condition

Midwifery Management and Care
- Careful booking history including weight, BMI and dietary history
- Advice on a calcium- and vitamin-D-rich diet with *no* alcohol, referring to a dietician if indicated
- Calcium based antacids rather than magnesium based (see Section 9.4)
- Confer with medical staff over vitamin supplementation
- Take the mother's concerns seriously and do not dismiss pain as a minor disorder of pregnancy, UTI or even signs of labour
- Observe the mother's gait at every appointment, as anomalies may indicate hip or pelvic pathology
- Be alert for signs of infection (see above)
- Ascertain infant feeding expectations, preparing for the possibility of formula feeding
- Tailor antenatal education (parent-craft) accordingly

Labour Issues
- Labour will be managed according to the clinical circumstances. In the unusual circumstance of collapsed vertebra or fracture of pelvis occurring during labour appropriate management will need to be considered
- The level of vertebral collapse will influence the possibility or otherwise of regional anaesthesia. Anaesthetic review is therefore recommended
- There is increased risk of venous thrombo-embolism (VTE) if the mother has restricted mobility

Medical Management and Care

Osteoporosis associated with pregnancy
- If vertebral collapse is suspected or confirmed the mode of delivery needs review

Midwifery Management and Care
- Care with handling should lithotomy position be required
- TED stockings and gentle passive exercises may be necessary to address the VTE risk

Postpartum Issues
- If the diagnosis has not been confirmed then lateral spinal X-rays and bone mineral density investigations will be needed
- Vertebral fractures may present anytime after delivery up to a few weeks or a month or so; sudden onset of severe and persistent back pain should be therefore considered carefully

Future pregnancies
If no cause is found, recurrence of spinal osteoporosis is not usual but osteoporosis of the hip can recur. Careful review and advice will need to be given.

Medical Management and Care

Osteoporosis associated with pregnancy
- Calcium and vitamin D supplementation will need to be considered
- Specialist advice will need to be sought about starting bisphosphonate or other specific therapy for osteoporosis
- If this problem arises after delivery, then X-rays and other management issues discussed above will need to be considered

Pregnancy-related osteoporosis of the hip
- X-ray bone densitometry
- Specific therapy requires specialist input
- Physiotherapy will normally be helpful

Midwifery Management and Care
- Controlling pain postpartum
- Breast-feeding needs careful assessment and may not be advisable
- Address practical issues, such as picking up the baby and self-care

9 Musculoskeletal Disorders

PATIENT ORGANISATIONS

The Pelvic Partnership
26 Manor Green
Harwell
Oxon. OX11 OEL
www.pelvicpartnership.org.uk

Disability, Pregnancy & Parenthood International
National Centre for Disabled Parents
Unit F9, 89-93 Fonthill Road
London N4 3JH
www.dppi.org.uk

Association to aid the Sexual and Personal Relationships of People with a Disability (SPOD)
www.spod-uk.org

National Osteoporosis Foundation USA
1232 22nd Street NW
Washington DC, USA
www.nof.org

National Osteoporosis Society
Camerton
Bath BA2 OPJ
www.nos.org.uk

Brittle Bones Society
Grant Patterson House
30 Guthrie Street
Dundee DD1 5BS
www.brittlebone.org

Strongbones Children's Charitable Trust
SCCT House
Kemp Road
Dagenham
Essex RM8 1ST
www.strongbones.org.uk

Women's Health (UK)
52 Featherstone Street
London EC1Y 8RT
www.womenshealthlondon.org.uk

Food Standards Agency
Aviation House
125 Kingsway
London C2B 6NH
www.food.gov.uk

The British Pain Society
Churchill House, 35 Red Lion Square
London WC1R 4SG
www.britishpainsociety.org

ESSENTIAL READING

Brayshaw, E. (2003) **Exercises for Pregnancy and Childbirth: A Practical Guide for Educators**. London; Books for Midwives/Elsevier.

Campbell, G., Compston, J. and Crisp, A. (1993) **The Management of Common Metabolic Bone Disorders**. Cambridge; Cambridge University Press.

Compston, J.E. and Rosen, C.J. (2004) **Fast Facts – Osteoporosis**, 4th Edn. Oxford; Health Press.

Fordham, J. (2004) **Your Questions Answered: Osteoporosis.** London; Churchill Livingstone/Elsevier.

Fry, D., Hay-Smith, J., Hough, J., McIntosh, J., Polden, M., Shepherd, J. and Watkins, Y. (1997) Symphysis pubis dysfunction – a guideline. **Physiotherapy, 83**(1).
NB: Currently under review (2007), and available from The Association of Chartered Physiotherapists in Women's Health.

Jain, S., Eedarapalli, P., Jamjute, P. and Sawdy, R. (2006) Review – Symphysis pubis dysfunction: a practical approach to management. **The Obstetrician and Gynaecologist, 6:**153–6.

NOS (2003) **Osteoporosis associated with pregnancy.** Bath; National Osteoporosis Society.

RCOG **Exercise in Pregnancy** (2006) Statement No. 4 http://www.rcog.org.uk/resources/Public/pdf/exercise_pregnancy_rcog_statement4.pdf

Roche, S. and Hughes, E.W. (1999) Pain problems associated with pregnancy and their management. **Pain Reviews, 6:**239–261.

Sutcliffe, A. (2006) **Osteoporosis: A guide for health professionals**. Chichester; Whurr/John Wiley.

Wainwright, M., Fishburn, S., Tudor-Williams, N., Naoum, H. and Garner, V. (2003) Symphysis pubis dysfunction: improving the service. **British Journal of Midwifery, 11**(11):664–667.

GASTROINTESTINAL DISORDERS

10

Manjiri Khare, Rosemary Lydall, Caroline Farrar and S. Elizabeth Robson

10.1 Gastro-oesophageal Reflux and Hiatus Hernia

Incidence	Risk for Childbearing
Heartburn: 20–40% adults[1] and >80% pregnant women[2] Hiatus Hernia: 20% of endoscopy patients[3]	Low Risk

EXPLANATION OF CONDITION

Heartburn

Heartburn is a burning sensation experienced in the region of the heart and in the throat[4] usually resulting from gastro-oesophageal reflux[5].

Gastro-oesophageal Reflux

Gastro-oesophageal reflux arises from a neuromuscular weakness in the lower oesophageal sphincter of the stomach. This results in the stomach contents regurgitating into the oesophagus[4]. As the stomach contents contain hydrochloric acid, the mucosa of the oesophagus is easily irritated resulting in the burning sensation of heartburn. **Dyspepsia** may result, entailing pain and discomfort after eating, sometimes accompanied by flatulence or belching, and is commonly known as 'indigestion'.

Reflux and heartburn are a particular problem in pregnancy, where progesterone reduces the muscle tone of the lower oesophageal sphincter, resulting in impaired competence with regards to closure[6]. The effects are elaborated on the next page.

Gastro-oesophageal Reflux Disease (GORD; GERD in USA)

After repeated reflux episodes **oesophagitis** can result. When combined with the cardinal symptom of heartburn[1], it becomes a disease with significant morbidity. Over time[1] insomnia and disturbed eating patterns may develop. Fortunately the mortality rate is low at 1:100,000[1].

Risk of developing GORD increases with age, noticeably once over 40 years of age[1]. It is associated with cigarette smoking, heavy alcohol consumption and increased intra-abdominal pressure[7] often associated with obesity or pregnancy.

Hiatus Hernia

Weakness of the diaphragmatic sphincter enables the lower oesophagus and upper part of the stomach to rise up through the diaphragm into the thorax[8]. This can take up to two years to develop[3] and is associated with obesity[9]. Gastro-oesophageal reflux may, or may not, accompany this[8] and impaired oesophageal emptying may ensue[10]. There are two forms:

1. **Sliding hiatus hernia**, in which the gastro-oesophageal junction literally 'slides up' through the hiatus (opening in the diaphragm) to lie just above the diaphragm but *below* the oesophagus[11]. It is more common in those aged >50 years, with oesophageal reflux usually the sole symptom[11]
2. **Rolling hiatus hernia**, in which part of the top of the stomach (fundus) literally 'rolls up' and herniates through the hiatus to lie *alongside* the oesophagus. The gastro-oesophageal junction stays below the diaphragm and remains competent[7,11]. There can be severe pain from volvulus or strangulation, usually necessitating surgery[11]

Investigations comprise barium swallow or endoscopy to identify the hernia and exclude other causes of symptoms[8].

COMPLICATIONS

- Altered weight
  - *weight gain* – as symptoms may be temporarily relieved by eating high carbohydrate or starch-based food
  - *weight loss* – due to dysphagia and dyspepsia[11]
- Dysphagia – difficulty with swallowing
- Oesophageal ulcers – can result with risk of bleeding[12]
- Barrett's oesophagus
  - acid reflux causes the squamous epithelium to be replaced by columnar epithelium
  - this neoplasia is a pre-malignant condition[12]

NON-PREGNANCY TREATMENT AND CARE

About 80% of people with reflux self-medicate with antacids, and only consult their GP once symptoms are prolonged and troublesome[5]. Appendix 10.1 algorithm outlines treatment from over-the-counter medications to referral.

First-line Management (lifestyle and diet)

- Measures to reduce obesity[5,7,8]
- Smoking cessation, and reduction of alcohol consumption[55]
- Avoidance of reflux-inducing foods, e.g. greasy, spicy foods, acidic products and carbonated drinks[5]
- Postural measures, such as raising the head of the bed and avoiding lying down for three hours after eating[5,8]
- Antacids for immediate relief, purchased over-the-counter[5]

Second-line Management (see Appendix 10.2 algorithm)

- Histamine$_2$-receptor antagonists (H$_2$RA)[5] to heal oesophagitis, e.g. cimeteidine or ranitidine[12]
- Proton-pump inhibitors[5] to inhibit gastric secretion[12], e.g. esomeprazole[14]
- Prokinetic drugs to increase oesophageal sphincter tone and enhance gastric emptying, e.g. metoclopramide

Third-line Management and Surgery

- Surgical repair of hernia in extreme cases[12,14]
- Emergency surgery may be needed for volvulus
- Malignancy investigation of Barrett's oesophagus

PRE-CONCEPTION ISSUES AND CARE

- High dose aluminium-based antacids can cause osteomalacia (rickets) in children[5], so a calcium-based alternative needs consideration for mothers at risk of osteomalacia or osteoporosis (see Sections 9.4 and 9.5)
- H$_2$RAs require review; ranitidine is preferred for pregnancy[15]
- Proton-pump inhibitor drugs are currently not recommended in pregnancy[14,15]. In intractable cases, this may be continued following careful counselling of the woman, with the current evidence published in literature
- If a woman is pending surgery she should be advised to delay conception until a full post-operative recovery has been made

Pregnancy Issues

- Pregnancy might be the first time that a woman experiences heartburn and reflux
- Reflux and heartburn are common problems in pregnancy, due to progesterone reducing the muscle tone of the lower oesophageal sphincter[6]
- Traditionally described as *minor disorders of pregnancy*[16] reflux and heartburn are considered a normal occurrence in a healthy pregnancy[15]
- Symptoms in pregnancy do not differ from the non-pregnant period[15], although they are exacerbated with multiple pregnancy
- The symptoms are likely to worsen in pregnancy[15] as both the progesterone level and intra-abdominal pressure increase
- Psychological support is necessary as many women feel 'miserable' with the symptoms as they worsen over pregnancy
- Serious reflux complications are rare in pregnancy; invasive diagnostic tests are infrequently needed[15]
- Pregnancy increases the chance of developing hiatus hernia as the rising progesterone level and mechanical effect of the expanding uterus cause the lower oesophageal sphincter to rise and become intrathoracic[6]; 10–20% of women are affected by late pregnancy[17]
- As hiatus hernia is age related, more women in the future could potentially present with this as a pre-existing condition if the average maternal age continues to rise

Medical Management and Care

Pre-existing condition
- Aluminium- or magnesium-containing antacids are considered safe in pregnancy[15]
- Avoid antacids containing sodium bicarbonate as they cause maternal or fetal metabolic alkalosis and fluid overload
- If on histamine$_2$-receptor antagonists, e.g. cimetidine, switch to ranitidine[5] for theoretical risk of interaction of cimetidine with androgen receptors; metoclopramide is also considered safe[2,15]
- Although proton-pump inhibitors are more effective in reducing gastric acid secretion these should be reserved for intractable cases not responding to H$_2$ receptor antagonists; a meta-analysis of 600 women with first trimester exposure to PPI did not show increased risk of teratogenicity[18]

Condition presenting in pregnancy
- Advise antacids as above
- See Appendix 10.1 algorithm for treatment options
- If there is dysphagia, bleeding, frequent vomiting or excessive weight loss refer for diagnostic evaluation[5]
- Endoscopy for diagnosis in cases with intractable reflux or atypical cases should not be delayed due to pregnancy as this can be performed safely under sedation[15]

Midwifery Management and Care
- Accurate booking history to determine and record previous treatment, and to identify current management and medication
- If a woman is taking Histamine$_2$-receptor antagonists or proton-pump inhibitors (Appendix 10.2) refer her to a doctor
- Heartburn and reflux without any other complications should not preclude a woman from low-risk midwifery care schemes
- Calculate the body mass index (Appendix 13), and if appetite is poor consider weighing the mother at each antenatal visit
- Reinforce lifestyle advice and use of antacids suitable for pregnancy
- The midwife should take the mother's concerns seriously and not dismiss them because of the 'minor disorders' categorisation
- Be aware that extreme symptoms of dysphagia or bleeding or frequent vomiting or excessive weight loss are suggestive of hiatus hernia and also complications such as 'strangulated hernia'. Therefore, such mothers require prompt medical review

Labour Issues

- The mechanical changes to the abdomen and thorax during labour may exacerbate symptoms
- It is preferable to avoid eating in labour as there is a potentially increased chance of reflux, with a theoretical risk of Mendelssohn's syndrome if general anaesthesia is undertaken

Medical Management and Care
- Avoid prolonged straining or pushing in second stage in women with known hiatus hernia
- Prophylactic ranitidine for women at risk, especially caesarean section under general anaesthesia, obese women and those with known GORD

Midwifery Management and Care
- In the absence of any significant complications, the labour can be managed normally by the midwife
- Prompt administration of ranitidine and allow water/isotonic drinks
- Additional antacids *might* be useful in this circumstance
- Have a vomit bowl discreetly near the mother throughout labour

Postpartum Issues

- Aluminium- and magnesium-based antacids are not concentrated in breast milk and are considered safe for breast-feeding mothers
- Histamine$_2$-receptor antagonists, such as ranitidine, pass into breast milk in small concentrations with an unknown effect on the baby[15] so they are used with caution
- Proton-pump inhibitors are not recommended for use in breast-feeding[15]

Medical Management and Care
- If iron is required postnatally as well as antacids, it is best to advise that they be taken at different times to allow absorption of the iron

Midwifery Management and Care
- Encourage breast-feeding; the mother should not return to her pre-pregnancy drugs without medical review, especially if breast-feeding; here advice on formula milk feeds may be necessary
- Explain that symptoms should improve as placental hormones diminish
- Reinforce the advice of first-line treatment (see previous page)
- Advise the mother to consult her general practitioner if her symptoms persist significantly after the puerperium

10.2 Coeliac Disease

Incidence	Risk for Childbearing
Active or symptomatic coeliac disease is approximately 1 per 1000 in Europe[1]	Variable Risk

EXPLANATION OF CONDITION

Coeliac disease is an inflammatory condition of the mucosa of the small bowel, which has been induced by gluten, a protein in cereals, wheat, rye and barley.

The inflammation, caused by gluten, leads to malabsorption in the proximal small bowel due to atrophy of the villi, which is associated with a decrease in the activity and amount of enzymes present in the surface epithelium. Injury caused to the intestinal villi is by an abnormal immune response to gliadin, a component of gluten. The precise cause of this condition still remains unknown but is related to a combination of genetic predisposition and environmental factors[2]. Factors such as the amount of gluten ingested, stress of a pregnancy or operation, or a gastrointestinal infection can exacerbate the condition, and if such stress factors are relieved the mucosa may return to normal.

Diagnosis of coeliac disease is made by small bowel biopsy together with serological tests for antigliadin and endomysial antibodies. It is becoming increasingly diagnosed with the use of serological screening tests that reveal cases of occult enteropathy[3].

Clinical features of this disease may become apparent during infancy and childhood but also in adulthood.

Infancy/childhood	Adulthood
Failure to thrive	Diarrhoea
Muscle wasting	Malabsorption
Diarrhoea	Anorexia
Abdominal distension	Weight loss
Short stature	Lethargy
Anaemia	Anaemia
	Infertility
	Abdominal pain
	Early menopause
	Recurrent miscarriage

COMPLICATIONS

There are many complications associated with coeliac disease if a gluten-free diet is not adhered to. Anaemia, osteoporosis, short stature and reproductive problems are associations secondary to malabsorption from coeliac disease. Some of the associated autoimmune disorders, cancer and neurological complications are more complex associations and cannot be explained by diet alone[4].

Malignant disease, such as small intestinal lymphoma, is increased as well as carcinoma of the small bowel. There are some reports related to an increased risk of squamous cell carcinoma of the oesophagus and pharynx[1].

Infertility is another associated complication of coeliac disease, including delayed menarche, relative infertility in men and women and premature menopause. Fertility will improve with treatment which includes a gluten-free diet and correction of nutritional deficiencies.

Other associations include **autoimmune** diseases, such as insulin dependent diabetes, thyroid disease and neurological syndromes. Another complication, which can affect up to 90% of patients, is **dermatitis herpetiformis**[1].

NON-PREGNANCY TREATMENT AND CARE

It is essential to follow a gluten-free diet (GFD) by avoiding products made from wheat, barley and rye. Some literature suggests oats should be initially avoided, especially if possibly contaminated by wheat flour[1]. If oats have not been contaminated by wheat flour they can be re-established safely into the diet.

A response is noticeable within at least three months in adults, and is clearly evident in children within a few weeks.

To be able to optimise care and ensure correct management, review of nutritional status of each patient is essential, together with regular follow-up appointments. It is important to consider this as a life-long condition that requires a gluten-restricted diet for life. If there is no improvement within three months this is usually due to non-compliance either intentional or accidental.

PRE-CONCEPTION ISSUES AND CARE

Gastrointestinal symptoms that may have been experienced in childhood may be seen again in pregnancy. This needs to be highlighted to the patient to ensure an awareness of the importance of a gluten-free or gluten-restricted diet and adherence to this as well.

Due to the nutritional requirements of pregnancy, referral to a dietician prior to pregnancy may alleviate any fears or anxieties the patient may have. Consequently, dietary advice can be discussed and monitored and any nutritional deficiencies can be addressed accordingly with dietary supplements if necessary.

As women with this condition have a predisposition to folate malabsorption, they should be advised to take higher doses of folate (5 mg) pre-conceptually, in order to optimise their levels of folic acid.

If the prospective mother has any other associated autoimmune diseases, issues surrounding the management of these conditions should be addressed on an individual basis.

Pregnancy Issues

Women who have been diagnosed with coeliac disease can experience an aggravated response during pregnancy and the puerperium.

Haematological disorders, for example megaloblastic and iron-deficiency anaemia, can present during pregnancy (see Sections 14.1 and 14.2).

Some studies have shown coeliac disease that is left untreated appears to carry an increased risk of miscarriage, fetal growth restriction and lower birth weight babies[5].

A gluten-free diet and further vitamin and mineral supplementations need to be given, especially folic acid, to aid protection against neural tube defects.

In the UK people with coeliac disease are able to obtain certain gluten-free dietary products on NHS prescription, however they usually have to pay prescription charges which can have an influence on dietary adherence.

Medical Management and Care

- Strict adherence to a gluten-free diet should be advised throughout pregnancy
- Anaemia can be associated as a common disorder in coeliac disease, therefore iron, folate and possibly vitamin B_{12} supplementation should be monitored and used appropriately
- Unexplained iron-deficiency or anaemia not responding to oral iron therapy, folate deficiency or vitamin B_{12} deficiency during pregnancy should be investigated to exclude coeliac disease
- Base-line calcium level measurement should be arranged at booking, and appropriate calcium supplementation given if hypocalcaemia is diagnosed
- Serial fetal growth scans should be arranged for pregnant women with coeliac disease

Midwifery Management and Care

- Ascertain if folic acid was initiated peri-conceptually, if not this needs to be implemented promptly in the first trimester
- Consideration should be given to vitamins and minerals within the diet, these include: vitamin B_{12}, folic acid, iron and trace elements such as zinc
- Encourage pregnant women to adhere to a gluten-free diet, because pregnancy has additional nutritional demands
- Prompt issuing of certification of pregnancy that entitles a mother to free prescriptions during pregnancy, because prescription charges for coeliac dietary products can impose a financial burden in pregnancy
- If a referral to a dietician is necessary this should be initiated promptly to appropriately consider any nutritional corrections that are required; such referrals are important if diabetes mellitus co-exists
- The consideration of increased folic acid is especially significant, due to the risk factor of neural tube defects; a nutritional assessment is required for both diet and supplements
- Ask about bowel motions as the mother is at risk of constipation, especially if taking iron tablets, and laxatives might be required

Labour Issues

Anaemia can be considered an issue in labour and therefore it is important to be aware of the woman's haemoglobin status in view of blood loss at delivery.

Medical Management and Care

- Intrapartum care should reflect the increased awareness of anaemia and consequences in labour

Midwifery Management and Care

- Discuss with the medical team if a FBC should be taken when the woman is admitted in labour, and if samples should be taken for group and save
- In view of a low haemoglobin status, active management of the third stage may be initiated, reducing the risk of a postpartum haemorrhage

Postpartum Issues

Breast-feeding appears to offer protection and decrease the risk of the development of coeliac disease in the newborn. This is dependent on breast-feeding[6] exclusively and also continuing to breast-feed during the introduction of gluten within the diet[7].

Other protective benefits conferred by breast-feeding are against gastrointestinal and respiratory infections[8].

Medical Management and Care

- Appropriate management of nutritional anaemia and continued emphasis on adherence to gluten-free diet should be an integral part of the care that these women receive from health professionals
- Encourage breast-feeding for its added benefits to the baby

Midwifery Management and Care

- If a woman's choice is to breast-feed exclusively this may act as a protective feature in the delay of onset of coeliac disease for the child, as symptoms usually occur at the time of weaning; hence the midwife should encourage and support breast-feeding
- The mother may worry that the baby could inherit the condition so any necessary follow-up appointments should be made, and the mother encouraged to seek the advice of the specialist public health nurse (health visitor) and attend child wellbeing clinics where weaning and infant feeding advice are given

10.3 Ulcerative Colitis

Incidence	Risk for Childbearing
60,000–120,000 in the UK – approximately 1:600 Most common age 15–35[1]	Variable Risk

EXPLANATION OF CONDITION

Ulcerative colitis (UC) is a chronic autoimmune disease of the bowel, characterised by mucosal inflammation in the colon. UC can be distal disease, confined to the rectum (proctitis), as in 95% of cases[2], or rectum with sigmoid colon (proctosigmoiditis). Alternatively, the disease can be more extensive, affecting parts of, or the whole colon[3]. A severe attack of UC is still a potentially life-threatening illness, due to the risk of haemorrhage caused by widespread mucosal ulceration or toxic megacolon causing perforation. If this happens, emergency colectomy must be performed immediately[3,4].

UC is diagnosed by stool examinations and sigmoidoscopic biopsies, which exclude Crohn's disease or infection.

Of patients with ulcerative colitis:

- 50% will have a relapse each year
- 20–30% will need a colectomy; however this is curative[3]

Symptoms include:

- Bloody diarrhoea
- Continence problems
- Abdominal pain

Aetiology is unknown. Smoking is known to decrease the risk of UC, although it is not known why[3].

COMPLICATIONS

In addition to the risk of perforation or toxicity, the symptoms and complications all lead to a poor quality of life and body image as follows:[5]

- Weight loss has an adverse effect on body image and self-esteem[6]
- Medical treatments such as corticosteroids or immunosuppressive drugs have their own unpleasant side effects, e.g. weight gain, Cushingoid features, osteoporosis, glaucoma, cataracts, infections[3]
- Ocular, oral, joint or skin changes are noted in some patients[2]
- Children may experience delays in onset of puberty
- Young adults may have trouble in forming intimate relationships
- Dyspareunia and recurrent vaginal candidiasis are more common than in healthy women[7]
- Increased risk of colonic carcinoma, particularly after about 8–10 years of disease
- Frequent laboratory and bowel investigations are necessary, mostly in the second decade of disease[3]

NON-PREGNANCY TREATMENT AND CARE

Treatment is based more on clinical severity of the attack than histology.

Treatment is primarily medical. The most common types of drugs used are aminosalicylates and corticosteroids. The combination of oral and topical aminosalicylates is more effective than monotherapy[2]. Aminosalicylates should be used in treatment of mild disease and steroids should be used for active disease. Long-term use of steroids is undesirable due to the side effects

For those patients with long-term chronic disease, or who are steroid dependent, azathioprine or 6-mercaptopurine (immune suppressants given to transplant recipients), are recommended. Newer agents are reserved for refractory disease (i.e. disease resistant to treatment).

Surgery is considered when a patient with UC does not respond to medical therapy. It is a decision that is made between the patient, the gastroenterologist and the colorectal surgeon. Surgery is also necessary if colonic carcinoma develops. Resection of the colon is then performed to form an ileostomy.

A rectal stump is left in some patients who may be considering the construction of an ileoanal pouch later. This involves removal of the colon and rectum, using the end of the ileum to form a new rectum or reservoir. If pouch surgery is not an option, due to poor sphincter efficiency or anal disease, a total pan-proctocolectomy may be considered, which includes removal of the rectum and closure of the anus[3].

PRE-CONCEPTION ISSUES AND CARE

- Fertility is not adversely affected by UC, with the possible exception of severely active disease.[8] However, voluntary infertility can be high, particularly if patients have had previous gastrointestinal surgery
- Preconceptual assessment for clinical activity of disease should be performed in liaison with gastroenterologist. This should include a full blood count, c-reactive protein, erythrocyte sedimentation rate, liver enzymes and albumin
- Sulfasalazine is in a group of drugs known as folic acid antagonists that have the potential of causing neural tube defects and other congenital abnormalities. Consequently, pre-conceptual folic acid supplementation is advised and a change to an alternative aminosalicylate preparation, such as mesalazine, that is considered safe in normal doses
- Conception during remission is advisable

Pregnancy Issues

As UC often occurs in young adults, managing the disease in pregnancy is not unusual. The risks of infertility are no different to those for a woman who does not suffer from UC[6,8], and 25% of women with UC will conceive following diagnosis[3].

Control during pregnancy is crucial for fetal and maternal health. Women may need to remain on medication to remain in remission, rather than risk an acute flare-up, which could hold more dangers for feto-maternal well being.[3]

Risks to pregnancy
- No significant increase in the rate of spontaneous miscarriage when compared with the normal population[8]
- An increased risk of pre-term birth, IUGR and caesarean section with active disease[9]
- If the woman has an ileostomy, there is a significant risk of a hernia or stomal prolapse developing, due to the increased strain on the weak abdominal walls
- Vomiting in pregnancy can also cause herniation of the small bowel

Medical Management and Care

In the event of acute flare-up:
- IV access with fluid and electrolyte replacement to prevent any dehydration or electrolyte imbalance
- FBC, ESR or CRP, serum electrolytes and liver function tests should be measured every 24–48 hours to monitor the severity of flare
- Flexible sigmoidoscopy can be used safely in pregnancy[6]
- Do not manage acute UC any differently than in non-pregnancy
- Azathioprine and corticosteroids to be continued as risks to fetus from disease outweigh risks from the continued therapy
- Emergency colectomy is not encouraged during pregnancy
- An intrapartum care plan to be agreed between the woman and the multi-disciplinary team (MDT) and documented in the notes

Midwifery Management and Care

- Involve the Inflammatory Bowel Disease nurse specialist (if available) as teamwork is fundamental to effective care
- Be aware that severe disease will require hospital admission, mild or moderate disease can be managed as an outpatient
- If hospital admission occurs, monitor the following:
  - stool frequency and condition
  - blood, mucous and consistency
  - four-hourly vital signs[3]
  - levels of abdominal pain and tenderness
- Due to the degree of 'urgency' UC women experience, it is essential that they have easy access to toilet facilities
- These women are prone to malnutrition, and may need referral to a dietician during pregnancy
- Regular weighing is essential

Labour Issues

Mode of delivery should be carefully planned and options discussed with the woman. This discussion will incorporate the multi-disciplinary team (MDT), so the woman can make an informed decision. Aim for vaginal delivery in most cases, unless severe or chronic disease is present. In these instances, a caesarean section may be offered in order to protect the anal sphincter from damage.

If the woman has already undergone gastrointestinal surgery, e.g. ileoanal pouch formation[3], or has an ileostomy, an elective LSCS may be offered, as an emergency LSCS would be very complex due to the scar tissue from previous surgery.

Medical Management and Care

- Aim for vaginal delivery unless disease is active
- Active disease – consider LSCS to protect the anal sphincter
- Prolonged second stage and difficult instrumental deliveries should be avoided to prevent anal sphincter damage, particularly if future surgery for ileoanal pouch is contemplated
- A senior obstetrician should perform caesarean if there is a history of previous gastrointestinal surgery, as there is a higher risk of bowel damage from previous adhesions

Midwifery Management and Care

- Quiescent disease – normal midwifery management of labour
- Keep woman well hydrated in labour
- Easy access to toilets, or alternative, is essential in labour
- There is no need for the midwife to have any concerns over bag management, if a woman with an ileostomy is labouring normally; assistance may be needed in emptying the appliance if the woman has an epidural and cannot get to the toilet

Postpartum Issues

- Anaemia may result from rectal bleeding, which is a symptom of active disease
- With haemoglobin already compromised, even the 'normal' bleeding at delivery may be detrimental to the woman's health
- If the disease remains quiescent, there are no significant postpartum issues
- With active disease, the mother may suffer from extreme tiredness; giving birth is a demanding experience, even without a chronic condition causing exhaustion
- Immunosuppressant drugs may be either contraindicated with breast-feeding, or used on a risk–benefit assessment basis, especially azathioprine (see Appendix 11)

Medical Management and Care

- Treat any anaemia
- If breast-feeding while taking azathioprine or 6-MP it is advisable for the baby to be monitored for clinical signs of immunosuppression and regular complete blood counts should be taken[10,11]
- A four-hour delay in breast-feeding following oral corticosteroid use is recommended by most manufacturers; this has practical implications and, after observation, steroids appear to be safe[6]

Midwifery Management and Care

- Support the mother in her choice of infant feeding, and deflect any guilt she may feel if she is not breast-feeding
- Be aware of the extreme tiredness and assist as needed
- Ascertain if the woman has any help at home
- Ensure that the mother and her relatives understand the need for rest
- Advise the mother:
  - that housework is not essential
  - to rest when the baby rests

10.4 Crohn's Disease

Incidence	Risk for Childbearing
50–100 per 100,000 Affects men and women equally Most common age 15–25[1]	Variable Risk

EXPLANATION OF CONDITION

Crohn's disease (CD) was identified in 1932 by Dr Burril Crohn. It comprises chronic inflammation, ulceration and scarring anywhere from mouth to rectum, but most commonly the small intestine. It is characterised by patchy inflammation that passes through the wall of the intestine, affecting each layer[2].

Symptoms include[1,2]:

- Colicky abdominal pain
- Urgent diarrhoea, leading to dehydration and nutritional deficiencies
- Severe tiredness
- Weight loss
- Malaise, anorexia and fever

Although the aetiology is unknown at present, it is considered that the condition is in response to environmental triggers, such as infections and drugs. Research shows a familial link with first degree relatives who have inflammatory bowel disease (IBD), but not necessarily the same IBD – some may develop ulcerative colitis (UC), others CD[3,4].

COMPLICATIONS

The symptoms can be embarrassing and cause poor self-esteem, leading to loss of education in the young and difficulties in gaining employment in adults[5]. CD causes greater disability than UC as only 75% of patients are fully capable of work in the year following diagnosis[2].

The main complications comprise:

- Intestinal obstruction caused by adhesions or by visceral distension in the presence of dilation
- Fissures in the anal canal
- Fistulas can develop as the inflammation affects all layers of the bowel
- Abscesses in the pelvis, abdomen or ischiorectal area
- Increased risk of gall stones, renal calculi and chronic pancreatitis
- Arthritis, iritis and painful skin complications often associated with the flare-ups themselves
- Increased risk of bowel carcinoma

NON-PREGNANCY TREATMENT AND CARE

- As there is no known cure, treatment is symptomatic
- Care should always be offered by a gastroenterologist who specialises in IBD
- An individual's own knowledge of their condition should always be respected
- After taking a full history, a general assessment of wellbeing, including BP, pulse, temperature, blood investigations, hydration, weight loss and abdominal examination is needed
- Discourage smoking, as this aggravates the condition[2]

- Colonoscopy is useful in endoscopic and histological assessment of large bowel and distal ileum
- MRI can be performed for assessment of perianal fistulating disease
- Stool culture and microscopy to exclude infective aetiology and rule out concurrent *Clostridium difficile* infection
- ESR and CRP to monitor severity of inflammation

Medical Management

Medical management will depend on the site of disease, activity, course of disease, previous responses to drugs and extra-intestinal manifestations and hence this needs to be individualised:

- Anti-inflammatory drugs containing mesalamine (sulfasalazine) are commonly used as first-line management; steroids are used in tapering doses to treat flares
- Other drugs used are:
  - immunosuppressors such as 6-mercaptopurine (6-MP) or azathioprine
  - infliximab is an anti-inflammatory drug approved for use in the treatment of moderate to severe disease that is not responding to standard treatment
- Commonly used antibiotics, which may be indicated in stricture or fistula infection, are:
  - ampicillin
  - cephalosporins
  - tetracycline
  - metronidazole
- Non-steroidal anti-inflammatory drugs (NSAIDs) should be avoided as they can cause inflammation and bleeding in the small intestine

Surgical Management

Surgery may be required to remove damaged parts of the intestine[1]. However, it is not a cure as with UC, and should only be used in symptomatic disease not responding to medical treatment or for complications such as abscess, perforation, strictures or bleeding in the bowel.

Common types of surgery include:

- **Bowel resection**: removing the affected part of the intestine, usually conservative
- **Strictureplasty**: opening up narrowed sections of bowel
- **Colectomy** and **ileostomy:** the complete removal of the colon and creating a stoma for waste elimination

PRE-CONCEPTION ISSUES AND CARE

- Fertility is generally not affected unless active disease is present[6,3,7]
- Due to complications during pregnancy from having active Crohn's disease at conception, planning to conceive when disease is quiescent is very important[3,7]
- Crohn's disease causes folate deficiency, as does the use of sulfasalazine, which is a folate antagonist
- Folic acid supplements of 5 mg daily rather than the usual 400 micrograms are needed[3] and supplements should continue throughout the pregnancy

Pregnancy Issues

- One third of women with inactive disease at conception can expect to relapse during the pregnancy or puerperium; relapse rate similar for non-pregnant patient[3]
- Conception during remission is advised:
  - If conception occurs during active disease, two thirds of women will continue to have disease activity and two-thirds of these will deteriorate[8]
  - Active disease is associated with miscarriage, IUGR and prematurity[3]
- Control of the disease during pregnancy is important, therefore drug therapy should not be discontinued; disease activity is more dangerous than the drugs used
- Any exacerbation of Crohn's disease should be investigated and treated promptly
- Anaemia is common and may be due to iron, folate or vitamin B_{12} deficiency as a result of malabsorption
- Emergency surgery in pregnancy is associated with high fetal loss (60%) and any necessary elective surgery should be deferred until after pregnancy[3]

Medical Management and Care

- Due to the adverse effect on the fetus and pregnancy from active disease, it is important to continue maintenance therapy and respond promptly to any flare-ups of Crohn's disease
- Prompt investigation with serum electrolytes, liver function tests and C–reactive proteins should be performed to assess clinical condition in case of flare of disease
- Corticosteroids can be used orally, intravenously or as rectal enemas as required in case of flare of disease; oral and local forms of 5-aminosalicylic acid derivatives and Salazopyrin compounds are considered safe in pregnancy; metronidazole is used to treat anal fistulas
- Monthly full blood count, serum folic acid and vitamin B_{12} levels should be monitored during pregnancy, as there is increased risk of nutritional anaemia due to malabsorption
- Folic acid 5 mg daily supplementation to continue throughout pregnancy, as folate deficiency can arise with Crohn's disease
- Oral or parental iron therapy or blood transfusion may be required depending on the degree of anaemia
- Sigmoidoscopy can be performed safely during pregnancy but colonoscopy may be deferred until the puerperium; in case of life-threatening complications requiring surgery, the management should be the same as for non-pregnant women[2]

Midwifery Management and Care

- Nutrition is a major component in the treatment of CD as malnutrition is common, so referral to a dietician is advisable
- Involve the IBD nurse specialist who is an expert that can liaise with the mother and the multi-disciplinary team

Labour Issues

- Vaginal delivery is not contraindicated unless there is active perianal disease or an ileoanal pouch
- There is evidence that there is a risk of perianal Crohn's disease developing following vaginal birth and episiotomy; if a woman already has perianal CD then delivery by LSCS is more appropriate[9,10]
- Generally the section rate is increased compared to non-sufferers of CD (15% compared to 10%)[3]

Medical Management and Care

- Mothers with either colostomy or ileostomy can deliver vaginally
- Good intrapartum care of the perineum should be encouraged and perineal trauma should be minimised
- A senior obstetrician should perform caesarean section in cases with previous bowel surgery as there is increased risk of injury to bowel, bladder or other viscera due to previous adhesions
- If necessary, a surgeon should be available

Midwifery Management and Care

- An experienced midwife should care for the woman in labour
- Perineal trauma should be minimised

Postpartum issues

- There are no known problems when Crohn's disease is quiescent

Medical Management and Care

- Sulfasalazine, oral or topical mesalazine and corticosteroids are considered safe in breast-feeding[8]
- As very small amounts of azathioprine and 6-mercaptopurine metabolites appear in breast milk this should be discussed on an individual basis and babies should be monitored clinically and haematologically for signs of immunosuppression[11,12]
- Ciclosporine and infliximab should be avoided when breast-feeding, as there is no safety data available[8]

Midwifery Management and Care

- Breast-feeding should be encouraged for its benefits (mothers may be concerned if they are currently receiving medication)
- If breast-feeding while taking azathioprine or 6-mercaptopurine, it is advisable for the baby to be monitored for clinical signs of immunosuppression and regular full blood counts should be taken[11,12]

10.5 Irritable Bowel Syndrome

Incidence	**Risk for Childbearing**
10–15% of adult population in the UK[1]	Low Risk
86% of those affected are women[2]	

EXPLANATION OF CONDITION

Irritable bowel syndrome (IBS) is a functional disorder of the intestines. IBS appears to be the result of motor disturbances in the intestine that respond to certain stimuli[3]. As there is no clear 'disease' or pathology with IBS, it is diagnosed by excluding other bowel disorders and by ensuring the absence of certain 'red flag' features[1]:

- Rectal bleeding
- Anaemia
- Weight loss
- Late age of onset or acute onset
- Family history of bowel cancer or IBD
- Signs of infection

A detailed medical history is taken using the 'Rome criteria'. This is a symptom-based classification system that assists clinicians in examining the symptoms before coming to a diagnosis[4] (see Appendix 10.3).

Symptoms

- Abdominal pain related to defecation
- Altered bowel habits, ranging from diarrhoea to constipation to 'normal'
- Abdominal bloating
- A feeling of incomplete evacuation and mucous in the stools[2]

COMPLICATIONS

- All the symptoms of IBS can erode quality of life and influence relationships with family and friends and cause absenteeism from work
- Diarrhoea or constipation can aggravate or cause haemorrhoids

NON-PREGNANCY TREATMENT AND CARE

IBS cannot be cured, but patients will have periods of remission between the bouts of disease activity[2]. The most effective way to manage IBS is to remain patient centred.

Maintaining a stool chart that also describes the stools, will aid the doctor in treating the symptoms[2].

Dietary Management

Keeping a dietary history may also reveal problem areas that can be addressed by altering habits. A fibre-rich diet may be advised when the stool requires 'bulking out' or constipation is present, although for some patients this can make their symptoms worse. Caffeine, alcohol, fat and sorbitol-rich foods (e.g. ice cream, chewing gum, honey and jam) are known to aggravate IBS and should be taken in moderation[2].

IBS can be exacerbated by dietary habits rather than specific foods, e.g. large, rushed or irregular meals[2] are also predictors of symptom intensity, with the absence of stress manifesting improved symptoms[5].

Psychological Therapy

It has been identified that IBS patients respond positively to the placebo effect of a caring physician. As there are psychological influences on IBS, the most important aspects of treatment are to listen, validate the symptoms, educate the patient and identify reinforcing and coping strategies with each individual[6].

Psychosocial factors such as a history of abuse should be addressed by the physicians caring for these women in a sensitive manner. Some women may require additional psychiatric or psychological intervention. Some of these include relaxation therapy, hypnosis, cognitive behavioural therapy and biofeedback techniques.

Pharmacological Treatment

Psychotropic agents can modify the symtoms of IBS by their action in modulating psychosocial factors, e.g. antidepressant medications (tricyclic antidepressants) in women who have major depression as co-morbidity with IBS. They can also modify the pain threshold in these patients.

The choice of antidepressants will depend on the main presenting complaints and side-effect profiles for the individual patient. Tricyclic antidepressants are likely to be more effective in cases of diarrhoea and abdominal pain, due to its anticholinergic activity. A sedating tricyclic antidepressant may be useful when there are associated sleep problems, whereas selective serotonin re-uptake inhibitors (SSRI) such as fluoxetine may help in cases that have constipation or bloating[7].

Anticholinergic medications such as diphenoxylate can be used to control pain and diarrhoea. Antidiarrhoeals like loperamide and cholestyramine are used if diarrhoea is a dominant symptom. Constipation may be treated with Lactulose.

Antibiotics must be used with caution as some, e.g. erythromycin, can exacerbate IBS[1].

PRE-CONCEPTION ISSUES AND CARE

The individual may find pregnancy easier to cope with if her IBS symptoms are not too severe. Avoiding stress, using individualised coping mechanisms and following dietary advice may all assist in keeping the IBS in abeyance.

Pregnancy Issues
- Normal hormonal changes in pregnancy can alter bowel habits even in the absence of irritable bowel disease
- IBS is not debilitating even though the mother's quality of life is affected

Medical Management and Care
- Diagnosis of IBS during pregnancy is difficult due to the normal physiological changes in the bowel
- Exacerbation of known IBS could also be difficult to diagnose for the same reasons
- Avoid foods that trigger the symptoms
- Antidepressants are sometimes used in the treatment of non-pregnant women for severe pain
- Selective serotonin re-uptake inhibitors (SSRIs) have not been shown to cause any major fetal problems other than irritability in neonates, thought to be due to withdrawal from the drug[3]
- Adequate fluid intake and bulking agents are used to manage constipation
- Loperamide has been used for treatment of diarrhoea in one prospective multi-centre study: no significant differences were found in the rate of major or minor malformations with matched controls following exposure in the first trimester[8]

Midwifery care
- Give dietary advice as usual, responding to each bowel symptom
  - high fibre diet
  - multiple smaller meals
  - drink plenty of water
  - avoid stimulant drinks, e.g. caffeinated tea and coffee
  - avoid gas-producing food
- Psychological support is paramount, rather than drug therapy in pregnancy

Labour Issues
- There are no significant labour issues with IBS

Medical Management and Care
- There are no specific issues related to IBS although offering early pain relief may help to reduce the stress related to painful labour

Midwifery care
- Supportive care in labour

Postpartum Issues
- No postpartum issues other than to continue with dietary advice and psychological support
- As stress is a major factor in IBS, this could influence symptoms either way, depending on how the individual approaches the experience of having a newborn:
  - some sufferers may be so preoccupied with caring for the new baby that the focus is removed from their own symptoms and consequently they improve
  - other women may find the experience so traumatic, that it has a negative influence on their IBS

Medical Management and Care
- Debriefing individuals who may have had difficult or traumatic birth experiences and dealing with those at risk of postpartum depression may reduce the trigger factors for worsening of pre-existing IBS

Midwifery care
- Continue with psychological support, demonstrating a caring positive demeanour
- Be ready to acknowledge and validate any symptoms
- Persist with dietary advice

10.6 Haemorrhoids

Incidence	**Risk for Childbearing**
50% of adult UK population at some stage in their life More frequent in pregnancy[1]	Low Risk

EXPLANATION OF CONDITION

Within the anal canal lie three vascular, fibrovascular cushions of submucosal tissue, which are suspended by connective tissue arising from the internal anal sphincter and the longitudinal muscle of the anal canal. The role of these cushions is to maintain continence. If this connective tissue breaks down, prolapse will occur. Once this has happened the venous pressure will increase and the venous return will be impaired, the cushions then become engorged and dilated[1].

Classification of Haemorrhoids
- First degree – haemorrhoids bleed but do not prolapse
- Second degree – haemorrhoids prolapse on straining but then return spontaneously
- Third degree – haemorrhoids prolapse on straining but then require manual reduction
- Fourth degree – haemorrhoids remain prolapsed and cannot be reduced manually

Rarely, an external haemorrhoid can develop on the outside edge of the anus – this is sometimes called a perianal haematoma.

Predisposing Factors[2]
- Straining to defecate, as with constipation or, by contrast, with chronic diarrhoea
- Pregnancy, due to poor venous return and relaxation of the smooth muscles
- Obesity
- Low-fibre diet
- Weakened pelvic floor[3]

Symptoms[2]
- Rectal bleeding
- Itching round anus
- Pain/discomfort on defecation
- Mucous discharge
- Feeling of incomplete evacuation

COMPLICATIONS

Complications include[4]:

- Strangulation – when the prolapsed haemorrhoid swells considerably so prevents venous return
- Thrombosis – if the blood in the swollen haemorrhoid clots, forming a thrombosed haemorrhoid
- Gangrene, if haemorrhoid blood supply is reduced
- Infection, leading to an abscess

NON-PREGNANCY TREATMENT AND CARE

Investigations are needed for correct diagnosis and exclusion of other disorders with rectal bleeding. Haemorrhoids are not always felt by performing a rectal examination; hence proctoscopy or sigmoidoscopy may be undertaken by the doctor. These investigations may need to be performed by a general or colorectal surgeon. Treatment is based on severity of symptoms, and the best treatment is prevention[5].

Conservative Treatment

Mostly treatment is conservative and includes[4]:

- High-fibre diet, including fibre supplements
- Remain well hydrated – at least two litres water per day
- Avoid codeine based analgesics, which are constipating
- Ice packs may be held in place for 15–20 minutes for immediate relief
- Warm baths to relieve itching
- Re-education in toileting habits:
  - Do not suppress the need to evacuate
  - Do not strain
  - Do not spend too long sitting on the toilet

Medical Treatment[1]
- Ointments and creams may ease the symptoms, but are not curative; a plain ointment may ease the itch
- Anaesthetic based creams may relieve the pain
- A steroid based cream, if there is inflammation
- Strong analgesia for an acute attack or complication

Surgical Treatment[1,6]
- Rubber band ligation: a band is placed around the haemorrhoid's base, causing it to become necrotic and fall off
  - usually performed as an outpatient
  - 79% successful with first- to third-degree haemorrhoids[1]
- Sclerotherapy: an injection of phenol into the pedicle causes tissue necrosis and can be used as an alternative to banding in outpatients for first- and second-degree haemorrhoids
- Cryosurgery: freezing causes the haemorrhoids to shrink and fall off
- Haemorrhoidectomy is recommended for fourth-degree haemorrhoids, or third-degree unresponsive to banding
- Stapled haemorrhoidopexy involves excising a section of anal mucosa, blocking the blood supply so that the haemorrhoids shrink[7]
  - has superseded haemorrhoidectomy: more rapid recovery and reduction in post-operative pain

PRE-CONCEPTION ISSUES AND CARE

- Avoid trying to conceive soon after haemorrhoid surgery as extra pressure on the pelvic floor could cause strain on the rectum
- Any conservative treatment would be safe in pregnancy
- Most medical treatments would be safe, with the exception of strong analgesia – this would need further discussion with the pharmacist or GP
- Surgical treatment may be avoided until the postnatal period, in order to assess the extent of the damage

Pregnancy Issues

As it enlarges, the uterus puts pressure on the pelvic veins and the inferior vena cava. This slows the return of blood from the lower half of the body, increasing the pressure on the veins below the level of the uterus and causing them to become more dilated or swollen. This makes the woman more prone to haemorrhoids – possibly her first experience.

- Management will depend on the severity of the condition
- As with non-pregnant treatment, it is necessary to confirm diagnosis and exclude any other more serious disorders e.g. Crohn's disease and ulcerative colitis

Medical Management and Care

- Antenatal management should be conservative as far as possible with diet modification, local creams and analgesia
- Urgent referral should be arranged for evaluation by surgeons in women with prolapsed haemorrhoids or any rectal bleeding
- Surgical intervention in pregnancy should be performed only in intractable cases
- Although there are studies published regarding efficacy of rutosides in reducing symptoms in pregnant women with first- and second-degree haemorrhoids, there is insufficient safety data at present; it is advisable to avoid these during pregnancy until further data is available[8]

Midwifery Management and Care

- Conservative treatment may continue, giving the same advice as for a non-pregnant woman – laxatives and high-fibre diet[1,8,9]
- Medical referral if this is the first episode or if the haemorrhoids become more severe
- It is unlikely that any operative measures will be undertaken, as the haemorrhoids may improve after delivery
- Encourage pelvic floor exercises, because the pelvic floor will be weakened as a result of pregnancy which will exacerbate the severity of the haemorrhoids
- Give advice on measures to avoid constipation

Labour Issues

- Haemorrhoids may prolapse with pushing in the second stage

Medical Management and Care

- In women with symptomatic haemorrhoids, avoid a prolonged second stage

Midwifery Management and Care

- Avoid prolonged active pushing in the second stage
- If the haemorrhoids prolapse, applying a cream may soothe any discomfort

Postpartum Issues

- One third of women will have exposed thrombosed haemorrhoids following delivery[10]
- Most cases of haemorrhoids in pregnancy will improve by six weeks after the birth, but they can still be troublesome and painful in the immediate postnatal period
- They must not be dismissed as a *minor disorder*: the woman suffering from the haemorrhoids will be quite distressed at the discomfort and need advice and support in managing the condition

Medical Management and Care

- Infected episiotomy, constipation and prolonged second stage can exacerbate haemorrhoids and can lead to thrombosis, strangulation or rectal prolapse; prompt treatment with antibiotics and encouraging plenty of hydration and high-fibre diet would help to reduce this risk
- Careful inspection of the perineum and assessment of the haemorrhoids is required to avoid complications and arrange appropriate referral in cases that may need surgical management

Midwifery Management and Care

- The routine postnatal examination by the midwife should include inspection of the perianal area
- Mild creams can be administered, e.g. Anusol
- Warm baths, without added bath products, might ease discomfort
- Ice packs or cold compresses will give some immediate relief
- Avoid post-delivery constipation with advice on diet and fluid intake
- Laxatives may be necessary to ensure a soft stool
- A woman with perineal sutures may be wary of opening her bowels
- Encourage defecation when the urge occurs, as to ignore the urge will increase the impaction of faeces within the bowel making it more difficult to defecate
- Equally, discourage straining to defecate
- Analgesia to be given as needed, but avoid codeine-based analgesics, e.g. cocodamol, due to their constipating effect; NSAIDs (if not contraindicated) will be the best form of analgesia
- Reinforce advice on pelvic floor exercises
- Advise the woman to mention any remaining haemorrhoids to the GP at her six-week postnatal examination; the GP can then make any necessary referral to a colorectal surgeon
- The GP will also need to know if the woman is able to perform a pelvic floor contraction: if this still has not been seen by this stage, a referral to the obstetric physiotherapist can be made

10.7 Anal Sphincter Disorders

Incidence
2% of adult population[1]
Obstetric anal sphincter injury: 0.6–9% of vaginal deliveries
Occult injury: 36% diagnosed following childbirth[2]

Risk for Childbearing
Low Risk

EXPLANATION OF CONDITION

Anal Sphincter Damage

Anal sphincter damage may be muscular or neurological in origin[3], often leads to faecal incontinence and is most commonly caused by[4]:

- Pelvic floor denervation
- External sphincter weakness
- Degeneration of the smooth muscle of the anal sphincter as a result of trauma, as in abuse
- Damage following surgery, e.g. haemorrhoidectomy or other sphincter surgery
- Spinal cord injury
- Diabetes, multiple sclerosis
- Structural damage, e.g. obstetric anal sphincter injury (OASI)

Obstetric Anal Sphincter Injury (OASI)

Obstetric anal sphincter injury may be classified as a third- or fourth-degree tear and includes injury to the perineum involving the anal sphincter complex (external or internal anal sphincter) and/or to the rectal mucosa[2].

Risk factors for OASI are:[2,5]

- Instrumental assistance, particularly at first delivery (<7% of OASI)
- Prolonged second stage (<4% of OASI)
- Persistent occipito-posterior position (<3% of OASI)
- Episiotomy (<3% of OASI); risk higher if midline[6]
- Previous sphincter damage at first delivery[7]
- High infant weight (over 4 kg) (<2% of OASI)
- Nulliparity (<4% of OASI)
- Rectal compromise due to illness, e.g. ulcerative colitis or Crohn's disease

As many of these risk factors are unpreventable, OASI is therefore difficult to avoid.

The damage can be overt (seen) and identified at delivery. Frequently (36%) damage is covert (hidden) and diagnosed during a postpartum endo-anal ultrasound for the investigation of incontinence[8]. Lack of understanding of the perianal anatomy by midwives and doctors is considered a contributing factor for increase in occult OASI[9].

COMPLICATIONS

The complications of anal sphincter damage are:

- Faecal/flatus incontinence, necessitating use of a pad
- Repeated contact with stools can be irritant to the perianal skin causing pain, itching and sores (ulcers)
- Urgency of defecation
- Lifestyle alterations and social embarrassment

NON-PREGNANCY TREATMENT AND CARE

Due to the embarrassment felt, only one third of those with damage are thought to present to their GP with symptoms[8].

A detailed history, anal endosonography, anal manometry will comprise part of the process to diagnose cause of the symptoms, and give advice on treatment. Treatment may involve correction of any predisposing factors.

Medical Treatment

- **Loperimide** will reduce the force of any bowel contractions, also reducing the amount of liquid in the stools that may lead to leakage
- **Topical phenylephrine** is being researched to see if the resting anal tone is increased; early results are encouraging[10]

Surgical Treatment

- **Sphincteroplasty**: overlapping of the anal sphincter muscles when caused by OASI[11]; long-term results not always satisfactory[12]
- **Artificial bowel sphincter**: can be created, or the gracillis muscle can be repositioned round the anal canal to form a new anal sphincter; these two surgical options still have considerable morbidity attached to them[11]
- **Colostomy**: may be performed as a last resort

Other Treatments

- **Behavioural techniques** and **biofeedback** teach patients how to control their bowel habits and use their pelvic floor muscles; physiotherapist is able to teach these techniques in an outpatient situation[13]
- **Nerve stimulation** of the damaged pudendal nerve is another treatment that provides good functional outcome and has minimal morbidity[14]

PRE-CONCEPTION ISSUES AND CARE

The type of pre-conception counselling will vary depending on the nature of treatment the patient has been receiving. This can entail:

- Advice regarding the safety of any medication in pregnancy, especially loperamide and phenylephrine
- The safety of proceeding with any sacral nerve stimulation
- The safety of biofeedback in pregnancy, as this involves a probe being inserted into the vagina to assist with stimulating the pelvic floor
- Women who have experienced OASI need specific counselling regarding future pregnancies and vaginal deliveries

Pregnancy Issues

Maternal concerns about vaginal delivery must be addressed early in the antenatal period.

The higher morbidity associated with caesarean section has to be considered, along with the symptoms the woman is experiencing. However, women who have experienced anal incontinence, required a repair for an occult OASI or are found to have significantly abnormal manometry results are at greater risk of further injury from a vaginal delivery, and should be offered a caesarean section[8,15].

Bowel habits often change frequently in pregnancy, due to hormonal changes. Hence, bowel function becomes a priority issue that requires particular attention to avoid the previous symptoms.

Medical Management and Care
- A plan of care must be discussed and clearly documented at booking
- The degree of anal incontinence and previous treatment will influence the decision regarding mode of delivery
- There may be a need for combined care between the colorectal team and the obstetrician

Midwifery Management and Care
- Accurate booking history to identify past obstetric problems including perineal trauma and treatment; it may be necessary to obtain medical records from other areas
- Referral to a consultant unit is crucial in order to plan care and the mode of delivery
- The woman will have many concerns about the impending birth and will need frequent reassurance and support from the midwife
- A focus on dietary needs in pregnancy is important to maintain healthy bowel function
- As iron tablets often disrupt bowel function, advice is needed in relation to foods high in iron, in an attempt to avoid anaemia and the need for iron supplementation
- Folic acid supplementation should be encouraged, as this aids the absorption of any natural iron in the diet

Labour Issues

Unless the caesarean section rate is increased dramatically, OASI will remain difficult to prevent, despite knowing the risk factors involved. Performing caesarean sections purely to protect the perineum, would lead to other risks associated with surgical morbidity. However, for those at greater risk of anal incontinence, elective caesarean section should be recommended[16].

For any overt OASI, experience of the practitioner is an important factor in management of these cases. A junior doctor should not be managing this without supervision.

There is evidence that midwives are poor at recognising third- and fourth-degree tears[8]. There is a need for further education on these issues to improve the recognition of the degree of perineal trauma.

Medical Management and Care
- Clear documentation of the degree of perineal and sphincter trauma from previous deliveries should be highlighted in the notes
- Intrapartum care plan should be documented clearly
- Recommendations for care for repair comprise[2,8]:
  - approximation (end to end), or overlapping of the anal sphincter muscles, can be used as a technique
  - polydioxanone sutures have a longer half-life and less chance of causing infection than polypropylene (Vicryl) and are therefore considered preferable
  - the operator must be skilled in the repair technique
  - broad-spectrum antibiotic cover should be prescribed

Midwifery Management and Care
- There is no evidence that a prophylactic episiotomy is of any benefit as was previously thought
- If an episiotomy is necessary, a mediolateral rather than a midline incision must be made[6,17]
- Perineal trauma is not influenced by whether or not the midwife practises perineal protection in the second stage
- It has been found that there is no difference in perineal outcome between the expectant ('hands off') or interventionist ('hands on') technique[18]
- As a third of OASIs are not identified at delivery, it is important to seek more experienced advice if there is any level of uncertainty with regard to the degree of perineal trauma

Postpartum Issues
- Increased awareness of need to question women directly about symptoms of faecal incontinence and dyspareunia following childbirth
- Short-term sequelae of anal sphincter injury include pain, infection, constipation and sexual dysfunction[15]

Medical Management and Care
- One third of coloproctologists recommend a defunctioning colostomy for fourth-degree tears[8]
- The woman should be debriefed about the risks of faecal incontinence following anal sphincter injury before discharge from hospital
- A follow-up period of 6–12 months with an expert practitioner
- Anal endosonography is to be recommended following any OASI[19]
- Address any issues regarding anxiety and effects of the injury on continence, body image and sexual function

Midwifery Management and Care
- As the perineum will feel particularly uncomfortable following anal sphincter injury adequate analgesia and assistance with positioning during breast-feeding will be needed
- Dietary advice is essential in order to avoid constipation
- Laxatives to be prescribed, as passage of a hard stool may disrupt the repair

10.8 Obstetric Cholestasis

Incidence	Risk for Childbearing
0.7% in multi-ethnic populations in England[1] 1.2–1.5% Indian-Asian or Pakistani-Asian origin[2]	High Risk

EXPLANATION OF CONDITION

Obstetric Cholestasis (OC) can also be known as **intrahepatic cholestasis of pregnancy** (ICP).

The condition was first reported by Aslfield (1883), later by Eppinger (1936), further reported by Thorling (1954) and by the late 1950s clinical features were described by several documented reports[3]. It is thought to be a rare liver disorder that only occurs in pregnancy[4]. Cholestasis is the term used to characterise the disruption and reduction of bile products from the liver and its flow to the intestine[5].

The cause of this condition is unclear[6]. However, current findings suggest a multifactorial phenomenon, with the involvement of genetic, environmental and hormonal factors[6]. One theory suggests the liver is unable to cope with high levels of sex steroids during pregnancy[7] therefore causing elevation of liver enzymes and potential for total hepatic failure.

The condition usually occurs after the 28th week of pregnancy[8] and ceases 1–2 weeks postpartum[9]. During this time the woman can suffer physiologically, psychologically and emotionally from the side effects of this condition.

Increased risk factors include:

- Environmental factors[10] and seasonal dietary requirements due to climate changes[11]
- Multiple pregnancies[8]
- Genetic trait – in some ethnic groups[11] such as, descendants of Araucanian Indians[12] in Chile and Quechaun Indians in Bolivia[13]
- Subsequent pregnancies are susceptible, manifesting earlier and more severely if jaundice was apparent during the first pregnancy[8]
- Symptoms could recur during menstruation and using the combined oral contraceptive pill[11]

Signs and symptoms of the condition are:

- Intense pruritus which mainly affects hands and soles of feet, but can affect face, back, chest and legs and, in rare cases, ears, eyelids and oral cavity
  - itching is more severe at night
  - no visible rash except from excessive itching, which is thought to be from increased levels of bile acids in the blood and liver[9]
- Urinary tract infections
- Pale stools
- Possible jaundice[4]

The diagnosis of OC is confirmed if abnormal liver function tests and/or raised serum bile acids are found and other causes for these results have been excluded.

COMPLICATIONS

This condition causes severe liver impairment and may cause liver failure in the woman, but also has effects on the fetus. These may include:

- Premature delivery, spontaneous/iatrogenic
- Fetal distress
- Intrauterine death

Therefore, the monitoring of fetal growth and wellbeing throughout the pregnancy is paramount. Such investigations can be carried out by regular ultrasound scans and biophysical profiles. Observation by the woman of her baby's activity and movements on a daily basis is important to illustrate any fetal compromise. Regular CTG should be carried out at each antenatal visit.

The associated maternal morbidity can be of significance, with severe pruritus and consequent sleep deprivation[14].

The most serious risk to maternal health is the increased risk of a primary postpartum haemorrhage. This is caused by altered coagulation due to a deficiency of vitamin K resulting from a lack of intestinal bile[15].

Obstetric cholestasis needs to be considered if a woman complains of a prolonged period of pruritus, which may be apparent after delivery if she had an epidural with opiates. If such symptoms persist for more than three months, investigations need to be carried out and the woman should be referred to a hepatologist.

PRE-CONCEPTION ISSUES AND CARE

Unless obstetric cholestasis occurred in a previous pregnancy there is no further management required. If there has been evidence in previous pregnancies the woman should be counselled for the chance of recurrence. There is a greater than 90% chance of recurrence in the UK population[16].

Hepatobiliary ultrasonography should be arranged to investigate cholelithiasis and/or other liver disease[17].

Pregnancy Issues

Women with OC are not generally unwell. The main symptom tends to be the intense pruritus that presents itself mainly at night and without the presence of a rash. Pruritus is thought to arise from elevated levels of bile acids and histamine released mainly in the areas of the soles of the feet and the palms of the hands[18]. Sleep deprivation could occur if pruritus is intense and prevents the woman from sleeping.

- An increased level of bile acids is associated with a higher incidence of premature birth and stillbirth; has been postulated to be due to the toxic effect on the myocytes
- Risk of stillbirth does not correlate with the onset of pruritus and the association of gestational weeks[19]
- The community midwife is generally the first professional to suspect the possibility of obstetric cholestasis
- There is no single biochemical test to prove the state of the condition or the risks to the fetus[7]

Medical Management and Care

Investigations
- Other causes for abnormal LFT and/or bile acids should be excluded
- Blood tests to exclude: CMV, hepatitis A, B, C and Epstein Barr virus infection
- Autoantibody screen to check for primary biliary cirrhosis and chronic active hepatitis should be performed

Symptomatic Treatment
- Topical treatment with Diprobase, calamine lotion and aqueous cream with menthol may be used; there is no evidence for or against use in pregnancy but they are considered safe and may provide transient symptomatic relief from pruritus
- Chlorpheniramine may be used for sedation at night but does not relieve pruritus
- Ursodeoxycholic acid may act by displacing bile salts and protect the hepatocyte cell membrane from the toxic effects of bile salts. Although commonly prescribed, there is inadequate evidence to recommend its use to improve pruritus and protect against stillbirth
- Vitamin K, 10 mg orally daily, should be prescribed from diagnosis of OC to delivery to reduce the risk of postpartum haemorrhage and fetal or neonatal bleeding
- Monitor pregnancy with weekly LFT once diagnosis of OC is made

Midwifery Management and Care
- A detailed history is paramount to highlight any previous history of OC
- Requires management as a high-risk pregnancy with complementary midwifery care, so transfer to a consultant unit may be required
- Measure fetal movements daily[22], with emphasis on pattern of movement for that pregnancy instead of a strict fetal kick count alone
- Regular cardiotocography may be performed although there is no evidence to suggest which pregnancies are most at risk of fetal distress or IUFD[23]
- There is a possibility of a pre-term delivery; an opportunity for the woman to view the neonatal unit would be advisable
- Direct the mother to appropriate support groups

Labour Issues
- It is recommended that women with OC be delivered at 37–38 weeks' gestation[20] as neonatal respiratory distress syndrome is not usually found at this stage of gestation
- Associated risk with pre-term delivery, intrapartum fetal distress and meconium-stained liquor
- If these incidences are not considered, perinatal mortality can range from 11–20%[21]

Medical Management and Care
- Timing of delivery should be individualised as there is no evidence to support or refute early induction of labour at 37–38 weeks
- Continuous electronic fetal monitoring, because of the increased incidence of meconium-stained liquor, abnormal CTG findings and prematurity

Midwifery Management and Care
- Labour should be managed from a midwifery perspective with additional implementation of prescribed treatment and care
- Active third stage management is recommended due to the high risk of postpartum haemorrhage

Postpartum Issues
- Symptoms generally resolve within 1–2 days postnatally
- Persistent abnormalities should be further investigated to determine if there is any underlying liver disease
- There is a high possibility of recurrence in subsequent pregnancies

Medical Management and Care
- Ensure liver function test results return to normal; due to raised levels in normal pregnancy[24] it is advised to defer these tests for ≥10 days[14]
- Women should be advised of the recurrence risk of OC, which can be as high as 90%[19]
- Contraceptive advice to avoid oestrogen-based preparations

Midwifery Management and Care
- Ensure that the mother has full understanding of the implications of OC and the possibility of recurrence, and encourage her to seek preconception care prior to a future pregnancy
- Advise the mother of the possibility of OC arising in family members[25]

10.9 Gall Bladder and Pancreatic Disease

Incidence	Risk for Childbearing
Cholelithiasis: about 15% of women ≥35 years of age[1]	Variable Risk

EXPLANATION OF CONDITION

Gall Bladder and Gallstones

The biliary system has a major role to play within the body by storing a liver product called bile. Bile is an alkaline fluid that is secreted by the liver and stored in the gall bladder. Bile pigments and bile salts are excretory products of bile. The bile salts assist in the emulsification of fats in the duodenum so that they may be more easily digested by the pancreatic enzymes.

Disorders within the biliary system generally present in middle age and are more common in women than men. However, the incidence after the age of 50 is equal for men and women[2]. There are five types of biliary tract disorder:

1. **Cholelithiasis** (gallstones) – two types, cholesterol stones and pigment stones

Risk factors associated with gallstones:

Cholesterol Gallstones	Pigment Gallstones
Female	Rising age
Rising age	Chronic haemolysis
Pregnancy/oral contraception	Alcohol abuse
Obesity	Biliary infection
Stasis of the gall bladder	Total parenteral nutrition
Spinal injury	Stasis of the gall bladder[3]

2. **Acute cholecystitis** – gallstones that can irritate the mucus membrane of the gall bladder or block the opening to the gall bladder causing inflammation
3. **Choledocholithiasis** – gallstones that are present in the common bile duct or hepatic duct
4. **Cholangitis** – obstruction within the bile duct that is associated with a bacterial infection
5. **Carcinoma of the biliary tract** – a rare cause of biliary tract disorder; may also involve the gall bladder

In addition, it is apparent that there is a close correlation between gallstones and pancreatitis. Alcohol abuse and gallstones in non-pregnant women have been allied as the result of pancreatitis[4].

Pancreatic Disease

Pancreatitis is the inflammation of the pancreas which usually results from obstruction of the pancreatic duct. Pancreatitis can be either an acute or chronic problem.

- Acute pancreatitis – an emergency situation that is commonly caused by alcohol abuse, abdominal trauma and gallstones, or it can occasionally be idiopathic
- Chronic pancreatitis – related to acute pancreatitis but usually caused by extreme alcohol abuse

The symptoms may be mild, moderate or severe and include:

- Nausea and vomiting
- Severe upper abdominal pain

COMPLICATIONS

The symptoms may be associated with:

- Shock
- Pyrexia
- Jaundice
- Substantial weight loss

The main complication of any biliary disorder is the obstruction or inflammation of the gall bladder. Therefore, by surgically removing the gall bladder the symptoms may be cured.

In the case of acute and chronic pancreatitis, there is inappropriate activation of enzymes in the pancreas, which can result in the destruction of the pancreas, having catastrophic consequences. These include infection, respiratory distress, pseudocyst, abscess or pancreatic fistula formation and extremely brittle diabetes.

NON-PREGNANCY TREATMENT AND CARE

Often investigation of biliary disorders may require endoscopic retrograde cholangiopancreatography (ERCP). This may also form part of the treatment. However, the majority of gall bladder cancers are treated palliatively[2].

Acute and chronic pancreatitis is usually treated conservatively, with the exception of pancreatic cancer, which may be treated surgically.

One of the key roles with treatment is the information and support offered by the multi-disciplinary team. Good pain relief, antibiotics and fluid resuscitation are key aspects of care.

PRE-CONCEPTION ISSUES AND CARE

It is suggested that, if any gall bladder or pancreatic disease is evident prior to conception, it would be advisable to seek medical opinion so that treatment may be instituted to optimise symptoms prior to pregnancy.

A low cholesterol diet and limited alcohol consumption should be considered prior to conception. Literature suggests that although pregnancy does not predispose to gastrointestinal disorders such as cholecystitis or pancreatitis, pregnancy does increase the risk of cholelithiasis and biliary sludge[5].

Pregnancy Issues

Over all, gall bladder and pancreatic disease impacts on perinatal mortality and morbidity by increasing the incidence of premature delivery[4]. It is therefore vital to have some understanding of the disease process to ensure optimum outcome for mother and fetus.

The symptoms previously mentioned in association with gall bladder disease in a non-pregnant state are mirrored in a pregnancy state. However, acute epigastric pain in pregnancy is a common symptom which can delay diagnosis and management of the condition. Other differential diagnoses include dyspepsia, pre-eclampsia, HELLP syndrome (haemolysis, elevated liver function, low platelets) and fatty liver disease.

- Pregnancy does alter the function of the gall bladder as there is delayed gastric emptying and reduced gastrointestinal motility
- Gall bladder disease is the second most frequent indication for surgery in pregnancy, after appendicitis[6]

Medical Management and Care

- A past medical history may reveal previous gall bladder disease or episodes of pancreatitis
- Laboratory diagnosis of gall bladder disease may be suggested by elevated white cell count and elevated liver function tests
- Serial amylase and lipid level tests should be performed to confirm the diagnosis of pancreatitis during pregnancy
- Diagnostic tools such as ultrasound are approximately 95% effective at diagnosing gall bladder problems, avoiding the exposure to radiation with X-rays[7]
- Conservative medical management is primarily used to reduce the risk of spontaneous miscarriage within the first trimester, and pre-term labour within the second and third trimesters. Management includes intravenous hydration, correction of hyperglycaemia, and electrolyte imbalance (mainly hypocalcaemia), analgesia, broad-spectrum antibiotics and a fat-restricted diet
- Women with acute pancreatitis should be managed in an intensive care unit

Surgery

- If possible, surgery should be postponed until after delivery
- Cholecystectomy, laparoscopic cholecystectomy and endoscopic retrograde cholangiopancreatography (ERCP) have been performed in pregnancy with varying degrees of success[8]
- The choice of the procedure will vary depending on operator skills, gestational age and severity of symptoms
- Indications for surgery include: ascending cholangitis, obstruction of the common bile duct or the development of severe pancreatitis and persistent biliary colic
- If laparoscopic surgery is performed during pregnancy, open laparoscopy technique is recommended to avoid injury to the uterus

Midwifery Management and Care

- A detailed history is important to ascertain any previous or relevant history that requires further attention
- Advise a low fat, low cholesterol diet and no alcohol
- It is essential to be alert to all the signs and symptoms that are related to gall bladder and pancreatic disease to ensure an urgent referral is made to expedite assessment and treatment
- Prompt identification and hospitalisation of women suffering from acute pancreatitis has been related to a reduction in both maternal and perinatal morbidity and mortality

Labour Issues

- There is a risk of iatrogenic pre-term labour following cholecystectomy and this would need surveillance by the midwives and doctors caring for these women

Medical Management and Care

- The decision to interfere surgically is dependent on an individual basis, taking into account the history of episodes of acute pancreatitis and gestational age

Midwifery Management and Care

- Supportive care in labour is clearly essential
- If cholecystectomy has been performed anticipate, and if necessary prepare for, a pre-term birth

Postpartum Issues

- There are no relevant postpartum issues to take into account for the mother unless cholecystectomy is to be considered
- If the birth was pre-term, then care of the mother with a baby on the neonatal unit should be implemented (see Chapter 1)

Medical Management and Care

- Cholecystectomy might be considered postpartum dependent upon symptoms and condition

Midwifery Management and Care

- Supportive care, with the assistance of the general practitioner, is required during the postnatal period

10 Gastrointestinal Disorders

PATIENT ORGANISATIONS

Living with Reflux
www.livingwithreflux.org

Irritable Bowel Syndrome Network
Unit 5
53 Mowbray Street
Sheffield S3 8EN
www.ibsnetwork.org.uk

National Association for Colitis and Crohn's Disease
4 Beaumont House
Sutton Road, St Albans
Herts. AL1 5HH
www.nacc.org.uk

Crohn's in Childhood Research Association (CIRCA)
Parkgate House
356 West Barnes Lane
Motspur Park
Surrey KT3 6NB
www.cicra.org

Coeliac UK
Suites A–D, Octagon Court
High Wycombe
Buckinghamshire HP11 2HS
www.coeliac.org.uk

Colostomy Association
15 Station Road
Reading RG1 1LG
www.colostomyassociation.org.uk

Ileostomy and Internal Pouch Support Group
(formally The Ileostomy Association)
Peverill House
1–5 Mill Road
Ballyclare, Co. Antrim
Northern Ireland BT39 9DR
www.the-ia.org.uk

National Advisory Service to Parents of Children with a Stoma (NASPCS)
51 Anderson Drive
Darvel, Ayrshire KA17 0DE
www.naspcs.co.uk

British Liver Trust
Portmann House
44 High Street
Ringwood BH24 1HY
www.britishlivertrust.org.uk

Obstetric Cholestasis Support
www.ocsupport.org.uk

ESSENTIAL READING

Alaedini, A. and Green, P.H.R. (2005) Narrative review: Celiac disease: understanding a complex autoimmune disorder. **Annals of Internal Medicine 142**(4):289–298.

De Swiet, M. (Ed.) (2002) Disorders of the liver, biliary system and pancreas; Disorders of the gastro-intestinal tract. **Medical Disorders in Obstetric Practice**, 4th Edn. Oxford; Blackwell/Wiley.

Lancaster Smith, M. (2004) **Gastrointestinal Problems**. Kent; Magister Consulting.

McLatchie, G.R. and Leaper, D.J. (2002) **Oxford Handbook of Clinical Surgery**, 2nd Edn, pp. 293–294. Oxford; Oxford University Press.

Simon, C., Everitt, H., Birtwistle, J. and Stevenson, B. (2002) **Oxford Handbook of General Practice**, pp. 528–529. Oxford; Oxford University Press.

Smith, M.L. (2004) **A General Practice Guide to Gastrointestinal Problems**. Dartford; Magister Consulting Ltd.

Thompson, W. and Heaton, K. (2003) **Fast Facts: Irritable Bowel Syndrome**, 2nd Edn. Oxford; Health Press.

11
AUTOIMMUNE DISORDERS

S. Elizabeth Robson and Sheena Hodgett

11.1 Rheumatoid Arthritis

Incidence
36:100,000 women in UK [1]; 14:100,000 men in UK [1]
Prevalence
0.8% of adult UK population[1]

Risk for Childbearing
Variable Risk

EXPLANATION OF CONDITION

Rheumatoid arthritis (RA) results from IgM autoantibodies *(rheumatoid factor)* activating the complement system to inflame the synovial membrane of joints, tendons and bursae, and, in 35% of cases, the pericardium of the heart[2]. The T4 lymphocytes initiate an immune response, causing the synovial membrane to thicken *(hyperplasia)* and be thrown into folds *(pannus)* with a subsequent increase of synovial fluid, causing painful swelling and restriction of joint movement[3].

The small joints of the hands and feet are most commonly affected, symmetrically, with later involvement of larger synovial joints[4]. Subsequently, the cells of the synovial membrane (synoviocytes) invade the joint cartilage where they secrete enzymes initiating destructive changes in bone and cartilage[3].

Onset is either chronic, over several weeks, with early morning stiffness, swelling of joints and progressive joint pain, or acute, with fever and generalised illness[4]. Sometimes a *palindromic* pattern presents, where there is pain and inflammation in one or two joints that resolves, and then the symptoms appear in previously unaffected joints, in a 'flitting' pattern that can be misdiagnosed with more trivial aches and pains[5]. There are usually periods of remission and relapses[6].

RA usually presents in the child-bearing years, but can occur in children. Formerly known as Still's disease, it is now called juvenile idiopathic arthritis (JIA) or juvenile rheumatoid arthritis (JRH)

Risk factors include genetic predisposition, adverse pregnancy outcome, smoking, obesity and recent infections[7]. The oral contraceptive pill may offer protection or delay the onset[8]. Onset is associated with the puerperium, especially with women who breast-feed after their first delivery[9].

Diagnosis is confirmed by clinical examination and investigations indicating a raised ESR or inflammatory markers, and a positive rheumatoid factor in some cases[10]. Prognostic criteria are under review[11] but currently, with modern management, 20% have mild disease, 75% moderate disease with relapses and remissions and 5% have severe destructive disease[6].

COMPLICATIONS

- Wasting of small muscles of the hand
- Diminished movement of the affected joints
- Swelling of soft tissue around the joints
- Ruptured tendons or joints (Baker's cysts)
- Spinal cord compression
- Neuropathy
- Infection (secondary to steroids)
- Secondary anaemia
- Sjögren's syndrome (dry eyes)
- Secondary Raynaud's phenomenon (see Section 11.2)
- Scleroderma (see Section 11.2)
- Lungs develop pleural effusion and nodules
- Heart develops asymptomatic pericarditis
- Reduced life expectancy from cardiac complications[5]

When JIA was followed up in adulthood[12], 83% of those affected were sexually active, but affected by:

- Relationship instability
- Detrimental effect on body image
- Short stature (associated with caesarean section)
- Reduced hip mobility (associated with caesarean section)
- Sexual problems, both physical and psychological

NON-PREGNANCY TREATMENT AND CARE

Modern management entails an aggressive treatment approach with disease-modifying anti-rheumatic drugs (DMARDs) at disease onset[13] to control disease activity, reduce joint erosions, reduce cardiovascular mortality and improve quality of life[14]. Examples of treatment include:

- **DMARDs** to modify disease
  - azathioprine (Imuran)
  - ciclosporine (Neoral)
  - gold (Myocrisin®, Ridaura)
  - hydroxychloroquine (Plaquenil)
  - leflunomide (Arava)
  - methotrexate (Maxtrex)
  - penicillamine (Distamine)
  - sulfasalazine (Salazopyrin)
- **TNF inhibitors** to suppress the immune response
  - etanercept (Enbrel)
  - infliximab (Remicade®)
- **NSAIDs** to control symptoms
  - aspirin
  - ibuprofen (Brufen, Nurofen)
  - naproxen (Naprosyn)
  - indomethacin (Indomod)
  - phenylacetic acid (Diclofenac)
  - ketoprofen (Ketocid™)
- **Steroids** to reduce inflammation
  - prednisolone (Deltacortril)
- **Diet**: there is no evidence to support specific diets, and fasting followed by a vegetarian diet risks malnutrition[15]
- **Physiotherapy**
  - re-education with provision of aids to assist mobility
  - exercises to improve and maintain joint function and muscle power
  - hydrotherapy
  - splints to rest joints during flare-up or for doing everyday tasks
- **Advice**: pre-conception care is essential, as drugs, especially DMARDs, are often contraindicated in pregnancy (see Appendix 11)

PRE-CONCEPTION ISSUES AND CARE

Refer back to rheumatologist where the disease state is assessed and a risk benefit analysis made on maintaining or altering drug therapy. DMARDs are replaced with other drugs such as NSAIDs[16] or steroids. Paracetamol is given for pain relief[17]. Leflunomide should be stopped, with contraceptive cover, for two years prior to conception or until plasma levels fall below 0.02 mg/l[18] (see Appendix 11).

Assess diet and weight. Encourage a vitamin- and iron-rich diet (see Appendix 1.3) and reduction of obesity. Folic acid 0.4 mg is important, as folate deficiency results from long-term DMARD usage[19]. Promote smoking cessation, and regular exercise.

Pregnancy Issues
- Young women receiving modern therapy have improved health, fertility and sex life, hence a risk of unplanned pregnancy with drug-related teratogenic risk to the fetus[20]
- NSAIDs in the third trimester are associated with fetal or obstetric complications (see Appendix 11)
- Consider existing complementary therapies, which are unlikely to have been sanctioned for use in pregnancy
- Mothers may be on a favoured diet to '*control*' their condition
- 75% of women experience improvement or remission during pregnancy[19]
- Existing complications of anaemia or infection could be exacerbated by pregnancy
- Rheumatoid joints become unstable due to joint loosening and altered weight distribution[21]
- Risk of subluxation of cervical vertebrae, especially[21] of C1–2; this is usually under-recognised
- Psycho-social issues arise as the woman faces motherhood with concerns of a prospective disability

Medical Management and Care
- Shared care with obstetrician and rheumatologist
- DMARDs are replaced by other drugs such as NSAIDs[16] or steroids if this has not already been done; paracetamol is given for pain relief[17]
- NSAIDs are prescribed with caution in third trimester (see Appendix 11)
- Additional screening for fetal congenital abnormalities may be required for women who conceive whilst on DMARDs

Midwifery Management and Care
- Thorough booking history, with identification of past/present drugs
- Assess expectations and share ideas on a model of care
- Book for consultant unit care and hospital confinement
- Support medical treatment prescribed by the doctor
- Give positive but realistic encouragement and take woman's concerns seriously
- Education in relation to RA and altered state of health in pregnancy
- Involvement of the multi-professional team, such as OT, to assess if specific aids are needed for the home
- Counselling in relation to fetal abnormality screening if the mother conceived whilst on DMARDs or TNF drugs
- Ascertain current diet and advise a well-balanced, iron- and folate-rich diet; discourage unorthodox nutritional practices which could potentially be harmful[23]
- If there has been a history of anaemia, regular haematinic investigations, especially FBC, to detect falling Hb levels and the potential for treatment with iron, B12 and folate tablets
- Assess ability to self-care, based on activities of daily living, and prospective ability to care for the baby
- Consider home antenatal or parent-craft visits for serious disability

Labour Issues
- Mobility issues, and theoretical risk of DVT for immobile mothers
- Problems with abduction of hips, especially a problem for lithotomy position
- Potential problems for iv cannulation, especially if there is scleroderma (see Raynaud's phenomenon, Section 11.2)

Medical Management and Care
- Consider use of additional steroid cover in labour
- Avoid lithotomy position whenever possible

Midwifery Management and Care
- Passive leg exercises to prevent DVT
- Consider left lateral position for delivery
- Partner to support mother's limbs
- Care and patience if mother has to be put into lithotomy position
- Aside from the above, labour should be made as normal as possible

Postpartum Issues
- Risk of acute and severe return of symptoms in the majority of cases[22], which can be accompanied by depression
- Neonate has theoretical risk of premature closure of ductus arteriosus if the mother is on NSAIDs[18]
- Mother may be cautious about breast-feeding as this would delay her return to pre-pregnancy drug regimen
- Restrictions of the condition may impede maternal coping skills with handling and feeding the baby
- Mothers with poor mobility are at risk of VTE disease postpartum (see Section 15.1)

Medical Management and Care
- Liaison with rheumatologist who is likely to reduce the steroid dosage slowly and return to pre-pregnancy drug regimen, unless breast-feeding
- Breast-feeding mothers are kept on steroids
- Neonatal examination to be conducted by a doctor if mother has received NSAIDs or other drugs with a potential effect on the neonate
- Those with poor mobility require VTE risk assessment (see Appendix 15.1)

Midwifery Management and Care
- Advise mother about likely sudden exacerbation of RA, and to contact the rheumatologist at earliest sign of joint symptoms
- Encourage and assist with mobility
- Assess ability to care for self and baby on activities of daily living
- Help with handling baby whilst in hospital
- If necessary ask the physiotherapist to visit on the postnatal ward
- Arrange drugs to take home and a rheumatology out-patient appointment
- Promote breast-feeding in a realistic manner
- Contraceptive advice
- Be alert for signs of depression

11.2 Raynaud's Phenomenon

Incidence
3–20% adults worldwide[1]
80% cases are women, mainly <35 yr[2]

Risk for Childbearing
Primary phenomenon: Low Risk
Secondary phenomenon: Variable Risk

EXPLANATION OF CONDITION

Raynaud's phenomenon was first described by M. Raynaud in Paris, 1862[3], and under-recognised, as many sufferers do not consult a doctor[4]. Peripheral blood circulation is congested due to arteriolar spasm under autonomic nervous control on exposure to a cold temperature or stress[5]. The aetiology of this is unknown[6], but it results in ischaemic type pain in the peripheries, especially ears, tip of nose, toes and the middle fingers of each hand. Classic triphasic colour changes comprise:

- **White** and very painful due to ischaemia
- **Blue** and numb due to cyanosis
- **Red** and painful when reperfusion occurs[7]

Attacks usually last minutes[2], but sometimes hours. There are two types of condition: primary and secondary.

Primary Raynaud's Phenomenon

- Mainly affects young women[7]
- Possibly familial if age of onset <30 yr[8]
- Nailform and autoantibody tests are normal allowing 'robust reassurance'[9]
- Exists as a condition alone, in the absence of connective tissue disease[10], accounting for 90% of cases[11]
- Usually benign
- Mild symptoms and good long-term outlook[1,9]
- Generally managed by GP[10] with advice and usually without drug treatment[12]

Secondary Raynaud's Phenomenon or Syndrome

Usually presents later in life and requires specialist referral[10] as it arises from another medical condition. The most commonly associated conditions are[1,12]:

- Scleroderma (also known as *scleroma, systemic sclerosis*)
- Rheumatoid arthritis
- Systemic lupus erythematosus (SLE)
- Sjögren's syndrome (dry eyes and mouth)
- Other connective tissue diseases
- Repetitive vibration injuries (white finger)

COMPLICATIONS

Most at risk of an attack or complications are those chronically ill with the secondary phenomenon, and the elderly who are unable to move voluntarily from the cold.

Complications are more likely to arise with the secondary phenomenon[1], and it may be difficult to differentiate whether the complications are attributed to Raynaud's phenomenon or to the co-existing condition. Such complications include[11]:

- Migraine
- Ischaemic pain in body extremities
- Chilblains
- Skin and mouth ulceration
- Skin rashes
- Joint inflammation and pain

NB: The midwife is most likely to encounter mothers with primary Raynaud's phenomenon and minimal complications.

Associated Conditions:

- *Scleroderma* (scleroma, systemic sclerosis)
  - skin becomes taught and 'leather-like' with a waxy appearance due to swelling of collagen fibres and constriction of the peripheral capillary networks
  - it is preceded by oedema[13]
  - hard plaques of skin become noticeable
  - in extreme cases this hard skin can result in claw-shaped hands
  - risk of renal disease in pregnancy[14]
  - rare in children, but if it occurs there is a risk of growth defects[1]
- Rheumatoid arthritis (see Section 11.1)
- Systemic lupus erythematosus (see Section 11.3)

NON-PREGNANCY TREATMENT AND CARE

This condition can herald connective tissue disease in 5% of cases[12], so investigations are required, primarily:

- Nailform capillary test with an ophthalmoscope
- Blood tests for FBC, ESR, autoantibody screen[1]
- If the latter two are abnormal, underlying connective tissue disease is implied – consider referral to a specialist centre[10]
- The woman is advised to:
  - cease smoking and minimise caffeine intake
  - avoid extremes of temperature
  - take sensible precautions, e.g. wear hat, gloves and socks in cold times, and use gloves in a deep freeze
  - Mention she has this condition when seeking contraceptive advice – the combined pill (COCP) is sometimes contraindicated
  - Seek pre-conception advice
- Put an alert note on case notes, as she should not take beta-adrenoceptor antagonists or vasoconstrictor drugs

Cases of the secondary phenomenon usually require treatment[8] with a vasodilator, such as nifedipine (Adalat, Tenif). Treatment depends on the underlying condition.

PRE-CONCEPTION ISSUES AND CARE

Primary Raynaud's

- Risk–benefit assessment for cessation of nifedipine[10] and other drugs peri-conception[15,16,17]
- Advise to cease smoking
- Advise that the phenomenon is unlikely to affect a forthcoming pregnancy and that placental blood flow is unlikely to be impaired
- COCP may be contraindicated

Secondary Raynaud's

As above, plus:

- Management and implications for childbearing will depend upon the co-existing condition
- Those with symptoms of Sjögren's syndrome should be investigated for anti-Ro/-La antibodies, because 90% have antibodies which cross the placenta with a 10% risk of neonatal lupus syndrome (see Section 11.3)

Pregnancy Issues

Primary Raynaud's
- No known adverse effect on placental blood flow so fetal growth should be normal

Secondary Raynaud's
- Problems depend upon the co-existing condition

Scleroderma associated with[17]:
- Miscarriage
- IUGR
- Renal disease

Generally
- Symptoms may improve due to:
  - vasodilatation from a relaxing effect of progesterone on the blood vessel walls[17] reducing arteriolar spasm[18]
  - blood volume increase
  - rise in maternal core temperature as the fetus enlarges, which increases blood flow to the periphery and encourages vasodilatation to assist with heat loss[18]
- Raynaud's attack on the nipple has been reported in pregnancy[19] and breast-feeding[20,21]
- Mothers may be using complementary therapies, e.g. evening primrose or fish oils[1]; an RCT with *Gingko biloba* showed a reduction in frequency of attacks in primary Raynaud's but no change in blood values[22] and no indication of its safety in pregnancy

Medical Management and Care
- **Primary Raynaud's**: standard antenatal care
- **Secondary Raynaud's**: treatment in tandem with the co-existing condition; the woman is likely to require antenatal care at a combined or specialist clinic
- Risk–benefit assessment for the first trimester use of nifedipine and other drugs[15,16,17]
- **Sjögren's syndrome**: test for anti-Ro and anti-La antibodies
- **Scleroderma**: care depends upon what is affected and these complex variables are outside the scope of this book

Midwifery Management and Care

Primary Raynaud's
Mother can have low-risk care and the phenomenon is not a contraindication for home confinement. The midwife should:
- Reinforce the general advice of the pre-pregnant state
- Advise on avoidance of complementary therapies due to lack of evidence on safety in pregnancy
- Encourage smoking cessation
- Advocate minimal caffeine products
- Advise on avoidance of extremes of temperature
- Encourage regular, well-balanced meals and hot drinks
- Advise about the risk of Raynaud's 'attack' on the nipple
- Promote breast-feeding
- Use astute observational skills to identify the potential for other co-existing conditions, then refer to an appropriate doctor

Secondary Raynaud's
Antenatal care is given in conjunction with physicians, according to the co-existing conditions. The midwife needs to:
- Give advice and care as for primary Raynaud's above
- Reinforce any medical advice and treatment given
- Seek information on recent treatments
- Advise on potential side effects of drugs
- Observe to identify deterioration of the co-existing condition

Labour Issues

Raynaud's
- No known effect from Raynaud's itself on placenta, fetus or neonate

Scleroderma – risks of:
- Premature labour[17]
- Difficulties with iv cannulation[17]
- Problems with intubation[17]

Medical Management and Care
- **Primary Raynaud's:** labour can be managed normally by the midwife
- **Secondary Raynaud's:** as per the co-existing condition
- **Scleroderma**: anaesthetist to assess mother in advance

Midwifery Management and Care
- Labour should be managed from a normal perspective
- Implement any prescribed treatment and care for a co-existing condition
- Oxytocin for active third stage management; Syntometrine and ergometrine are vasoconstrictive, and should not be used routinely[18]

Postpartum Issues
- Severe, throbbing nipple pain from a Raynaud's attack may be misdiagnosed as thrush and contribute to breast-feeding failure[23]
- Maternal blood volume will return to its pre-pregnancy state and the symptom relief of pregnancy will subside
- If the mother enquires, there is an increased theoretical risk of the neonate developing Raynaud's in later life
- Childhood Raynaud's usually presents at 5–16 years[24] but has been reported in one-year-olds[25], hence a mother could worry the baby could be affected

Medical Management and Care
- Consider re-commencement of pre-pregnancy drugs after breast-feeding has finished
- If the mother has symptoms of Sjögren's syndrome be alert for neonatal lupus, which usually presents in the baby as a florid facial rash with an 'owl eyes' appearance and carries a risk of congenital heart block[26]
- Neonatal features may initiate maternal diagnosis[27]

Midwifery Management and Care
- Do not use ice cube or cold compress on or near the nipple
- Examine nipples if pain is reported, and do not dismiss as thrush
- The mother should be advised:
  - that her old symptoms will return
  - that the baby should be dressed sensibly in warm baby clothing for outdoors, including hat and mittens, as would any other baby
  - to avoid a reactionary tendency to over-wrap and over-heat the baby giving a theoretical increased risk of SIDS (see Appendix 16.1)

11.3 Systemic Lupus Erythematosus

Prevalence	**Risk for Childbearing**
0.12% UK population[1] with a female dominance, affecting 1:2,000 UK women[2] More common in Asian, Afro-Caribbean and Chinese women[2]	High Risk

EXPLANATION OF CONDITION

Lupus erythematosus, commonly known as *lupus,* is a serious disorder whereby the body produces autoantibodies against its own connective tissue. Two main types exist:

1. **Discoid lupus erythematosus** (DLE): skin alone is affected, with defined, red scaly patches on the face and neck and alopecia leading to scarring on the scalp, both aggravated by sunlight[3]; treatment is by avoiding sunbeds or intense sunlight[3] and applying topical corticosteroids or hydroxychloroquinine[4]
2. **Systemic lupus erythematosus** (SLE): this condition extends beyond the skin to the organs, with enlarged lymph glands and various other manifestations[2]; can be fatal, especially if the kidneys are involved
    a. fetus is of great concern in pregnancy, as the condition often worsens, and 10% of affected mothers will transfer anti-Ro or anti-La antibodies to the fetus resulting in **neonatal lupus syndrome** (NLS)[2]

In 75% of cases, SLE first presents[5] with:

*   Fatigue and headaches
*   Arthralgia (joint pain without swelling)
*   Fever with flu-like symptoms
*   Weight loss
*   Malar (butterfly) rash on cheeks (33% of cases)

Diagnosis is based upon clinical criteria (currently under review)[6] and investigations. One is a skin biopsy to detect SLE autoantibodies reacting with its complementary antigen[7]. Patients usually test positive for antinuclear antibody (ANA) and often DNA antibodies. A raised erythrocyte sedimentation rate (ESR) is common, and a positive rheumatoid factor is found in 25%. A false positive test for syphilis is found in 33%[8] and some have antiphospholipid antibodies[9], which can result in a co-existing antiphospholipid syndrome[2] with thrombo-embolic sequelae[9].

The disease has periods of remission, and when active is termed 'lupus flare' which is often triggered by infection, exposure to sunlight or oestrogen increase – as may occur when prescribed the oral contraceptive pill. It can be difficult to differentiate between a flare and infection[2].

Urinalysis is performed regularly, as blood or protein can indicate a lupus flare with renal involvement. Five-year survival is over 95% with modern treatment regimens unless there is renal involvement[5]. Death usually results from generalised disease, infection or cardiovascular disease[5].

COMPLICATIONS

Some of the following manifestations may be experienced[2]:

*   Fatigue and myalgia (muscle pain)
*   Nausea, vomiting and diarrhoea
*   Photosensitivity
*   Arthritis and sometimes early morning stiffness
*   Secondary Raynaud's phenomenon (see Section 11.2)
*   Sjögren's syndrome (dry eyes/mouth) (see Section 11.2)
*   Alopecia (hair loss)
*   Ulceration of mouth, nose and vagina
*   Acute and chronic infection

*   Jaccoud's arthropathy (deformed joints due to lax ligaments)
*   Renal Disease
*   Pleurisy (often asymptomatic)
*   Pericarditis (often asymptomatic)
*   Ischaemic heart disease
*   Pulmonary hypertension
*   Leucopenia (reduced leucocyte count)
*   Thrombocytopenia
*   Anaemia – as a result of chronic infections[7]
*   Neuro-psychiatric states, e.g. cerebrovascular accident[2], migraine, epilepsy[10] and depressive or manic symptoms[11] and dementia[10]

NON-PREGNANCY TREATMENT AND CARE

Advice for the Woman

*   Avoid sunlight and use sun block
*   Avoid infection if possible
*   Avoid unplanned pregnancy and seek pre-conception care
*   Avoid stress and get adequate rest (may need to adapt job)
*   Use analgesics as needed
*   Protect against cold if Raynaud's occurs
*   Eat a well-balanced diet
*   Have a positive self-image (e.g. camouflage make-up)

Monitor

*   Regular blood pressure measurement
*   Urinalysis for blood and protein (indicates renal disease)
*   Blood tests for FBC, ESR, WBC, U&E, creatinine, C3 and C4 complement and anti-DNA titre[5]
*   LFT if taking azathioprine
*   Screening for diabetes
*   Assessing osteoporosis risk (from prolonged steroid use)
*   Investigations for antiphospholipid (Hughes) syndrome

Medical Treatment

*   Corticosteroids for disease flare, e.g. prednisolone[8]
*   NSAIDs for pain, fever and arthritis[8]
*   Antimalarial drugs (e.g. hydroxychloroquine) for skin disease, fatigue and arthralgia[8]
*   DMARDs to arrest disease progression
    –   methotextrate
    –   cyclophosphamide[2]
    –   azathioprine
    –   mycophenolate
*   Artificial tears for Sjögren's syndrome[2]

PRE-CONCEPTION ISSUES AND CARE

*   Fetal loss increases if conception occurs during disease flare, so aim for the woman to conceive during remission
*   Refer to rheumatologist for screening of organ involvement and risk–benefit analysis on altering drugs
*   Avoid the oestrogen-based contraceptive pill
*   DMARDs are usually replaced by NSAIDs or steroids (see Appendix 11)

Pregnancy Issues

- Fetal loss has reduced from 50% to 20% with modern management, but there is still an increased risk[12] of:
  - IUGR
  - pre-term labour
  - IUFD
  - miscarriage
  - risk of congenital abnormalities – linked with some drug treatment (see Appendix 11)
- 50% chance of a lupus flare in pregnancy or postpartum[13]
- Can be difficult to differentiate between body changes of pregnancy and mildly active lupus[14]
- Flare is associated with premature delivery[15]
- Pre-existing renal disease may worsen and active nephritis is a factor for fetal mortality[15]
- There is an increased risk of hypertensive disease of pregnancy[16]
- Pre-eclampsia may be difficult to differentiate from a renal flare[17]
- Risk of fetal loss is increased with hypertensive disease and a raised antiphospholipid antibody titre[17]
- Hazards to the mother are reduced if the lupus is mild or stable[14]
- Pseudocyesis (phantom pregnancy) has been reported[18,19]

Medical Management and Care

- DMARDs are replaced by other drugs, such as NSAIDs or steroids, if this was not done pre-conception; paracetamol is given for pain relief
- Additional screening for congenital abnormalities may be required for women who conceived on DMARDs or TNF therapy
- Serial scans to detect IUGR
- Blood tests for anti-DNA antibodies, anti-Ro and anti-La antibodies, FBC, platelets, complement and LFT
- Women with anti-Ro/-La antibodies have a 2–5% chance[9,22] of their first child having congenital heart block (CHB), rising to 16% with subsequent pregnancies[13,23]; fetal monitoring with echocardiography is advocated[9] and corticosteroid use is debated[22,23]
- Consideration of elective pre-term delivery at earliest suggestion of flare, renal deterioration or significant pre-eclampsia

Midwifery Management and Care

This is a high-risk pregnancy, and the mother must be booked for antenatal care by the multi-disciplinary team at a combined clinic[21] and for delivery at a hospital with a neonatal unit. The midwife should also:

- Take a detailed booking history, noting all manifestations of the condition and current medication
- Advise false positive result for syphilis possible if Wassermann test is used
- Advise risk of miscarriage or pre-term delivery, and the necessity to contact delivery suite for any signs of labour
- Take the mother's concerns seriously and accept she has insight into her condition and will be the first to recognise altered body function
- Be vigilant with observations at each antenatal visit, especially with urinalysis and blood pressure
- Refer to hospital and inform medical staff if proteinuria is detected, as this may be first indication of renal flare
- Encourage a well-balanced, iron-rich diet to prevent anaemia
- Advocate gentle exercise to reduce risk of DVT

Labour Issues

- Most women with SLE should be able to deliver vaginally[12] in the absence of obstetric complications or lupus flare
- Condition remains a high-risk pregnancy and labour

Medical Management and Care

- Consider the need for additional steroids to cover delivery
- TED stockings for operative delivery

Midwifery Management and Care

- Continuous EFM is indicated
- Normal, term, vaginal deliveries can be performed by the midwife

Postpartum Issues

- 5% of neonates born to anti-Ro or anti-La positive mothers risk neonatal lupus[9], which may present with a discoid, facial 'owl eyes' rash and 2% risk of congenital heart block[13]
- Lactation might be suppressed by corticosteroids and disease activity[20]
- Drugs pass into breast milk, and breast-feeding exacerbates maternal fatigue
- Prolactin released may lead to exacerbation of the condition[12]
- A neuro-psychiatric state could be wrongly identified as postnatal depression
- The mother may need prompt return to pre-pregnancy drug regimen

Medical Management and Care

- Steroids are increased for 'postpartum flare' and breast-feeding
- Bottle-feeding mothers are returned to pre-pregnancy drug regimen
- Avoid the oestrogen-based contraceptive pill
- MRI scan if symptoms of neuro-psychiatric lupus are reported
- Neonatal examination prior to discharge by paediatrician not midwife
- Post-delivery ECG for babies born to Ro and La positive mothers

Midwifery Management and Care

- Continue maternal observations for ten postnatal days, and assess need to continue home visits beyond ten days postpartum
- Report any neonatal facial rashes promptly, and be alert for the baby experiencing any cardiopulmonary problems
- Reinforce advice, treatment and contraception advocated by doctors
- Seek paediatric/pharmaceutical advice on drugs and breast-feeding
- Promote breast-feeding in a realistic manner and deflect maternal 'guilt' if she ceases breast-feeding or uses complementary feeds
- If any psychiatric symptoms present, refer promptly to medical staff and do not dismiss as the 'baby blues'
- Advise mother about risk of neonatal lupus, and to avoid excess sunlight exposure for the baby

11.4 Antiphospholipid (Hughes) Syndrome

Incidence	Risk for Childbearing
1% adults have antibodies without disease[1]	High Risk
27% of patients with SLE have antibodies[2]	
15% women with recurrent miscarriage have antibodies[3]	

EXPLANATION OF CONDITION

Antiphospholipid syndrome (APS) was originally observed in patients with systemic lupus erythematosus (SLE) and first described by Graham Hughes[4], hence its alternative name, **Hughes syndrome**. The condition was originally associated with thrombo-embolic disorders, recurrent miscarriage and neurological associations[5]. It mainly occurs in young and middle-aged adults and there is no defined racial predominance[1].

Phospholipid is a component of cell membranes. In APS, autoantibodies called antiphospholipid antibodies (APA) are produced. APA is an umbrella term for the presence of one or both of two autoantibodies: lupus anticoagulant (LA) and anticardiolipin antibodies (aCL)[6]. Cardiolipin is a component of the Wasserman reaction which tests for syphilis[7], so APS patients may get a false positive result for syphilis in areas still using this test.

The autoantibodies (aCL and/or LA) bind to phospholipid-binding proteins[7] and any body organ or vessel can be affected[8]. When blood platelets are involved a state of hypercoagulability results[7], or, put colloquially, the sufferer has 'sticky blood'[8]. The presence of antibodies predisposes a person to thrombotic disorders.

Diagnosis is based on the Sapporo criteria[9] entailing the presence, in each category, of at least one of:

- *Clinical:*
  - vascular thrombosis
  - pregnancy morbidity
- *Laboratory:*
  - aCL antibodies
  - LA antibodies

Two positive antibody results, six weeks apart, are required for accurate and reliable diagnosis.[3]

This thrombotic disease can manifest in several forms:

Primary Antiphospholipid Syndrome (PAPS)

This syndrome occurs in isolation[10] and manifests as one of:

- Arterial or venous thrombo-embolic disease
- Endocarditis
- Recurrent pregnancy failure[11], which is associated with thrombocytopenia (see Chapter 14) in 20–40% of cases[12]

Secondary Antiphospholipid Syndrome (SAPS)

This condition is associated with infection or autoimmune disease, especially SLE[10,5] and thrombocytopenia[13]. It manifests as above, as one of:

- Arterial or venous thrombo-embolic disease
- Endocarditis
- Recurrent pregnancy failure[11]

Catastrophic Antiphospholipid Syndrome (CAPS)

This is rare, but develops rapidly, with small vessel thrombosis causing multi-organ failure, DVT, pulmonary embolism and stroke, resulting in a high mortality rate.[14] In 50% of cases patients had PAPS and 45% SLE[14]. Six percent of cases present in pregnancy or the puerperium[15].

COMPLICATIONS

- **Thrombosis** – arterial or venous[5]
- **Cerebrovascular disease** – atherosclerosis, transient ischaemic attack and stroke[16,5]
- **Cardiac disease** – valve thickening, ventricular dysfunction, myocardial infarction[16], pulmonary hypertension[17]
- **Anaemia** – haemolytic
- **Renal disease** – nephropathy[18], glomerulonephritis[19]
- **Neurological disorders** – especially migraine, chorea, epilepsy and stroke[5]
  - 15% of neurological outpatients have APA[21]
  - Controversially, some cases of APS may have been misdiagnosed as multiple sclerosis[5]
- **Cognitive dysfunction** – poor memory or concentration[5]
- **Psychiatric conditions** – depression, dementia and psychosis[5]
- **Skin problems** – especially livedo reticularis and ulcers[21]
- **Pregnancy problems** – IUFD, IUGR, miscarriage, APH, pre-eclampsia and HELLP syndrome (see below)

NON-PREGNANCY TREATMENT AND CARE

Medical Treatment

For thrombotic manifestations:

- Daily aspirin[9]
- Low-molecular-weight heparin (LMWH) sc injection
- Warfarin tablets

Management

- Monitor platelet count regularly if heparin is used[10]
- Patients with recurrent thrombotic episodes require life-long anticoagulation[1]

PRE-CONCEPTION ISSUES AND CARE

All women with SLE should be screened for APS[2].
Women already diagnosed with APS should:

- Be informed of risks:
  - thrombosis
  - stroke
  - pre-eclampsia
  - IUGR
  - placental abruption
  - miscarriage
  - pre-term delivery and consequent neonatal morbidity[6]
- Have rubella status checked, and commence folic acid[6]
- Have antibody levels confirmed[6]
- Be assessed for anaemia, thrombocytopenia, SLE and underlying renal disease[6]
- Take low dose aspirin (75 mg) pre- and post-conception.
- Commence LMWH, if required, with a positive pregnancy test
- Discontinue warfarin and commence LMWH, as warfarin is teratogenic at 6–12 weeks of pregnancy[6]

Pregnancy Issues

- Untreated APS risks fetal morbidity, classified under the Sapporo criteria[10] as:
  A: Recurrent miscarriage <10 weeks
  B: Death of an apparently normal fetus ≥10 weeks gestation
  C: Premature labour ≤34 weeks gestation
- The rate of fetal loss is directly related to the antibody titre[6]
- Untreated the chance of a successful pregnancy is around 20%, with treatment the chance of a live birth increases to 70%[6]
- Those treated are still susceptible to pre-eclampsia and IUGR[24], and thrombocytopenia may worsen[6]
- Although rare, catastrophic APS can be triggered by infection, anticoagulation withdrawal, surgery, neoplasia and lupus 'flares' in pregnancy or the puerperium[15]
- Warfarin is avoided in the first trimester as it is teratogenic, and second/third trimester use should be justified on clinical grounds[6]

Additional complications[6,7,22,23]:
- IUGR
- Placental abruption
- Thrombosis in any organ or tissue
- Pre-eclampsia
- HELLP syndrome
- Treatment side effects – e.g. osteoporosis risk with LMWH

Medical Management and Care

- Early dating scan[6], and regular/serial scans to detect IUGR
- Uterine artery waveforms[6] at 20 and 24 weeks – if normal consider cessation of heparin
- Liaison with haematologists or immunologists[22]
- Aspirin and/or LMWH to improve pregnancy outcome (heparin blocks complications by suppressing complement action[28])
- Blood tests – FBC and platelet count
- Anti-factor Xa activity may be monitored to adjust LMWH dose
- Heparin, or second/third trimester warfarin, to prevent thrombosis in women with previous thrombotic complications
- Corticosteroids are no longer recommended[6] unless a co-existing condition such as ITP or SLE necessitates their use
- Immunoglobulin, as IVIG, might be tried in specialist centres[6] for women with previously poor outcomes on aspirin and LMWH
- Prompt identification and treatment of infection
- Discuss and arrange an intrapartum care plan with the mother and members of the multi-disciplinary team
- Counselling – prognosis of pregnancy, chance of pre-term delivery and potential for further medical complications

Midwifery Management and Care

- An accurate booking history should be taken, and the mother booked for care at a consultant unit with specialist maternal medicine clinics
- Educate mothers to self-administer heparin injections correctly and encourage them to persevere with therapy[18]
- Midwives need to understand the condition to collaborate with doctors in explanations or to support potentially grieving parents[18]
- Encourage regular clinic attendance, with close surveillance of blood pressure and urinalysis to detect pre-eclampsia promptly[6]
- Get the mother fitted for TED stockings in readiness for labour
- Mother to have midwifery contact within a high-risk clinic situation

Labour Issues

- Use of aspirin in pregnancy does not affect intrapartum use of regional anaesthesia[6]
- Women who are admitted in spontaneous labour, or for a planned delivery, will have been advised to omit their LMWH injection at the onset of contractions to avoid the problem of having an anticoagulant effect at the time of delivery and facilitate the use of epidural anaesthesia
- The fetus risks intrapartum asphyxia[25]

Medical Management and Care

- Omit heparin to allow for regional analgesia

Midwifery Management and Care

- Ensure that the woman is seen by an anaesthetist early in labour
- TED stockings throughout labour
- Encourage mobility and leg care
- Ensure adequate hydration and IVI may be necessary
- Continuous fetal heart monitoring
- Active management of third stage after vaginal delivery
- Prompt and expert suturing of perineal tears or episiotomy

Postpartum Issues

- APS itself is rare in neonates[26] and the effect of maternal disease on the neonate is debated, hence some centres recommend that such infants have paediatric follow-up until transplacentally-acquired antibodies are undetectable[27]
- The baby may well be small for gestational age or pre-term, with chance of admission to a neonatal care unit
- The postpartum period is a risk time for thrombosis for normal mothers, and the risk is increased with APS

Medical Management and Care

- Those previously on long-term warfarin need this recommenced and LWMH stopped once the international normalised ratio is >2.0[23]
- Mothers with previous thrombosis need heparin or warfarin for six weeks[23]
- Mothers without previous thrombosis need heparin for five days[23]
- Avoid COCP because of thrombo-embolic risk[29]

Midwifery Management and Care

- Early mobilisation, being alert for thrombosis and catastrophic APS
- Be aware that not all mothers are for early discharge
- If the baby is on NNU additional support is needed for the mother
- Advise that it is safe to breast-feed on warfarin or heparin therapy having first conferred with the paediatrician and or pharmacist
- Make sure that appropriate maternal and neonatal follow-up appointments have been made prior to discharge and that above anti-coagulants have been obtained to take out

11 Autoimmune Disorders

PATIENT ORGANISATIONS

ARC–Arthritis Research Campaign
www.arc.org.uk

Arthritis Care
18 Stephenson Way
London NW1 2HD
http://www.arthritiscare.org.uk

NRAS – National Rheumatoid Arthritis Society
11 College Avenue
Maidenhead, Berks. SL6 6AR
www.rheumatoid.org.uk

Raynaud's and Scleroderma Association Trust
112 Crewe Road, Alsagar, Cheshire ST7 2JA
www.raynauds.org.uk

Lupus UK
St. James House
Eastern Road
Romford
Essex RM1 3NH
www.lupusuk.com

St. Thomas's Lupus Trust
St. Thomas's Hospital
London SE1 7EH
www.lupus.org.uk

Hughes Syndrome Foundation
Louise Coote Lupus Unit
Gassiot House
St. Thomas's Hospital
London SE1 7EH
www.hughes-syndrome.org

ESSENTIAL READING

Graves, M., Cohen, H., Machin, S.J. and Mackie, I. (2000) Guidelines on the investigation and management of the antiphospholipid syndrome. **British Journal of Haematology**, **109**(4):704–715.

Hakim, A., Clunie, G. and Haq, I. (2006) **Oxford Handbook of Rheumatology**, 2nd Edn. Oxford; Oxford University Press.

Isaacs, J. and Moreland, L. (2002) **Fast facts: Rheumatoid Arthritis.** Oxford; Health Press.

Isenberg, D. and Morrow, J. (1995) **Friendly Fire: Explaining Autoimmune Disease.** Oxford; Oxford University Press.

Khare, M. and Nelson-Piercy, C. (2003) Acquired thrombophilias and pregnancy. **Best Practice and Research in Obstetrics and Gynaecology, 17**(3):491–507.

Lupus UK (undated) **Lupus in Young Women: A guide to living with systemic lupus erythematosus**. Romford: Lupus UK. (direct from Lupus UK www.medical.lupusuk.org.uk)

Moots, R. and Jones, N. (2004) **Your Questions Answered: Rheumatoid Arthritis**. London; Churchill Livingstone.

Nelson-Piercy, C. (2002) **Handbook of Obstetric Medicine**. London; Martin Dunitz.

Norton, Y. (2000) **Lupus: A GP guide to Diagnosis.** Romford; Lupus UK.
(direct from Lupus UK www.medical.lupusuk.org.uk)

Ostensen, M. and 28 authors (2006) Anti-inflammatory and immunosuppressive drugs and reproduction. **Arthritis Research & therapy, 8**:209–228.
http://arthritis-research.com/content/8/3/209

Snaith, M. (2004) **ABC of Rheumatology**. Oxford; BMJ Books – Blackwell.

Vials, J. (2001) A Literature Review on the antiphospholipid syndrome and the effect on childbearing. **Midwifery, 17**: 142–149.

http://www.bnf.org

http://www.prodigy.nhs.uk

http://www.raynauds.demon.co.uk

INFECTIOUS CONDITIONS*

12

Karen Watkins, Veronica Johnson-Roffey and Juliet Houghton

*Other viral and bacterial infections can be found in Appendix 12.2

12.1 Viral Hepatitis

Incidence	Risk for Childbearing
HCV – estimated at 250–500 million worldwide HBV – over 350 million worldwide are carriers[1,2]	Variable Risk: *In utero* and peripartum transmission both possible for hepatitis B and C

EXPLANATION OF CONDITION

The description viral hepatitis describes a group of blood-borne viruses denoted as A, B, C, D or E, which can cause hepatocellular necrosis and inflammation (see Appendix 12.1). The infections can be either acute or chronic in nature. The most important of these to health workers are hepatitis B and hepatitis C.

These viruses are found in blood, but can also be found in other bodily fluids (including semen and saliva). They are most commonly transmitted through unprotected sexual intercourse, by sharing injecting equipment or from a mother to her infant *in utero* or during delivery – known as vertical transmission. Breast-feeding poses a low risk if nipples are not cracked or bleeding[3].

Both viruses can lead to serious illness, including cirrhosis of the liver and even death, but this is more commonly seen with hepatitis B. Both infections may also resolve spontaneously and have no adverse effects.

Treatments for hepatitis B include interferon or lamivudine, but prevention of infection remains the primary aim and can usually be achieved through immunisation. Prevention of infection with hepatitis B for the majority of newborns can be effectively instituted through immunisation commenced at birth. There is no immunisation against hepatitis C, but new treatments are proving to be successful in eradicating the virus.

COMPLICATIONS

The key complication associated with hepatitis B is *chronic hepatitis*, the key features of which include:

- Chronic liver disease including:
  - spider naevi
  - finger clubbing
  - jaundice
  - hepatosplenomegaly and ascites
  - skin bruising[4]
- Liver cirrhosis
- Liver failure
- Hepatocellular carcinoma

Fulminant hepatitis is rare in hepatitis C infection[5,6], but occurs more commonly with co-infection with hepatitis A[7]. Vertical transmission (*in utero* or peripartum) is a complication for acutely infectious hepatitis B carriers, as, in this situation, over 90% of infants born to HBV infectious mothers will become chronic carriers unless immunised[8,9]. They then risk developing cirrhosis and hepatocellular carcinoma.

The risk of vertical transmission of hepatitis C infection is currently around 5–6%, and is related to the amount of hepatitis C virus the mother has in her bloodstream during pregnancy and delivery[10].

NON-PREGNANCY TREATMENT AND CARE

- All women with HCV or HBV require ongoing medical care to monitor for any progressing liver disease
- Women should be advised to stop or reduce alcohol consumption, and to avoid taking over-the-counter or herbal medicines without first seeking medical advice
- Women identified as HBV infected should be offered assessment and immunisation for previous and current sexual partners and close family contacts
- Barrier methods of contraception should be advocated until immunisation of the sexual partner is complete
- Detailed explanation of the condition should be given, with emphasis on routes of transmission
- Carriers should be advised not to donate blood or organs

There are now effective treatments for chronic hepatitis C, primarily the use of pegylated interferon in combination with ribavirin. This treatment is successful in clearing infection in up to 55% of patients[11].

Hepatitis B and acute hepatitis C are both notifiable diseases in the UK. Notification forms are completed by a doctor.

PRE-CONCEPTION ISSUES AND CARE

Any woman found to have either HBV or HCV should be advised to seek specialist opinion prior to conception, to ensure that she is in optimum health for pregnancy.

When a woman is known to have HBV prior to conception, it is important to identify whether she is chronically infected or acutely infectious. Those women in whom hepatitis B e-antigen (HBeAg) is detected are most infectious[12]. Those with antibody to HBeAg (anti-HBe) are generally of low infectivity.

Mothers should be counselled of the importance of immunisation of their newborn and, if they are HbeAg positive, the need for hepatitis B immunoglobulin (HBIG). It has been established that the administration of immunisation and HBIG in high risk infants reduces the vertical transmission risk by 90%[13]. There is no vaccine to prevent HCV infection.

- Women known to have HCV prior to conception should have their general health and lifestyle assessed (including liver function), and immunisation against hepatitis A and B should be offered
- Screening of sexual partners and existing children should be initiated
- Increasing migration to the UK from high prevalence countries is increasing the rates of hepatitis infections seen here
- Vaccination for Hepatitis A and B are often required for travel to high prevalence countries and should be administered prior to pregnancy
- Vaccination differentials are outlined in Appendix 12.1

Pregnancy Issues

- All pregnant women are routinely screened for hepatitis B and this might be how it is first diagnosed
- Women deemed to be at higher risk for hepatitis C (i.e. partners of carriers, those from high prevalence areas, intravenous drug users and sex workers) should be tested for this and results clearly documented in maternity notes/hand-held records
- Women with a positive result should be counselled about the risk to sexual partners, other family members and their baby; written information should also be provided
- Consent for immunisation against hepatitis B (and the need for HBIG where appropriate) should be negotiated and agreed prior to delivery
- Vaccine (+/− HBIG) should be ordered in advance and stored in the labour ward fridge

Medical Management and Care

Hepatitis B
- Establish high- or low-infectivity of the client
- Counsel for risks to partner, children and infant
- Obtain consent for hepatitis B immunisation (+/− HBIG)
- Document delivery and immunisation plan in maternal notes

Hepatitis C
- Counsel for risks to partner, children and infant
- Explain screening for partner, children and infant
- Document delivery plan in maternal notes

Midwifery Management and Care

Hepatitis B
- Counsel for risks to partner, children and infant
- Ensure the mother is informed of risks and benefits of immunisation (+/− HBIG)
- Advise of safety of breast-feeding (including abstinence if nipples are cracked or bleeding)

Hepatitis C
- Counsel for risk to partner, children and infant
- Stress importance of follow-up care for all
- Advise of safety of breast-feeding (including abstinence if nipples are cracked or bleeding)

Labour Issues

- Labour and delivery should be planned and instigated with adherence to 'Control of Infection' guidelines provided by the hospital
- Invasive procedures, such as use of fetal scalp electrodes or fetal blood sampling, pose a significant risk of vertical transmission to the fetus
- Consideration of patient confidentiality should be paramount at all times to prevent inappropriate disclosure of diagnosis or undue anxiety during labour and delivery

Medical Management and Care

Hepatitis B and C
- Avoid fetal blood sampling due to the risk of vertical transmission
- No clear benefit of caesarean section
- Apart from the infection issues the labour can otherwise be managed normally by the midwife

Midwifery Management and Care

Hepatitis B and C
- The woman and her birth partner should be reassured about planned interventions and the rationale for these and kept informed and reassured throughout labour
- Avoid fetal scalp electrode use due to the risk of vertical transmission
- Ensure that 'Control of Infection' guidelines are adhered to

Postpartum Issues

- No evidence that HCV or HBV are transmitted via breast milk, so breast-feeding should still be promoted
- Transmission of infection occurs via blood, so breast-feeding mothers with cracked or bleeding nipples present a significant transmission risk to the neonate
- Infants born to HBV-infected mothers should be immunised with the accelerated immunisation schedule (at birth, one month, two months and twelve months of age)
- If the mother is hepatitis B e-antigen (HBeAg) positive, hepatitis B immunoglobulin (HBIG) should also be given to the infant
- Bathing the infant immediately after birth will further decrease the transmission risk

Medical Management and Care

- Ensure referrals to appropriate services are in place to provide follow-up for the mother and her infant
- Communicate with relevant health professionals with consent

Midwifery Management and Care

- Bathe the infant shortly after delivery
- Provide support for successful initiation of breast-feeding (if wished)
- Examine the breast-feeding mother's nipples daily to detect cracking
- If cracked or bleeding nipples occur, mothers should temporarily abstain until healing has occurred

Hepatitis B
- Ensure that first vaccine (+/− HBIG) is administered to the infant before transfer to the postnatal ward or discharge home

12.2 Human Immunodeficiency Virus

Incidence	Risk for Childbearing
58,003 known cases in the UK, of which 1,650 are children (to end of 2004)[1]	Low Risk – with interventions/no breast-feeding Variable Risk – without interventions plus breast-feeding

EXPLANATION OF CONDITION

Human immunodeficiency virus (HIV) is a retrovirus that is transmitted sexually (through unprotected sexual intercourse), parenterally (via shared injecting equipment or blood transfusion/organ receipt) or from a mother to her infant through vertical transmission (during pregnancy, delivery or breast-feeding). HIV infects the CD4 T-lymphocytes (an essential component of the immune system) rendering them ineffective at fighting infections, and leads to a gradual deterioration in immune function. This leaves the body susceptible to any form of infection, including those commonly present in the body that are usually contained by the immune system (known as opportunistic infections).

The advent of antiretroviral therapy has enabled the replication of HIV to be suppressed to such a level that the CD4 count can recover. HIV is therefore now viewed as a chronic infection that is manageable with medication[2].

COMPLICATIONS

HIV may take many years to damage the immune system, but if untreated it will ultimately lead to the development of AIDS (acquired immune deficiency syndrome), a collection of diseases (including opportunistic infections) that ultimately may result in the premature death of the woman[2]. Early identification of women with HIV allows for the preservation of the immune system and the introduction of antiretroviral therapy before she becomes unwell.

HIV positive women have a small increased risk of adverse effects during pregnancy, including:

- Miscarriage
- Stillbirth
- Fetal abnormality
- Perinatal mortality
- Neonatal death
- Intrauterine growth retardation (IUGR)
- Low birth weight
- Premature delivery[3,4]

NON-PREGNANCY TREATMENT AND CARE

HIV is now viewed as a chronic disease, and many women do not require drug therapy for many years after contracting HIV. Regular monitoring by their specialist team will ensure that their immune function is monitored, and treatment initiated when their clinical or immunological condition dictates.

Standard treatment for non-pregnant women is three antiretroviral medicines (known as combination therapy), usually started once the CD4 count is 200–350 cells/mm^3 or the patient displays signs of advancing clinical disease[2].

Sexually active women are also advised to seek routine cervical screening, as they are at increased risk of cervical cancer[5].

Psychological and emotional support remains a key aspect of routine HIV care, along with ongoing education about the illness and the importance of adhering to the antiretroviral therapy prescription.

PRE-CONCEPTION ISSUES AND CARE

The three key aspects to consider are:

1. Minimising the risk of HIV transmission between discordant couples
2. Management of any fertility issues
3. Health and medication needs

Couples wishing to conceive should be advised against unprotected sexual intercourse (regardless of the man's HIV status). They should be provided with quills, syringes and sterile containers, with advice on self-insemination techniques during the fertile period of the menstrual cycle. Guidelines for the fertility management of discordant couples are available from the British Fertility Society[6].

There is limited data on genital infections among HIV positive women[7] but sexually-transmitted infection rates in sub-Saharan Africa (where the majority of UK HIV infections originate) are known to be high[8]. Women are therefore advised to seek regular check-ups at a genito-urinary medicine clinic, as *Chlamydia trachomatis*, *Neisseria gonorrhoeae*, *Ureaplasma urealyticum*, and bacterial vaginosis are all associated with chorioamnionitis[9,10], which may lead to premature rupture of membranes, premature delivery[9,11] and an increased risk of vertical transmission of HIV. Ideally, these infections should be identified and treated before conception.

Where infections are diagnosed, sexual partners should be screened and treated as required.

Other viral and bacterial infections are outlined in Appendix 12.2.

Pregnancy Issues
- All HIV positive women should be routinely screened for sexually transmitted infection at presentation and in the third trimester[2]
  - cervical cytology should routinely be performed
  - *Treponema* serology should also be repeated in the third trimester
- A full assessment of the psycho-social issues should be undertaken to ensure adequate and appropriate support
- Disclosure of HIV to partners is advised, but is often challenging and complex and should therefore be viewed as a process rather than an event; never assume that anyone other than the woman knows her HIV status
- Sensitive handling of exclusive formula feeding must be provided
- Disclosure of HIV infection to other health care professionals is on a 'need to know' basis, and rationale for disclosure should be provided and consent sought (where appropriate)
- Support of adherence to antiretroviral medication is crucial if medications are to be taken correctly

Medical Management and Care
- Sexually transmitted infection screen at presentation and in the third trimester
- Cervical cytology should also be performed
- *Treponema* serology should be repeated in the third trimester
- Genotypic resistance testing is recommended before starting zidovudine and prior to delivery to identify viral mutations
- Referral to paediatric team and other services as required
- Initiate and continue dialogue around disclosure of HIV diagnosis to partner and/or health care professionals

Midwifery Management and Care
- Promote attendance for sexually-transmitted infection screening
- Provide sensitive advice around risk of HIV transmission through breast-feeding, and advise exclusive formula feeding to all HIV positive mothers
- Refer to available services for assistance with the purchasing of infant formula (where available)
- Ensure documentation is maintained around all aspects of pregnancy care, including who their HIV diagnosis has been disclosed to
- Provide support and monitoring of antiretroviral medication and promote adherence

Labour Issues
- All women should have a plan for their expected mode of delivery; invasive fetal monitoring should be avoided due to the risk of transferring maternal HIV infection to the baby
- Prophylactic intravenous antibiotics should be considered to reduce the incidence of chorioamnionitis or post-caesarean infection
- Sensitivity around inadvertent disclosure of diagnosis is crucial (through notes, prescriptions, etc.) and local control of infection guidelines must be followed correctly

Medical Management and Care
- Elective vaginal delivery is an option for women with an HIV viral load <50 cps/ml
- Elective caesarean section should be planned for 38 weeks
- Avoid invasive procedures (including fetal scalp monitoring and artificial rupture of membranes)
- Consider intrapartum antibiotics

Midwifery Management and Care
- Home confinement not advised
- Avoid invasive procedures (see above)
- Follow control of infection guidelines
- Administration of intravenous zidovudine as indicated
- Bathe the baby immediately after delivery
- Maintain discretion around HIV diagnosis

Postpartum Issues
Postnatal depression is a risk for HIV positive women due to compounding pressures associated with HIV, housing or financial difficulties, immigration uncertainties or social isolation. Early referral to appropriate psychology or mental health services is advised.

Many women discover their HIV infection during antenatal screening, and pregnancy becomes a stressful and medically invasive process. Supporting women to remain in health care during and following their delivery is therefore crucial for their long-term wellbeing.

Medical Management and Care
- Short-term antiretroviral therapy should be discontinued after delivery when viral load <50 cps/ml
- Consider the half-life of each drug prior to discontinuation to avoid inadvertent monotherapy
- ART commenced prior to pregnancy should continue postnatally
- Liaise with health professionals to ensure maternal and neonatal HIV follow-up is arranged

Midwifery Management and Care
- Ensure neonatal antiretroviral therapy prescription is completed and administered within six hours of delivery
- EDTA blood from both mother and baby (*not* cord blood) on first or second postpartum days
- Ensure postnatal HIV appointments have been arranged

12.3 Malaria

Incidence	Risk for Childbearing
Estimated 300–500 million cases worldwide >1 million deaths annually, mostly children <5 yrs and pregnant women[1,2]	Variable Risk – uncomplicated malaria High Risk – severe malaria

EXPLANATION OF CONDITION

Malaria is a protozoal infection that is potentially fatal. Transmission occurs mainly in tropical and sub-tropical countries, especially in Africa. More than 2000 cases of malaria are imported into UK annually[1,6].

Malaria is caused by four protozoal species: *Plasmodium falciparum, P. malariae, P. ovale* and *P. vivax. P. falciparum* is present in most of the endemic areas and is associated with most deaths; the remaining three being more localised[1,5]. Those people residing in, or travelling to, a malaria area risk infection. Partial immunity develops with repeated attacks but is lost with lack of exposure, especially after emigration. Sickle cell trait offers some protection, with those affected by *P. falciparum* more likely to survive acute illness if they have sickle cell trait[3,4].

Malaria parasites in the infected *Anopheles* mosquito saliva are transmitted from person to person by its bite. Transmission can also occur by infected blood transfusions, organ transplant, sharing contaminated needles and, rarely, from mother to baby during delivery[3,9]. Parasites within a victim's blood are carried to liver cells where they invade, grow and multiply. Eventually parasites are released back into the circulation to infect and destroy red blood cells[5].

Incubation period varies and symptoms can occur in the first week of exposure; *P. falciparum* has the shortest incubation period. Suspect malaria in anyone who has travelled to a malaria area in the previous year and exhibits symptoms. *P.ovale, P. malariae* and *P.vivax* produce dormant stages, thus may be symptomatic over a year after exposure[5,6].

Symptoms of uncomplicated malaria comprise:

- Sweats
- Periodic fevers
- Headache
- Malaise
- Aching muscles
- Joint pain
- Rigors
- Vomiting
- Enlarged spleen
- Mild jaundice[1,5]

Symptoms may be misdiagnosed for other conditions such as meningitis. Correct diagnosis is made using a microscope to demonstrate *Plasmodium* parasites in peripheral blood samples ideally taken at the height of a fever[7,8].

COMPLICATIONS

P. falciparum infection in immunosuppressed, young and pregnant patients leads to severe (complicated) malaria, often presenting within days of the initial symptoms. Complications occur singly or in combinations[1], as:

- Coma (cerebral malaria)
- Severe anaemia and jaundice
- Pulmonary oedema and respiratory distress
- Renal failure
- Hypoglycaemia and convulsions
- Disseminated intravascular coagulation
- Hyperpyrexia
- Hyperparasitaemia
- Malarial haemoglobulinurea

NON-PREGNANCY TREATMENT AND CARE

Due to antimalarial drug resistance, specialist expert medical advice should be sought before treatment, e.g. from the *HPA Malaria Reference Laboratory – 020 7636 3924*.

Treatment in the UK usually commences after diagnosis is confirmed by blood test. However, if severe malaria is strongly suspected treatment might have to commence before laboratory diagnosis. Treatment is with the appropriate antimalarial drug, and choice of drug treatment is dependent on the woman's clinical status, the infecting *Plasmodium* species and its drug susceptibility[6,10,16]. In the UK, hospitalisation is usually advised until the strain of malaria is identified. Patients with *P. falciparum* malaria will usually require longer hospitalisation due to potential manifestation of severe complications.

Currently the drugs used in the UK for the treatment and prophylaxis of malaria include:

- Quinine
- Malarone
- Doxycycline
- Chloroquine
- Primaquine
- Riamet®
- Mefloquine

These drugs can be used individually or in combination, orally, im or iv[10].

Good patient care includes monitoring vital signs, intake/output, blood glucose and general conditions of the patient to observe for the signs of severe malaria, which will need specialist treatment. Ensure adequate patient follow-up after discharge.

NB: *Delay in diagnosis and treatment could be fatal.*

PRE-CONCEPTION ISSUES AND CARE

Anyone travelling to a malaria endemic area should pay particular attention to preventative measures. Awareness of risk, avoiding mosquito bites, taking appropriate prophylaxis and seeking immediate medical attention if symptoms develop within and up to a year after travel[11,12].

Prophylaxis is dependent on the areas to be visited, so encourage compliance with treatment. At-risk groups include anyone originating from an endemic area, recent immigrants and long-term travellers such as those in the forces[11,12].

Pregnant women are at greater risk of developing severe malaria with adverse effects of drugs on a developing fetus, so advise women to avoid conceiving for up to 12 weeks after completing prophylaxis. Those wishing to conceive sooner should consider whether their travel to a malaria area is necessary[12].

Advise avoidance of insect bites by:

- Using insect repellents
- Sleeping under a pyrethroid-impregnated mosquito net
- Using knockdown insecticide sprays in room at night
- Wearing long sleeves, trousers and socks[11,12]

Pregnancy Issues

In pregnancy, immunity is reduced, rendering the mother susceptible either to infection or to a relapse. This is especially so during a first pregnancy, but also the second trimester of all pregnancies. *P. falciparum* in particular can have a significant impact on maternal, fetal and neonatal health and is a medical emergency.

Even if no clinical symptoms are shown women can still develop placental parasitaemia, and relapses of *P. vivax* and *P. ovale* can also occur in pregnancy[12,13,15].

Adverse effects of malaria on pregnancy are:
* *Maternal effects* – complications as mentioned above
  – anaemia makes woman more susceptible to other infections
  – women with co-existing HIV are more likely to suffer maternal and fetal complications and malaria infections in placenta may increase fetal transmission of HIV[14]
* *Fetal effects*
  – miscarriage
  – stillbirth
  – low birth weight
  – prematurity
  – fetal acidosis
  – congenital malaria
  – neonatal death[14,15,17]
* Management in pregnancy involves treating the malaria, monitoring for and managing any complications, surveillance of fetal wellbeing and management of labour[17]

Medical Management and Care

Prevention of malaria in pregnancy
Advise not to travel to malaria area while pregnant but if necessary stress correct prophylaxis and give preventative advice. Some antimalarials contraindicated in pregnancy, therefore seek expert advice, e.g. from *HPA Malaria Reference Laboratory – 020 7636 3924* for the UK[6,10,16].

Management of malaria in pregnancy
* Confirm infection by demonstrating malaria parasites in peripheral blood on thick and thin films
* If symptomatic, admit immediately for prompt specialist management, treatment and monitoring of complications, such as anaemia, renal failure, hypoglycaemia and DIC[14,17]
* Fluid replacement should be carefully monitored because of the risk of pulmonary oedema
* 50% glucose may need to be given for hypoglycaemia and blood transfusion if anaemia causes cardiovascular compromise
* Treat pyrexia promptly as may cause pre-term labour
* Severe malaria is a medical emergency and should be managed in a HDU/ITU with multidisciplinary input
* Fetal surveillance
  – monitor for pre-term labour and give steroids for lung maturation if needed
  – monitor fetal wellbeing by CTG and ultrasound
* Induction of labour may be necessary if fetal and maternal health concerns

Midwifery Management and Care
* Booking history should always include travel and prophylaxis history
* Advise against travel to malaria areas unless strictly necessary
* Advise to seek immediate medical help if symptoms develop abroad or on return, as infection is possible even if prophylaxis was taken
* Be aware that some symptoms of malaria resemble pre-eclampsia
* Seek medical advice immediately for concerns about mother or baby

Labour Issues
* Monitoring for fetal distress in labour is important due to adverse maternal condition
* There is increased risk of postpartum haemorrhage[17] (PPH) and infection
* Pulmonary oedema, if not already present, can occur immediately after delivery if the woman is severely anaemic[17]

Medical Management and Care
* Manage according to medical condition
* Obstetric intervention may become necessary if fetal distress detected
* Fetal heart rate abnormalities may improve on correction of maternal pyrexia or hypoglycaemia, otherwise delivery may be required

Midwifery Management and Care
* Manage according to medical condition at time of labour
* Active management of third stage with regard to increased risk of PPH
* Careful observations of vital signs and temperature in mother
* Attention to strict infection control precautions
* Cord blood should be taken post-delivery and sent to the laboratory for a *blood smear* to diagnose or exclude congenital malaria

Postpartum Issues
* Risk of secondary postpartum haemorrhage (PPH)[17]
* Theoretical, but rare, risk of congenital malaria in the baby.[19]
* Possible complications associated with low-birth-weight infant
* Some antimalarial drugs are contraindicated in breast-feeding[20]

Medical Management and Care
* Be alert for signs of pulmonary oedema such as acute breathlessness, which could develop immediately after birth and should be treated
* Prompt medical intervention if PPH occurs
* Observe for anaemia and instigate prompt treatment if necessary

Midwifery Management and Care
* Manage according to medical condition
* Mother and baby are not for early discharge home
* Continue observation of mother's vital signs
* Observe for PPH
* Observations of neonate for signs of fever, respiratory distress or jaundice, which could be suggestive of congenital malaria[18,19]
* Care of possible low-birth-weight baby
* Confer with paediatrician and pharmacist about safety of maternal drugs whilst breast-feeding
* Paediatrician, not midwife, for the neonatal 'discharge' examination

12.4 Listeriosis

Incidence
Varies worldwide, but within European Union approximately 2–10 cases per million population reported annually[1]

Risk for Childbearing
High Risk

EXPLANATION OF CONDITION

In 2004 in England and Wales, 213 cases of listeriosis infections were reported to the Health Protection Agency, of which 20 were pregnancy related[2]. In Scotland, 15 cases were reported[3].

This is an uncommon but potentially serious infection in humans. It is caused primarily by eating food contaminated with the bacterium *Listeria monocytogenes*, a Gram-positive bacillus that has also been identified in natural environments, such as soil, water, intestinal tract of animals and sewage. Humans may be asymptomatic carriers in their intestinal flora. Human listeriosis was recognised in the late 1920s and demonstrated to be a food-borne infection in 1981. Food stored in a refrigerator can still be a hazard, as *L. monocytogenes*, can grow at low temperatures[4,5,6,7].

L. monocytogenes is found in a variety of raw foods, such as uncooked meats, raw fish, poultry and vegetables and in some processed foods that become contaminated after processing, i.e. cook–chill meats, salads, soft cheeses and pâté. Unpasteurised milk and food made from it has also been implicated[6,7]. Most cases are sporadic, however some outbreaks have been associated with contaminated food[8].

Transmission from person to person is rare *except* for vertical transmission from mother to fetus transplacentally or during delivery. Papular lesions may occur on hands and arms from contact with infectious material, i.e. sick or dead animals. A few cases due to hospital cross infection and nosocomial infection in nurseries have been reported[6,7,9,10].

L. monocytogenes infections are most harmful to pregnant women, newborns, the elderly and those with weakened immune systems due to HIV infection or cancer[6,11]. The incubation period varies widely, but is reported to be on average 21 days in adults, intrauterine infections 30 days and in neonates just a few days[6,7]. Infection can be asymptomatic, but if symptoms manifest in healthy adults these are usually mild and include fever, muscle ache, nausea or diarrhoea.

Isolating *L. monocytogenes* in cerebrospinal fluid or blood culture confirms the diagnosis. The bacterium may also be identified in meconium, amniotic fluid and placenta samples.

COMPLICATIONS

In the immunocompromised, elderly, or pregnant listeriosis can be more serious and can cause meningitis or septicaemia thus giving rise to symptoms such as headache, neck stiffness, loss of balance or confusion[6,12].

While infection in the mother might be asymptomatic or mild, in the fetus and neonate it is serious. Transplacental infections during the very early stage of pregnancy might lead to spontaneous abortion and fetal infection later in pregnancy may lead to premature birth, stillbirth or death in the first few days of life[6,13,14,15,16]. Neonatal listeriosis has two stages of clinical onset presentation.

Early Onset

- Birth is usually premature and the disease is due to intrauterine infection
- Symptoms occur within hours to first five days of birth and fatality is high

- Symptoms include:
  – meconium staining
  – respiratory distress
  – fever
  – rash
  – lethargy
  – vomiting
  – poor feeding
  – jaundice

Late Onset

- Most likely due to infection around birth
- Usually a term infant, well at birth, develops symptoms after 5–7 days presenting as meningitis or septicaemia
- Neurodevelopment delay and hydrocephalus have also been reported in those with meningitis[4,13,14,16,17]

NON-PREGNANCY TREATMENT AND CARE

Currently first-line treatment is with ampicillin, sometimes combined with gentamicin. Several other antibiotics are also available as second-line treatment[18].

Advise the woman to complete the course of antibiotics, get plenty of rest, good fluid intake and a healthy diet. Advise on good hygiene measures to prevent spread.

In the UK this is a notifiable disease if identified as food-borne 'food poisoning', which should be reported to the Health Protection Agency by the clinician.

PRE-CONCEPTION ISSUES AND CARE

All women preparing for pregnancy should be advised to maintain a healthy lifestyle, eat a well-balanced diet and avoid known infection risks. Additional advice should be given on avoidance of contracting listeriosis, and to report any symptoms of infection to the doctor immediately in order to aid investigation and early treatment. Women with a known infection should always make sure that the infection is treated successfully if possible before becoming pregnant.

Measures to reduce risk of listeriosis are:

- Completely cook raw meat and poultry before eating
- Wash all fruits and raw vegetables
- Keep uncooked meats separate from cooked foods, ready to eat foods and vegetables
- Avoid unpasteurised milk or foods made from it
- Wash hands, utensils and chopping boards after dealing with uncooked foods
- Eat ready-prepared and perishable foods as soon as possible while still in date
- If re-heating food make sure it is piping hot all through, cooking destroys this bacteria[4,6,12]
- Avoid eating *soft* cheeses such as brie, camembert, blue-veined and Mexican-style cheeses, meat spreads and pâté
- Avoid delicatessen-counter food unless thoroughly heated

Whilst they are not a main source of infection, it is still wise to avoid contact with sheep during lambing and aborted animal fetuses and silage on farms[4,6,12].

Pregnancy Issues

- Emphasis should be on prevention and early detection of listeriosis
- Prompt identification and treatment of listeriosis during pregnancy can lead to a successful pregnancy outcome[16]
- Maternal infection during pregnancy can lead to complications as discussed previously
- Diagnosis is made by culturing the organism from blood, placenta or liquor
- Maternal symptoms may be mild, can be overlooked and therefore go untreated, thus leaving fetus at risk of contracting infection *in utero*
- A child born to a woman diagnosed with *L. monocytogenes* infection during pregnancy could be at risk of developing early or late neonatal listeriosis (see earlier) so confinement in hospital consultant unit should be discussed with the mother to be

Medical Management and Care

- Be aware that any febrile illness in pregnancy, amnionitis or pre-term labour, particularly with meconium staining of liquor could be due to *L. monocytogenes* infection
- If diagnosed, the mother requires hospital admission for immediate intravenous antibiotic treatment and observation

Midwifery Management and Care

- There is no routine screening for listeriosis in the UK
- Women should be advised to seek medical advice immediately if they develop any flu-like symptoms during pregnancy
- Advise on which foods to avoid during pregnancy, good food and kitchen hygiene measures (as discussed under preconception care)
- If maternal listeriosis is suspected or diagnosed, there should be regular monitoring of maternal and fetal wellbeing throughout pregnancy to detect early any abnormalities such as signs of pre-term labour

Labour Issues

- There is an increased risk of premature birth or stillborn baby in mothers with listeriosis
- Characteristics of listeriosis infections in the neonate can be similar to those caused by group B streptococci
- Sometimes in neonatal *L. monocytogenes* infection there may be micro-abscesses seen on the fetal surface of the placenta as well as on the skin of the neonate[14,16]

Medical Management and Care

- Medical management as necessary if pre-term labour
- If mother and fetus well, and full-term pregnancy, midwife can manage labour; if maternal or fetal complications present or develop then manage accordingly

Midwifery Management and Care

- Summon medical aid immediately if any concern such as fetal compromise arises
- After delivery examine placenta and note any signs of chorioamnionitis (e.g. a yellow or green tint of membranes and chorion), or signs of micro-abscesses, all of which may indicate early onset infection in the neonate of a woman who has been treated for listeriosis
- Send samples for culture if abnormality present
- Observe newborn for signs of infection, respiratory distress or any other complications

Postpartum Issues

- Early and late onset listeriosis may become evident
- Signs of early onset occur within hours to five days of birth, and late onset from 5–7 days after birth (symptoms as described earlier)
- There have been reports of nosocomial infections of *L. monocytogenes* infections in nurseries[9,10]
- Breast-feeding is rarely contraindicated[19]
- Signs and symptoms of early and late onset listeriosis in the baby include those of meningitis or septicaemia:
  - fever
  - rash
  - irritability
  - lethargy
  - poor feeding
  - bulging fontanelle

Medical Management and Care

- Test baby for *L. monocytogenes* if mother was affected during, or immediately prior to, this pregnancy
- Commence antibiotic treatment if necessary

Midwifery Management and Care

- Observe for signs of early- and late-onset neonatal listeriosis, i.e. signs of respiratory distress soon after birth
- Advise parents what signs to look for
- Strict adherence to infection control precautions to prevent nosocomial infections in nursery
- If pre-term delivery, attention to the specialist care of such infants
- If mother intends to breast-feed, help to establish lactation promptly
- Support and keep parents/family informed
- Good communication between hospital and community staff on transfer home
- Continue observation for signs and symptoms of late-onset listeriosis, extending the period of home visits by the midwife if indicated

12.5 Toxoplasmosis

Incidence	Risk for Childbearing
Worldwide: 20–40% adults in developed countries affected[1] UK: 0.5%–1% of population affected annually[2]	High Risk: acute infection Variable Risk: chronic infection

EXPLANATION OF CONDITION

Toxoplasmosis is a common parasitic infection, caused by the protozoan parasite *Toxoplasma gondii*, which was discovered in 1908[2,3]. It is found in a wide variety of animals, but the reservoir is the cat and other felines in whose gut the parasite completes its sexual stage by producing oocysts (egg cysts). Cats acquire the infection by eating infected birds or rodents. For up to 2 weeks following primary infection they pass the oocysts, which remain viable in the soil for up to 18 months, in their faeces. If other animals and humans eat these oocysts they hatch and the parasite moves from the gut to invade tissues and cause toxoplasmosis.

Toxoplasmosis potentially poses a significant health risk to the fetus during pregnancy and to people with impaired immunity, i.e. HIV disease. It can cause congenital mental retardation, chorioretinitis and encephalitis[1,2,4,5,6].

Humans acquire the infection by:

- Ingestion of undercooked meat (mainly mutton or pork)
- Ingesting unwashed, uncooked vegetables and fruits
- Hand to mouth contact with faeces of infected cats
  - cleaning out litter tray
  - gardening
- Blood transfusion or organ transplant
- Drinking unpasteurised milk[1,4,5,6]

Person to person transmission does not occur except vertically from pregnant woman to the fetus or, rarely, by organ transplant or blood transfusion.

The incubation period is 10–25 days[1,6]. After the initial acute infection the parasite becomes inactive and remains dormant, giving lifelong protection, but can be reactivated if the immune system becomes impaired. Generally, reactivation in a seropositive woman carries very little or no risk of transmission to the fetus[4].

The majority of healthy sufferers have little or no symptoms or a mild flu-like illness, sometimes mistaken for glandular fever. These symptoms include:

- Headache
- Sore throat
- Fever
- Fatigue
- Swollen glands
- Night sweats
- Muscle aches

Diagnosis is confirmed by history of clinical symptoms and examination of blood or body fluid to detect IgG and IgM antibodies. Raised levels of IgG antibodies indicate past infection and raised IgM indicate current infection. Other means of diagnosis, such as demonstration of cysts in the placenta or lymph tissue, have also been used[1,2,4,6].

COMPLICATIONS

First and Second Trimester Acquired Infection

- Miscarriage
- Congenital hydrocephalus
- Mental retardation

- Deafness and blindness
- Growth problems

Third Trimester Acquired Infection

- Retinochoroiditis developing later[4,7]
- Stillbirth[4,7]

In about 40% of new infections in pregnancy the fetus is infected, with most cases occuring in the third trimester, in which case the baby can appear 'normal' at birth. The earlier in pregnancy the infection occurs the more severe the disease in the neonate.

NON-PREGNANCY TREATMENT AND CARE

Most cases are asymptomatic and patients make a full recovery requiring no treatment. However, some people, e.g. those who are immunocompromised, may develop severe symptoms and in these cases specialist treatment advice should be sought from a reference laboratory.

For those requiring treatment this is usually with a combination of pyrimethamine and sulfadiazine or clindamycin. Pyrimethamine is a folate antagonist, so weekly blood counts should be taken and folinic acid supplement given[8].

Advise patients to get plenty of rest, take medication as prescribed and report any unusual side effects of medication.

If maternal diagnosis is confirmed during early pregnancy, spiramycin may be given to the mother to try and reduce the risk of transmission to the fetus[4,7]. If there is concern that the baby may already be infected, and the woman is more than 15 weeks pregnant, then she may be offered amniocentesis, or cordocentesis at 20–22 weeks, both preceded by thorough counselling as to the implications.

If the fetus is affected, a termination of pregancy may be offered or alternatively continue pregnancy with treatment using pyrimethamine and sulfadiazine and folinic acid supplement. Unfortunately this may have side effects. Drug treatment will reduce the severity of infection in the fetus but won't reverse any harm which may already have occured[4,6].

PRE-CONCEPTION ISSUES AND CARE

Emphasis should be on prevention. In additon to the usual advice on maintaining a healthy lifestyle, healthy diet, folic acid supplement and avoiding infections, women should be educated about toxoplasmosis and methods of minimising the risk of contracting this infection before, during and after pregnancy by[1,2,3,4,5,6,7]:

- Avoid eating under-cooked meats
- Wash fruits and vegetables thoroughly
- Wash hands and utensils after preparing raw meat
- Feed cat with dry or canned food instead of raw meat
- Wash hands after handling cat, if necessary to handle cat litter tray wear gloves and wash hands afterwards
- Disinfect cat litter box with boiling water for 5 minutes
- Avoid handling stray or ill cats
- Wear gloves when gardening and wash hands afterwards

Women with an active infection should be advised to avoid becoming pregnant until treatment is completed.

Pregnancy Issues

Management of pregnancy is aimed at preventing vertical transmission.

During pregnancy spiramycin is used to treat toxoplasmosis as it reduces the risk of transmission of infection. It is not effective if the baby is already infected, however, so if tests reveal fetal infection and the pregnancy is to continue then pyrimethamine and sulfadiazine may be suggested[8].

Pyrimethamine can cause suppression of bone marrow, is a folate antagonist and terratogenic in animals. Sulfadiazine can cause macular papular rash and should be discontinued immediately should this occur[6,8].

At 20 weeks of pregnancy an ultrasound scan may also highlight any obvious physical abnormalities, such as hydrops or microcephaly in the baby. Termination of pregnancy is an option for some women, when an infected baby with severe abnormalities has been confirmed[7].

France and Austria conduct routine antenatal toxoplasma screening, but not the UK, where cost effectiveness is not proven[9] because prevalence is low.

Medical Management and Care

- Consider toxoplasmosis if a pregnant woman develops a glandular-fever-like illness; test for IgG and IgM antibodies
- Obtain specialist reference laboratory advice on treatment
- Consider congenital toxoplasmosis if mother has positive serology
- Discuss screening of fetus using amniocentesis or cordocentesis and implications with mother, including consideration of termination of pregnancy
- Fetal ultrasound may be used to demonstrate any abnormality such as IUGR, fetal hydrops, microcephaly, intracranial calcification or hepatosplenomegaly[7]
- Ultrasound examination should be performed at least monthly to monitor for any signs of fetal infection

Midwifery Management and Care

- Advise how to avoid toxoplasmosis exposure during pregnancy
- Advise woman to seek medical advice if they experience fever or flu-like symptoms or if concerned that she could have acquired infection
- If the toxoplasmosis infection is chronic, with no other fetal or maternal concerns, manage as a low-risk pregnancy
- If infection is acute, treat as high-risk pregnancy that will require intense fetal monitoring and treatment of mother to prevent vertical transmission to the fetus
- Women with acute infection, and hence an 'at risk' fetus, may decide to terminate the pregnancy and will require counselling and support[10]
- Some women will decide to continue pregnancy and have prophylactic antibiotics to try and prevent fetal infection; reinforce any advice and instructions regarding treatment
- If amniocentesis or cordocentesis or other investigation is to be carried out, reassure and support mother and ensure she understands procedures[10]
- If the fetus is not infected, and there are no other maternal or fetal complications, home confinement is not contraindicated

Labour Issues

Delivery should follow normal practice unless there are any gross abnormalities, such as hydrocephalus, which will necessitate medical intervention, or any other maternal or fetal concerns.

Medical Management and Care

- Normal midwifery care, unless any concerns arise requiring medical intervention for birth

Midwifery Management and Care

- Manage from normal perspective unless medical concerns arise
- Be aware that the parents may express anxiety, and want answers about the baby's prognosis immediately after birth; hence the baby may need to be seen by a paediatrician sooner rather than later

Postpartum Issues

Breast-feeding has not been demonstrated to be a means of toxoplasmosis transmission in humans[4]. However, if the baby is not infected, but the mother is receiving treatment, check compatibility of drugs with breast-feeding.

Babies born to women with confirmed toxoplasmosis in pregnancy will be monitored closely by paediatricians, with repeated investigations in first year of life. If still seropositive at one year of age, with abnormal clinical findings, then congenital toxoplasmosis is confirmed and therapy should continue[11].

Medical Management and Care

- Treatment of the neonate usually continues for the first year of life
- Consider congenital toxoplasmosis if mother had positive serology
- Refer to paediatricians for follow-up
- The neonate will need clinical, serological, neurological and ophthalmic assessment to rule out or confirm congenital infection[4]

Midwifery Management and Care

- Support prompt commencement of breast-feeding
- Reinforce any advice on medication given for mother and baby
- Care of baby according to condition
- If congenital toxoplasmosis confirmed, or suspected, initiate communication with health visitor or specialist nurse and the community team, because long-term follow-up will be necessary

12.6 Chickenpox

Incidence	Risk for Childbearing
Complicates 3 in 1,000 pregnancies[1]	High Risk

EXPLANATION OF CONDITION

Chickenpox, also known as **varicella**, is a common childhood illness caused by infection with *Varicella zoster* virus. This is a DNA virus from the herpes family. The mode of transmission is mainly via respiratory droplets or by direct contact and is therefore highly contagious. Reactivation of the virus, which has remained latent in the dorsal root or cranial nerve ganglion, causes shingles. This often occurs many years after the initial infection. Chickenpox may be acquired by contact with shingles but this is less common.

Clinical features of chickenpox include a mild febrile illness, associated with malaise and the development of a characteristic vesicular rash. The rash is pruritic, the vesicles appear in waves and typically vesicles, pustules and crusted lesions appear together. The illness usually lasts 7–10 days. There is increased morbidity and mortality in pregnancy compared with non-pregnant, especially as the pregnancy advances[2].

Shingles is characterised by an eruption of painful vesicles covering an area of skin corresponding to one or two sensory nerves, particularly the thoracic nerves, but may affect the cranial nerves, e.g. ophthalmic. If the dorsal root ganglion is affected then the rash may extend from the middle of the back to the chest wall.

The incubation period is 10–12 days, however the infective period extends from 48 hours prior to the appearance of the rash until all the vesicles have crusted over.

Immunity is solid and long-lasting and as the infection is so commonly acquired in childhood over 90% of the antenatal population is immune to the virus[3]. Of those with uncertainty regarding their immune status, 80% will have IgG antibodies on serum testing and will therefore be immune[4].

COMPLICATIONS

Chickenpox is generally a mild, self-limiting illness in childhood however it can be a much more serious condition in adults, with pneumonia being relatively common and encephalitis and hepatitis being other possible complications. Up to 10% of pregnant women with chickenpox develop pneumonia and it is associated with a higher mortality and morbidity than in the non-pregnant patient. The severity of the pneumonia increases as the pregnancy progresses[2] and many of these women will require hospital admission.

Fetal risks include the risk of *fetal varicella syndrome* (FVS) if the infection is acquired within the first 20 weeks of pregnancy, and *varicella infection of the newborn* (VIN) if the infection is acquired within the last four weeks of the pregnancy. Chickenpox has not been associated with an increased risk of miscarriage[6].

The risk of FVS is 1–2% if the infection is acquired in the first 20 weeks of pregnancy and is associated with:

- Skin loss or scarring
- Eye defects, including cataracts
- Hypoplasia of the limbs
- Neurological abnormalities[6,7]

Some features of FVS can be detected prenatally by ultrasound examination of the fetus and these include:

- Shortening of the long bones
- Hydrocephalus
- Microcephalus
- Intrauterine growth restriction[8]

There have been very occasional reports of FVS occurring at 20–28 weeks gestatation[9] however the risk is likely to be extremely small. At 20–36 weeks of gestation the risk is the possibility of the infant developing shingles, which may present subsequently in the first few years of his/her life.

VIN can occur when maternal infection is acquired within four weeks of delivery or immediately after. Approximately half of the babies born will be infected, with a quarter of them developing chickenpox. If, however, the delivery is within one week of the rash developing, or just prior to the onset of the rash, then passively-acquired antibodies in the baby are low and severe chickenpox infection, which may be fatal, can occur in the baby[10].

There does not appear to be any risk to the fetus of shingles in pregnancy[7].

NON-PREGNANCY TREATMENT AND CARE

As chickenpox in childhood is a mild, self-limiting illness all that is generally required is control of the pyrexia and pruritus, e.g. with paracetamol and antihistamines if necessary. Care needs to be taken to avoid secondary infection of the lesions, advice on hygiene should be given and antibiotics if secondary infection does occur. As adults tend to have a more severe illness, oral aciclovir may be given within 24 hours of developing the rash[11]. If complications develop then hospital admission may be required.

PRE-CONCEPTION ISSUES AND CARE

Although a safe and effective vaccine does exist for chickenpox it is not widely used in the UK. The vaccine is contraindicated in pregnancy and pregnancy should be avoided for three months after vaccination. The vaccine is not currently available to seronegative women in the UK planning a pregnancy. The UK Department of Health, however, recommends *Varicella zoster* vaccine to be given to seronegative health care workers who have direct contact with patients[11].

Women who have not had chickenpox should be advised to avoid contact with chickenpox in the peri-conception period, and to report any possible contact to their midwife or doctor.

Pregnancy Issues

Varicella zoster immunoglobulin (VZIg) should be used to prevent chickenpox in susceptible women who have had significant exposure. It should be given within ten days of exposure for maximal effect[12]. It has no place in treatment once chickenpox has developed.

Oral aciclovir decreases the duration and severity of symptoms in women who develop chickenpox in pregnancy. To be effective it needs to be given within 24 hours of the rash developing. It may also decrease the risk of serious complications[12].

Women with chickenpox in pregnancy should be alerted to the possible complications that may occur and should report any respiratory or neurological symptoms or any bleeding immediately so that hospital admission may be considered. Hospital admission may also be required if the mother is in the latter stages of pregnancy, if she smokes or is taking steroids or is immunosuppressed[13].

Neonatology involvement is very important and the mother should be given the opportunity to discuss possible neonatal complications and plans for investigation and treatment of the neonate, post delivery.

Medical Management and Care

- If a mother presents with chickenpox within the first 20 weeks she should be counselled regarding the risks of fetal varicella syndrome (FVS) (1–2%); discuss amniocentesis to determine whether the viral DNA is detectable in the liquor and arrange detailed ultrasound examinations to try to detect features of FVS
- If complications arise the mother should be managed in hospital by a multidisciplinary team involving obstetrician, virologist and neonatologist[12]

Midwifery Management and Care

If a women reports contact with chickenpox
- Ask if previous infection – if so, reassure
- If not, check if significant exposure – was the diagnosis definite; did exposure occur when uncrusted lesions were present or 48 hours prior to development of the rash; was there face to face contact with infected person?
- If yes – arrange for booking blood samples to be tested for *Varicella zoster* virus IgG or send serum for testing
- If IgG negative – arrange for VZIg to be given as soon as possible
- Inform the woman to notify her doctor or midwife if she develops a rash, irrespective of whether she had VZIg or not

If a woman presents with chickenpox in pregnancy:
- Arrange for her to be given oral aciclovir if >20 weeks gestation and if she has presented within 24 hours of the onset of the rash
- Consider whether factors indicating hospital admission are present, and discuss with obstetrician if in doubt
- Inform the woman to report any new symptoms immediately, e.g. chest symptoms, bleeding
- If the woman is less than 20 weeks pregnant, refer to obstetrician for counselling regarding the risks of fetal varicella syndrome
- Counsel her to avoid contact with anyone at risk of developing severe chickenpox, e.g. other pregnant women, including attending ANC
- Advise on use of topical soothing agents and possible use of antihistamines
- Ensure women who remain at home are reviewed regularly

Labour Issues

- Delivery should be avoided during the acute illness
- There is a risk of serious maternal complications including disseminated intravascular coagulation (DIC)
- For the neonate, there is the risk of severe varicella of the newborn, with significant morbidity and possible mortality[10]

Medical Management and Care

- Supportive treatment should be given if labour occurs in the viraemic period
- Intravenous aciclovir is recommended in this situation[12]

Midwifery Management and Care

- The woman should be closely observed for the development of the complications of chickenpox, in particular DIC
- Ascertain if the paediatrician is to review the baby post delivery

Postpartum Issues

The highest risk to the neonate is when delivery occurs within five days of maternal infection or if the mother develops chickenpox within two days of delivery. In this situation the baby should be given VZIg and monitored. If chickenpox does develop then the baby should be treated with aciclovir.[12]

- Any baby born to a seronegative mother who has significant exposure to chickenpox in the first seven days of its life should be given VZIg[12]
- Premature babies (less than 28 weeks gestation) are at risk of chickenpox because of inadequate transfer of maternal antibodies at this gestation; if exposure has occurred VZIg should be given[12]

Medical Management and Care

- If maternal infection occurred in the first 20 weeks of pregnancy then neonatal blood should be sent for *Varicella zoster* virus IgM antibody testing[12] and the baby should have a neonatal ophthalmic examination soon after birth
- If delivery occurred during the acute maternal illness the neonatologists should be involved to treat and observe the baby appropriately
- If severe maternal complications arise then the woman may require transfer to the intensive care unit for further monitoring and supportive treatment

Midwifery Management and Care

- The woman should continue to be monitored for complications
- If infective, woman and baby should be isolated from other mothers and babies on the ward but not from each other[14]
- Breast-feeding is not contraindicated and should be encouraged[14]

12.7 Herpes Simplex Virus

Incidence	Risk for Childbearing
Genital herpes in women has increased twenty-fold over the last 30 years[1]	High Risk
Neonatal herpes – 1.7 per 100,000 UK live births[2]	

EXPLANATION OF CONDITION

Herpes simplex virus (HSV) can manifest itself in a variety of different ways and can be due to primary infection, when the virus is first encountered, or reactivation of the latent virus.

The clinical manifestations of a primary infection include:

- **Gingivo-stomatitis** – vesicles appear on the inside of the mouth
- **Herpetic whitlow** – seen as a lesion on the fingers
- **Conjunctivitis** or **keratitis** (inflammation of the cornea)
- **Genital herpes** – as vesicular eruption on the genital area
- **Neonatal herpes** – as generalised infection (see below)

The virus then remains dormant in either the trigeminal or sacral ganglion, until reactivated, causing recurrent infection. This manifests itself in the form of cold sores (**orolabial herpes**), keratitis or recurrent genital herpes. Neonatal herpes is caused by transmission to neonate at or around delivery and is associated with a high morbidity and mortality[3].

Orolabial herpes is usually caused by HSV type 1. Genital herpes (GH) can be caused by HSV 1 or HSV 2[4]. Symptoms of GH include blistering and painful ulceration of the external genitalia, which may involve the cervix and rectum, systemic symptoms, e.g. myalgia, inguinal lymphadenopathy[4]. Symptoms are commoner in primary infection and often more extensive. Prior infection with HSV 1 modifies the clinical manifestation of HSV 2[4]. The patient may be asymptomatic or may only present with systemic symptoms. Reactivation can be provoked by stress, menstruation, and other viral infections.

The virus is spread by close person contact, kissing or sexual contact, and there is a peak in the incidence during adolescence due to kissing. Asymptomatic viral shedding occurs with genital HSV 1 and 2 but more so with HSV 2[4]. It occurs most commonly in the first year after infection and can cause transmission of the virus[4].

COMPLICATIONS

Urinary Retention

- Catheterisation may be needed if conservative measures (analgesics/topic anaesthetics) fail
- Suprapubic catheterisation is preferred to transurethral[4]

Herpes Hepatitis

- Most cases caused by primary HSV 2 infection
- Clinical features are:
  - fever
  - abdominal pain
  - abnormal liver transaminases
  - high mortality rate
- Treatment comprises iv antiviral therapy and hospitalisation[5]

Encephalitis/Meningitis

- This is a rare but serious complication
- Clinical features are:
  - fever
  - headache
  - confusion
- Treatment with iv antiviral therapy required

Neonatal Herpes

- Can be caused by HSV 1 or HSV 2 and is characterised by severe generalised infection in the neonate[6]
- Affected babies can present with:
  - jaundice
  - hepatosplenomegaly
  - thrombocytopenia
  - vesicular lesions on the skin
- Risk is greatest with primary GH during late pregnancy as the baby will not have acquired protective antibodies from the mother[3]

NON-PREGNANCY TREATMENT AND CARE

Primary herpetic gingivo-stomatitis is treated by soft diet, encouraging adequate fluid intake and analgesia, including the use of local analgesic mouthwashes. Chlorhexidine mouthwash will help to prevent secondary infection[7]. If the lesions are severe, an antiviral, such as aciclovir, may be used orally[7]. Aciclovir cream can be used for cold sores (recurrent orolabial herpes infection) and should be commenced at the first sign of an attack, ideally before vesicles appear[7].

For GH it is important that the diagnosis is made as this will have implications for women if an episode were to occur in a future pregnancy. Ideally it would be valuable to determine whether the infection was due to HSV 1 or 2 as it would then be possible to determine whether a future attack in pregnancy was a primary infection with that type or a recurrence[4]. The virus can be isolated and typed by swabs taken from the base of an ulcer, ensuring that the swab is sent rapidly to the laboratory. The diagnosis can also be made by serological testing but viral detection remains the method of choice[4].

Primary or secondary GH is usually treated by an oral antiviral drug, e.g. aciclovir, and should be started within five days of the onset of the episode[7]. These have been shown to decrease the severity and duration of the episode and are more effective than topical antiviral agents. General hygiene advice needs to be given also and includes the use of saline baths[4]. Analgesia, with or without topical anaesthetic agents, is often required[4] and the patient advised to seek advice if they are unable to pass urine. Hospitalisation may be required for complications.

If the patient experiences regular attacks of recurrent GH, suppressive antiviral therapy may be required, e.g. with aciclovir. This should initially be used for up to a year and then the recurrence frequency should be reassessed[4]. Patients should abstain from sexual contact during an attack.

PRE-CONCEPTION ISSUES AND CARE

- If women are known to have a history of genital herpes then reassurance should be given that the risk of transmission to the neonate with recurrent episodes is very small
- Women in whom there is no history of GH, but the partner has a positive history, are advised to abstain from sexual intercourse at times when he has a recurrence.[6] This will not completely prevent transmission to the woman, as asymptomatic viral shedding at times when there is no evidence of an attack can lead to transmission[8]. Use of condoms has been proposed but not formally assessed[4].
- Identifying women who are susceptible to acquiring primary GH in pregnancy by serological testing has not been found to be cost effective in the UK[9].

Pregnancy Issues

- Aims:
  - give symptomatic relief of infection
  - monitor for and treat any complications that arise
  - prevent neonatal herpes in the newborn
- Important to check for other sexually transmitted diseases in cases of primary herpes
- Aciclovir has been shown to be safe in pregnancy with no evidence of maternal or fetal toxicity[6]
- Oral or iv aciclovir should be used in standard doses in line with the clinical condition[4]
- A five day course of oral aciclovir should be used for uncomplicated primary genital herpes
- In women who have had their first episode of genital herpes in the first or second trimester or for women who have recurrent genital herpes, oral aciclovir taken for the last four weeks of pregnancy can be given to prevent recurrence at term[10]
- Determination of whether any episode is a primary infection or recurrence is extremely important and has implications for the mode of delivery (see below)
- Recurrences of genital herpes in pregnancy are likely to be brief and uncomplicated

Medical Management and Care

Primary genital herpes in pregnancy
- Swabs should be sent to confirm diagnosis and referral to a genitourinary physician made[4]
- A full screen for other sexually transmitted diseases should be undertaken
- The woman should be given counselling, support and written information[4]

Primary and chronic management of herpes in pregnancy
- Treatment with oral aciclovir should be considered and iv aciclovir used if the condition warrants this[4]
- The woman should be warned of the possible complications and to report any deterioration in her condition
- Consideration of daily aciclovir in the last four weeks of pregnancy should be discussed with the patient, along with the need for LSCS if infection has occurred within six weeks of delivery

Midwifery Management and Care

- A history of previous HSV should be obtained at booking and the woman warned to report any symptoms of genital herpes if they arise, in which case she should be referred for confirmation, treatment and counselling
- General hygiene advice and advice regarding pain relief should be given if an episode occurs
- Be aware of confidentiality issues including possibility of withholding details on patient-held records

Labour Issues

The mode of delivery depends upon whether the episode is primary or a recurrence and how near to delivery the primary infection was.

When the *first episode* of genital herpes occurs at the time of delivery and if the baby is delivered vaginally in the presence of active lesions, the risk of neonatal herpes is around 40%[6]. In view of this LSCS is recommended if primary genital herpes occurs at or up to six weeks prior to delivery.

LSCS may also be considered for women who develop primary herpes earlier in the third trimester[4].

For those women who opt for a vaginal delivery despite having a recent history of primary genital herpes, the risk of neonatal transmission should be minimised by avoiding invasive procedures and giving intrapartum iv aciclovir to the mother to reduce maternal viraemia[6]. The baby should also be treated with aciclovir after delivery[6].

If a woman has a *recurrence* around the time of delivery, the risk to the baby of neonatal herpes is small[11,12], and vaginal delivery is now considered safe[6]. Any woman considering caesarean section for recurrence of genital herpes at the time of delivery needs to be made aware of the increased morbidity associated with LSCS.

Medical Management and Care

- Discuss the benefits of caesarean section if primary genital herpes occurs at, or within, six weeks of delivery; not the case if the infection occurs in the first or second trimesters[4,6]
- If a woman has primary herpes during labour, or within the previous six weeks, and opts for a vaginal delivery, then iv aciclovir should be given in labour and invasive procedures such as fetal blood sampling, the use of fetal scalp electrodes and instrumental deliveries avoided[6]
- Women who have a recurrence of genital herpes in pregnancy should be reassured that vaginal delivery is safe and that in the absence of active lesions there is no indication for a LSCS
- If a woman has active lesions of recurrent genital herpes at the onset of labour then the mode of delivery should be discussed with her, but she should be informed that the risks to the baby are small and should be set against the risks of LSCS[6]

Midwifery Management and Care

- Examination of all women during vaginal assessment for any possible sign of genital herpes should be made at the beginning of labour[4] and the medical staff alerted if any concerns

Postpartum Issues

- The neonatologists' should be informed of any women who delivered within six weeks of primary genital herpes infection, irrespective of mode of delivery – and the baby observed and treated appropriately[6]
- Care of the perineum is important in the presence of active lesions
- There is a risk of postnatal transmission of HSV to the baby due to contact with HSV infection such as orolabial herpes or herpetic whitlow[6]

Medical Management and Care

- The baby should be assessed and the need for aciclovir in the baby determined

Midwifery Management and Care

- Advice on perineal hygiene should be given and ensure adequate bladder care
- Mothers, family members and health care worker with active HSV infection, including 'cold sores', should avoid contact with newborn babies[6]

12 Infectious Disease

PATIENT ORGANISATIONS

Children's Liver Disease Trust
36 Great Charles Street
Birmingham B3 3JY
www.childliverdisease.org

British Liver Trust
Ransomes Europark
Ipswich IP3 9GQ
www.britishlivertrust.org.uk

Hepatitis Foundation International
504 Blick Drive
Silver Spring, MD 20904, USA
www.HepatitisFoundation.org

Hepatitis C Trust
27 Crosby Row
London SE1 3YD
www.hepcuk.info

NHS Hepatitis C
www.hepc.nhs.uk

Human Immunodeficiency Virus
Children's HIV Association (CHIVA)
www.bhiva.org/chiva

Children with AIDS Charity (CWAC)
Lion House
3 Plough Yard
London EC2A 3LP
info@cwac.org

Terence Higgins Trust (THT)
52–54 Grays Inn Road
London WC1X 8JU
www.tht.org.uk

Tommy's Pregnancy Information Service
(Toxoplasmosis Support Network)
http://www.tommys.org/pregnancy-information/problems-in-pregnancy/toxoplasmosis.htm

International Herpes Alliance
www.herpesalliance.org

Group B Strep Support
PO Box 203
Haywards Heath
West Sussex RH16 1GF
www.gbss.org.uk

ESSENTIAL READING

Clinical Effectiveness Group (2001) **National Guideline on the Management of Genital Herpes.** Association of Genito-urinary Medicine and the Medical Society for the Study of Venereal Diseases.

Department of Health (2004) **Hepatitis C: Essential information for professionals and guidance on testing**. London: DoH. www.dh.gov.uk/publications.

Doroshenko, A., Sherrard, J. and Pollard, A. (2006) Syphilis in pregnancy care and the neonatal period. **International Journal of STD and AIDS, 17**(4):221–226 (reprinted in **MIDIRS, 16**(4):491–496).

Gilling-Smith, C. and Almeida, P. (2003) HIV, Hepatitis B and Hepatitis C and Infertility: Reducing Risk. Educational Bulletin by the Practice & Policy Committee of the BFS. **Human Fertility, 6**:106–122.

Health Protection Agency **Pregnancy and Tuberculosis.** www.hpa.org.uk/infections/topics_az/tb/menu.htm

James, D.K., Steer, P.J., Weiner, C.P. and Gonik, B. (Eds) (2006) Other infectious conditions; Parasitic infections. In: **High Risk Pregnancy Management Options**, 3rd Edn. London; W.B. Saunders.

Kennedy, J. (2003) **HIV in Pregnancy and Childbirth**, 2nd Edn. Hale; Books for Midwives Press/Elsevier.

Ratnaike, D. and Coutsoudis, A. (2006) Breastfeeding with HIV. **Midwives, 9**(11):422.

Royal College of Obstetricians and Gynaecologists Clinical Guidelines, **No. 13**: Chickenpox in Pregnancy; **No. 30**: Management of genital herpes in pregnancy; **No. 36**: Prevention of early onset neonatal group B streptococcal disease www.rcog.org.uk

The Cat Group Policy Statement No.6. **Cats and Toxoplasmosis** The Cat Group, High Street, Tisbury, Wilts. SP3 6LD. www.thecatgroup.org.uk

World Health Organisation (2000) **Management of Severe Malaria: A Practical Handbook**, 2nd Edn. Geneva; WHO. http://www.who.int/malaria/docs/hbsm.pdf

http://www.hpa.org.uk/infections/topics_az/malaria/guidelines.htm

http://www.who.int/topics/malaria/en/

http://www.cdc.gov/malaria/

http://www.dh.gov.uk/PolicyAndGuidance/HealthAndSocialCareTopics/Toxoplasmosis/fs/en

13 METABOLIC DISORDERS

Rowena Doughty and Jason Waugh

13.1 Obesity

Incidence	Risk for Childbearing
Obesity is an increasing phenomenon worldwide In pregnancy the incidence is around 18–19% in the UK[1]	High Risk – throughout the childbearing period, especially if complications occur

EXPLANATION OF CONDITION

In the past three years 15% of all UK maternal deaths have occurred in women with a BMI >35 (half of these with BMI >40). 52% of deaths occurred in women with a BMI >25[2]. Obesity is an increasing phenomenon worldwide, with non-pregnant rates of about 24% in the UK reported in 2006 by the Department of Health.

- Caused by excessive accumulation of fat within the fat cells – result of discrepancy between energy intake and energy expenditure
- A weight of 90 kg or above is considered obese, but this definition alone is limited[3], as an individual's height affects their level of obesity
- Generally, obesity is diagnosed using the body mass index (BMI) classification as recommended by NICE: weight in kilograms divided by the square of the height in metres (see Appendix 13)
- Obesity is defined as a BMI >30, with underweight as <18.5, normal weight 18.5–24.9 and overweight 25–29.9. Obesity can be further subdivided into obesity (BMI >30) and extreme or morbid obesity (a BMI >40)
- Of similar significance is the distribution of body fat, especially an increased waist-to-hip ratio; thought to be more valuable than weight alone and suggestive of disordered glucose tolerance[4]

Obesity is also associated with:

- Gender – more common in women than men
- Postcode – there are more cases in the north of the country than in the south of the UK
- Lifestyle – increasing sedentary occupations, reliance on the car, fast food, etc.
- Mental wellbeing – depression may be linked with obesity
- Social class – rates of obesity increase as the social class lowers
- Ethnicity – increased obesity seen in certain ethnic groups, e.g. Afro-Caribbean
- Genetics – some obesity has an inherited component, although this accounts for only a small proportion of cases

COMPLICATIONS

Obesity is a common risk factor in many conditions, especially:

- Metabolic (e.g. type 2 diabetes)
- Circulatory (e.g. cardiovascular disease)
- Degenerative (e.g. osteoarthritis)

These conditions are usually associated with advancing age, although with increases in childhood obesity the age of presentation of many of these conditions is lowering.

Many of these diseases have a negative effect on life expectancy and there are increased morbidity rates for individuals with obesity. The amplified health and social welfare costs for society in managing obesity-related conditions is also a concern, especially due to the shifting population demographics. Individuals with obesity also suffer from discrimination directly attributed to their size, which may lead to lower self-esteem and self-confidence; many individuals with obesity report an overall poorer quality of life.

For women, obesity increases the risk of gynaecological complications, e.g. endometrial cancer, infertility and menorrhagia through menstrual disturbances and ovulation disorders. Small babies may be at greater risk of cardiovascular disease in later life and this is compounded if the mother has a high BMI, although more research is needed[5]. Therefore, weight loss to achieve a normal BMI has short- and long-term health benefits.

NON-PREGNANCY TREATMENT AND CARE

The management aim is to attain a steady weight loss until the BMI is within the normal range. Slow weight loss is more sustainable in both the short- and long-term. This is achieved through education about what constitutes a healthy diet and eating patterns and lowered overall energy intakes.

Moderate exercise in combination with a well-balanced, energy-restricted diet has been shown to increase weight-loss success rates by:

- Increasing overall muscle mass (which consumes more energy than fat)
- Producing a sense of wellbeing
- Depressing the appetite
- Increasing the overall metabolic rate

Studies have also shown that behavioural and cognitive therapy combined with the above can augment success rates[6]. Group therapy, e.g. Weight Watchers©, is also thought to improve success rates.

Some obese individuals resort to surgery. There are two main types of surgical techniques: restrictive, e.g. gastric banding, and malabsorptive, e.g. stomach stapling. There has also been renewed interest in diet pills, e.g. orlistat (a lipase inhibitor) and sibutramine (a centrally-acting appetite suppressant), although these must be prescribed and supervised closely by the medical team and are contraindicated in pregnancy[7].

PRE-CONCEPTION ISSUES AND CARE

Because of the strong association with maternal death, and the problems outlined in this chapter, pre-conception advice should be available for all women with a BMI >30[2].

In the presence of sub-fertility, to increase the chances of spontaneous conception through regular menses or to increase the sensitivity of ovulation-induction techniques, women with obesity are recommended to achieve a moderate weight loss of at least 5%[8].

Pregnancy Issues

Obesity is a significant risk factor during pregnancy and increases the risk of many disorders that have a direct influence on pregnancy outcome:

- Early miscarriage
- Gestational diabetes and pregnancy hypertension/pre-eclampsia[9,10,11,12]
- Venous thrombo-embolism[3]
- Anaesthetic problems, e.g. tracheal intubation or epidural/spinal insertion[3]

Especially if maternal complications develop, the fetus/neonate is also at risk of:

- Neural tube defects[12]
- Late stillbirth[3] and neonatal death[13]
- Fetal macrosomia[14]
- Fetal trauma[3]
- Neonatal Unit admissions

Obesity creates issues pertaining to the value and reliability of certain aspects of care during the antenatal period:

- Difficulties in performing amniocentesis[3]
- Difficulties in achieving venous access
- Difficulties in performing an abdominal palpation[15]
- Difficulties in obtaining ultrasound data for fetal anomalies[16] and growth

Medical Management and Care

- It is important to identify those women who have a condition directly attributed to their obesity, in particular diabetes and hypertension
- The presence of related conditions will have a direct influence on their care needs; a multi-disciplinary team approach to management during pregnancy is advised[2]
- Follow local policies for antenatal anaesthetic referral
- Screening and management for conditions such as gestational diabetes and hypertension should be offered

Midwifery Management and Care

- All women have their BMI calculated as part of a full risk assessment performed at booking and women found to have a BMI >30 should be referred to a consultant for shared care and be encouraged to book to give birth in a consultant-led environment
- All women should receive advice about healthy eating in pregnancy[4], i.e. to be advised to 'eat for appetite', rather than 'eat for two'
- A referral to a dietician is important for obese women
- Weight gain in pregnancy should be restricted to around 6 kg
- *Strict dieting* should be avoided
- Moderate exercise should be encouraged, unless the woman is experiencing other signs or symptoms, i.e. dyspnoea[20]
- Individualised advice, especially options for screening, is important, taking into account the effects of weight on biochemical results
- Careful observation of the maternal and fetal status is important during pregnancy to detect complications
- Ascertain mobility, and assess risks of potential intrapartum moving and handling/environmental concerns in preparation for birth
- Midwifery support is important to foster self-esteem and self-confidence

Labour Issues

Obesity is a significant risk factor during the intrapartum period:

- Increased rates of prolonged labour[17]
- Risks associated with macrosomia, e.g. shoulder dystocia[3,9]
- Increased rates of operative birth[3,18] especially for primigravida[19]
- Difficulties in undertaking instrumental and operative procedures[3,9]
- Difficulty siting an epidural or spinal for labour or caesarean section[3]

Medical Management and Care

- Encourage birth in a consultant-led environment
- Strongly consider thrombo-embolic prophylaxis[21] (see Section 15.1)
- Consider the differences in labour progression in obese women before resorting to augmentation[17]

Midwifery Management and Care

- Effective midwifery support in labour is important
- Encourage changes in maternal position throughout labour
- Avoid dehydration in labour (risk of venous thrombo-embolism)
- Observe progress/use partogram closely throughout labour
- Consider a fetal scalp electrode if there is difficulty with auscultation of the fetal heart abdominally[3]

Postpartum Issues

Obesity has a direct influence on short and long-term health and wellbeing, especially:

- Venous thrombo-embolism[3]
- Longer post-operative recovery and increased rates of post-operative complications, e.g. infections of wound and urinary tract[3]
- Women who are obese during pregnancy exhibit a tendency to retain fat centrally on their abdomens postnatally, which may result in increased morbidity and mortality in later life[4]
- Contraceptive choices will be influenced by the presence of complications, and the combined pill may not be as effective in obese women

Medical Management and Care

- A multi-disciplinary approach to the management of conditions associated with obesity is recommended
- Obesity in the presence of two other persisting risk factors should prompt the need for thrombo-prophylaxis for 3–5 days[22]

Midwifery Management and Care

- May need increased post-operative analgesia[18]
- Encourage early mobilisation; continue thrombo-embolic prophylaxis until fully mobile[22]
- Encourage and support breast-feeding to help mobilise fat stores: tailor breast-feeding advice to meet individual needs; suggest underarm positioning at the breast
- Referral to a dietician for support and advice regarding weight reduction – but avoid strict dieting, especially if breast-feeding
- Consider referral for cognitive and behavioural therapy and consider providing extended midwifery postnatal care[23]

13.2 Phenylketonuria

Incidence	Risk for Childbearing
1 in 10,000 live births worldwide, but more common in Caucasian races[1]	High Risk – for pre-conceptual, antenatal and neonatal care Low Risk – for labour

EXPLANATION OF CONDITION

Phenylketonuria (PKU) is an autosomal recessively inherited metabolic disorder, caused by mutations in the gene for phenylalanine hydroxylase, found on chromosome 12. Phenylketonuria, as a disease, was first recognised in the 1930s, but maternal PKU syndrome as a complication was not documented until the 1950s[2].

There are two main types of phenylketonuria:

1. Classical phenylketonuria – the more serious form of the disease, discussed below
2. Hyperphenylalaninaemia – a less severe form, with lower serum phenylalanine levels and fewer complications

Phenylalanine hydroxylase is an enzyme produced by the liver that converts the amino acid phenylalanine, which is found in dietary protein, to another amino acid called tyrosine. Amino acids are important building blocks for proteins, which are vital for growth and wellbeing. In individuals with PKU, phenylalanine and its by-products accumulate in the body and will result in neurological symptoms and irreversible damage to nerve cells within the developing brain and nervous system.

As this is a recessively inherited disorder[3]:

- A woman with PKU whose partner does not carry the affected gene for PKU will produce unaffected children
  - the couple will always pass on the affected gene to their infants, who will be carriers
  - carriers do not exhibit signs of PKU – a child would need to inherit both affected genes to inherit and express symptoms of PKU
- A woman with PKU whose partner also carries an affected gene for PKU will have a 1 in 2 chance of having an affected child
- If a woman's partner also has PKU, all children conceived will have PKU
- Individuals who are both carriers of the PKU gene will have a 1 in 4 chance of conceiving a child with PKU

COMPLICATIONS

Complications will occur in affected individuals unless screening to detect the condition and management to control the condition is instigated. The earlier treatment begins the less affected the child will be; some limited evidence suggests that the diet should be modified within the first month of life for best results[4].

A neonate will appear normal at birth, as the mother will process phenylalanine through her bodily systems. Symptoms in untreated, affected infants will begin to appear from four months of age onwards. These include:

- Abnormal movements
- Developmental delay
- Decreased muscle tone
- Difficulty walking
- Microcephaly
- Learning disabilities
- Seizures
- Psychosis
- Reduction in IQ
- Skin conditions, e.g. eczema
- Pale skin

Attention deficit hyperactivity disorder (ADHD) is also associated with biological insults such as PKU; this is thought to be dose-related and associated with high levels both before birth and in the neonatal period[5].

NON-PREGNANCY TREATMENT AND CARE

All mothers of newborn infants are offered screening for the condition in their baby within the first week of life[1].

Treatment of affected infants consists of a low phenylalanine diet and a supplement of synthetic amino acids (protein substitutes) and vitamins, minerals and trace elements, with food exchanges. This modified diet should continue throughout childhood and some studies suggest this should continue into adulthood[6]. Foods that are naturally high in phenylalanine include meat, dairy produce and nuts, while foods that are low in phenylalanine are generally fruit and vegetables and are considered to be phenylalanine-free foods[7]. A traffic-light approach to foods is taken.

The diet is restrictive and studies have shown that it is difficult to adhere to[8]; social support has been shown to improve compliance so support by the midwife in pregnancy, as part of the multi-disciplinary team, is crucially important.

Gene therapy, as an alternative to dietary management, is in the experimental stage and may be available in the future[9].

PRE-CONCEPTION ISSUES AND CARE

To prevent maternal PKU syndrome women with PKU are advised to return to the restricted diet when planning to conceive or as soon as possible when pregnant.

This has been shown in many studies to prevent or lessen the effects on the neonate[10,11,12]. It can take 1–2 weeks to reduce phenylalanine levels to a therapeutic range of 60–200 mmol/l on commencing the diet.

As many pregnancies are unplanned the advice to remain on the restrictive diet during adulthood[6] is important for women of child-bearing age as the aim is to achieve low blood phenylalanine levels early, ideally pre-conception.

Pregnancy Issues

Women with PKU who have not continued on their low phenylalanine diet need to resume the diet ideally pre-conceptually or as early as possible antenatally[10,11,12]. This lessens the risk of maternal PKU syndrome, which can affect the fetus and increase the risk of:

- Congenital heart disease[13]
- Microcephaly
- Cranio-facial abnormalities
- Intrauterine growth restriction (IUGR)

The frequency and severity of abnormality rises with increasing phenylalanine levels[11].

- It is important to maintain blood phenylalanine levels at <200 µmol/l[3,8]
- Untreated levels of phenylalanine of 1200 µmol/l have been reported
- Women who are given increased support tend to attain earlier metabolic control[8]

The woman is allowed around 3–6 exchanges daily in the first 20 weeks, but this may be increased in the latter half of pregnancy, under dietetic advice. It is also essential that the woman with PKU eats significant calories to maintain metabolic control and avoids catabolism, where the body will breakdown protein and release phenylalanine[14].

Medical Management and Care

- Pre-conception care is essential to optimise maternal levels before conception
- In women with PKU who conceive on normal diets, early recourse to the restrictive diet has been shown to reduce fetal effects
- Referral to wider multi-disciplinary team as necessary, e.g. physician, dietician, geneticist, clinical nurse specialist
- Early booking facilitates first and second trimester screening for associated congenital abnormalities and appropriate counselling
- Serial ultrasound assessment to screen for IUGR

Monitoring of PKU status is advised

- Twice-weekly phenylalanine self-blood-testing by the woman
- Regular venous blood testing, i.e. Hb, FBC, copper, zinc, selenium, calcium, albumin, phosphates, ferritin, vitamin B_{12} and tyrosine
- Monthly 24-hour phenylalanine profile

Midwifery Management and Care

- Support by a known midwife may help dietary compliance rates and attendance at clinics, which will improve pregnancy outcomes[16]
- Shared care is necessary during the antenatal period
- Place of birth is dependent on presence of fetal complications, e.g. IUGR when birthing in a consultant-led environment with neonatal unit facilities would be advised
- If no complications develop by term then giving birth in a midwifery-led environment may be possible
- Full information on risks and management, both through discussion and in written format should be provided
- If antenatal in-patient care is needed, attendance to diet is vitally important, so seek advice from a dietician on admission

Labour Issues

There are no special requirements for women with PKU during labour. Place of birth and care in labour will depend on the presence of complications, e.g. IUGR.

Babies of women with PKU are not screened immediately after birth, as levels of phenylalanine are higher immediately after birth and would result in false-positive screening results[3].

Medical Management and Care

- No significant implications for delivery
- Babies will require neonatal assessment at delivery

Midwifery Management and Care

- Decisions about the place of birth are dependent upon the presence or absence of complications
- Complications should be managed in accordance with local unit guidelines
- Provide good-quality, midwifery-led care for low-risk women

Postpartum Issues

The routine screening of all neonates for PKU by the Newborn Blood Spot Screening Test began in 1969. The neonatal screening test that is offered to all babies between 5–8 days will detect almost 100% of the cases of PKU. As this is a screening test, any babies who screen positive will need diagnostic follow-up. Screening for all neonates has been shown to be cost-effective[15].

Breast-feeding of babies with PKU is not prohibited, but supplements of phenylalanine-free formula feeds are required to lessen the risk of neurological damage.

A low phenylalanine diet should be commenced within the first month of life to lessen the effects of the condition[4].

Medical Management and Care

- Re-affirm the need for pre-conception care ahead of any further pregnancies

Midwifery Management and Care

- Ensure all women are informed about the Newborn Blood Spot Screening Test – this subject should be discussed antenatally as well as pre-test, giving women and their partners adequate time to ask questions
- Women whose infants have PKU can still breast-feed and should be supported
- A small study suggests that alternate feeds of a phenylalanine-free formula feed, rather than at every feed, would allow for breast-feeding[17]
- If a woman with PKU chooses to revert to a 'normal' diet postnatally, this circumstance should not preclude her breast-feeding[3]
- Women with PKU should be reminded, in the late postnatal period, about the value of pre-conceptual care for a prospective pregnancy

13 Metabolic Disorders

PATIENT ORGANISATIONS

Weight Wise
www.bdaweightwise.com

The Obesity Awareness and Solutions Trust (TOAST)
The Latton Bush Centre
Southern Way
Harlow
Essex CM18 7BL
www.toast-uk.org.uk

The National Society for Phenylketonuria
(Charity Number: 373670)
www.nspku.org

PKU.com
www.pku.com

Children's PKU Network
www.pkunetwork.org

PKU Teens – It's all in the genes!
www.pkuteens.co.uk

USEFUL WEBSITES

Association for the Study of Obesity
www.aso.org.uk/portal.aspx

National Obesity Forum
www.nationalobesityforum.org.uk/

UK Newborn Screening Programme Centre
www.newbornscreening-bloodspot.org.uk

ESSENTIAL READING

Department of Health (2006) **Care Pathways for the Management of Overweight and Obesity** Adult Care Pathway (Primary Care)
www.dh.gov.uk/asserRoot/04/13/44/12/04134412.pdf

Lewis, G. and Drife, J. (2002) **CEMACH 6th report: Why Mothers Die 2000–2002** Confidential Enquiries into Maternal and Child Health. London; RCOG Press.

National Institute for Clinical Excellence. **Guidance on the Prevention, Identification, Assessment and Management of Overweight and Obesity in Adults and Children**
www.nice.org.uk/guidance/CG43/guidance/pdf/English/download.dspx

NICE (2003) **Antenatal Care Clinical Guideline** No. 6
www.nice.org

RCOG (2006) **Exercise in Pregnancy Statement** No. 4
www.rcog.org

RCOG (2004) **Thromboprophylaxis During Pregnancy, Labour and After Vaginal Delivery** – Guideline No. 37
www.rcog.org

RCOG (2001) **Thromboembolic Disease in Pregnancy and the Puerperium: Acute Management** – Green Top Guideline
www.rcog.org

HAEMATOLOGICAL DISORDERS

14

Abena Addo, S. Elizabeth Robson and Christina Oppenheimer

14.1 Iron Deficiency Anaemia

Incidence	Risk for Childbearing
5–10% pregnant women from industrialised countries[1]	Variable Risk

EXPLANATION OF CONDITION

Iron deficiency is the commonest cause of anaemia amongst women of child-bearing age and in particular pregnant women (51%) worldwide[2].

Symptoms vary from mild tiredness to potentially hazardous palpitations, breathlessness or symptoms of high-output cardiac failure. In humans, mineral iron is present in all cells and carries oxygen to the tissues from the lungs in the form of haemoglobin (Hb), facilitating oxygen use in muscles such as myoglobin, and also transportation of cytochromes within cells for enzyme reactions in tissues.

Women have approximately 2.3 g total body iron of which most (80%) is found in the red blood cell mass as haemoglobin (Hb). Total body iron is determined by intake, loss and storage of this mineral. Any iron not in use is stored as the soluble protein complex ferritin, present primarily in the liver, bone marrow, spleen and skeletal muscle. Normal absorption mechanisms in the gastrointestinal system of the body are required to maintain the balance between functional iron (Hb) and stored iron (myoglobin) levels. The body is able to absorb 1–2 mg iron daily from the diet, with the aid of absorption enhancers in the diet and a satisfactory rate of red blood cell production. The main factor controlling iron absorption is the amount of iron stored in the body and the type of iron in one's diet[3].

Anaemia results in a reduction in the oxygen-carrying capacity of the blood. Iron deficiency anaemia is defined by a low serum ferritin concentration of <30 µg/l and haemoglobin <11.0, 10.5 and 11.0 g/dl in the first, second and third trimesters respectively[2,4,5]. Red blood cells are microcytic and hypochromic on microscopic examination. Iron deficiency anaemia arises from an increase in iron requirements or inadequate iron absorption.

Iron requirements are increased to deal with:

- Growth
- Menstruation
- Blood loss/donation
- Pregnancy
- Haemolytic disorders
- Drugs that cause haemolysis (e.g. antiretrovirals)
- Genitourinary tract infections
- Hookworm infestation

Anaemia caused by inadequate iron absorption occurs from:

- Diet low in haem iron
- Malabsorption
- Gastric surgery
- Malaria infection resulting in poor use of dietary iron

The amount of functional iron in the body and the concentration of the iron-containing protein Hb in circulating red blood cells are measured by two simple blood tests, Hb and haematocrit and ferritin concentration.

Haemoglobin Concentration and Haematocrit

Haemoglobin and haematocrit (HCT) are both late indicators of anaemia. Haematocrit indicates the proportion of whole blood occupied by the red blood cells, and falls only after the Hb concentration has also fallen. Mean cell volume (MCV) is also important as it falls in iron deficiency, but needs further testing to distinguish from other causes of microcytosis (see Section 14.3 Thalassaemia).

Serum Ferritin Concentration

Serum ferritin concentration is an early indicator of the status of iron stores and the most specific indicator of depleted iron stores routinely available. A serum ferritin concentration of ≤30 µg/l confirms iron deficiency among women who test positive for anaemia on the basis of Hb concentration or haematocrit[6]. Serum ferritin can be raised in infection and may need repeating for a definitive diagnosis of iron deficiency. Caution is advised in interpretation of normal levels in pregnancy since a low normal level (30–50) may still indicate iron deficiency. Use of other tests should be confirmed with local laboratories.

COMPLICATIONS

Iron deficiency can interfere with vital body functions leading to morbidity and mortality including:

- Palpitations
- Tiredness
- Irritability
- Depression
- Breathlessness
- Poor memory
- Muscle aches
- Poor appetite
- Cardiac failure
- Increased vulnerability if small amounts of blood are lost

NON-PREGNANCY TREATMENT AND CARE

Encourage iron-rich foods in the diet and treat with iron supplementation 60–120 mg/day for four weeks[7]. If no response to treatment, investigate using other tests: reticulocyte count and serum ferritin concentration. Conditions such as sickle cell trait or thalassaemia minor in women of African, Mediterranean or Southeast Asian ancestry cause mild anaemia unresponsive to iron therapy. The normal Hb level for this group can be as low as 10 g/dl, however the lowest normal Hb in healthy non-pregnant women is defined as 12.0 g/dl[2]. Iron absorption can be increased in a vegetarian diet by careful planning of meals to include other sources of iron and enhancers of iron absorption[8].

PRE-CONCEPTION ISSUES AND CARE

A non-pregnant woman of reproductive age has an average iron requirement of 1.3 mg/day. This increases when pregnant by an extra requirement of 3.0 mg/day mainly for increases in maternal red cell mass, placental and fetal growth, blood loss at delivery, physiological intestinal blood loss and menstruating loss over the child-bearing years. A further iron requirement of 6–8 mg/day occurs after 32 weeks' gestation.

Provide culture-specific dietary advice with information on iron body stores and avoidance of absorption inhibitors, e.g. tea, bread and chapatti. A reliable system for investigation of anaemia and monitoring of response to treatment is paramount[2].

Pregnancy Issues

- **Prevention** of anaemia by early recognition of iron deficiency in those at risk is paramount
- Anaemia in the third trimester increases the risk of poor recovery from blood loss at birth, as well as tachycardia, shortness of breath and maternal exhaustion
- Parenteral iron, intravenous or intramuscular, is used in cases of non-compliance or malabsorption, but contraindicated in cases of allergy
- A rise in reticulocyte counts and Hb of 0.8 g/dl/wk occurs 5–10 days after starting oral iron treatment[9]; the increase in Hb is similar for parenteral iron[10]
- In pregnant women with severe anaemia, there may be an increase in the risk of pre-term delivery, low birth weight and a possible increased perinatal mortality rate
- Randomised controlled trials have been inconclusive on the effect of universal iron supplementation in pregnancy versus adverse maternal and fetal outcomes[11]

Medical Management and Care

- Assess cause of anaemia by adequate dietary and medical history and appropriate testing
- Prescribe ferrous sulphate 200 mg 2–3 times daily, or a proprietary combined iron and folate tablet with a higher elemental iron content until Hb normalises and thereafter to replenish stores
- If required, im or iv dose is calculated according to iron deficit and body weight
- Administer iron dextran or sucrose iv in 0.9% sodium chloride infusion as total or divided doses
- Consider blood transfusion only if severe anaemia in a situation with a high risk of blood loss (blood products and transfusion are outlined in Appendix 14.1 and refusal of transfusion in Appendix 14.2)

Midwifery Management and Care

- Severe/chronically anaemic women to be booked at consultant unit
- Encourage pregnant women to eat iron-rich foods and foods that enhance iron absorption, such as orange juice, and provide women with information on nutrition in pregnancy[12]
- Inhibitors of iron absorption include polyphenols (in certain vegetables), tannins (in tea), phytates (in bran) and calcium (in dairy products)
- Iron tablets should be taken one hour away from food, and with orange or apple juice
- Screen all women at booking visit and at 28 weeks' gestation[13]
- Women with known anaemia need testing at each antenatal visit
- Ensure anaphylactic emergency treatment is available during parenteral iron administration
- Treat selectively with iron[1,7] and folate preparations[14] and if needed reduce gastrointestinal complaints[15] with low dose[5] slow release oral preparations

Labour Issues

Risk of:
- Maternal exhaustion
- Exacerbation of anaemia by excessive blood loss:
  - multiple birth
  - prolonged labour
  - instrumental delivery
  - caesarean section
  - grand multiparity
- Shortness of breath
- Tachycardia

Medical Management and Care

- Group and save serum on admission to labour
- Assess risk factors for excessive blood loss

Midwifery Management and Care

- Care in consultant-led unit
- Active third stage of labour – Syntometrine and IVI of oxytocin
- Await FBC results before advocating eating and drinking in labour
- Vigilant monitoring of labour progress
- Prompt referral to obstetrician if slow progress develops
- Avoid directed pushing where possible
- All perineal trauma to be sutured

Postpartum Issues

Maternal considerations
- Mother is at risk of:
  - postpartum haemorrhage
  - infection
  - poor wound healing
  - postnatal depression
  - lethargy
  - breast-feeding difficulties
- Mother requires return of Hb to normal level before planning further pregnancies

Neonatal considerations
- Fetus obtains iron from placental transfer regardless of maternal iron stores, hence is unlikely to be anaemic
- Potential for IUGR or pre-term neonate with associated problems

Medical Management and Care

- Reassure mother that the baby is unlikely to be anaemic
- Continue the maintenance dose of oral iron for up to 3 months postpartum to replenish stores
- See algorithm for management (see Appendix 14.3)

Midwifery Management and Care

- Be alert for signs of postpartum haemorrhage, infection and side effects of iron supplementation
- Postnatal assessment – FBC to identify any extra requirements
- Promote breast-feeding realistically with options to rest, e.g. express breast milk so that baby can be fed by other family members
- Consider social circumstances and use support such as *Home Start*, family and friends for basic housework
- Reassure mother that baby unlikely to be anaemic and advise an iron-rich diet to improve iron stores (see Patient Organisations)
- Be alert for signs of postnatal depression and continue postnatal visiting if indicated
- Contraceptive advice to ensure adequate spacing of pregnancies

14.2 Megaloblastic Anaemia

Incidence	Risk for Childbearing
Complicates a third of pregnancies worldwide UK incidence is 0.2%–5%[1]	Variable Risk

EXPLANATION OF CONDITION

Megaloblastic anaemia is an acquired condition characterised by **macrocytosis** – the mean cell volume (MCV) of the red blood cells (erythrocytes) is above the normal range of 80–95 femtolitres (fl). It is called **megaloblastic** because the developing red blood cells in the bone marrow are larger than normal and have immature nuclei. A full blood count may reveal an increased number of immature red blood cells (megaloblasts) in the blood, reduced platelets and haemoglobin levels unresponsive to treatment with iron supplements, as well as the raised mean cell volume.

Megaloblastic anaemia is usually caused by deficiency of folic acid or vitamin B$_{12}$ (cyanocobalamin), but more rarely may be drug-induced or associated with myelodysplastic syndrome. It is also possible to see a non-megaloblastic macrocytic picture in liver disease, hypothyroidism and alcoholism. **In pregnancy a relative macrocytosis is common and normal.**

Folate deficiency is associated with nutritional and socioeconomic status[2] and may cause complications in pregnancy. Megaloblastic anaemia develops insidiously following:

- Poor dietary folate intake
- Excessive alcohol consumption[3,4]
- Increased cell turnover due to:
  - pregnancy (demands of mother and fetus)
  - chronic haemolytic anaemia (e.g. sickle cell anaemia, hereditary spherocytosis)
  - chronic inflammatory conditions
- Renal loss
  - chronic renal failure
  - dialysis
- Malabsorption disorders, e.g. gluten-induced enteropathy (coeliac disease)
- Drug-induced
  - some anticonvulsants
  - sulfasalazine
  - methotrexate

Mainly stored in the liver, cellular folates help to build DNA and protein in all tissues. This includes those required for growth of the fetus, placenta, maternal red cell mass and uterine development in pregnancy. Folate is found in beans, rice and green vegetables and some food stuffs have folic acid supplemented.

Vitamin B$_{12}$ deficiency is caused by veganism or poor-quality diet, pernicious anaemia, gastrectomy or ileal resection (as occurs with Crohn's disease).

COMPLICATIONS

The consequences of true megaloblastic anaemia include:

- Pallor and jaundice
- Increasingly severe anaemia
- Heart failure
- Pancytopaenia (low white cell and platelet counts)

Other complications of vitamin B$_{12}$ deficiency include:

- Neuropathy involving peripheral nerves and spinal cord
- Psychiatric disturbances
- Visual disturbance
- Fetal neural tube defects

Both deficiencies can cause epithelial disturbance, e.g. the smooth painful tongue (glossitis), and, if low serum homocysteine levels are present (part of this metabolic pathway), arterial obstruction and venous thrombosis.

NON-PREGNANCY TREATMENT AND CARE

Advise a diet rich in vitamin B$_{12}$ and folate, such as cheese, cereals, leafy green vegetables, fortified cereals, fruit and egg yolks. The recommended daily intake of folate is 3 micrograms per kilogram of body weight for non-pregnant and non-lactating women.

A daily intake of 5 mg folic acid is recommended for women with hereditary haemolytic disorders, epileptics on anticonvulsants and women of reproductive age with a family history of neural tube defects who are planning a pregnancy[4,5,6].

PRE-CONCEPTION ISSUES AND CARE

Estimated dietary requirements of folates in pregnancy are 100–600 micrograms/day with an average daily intake of 237 micrograms/day[7,8].

An association exists between periconceptual folic acid deficiency and neural tube defect, cleft lip and cleft palate in the fetus[5], hence the recommended folic acid supplementation of 400 micrograms/day for the first three months preconceptually and throughout the first trimester[4,9].

A daily oral supplementation of 5–15 mg folic acid is recommended for those with a previously affected fetus and family history of neural tube defects and to epileptics[4,10].

Other factors such as genetic factors, pre-conceptual diabetes and first trimester hyperglycaemia and drugs such as sodium valproate used for epilepsy also contribute to the development of megaloblastic anaemia. Also relevant are the increased demands of pregnancy, multiple pregnancy, grand multiparity or frequent pregnancies[3] which may exacerbate other factors or in extreme cases precipitate megaloblastic anaemia.

Pregnancy Issues

It is important to remember that both macrocytosis (raised MCV) and low B_{12} levels (normal range in pregnancy down to 150 micrograms/l) are most likely to be normal in pregnancy.

With megaloblastic anaemia the drop in haemoglobin and platelet levels is exaggerated, however serum ferritin can remain normal[2]. Leucopenia[1], which is worsened when there is infection, is present.

Folate deficiency is associated with:
- Cervical dysplasia
- Loss of appetite and maternal weight loss
- Glossitis
- Increased risk of neural tube defects
- Increased risk of fetal cleft palate
- Intrauterine growth restriction (IUGR)

Vomiting in pregnancy makes the increased demands of pregnancy worse, especially in the presence of multiple pregnancy, where there is more folate transfer from mother to fetus[11] leading to further depletion of folate stores.

Average daily folate requirements rise in pregnancy from 50 micrograms/day to 400 micrograms/day which can be met through a normal diet. However, note that folates are vulnerable to heat, being easily destroyed during cooking.

Medical Management and Care
- Full blood count – assess serum and red cell folate levels[9]
- Mild/moderate anaemia – synthetic oral folic acid 5–10 mg/day
- Folic acid oral or im supplement may be prescribed
- Vigilant screening for congenital abnormalities – ultrasound scan
- Further investigations for associated conditions if megaloblastic anaemia presents for the first time in pregnancy[4], but ensure this is true megaloblastic anaemia; obstetrician may need to liaise with physician/haematologist
- Infection screening may be indicated
- IUGR – consider serial ultrasound scanning
- NICE recommend routine supplementation of oral folic acid 400 micrograms/day prior to pregnancy and in the first trimester[9]

Midwifery Management and Care
- Midwife to take thorough booking history to identify any current treatment and co-existing conditions that may influence megaloblastic anaemia, e.g. haemoglobinopathies, dietary restriction
- All such mothers should be booked at a consultant unit
- Weigh at each antenatal appointment if there is any suggestion of weight loss or loss of appetite
- Conduct a nutritional assessment referring to a dietician if indicated
- Promote a folate-rich diet and taking of prescribed supplements
- Encourage attendance at antenatal parent education with an emphasis on food preparation
- Assess for signs of infection and refer for treatment promptly
- Severe anaemia is treated with folic acid 5–10 mg/day im, oral iron and blood transfusion
- Counselling about the increased risks of congenital anomalies is advised if confirmed folate deficiency
- Be alert for IUGR and refer as appropriate
- Be alert for APH and advise mother to seek prompt help if symptoms present, including giving of emergency telephone numbers
- Prepare mother for the possibility of blood transfusion in labour

Labour Issues
- Increased risk of prematurity and low birth weight in severe cases
- Risk of postpartum haemorrhage exists
- Maternal tiredness is more likely at the onset of labour

Medical Management and Care
- If symptomatic anaemia presents, repeat full blood count with cross-matched blood available if needed
- No specific recommendations in labour and birth if blood count is stable

Midwifery Management and Care
- Encourage mobilisation and maintain hydration to combat tiredness
- Actively manage third-stage labour to reduce blood loss at birth, especially if symptoms of anaemia persist
- Alert neonatal team if premature birth is imminent

Postpartum Issues
- Human milk has a folate content of 5 micrograms/dl, therefore red cell folate levels are further depleted in lactating women
- Women with folate deficiency diagnosed prenatally should continue supplementation for several weeks postpartum
- Adequate inter-pregnancy interval is advised to encourage woman to fully recover and maintain good folate reserves

Medical Management and Care
- Indices of folate metabolism return to pre-pregnant values within six weeks of delivery
- Haematological follow-up may be needed

Midwifery Management and Care
- Continue to promote a diet rich in folates
- Full blood count to determine haemoglobin status, red cell folate concentrations, reticulocyte count and blood film recommended if symptomatic anaemia occurs
- Provide contraceptive advice and consider further discussion with women suffering from epilepsy and malabsorption disorders
- Continuation of folate supplementation advised for those with hereditary haemolytic disorders and epilepsy

14.3 Thalassaemia

Incidence	**Risk for Childbearing**
Over 700 people in UK are estimated to have β-thalassaemia major[1,2]	High Risk – thalassaemia major Low or Variable Risk – all other thalassaemias

EXPLANATION OF CONDITION

Thalassaemia is an autosomal recessive inherited disorder of haemoglobin synthesis, prevalent in population groups that originate from Africa, the Caribbean, the Mediterranean, Southeast Asia and the Middle East[3].

Adult haemoglobin consists of two pairs of alpha (α) and beta (β) globin chains per haem complex. The α-globin chain production is controlled by four genes located on chromosome 16 and β-globin chain production is controlled by two genes located on chromosome 11. Individuals inherit two α genes and one β gene from each parent[4].

There are three types of haemoglobins present at birth, produced from the pairing of α, β, γ (gamma) or δ (delta) globin chains:

1. **Haemoglobin A** $(\alpha_2\beta_2) - 97\%$
2. **Haemoglobin A$_2$** $(\alpha_2\delta_2) - 2\%$
3. **Haemoglobin F** $(\alpha_2\gamma_2) - 0.5\%$

Thalassaemia is caused by the inheritance of a defective α- or β-globin gene. This results in a reduced rate of globin chain formation and red blood cells (RBC) with inadequate haemoglobin (Hb) content. The thalassaemias are classified by the defective gene inherited[3] and further sub-classified by the reduction of globin chains produced.

α-thalassaemias

Characterised by defective production and number of functional α-globin chains:

- **α-thalassaemia trait** (α-thal⁺)
    - inheritance of one defective α gene
    - clinically undetectable
- **α-thalassaemia intermedia**
    - inheritance of two defective α genes
    - mainly asymptomatic
    - α-thal⁰ trait: both defective genes inherited from one parent
    - homozygous α-thal⁺ trait: one defective gene is inherited from each parent
- **Haemoglobin H disease (HbH)**
    - inheritance of three defective genes resulting in rapid RBC haemolysis and mild/moderate anaemia
- **Thalassaemia major** (homozygous α-thal⁰)
    - all four α genes are absent and substituted by the four γ-globulin chains
    - the resultant Bart's haemoglobin (Hb Barts hydrops) is incapable of oxygen exchange at tissue level
    - this hydropic fetus requires intrauterine transfusions to survive and will be transfusion dependent for life

β-thalassaemias

Characterised by defective production of β-globin chains:

- **β-thalassaemia minor**
    - a carrier state caused by the inheritance of one defective β
    - characterised by a mild microcytic anaemia
- **β-thalassaemia intermedia**
    - moderate homozygous β-thalassaemia where both inherited genes are defective
    - individuals are less likely to require blood transfusions
- Clinical findings include:
    - enlargement of heart, liver and spleen
    - bone deformities due to bone marrow expansion

- **β-thalassaemia major**
    - inheritance of both defective genes resulting in a severe homozygous β-thalassaemia
    - severe haemolysis of red blood cells
    - life-threatening anaemia requiring chronic blood transfusion therapy

Diagnosis

Diagnosis is by identifying high risk groups[5] and performing:

- Full blood count – reveals low mean corpuscular haemoglobin (MCH <27 pg) and a low mean cell volume (MCV <75 fl)
- Bone marrow examination – reveals microcytic, hypochromic red blood cells
- Haemoglobin analysis – elevated HbA$_2$ levels

COMPLICATIONS

- Severe haemolysis and anaemia
- Bone marrow expansion
- Elevated cardiac output and severe cardiac impairment
- Endocrine, splenic and hepatic dysfunction
- Megaloblastic anaemia, iron overload in organs

NB: Those with 'trait only' have anaemia of variable severity.

NON-PREGNANCY TREATMENT AND CARE

Screening involves the identification of at-risk groups from history taking – ethnicity of woman, family origins, medical history, paternal screening, full blood count, haemoglobin analysis[1,5]. Further investigations include cardiology assessment, blood-borne infection screening, maternal antibody and iron overload levels.

Treatment

- Oral iron if low ferritin levels; avoid parenteral iron
- 5 mg folic acid daily
- Transfusion therapy for severe anaemia
- Iron chelation therapy with desferrioxamine (25–50 mg/kg) infusion pump overnight for 10–12 hours; removes iron from tissues and reduces organ damage caused by iron overload
- Desferrioxamine is given daily through the abdominal wall subcutaneously

PRE-CONCEPTION ISSUES AND CARE

- Accumulation of iron stores in the heart, pancreas and thyroid can lead to cardiomyopathy, type 1 diabetes and hypothyroidism, hence screening is indicated
- Levels of iron overload are measured through gall bladder and biliary tract assessments
- Those with major thalassaemia infertility problems caused by chronic iron overload in the ovaries and pituitary gland can be treated with ovulation induction
- Assisted conception, pre-implantation, prenatal diagnosis and surgical termination of pregnancy should be discussed
- Multi-disciplinary care from haematology, genetic counselling, physiotherapy and maternal–fetal medicine
- Iron chelation programme should be optimised

Pregnancy Issues

There is a 1:4 chance of a child inheriting a major condition from parents who are both healthy α, β or sickle cell carriers.

Diagnostic tests
Tests are offered to determine fetal risk and include:
- DNA analysis of chorionic villi
- Fetal blood sample or amniotic fluid[3]

Risk of pregnancy complications
- Thrombo-embolic disease
- Congestive heart failure caused by iron deposits in heart; increases maternal mortality by 50%[6]
- Damage to liver, renal and endocrine organs due to iron overload
- Diabetes more likely
- Increased transfusion requirements
- Haemolytic disease of the newborn
- Intrauterine growth restriction
- Spontaneous abortion caused by worsening de-oxygenation of placental tissue
- Maternal red blood cell allo-antibodies
- Anaemia
- Pre-eclampsia (Hb Bart's hydrops)

Medical Management and Care
- Counselling depends on whether the risks are fetal or maternal or both – discuss the potential perinatal outcomes of antenatal tests and available options for ongoing pregnancy and care
- Specialist haematologist involvement – discuss transfusion therapy for treatment of worsening Hb levels
- Iron chelation is contraindicated in pregnancy, therefore implement aggressive iron chelation programme prior to conception[7]
- Serial ultrasound assessments for fetal anaemia, growth and placental pathology[6,5]
- Maternal surveillance includes:
  - MRI scanning to assess iron overload in maternal organs[8]
  - echocardiography to exclude cardiomyopathy
  - regular assessment of blood antibody levels, liver and thyroid function tests
- Discuss risks for continuing pregnancy and birth options

Midwifery Management and Care
- Book at consultant unit, discussing high-risk care and birth options
- Assess for blood-borne infections, haemoglobin levels and full blood count to determine severity of maternal anaemia
- Assess for signs of pre-eclampsia – blood pressure measurements and urinary microscopy and culture
- Treat iron and folic acid deficiency anaemia as prescribed[9] to meet the increased demands of pregnancy and increased turnover of red blood cells in bone marrow; caution with the use of iron in β major is advised[7]
- Provide dietary advice to enhance folate intake (see Section 14.2)
- Be vigilant for signs and symptoms of a reaction to transfusion therapy, including an exacerbation of existing cardiac problems
- Physiotherapy may be required as chelation can cause arthritis
- Encourage full attendance to antenatal surveillance visits and provide stress-reduction strategies through supportive care and counselling of the couple

Labour Issues

Thalassaemia major mothers are at risk of:
- Pre-term labour
- Fetal hypoxia
- Maternal hypoxia and exhaustion
- Raised blood pressure
- Delivery difficulties – hydropic fetus and placenta and maternal bone deformities
- Potential for postpartum haemorrhage (PPH)

Medical Management and Care
- Individual plan of care based on outcomes of feto-maternal surveillance including maternal pelvic size

Midwifery Management and Care
- Adhere to above plan and local guidelines
- Continuous EFM and assess for signs of early fetal hypoxia
- Optimise oxygenation of mother and utero-placental perfusion through appropriate positioning
- Monitor blood pressure and fluid balance strictly to prevent cardiac compromise and maintain hydration using intravenous fluids
- Provide support and pain relief to avoid cardiopulmonary stress
- Active management of third stage of labour

Postpartum Issues

Neonate with thalassaemia major at risk of:
- Pre-term birth
- Low birth weight
- Fetal haemolytic anaemia
- Feeding problems
- Jaundice, enlarged liver and spleen
- Failure to thrive in first year

Mother at risk of:
- Poor wound healing
- Infection due to severe anaemia
- PPH and worsening of anaemia
- Depression

Medical Management and Care
- Individual plan of care based on outcomes of ongoing neonatal and maternal surveillance
- Multi-disciplinary team working with neonatal, haematology and counselling professionals

Midwifery Management and Care
- Mother and infant are not for six-hour discharge
- Affected neonate with failure to maintain body temperature, poor feeding or pallor is transferred to neonatal unit for investigation
- Universal newborn blood spot (Guthrie) screening test on sixth day[1]
- Monitor prescribed iv fluids and fluid balance/oral intake
- Provide supportive care and pain relief to prevent exacerbation of cardiopulmonary compromise
- Observe for signs of haemorrhage/infection with prompt referral
- Refer for appropriate types of counselling
- Arrange relevant maternal and neonatal follow-up[7]

14.4 Sickle Cell Disorders

Incidence	Risk for Childbearing
0.2% African–Caribbean in the United Kingdom, comprising 6000–10,000 people[1,2]	High Risk

EXPLANATION OF CONDITION

Homozygous sickle cell disease (HbSS) is an autosomal recessive disease in which sufferers are homozygous (inherited from both parents) for the mutant gene while individuals with a trait are heterozygous (HbAS).

Variants of the disease include sickle cell haemoglobin C disease (HbSC), sickle cell β^o thalassaemia (no normal β chains produced) and sickle cell β^+ thalassaemia (reduced amount of chains made). There are other, rarer variants of varying clinical significance.

HbSS results from an abnormality in the formation and quality of the adult haemoglobin molecule (HbA) caused by an error in the amino acid sequence. The amino acid glutamic acid is substituted for either valine (HbS) or lysine (HbC) on the beta globin chain.

HbSS is characterised by the distortion and slow movement of red blood cells which is exacerbated when oxygen levels drop, and leads to:

- Chronic haemolytic anaemia
- Metabolic acidosis
- Capillary stasis
- Increased blood viscosity
- Occlusion of blood vessels
- Resultant infarction and ischaemic necrosis of tissues in organs such as lungs, kidneys, spleen and bones[3]

Repeated deoxygenation of red blood cells (HbS) results in irreversible cell-membrane rigidity and damage and destruction within 17 days, compared with the 120-day lifespan of normal red blood cells (HbA). Damaged red blood cells are removed from the circulation by the reticulo-endothelial system (largely spleen and liver).

Acute episodes of deoxygenation in sickle cell disease can result in episodes called 'sickle cell crises', of which there are three types:

1. Sequestrative
2. Aplastic
3. Vaso-occlusive

Sickle cell crises are manifested by:

- Worsening of chronic anaemia (6.5–9.0 g/dl)
- Severe pain
- Breathlessness
- Weakness
- Pallor and fever[1]

HbSS is diagnosed by taking a thorough medical history, clinical examination and haemoglobinopathy investigations, which include:

- Hb electrophoresis
- Sickle-shaped red blood cells
- Hyperplastic, immature red blood cells in bone marrow aspirate if required

COMPLICATIONS

- Acute-on-chronic anaemia caused by blood loss, dehydration, cold or infection
- Excessive haemolysis and bone marrow suppression
- Acute chest syndrome, a life-threatening sickling in the lungs manifests itself with:
  - cough
  - severe chest pain
  - difficulty breathing
  - severe anaemia
  - fever[4]
- Thrombo-embolic events including:
  - pulmonary embolism
  - cerebrovascular accident
  - seizures
  - liver and splenic autoinfarction
  - sequestration
- Cardiac failure caused by chronic hypoxaemia and aplastic anaemia
- Vaso-occlusive or painful crisis exacerbated by stress, cold, infection, dehydration and exercise causing swelling to joints

NON-PREGNANCY TREATMENT AND CARE

Prophylactic penicillin V by mouth daily, folic acid 1 mg daily both long term. Other measures may include hyroxyurea to induce increased levels of fetal haemoglobin (HbF), exchange blood transfusion, anti-thrombotic measures, family history to determine the requirement for partner haemoglobinopathy screening and counselling. Pneumococcal vaccine may be given. Renal, hepatic and retinal function are assessed regularly.

Other requirements include human immunodeficiency virus, and hepatitis B or C screening following repeated transfusions[5].

PRE-CONCEPTION ISSUES AND CARE

- A thorough clinical and risk assessment; a family history of ancestors or relatives who originate from outside northern Europe is used as an indicator for screening; partners also require haemoglobinopathy screening and counselling
- The clinical assessment should identify immunisations to date, incidences of sickle cell crises (i.e. disease severity), past requirements for blood transfusion, iron status and levels of organ damage
- At-risk couples require information on: pre-implantation genetic diagnosis, which requires in-vitro fertilisation; prenatal diagnostic tests, such as chorionic villus sampling, amniocentesis and fetal blood sampling[6]
- Folic acid should be increased to 5 mg per day when planning a pregnancy and hydroxyurea and iron chelation discontinued 3–6 months prior to conception due to possible teratogenicity
- Discuss analgesia for sickle pains and penicillin prophylaxis throughout pregnancy

Pregnancy Issues

- Hydroxyurea and iron chelation agents are contraindicated in pregnancy[9]
- Red cell antibodies may be present if previous multiple transfusions
- Hyperemesis may cause dehydration and sickle crisis
- Pregnancy is contraindicated with pulmonary hypertension due to increase in maternal mortality by 30–50%[1]
- At risk of:
  - haemolytic anaemia, with or without iron deficiency
  - intrauterine growth restriction (IUGR)
  - sickle crisis secondary to infection (particularly of the urinary tract)
  - increased risk of miscarriage
  - increased risk of pre-eclampsia
  - increased risk of stillbirth
  - increased risk of maternal mortality

Appendix 14.4 gives an example of a management plan for pregnancy sickle crisis.

Medical Management and Care

- Women with pulmonary hypertension should consider termination of pregnancy because of high maternal mortality (see Section 4.9)
- Prescribe 5 mg folic acid per day orally
- Provide iron supplements only if indicated
- Baseline investigations – full blood count, blood group and antibody screen, reticulocyte count, serum ferritin levels, renal and liver function tests, HIV and hepatitis screening
- Ultrasound scans to confirm dates and for prompt detection of IUGR
- Monitoring of pregnancy – 2-4 weekly antenatal visits in first and second trimesters to assess blood pressure, urine microscopy and culture and a full blood count
- **Third trimester**: Serial growth scans, estimation of liquor volume, umbilical artery Doppler measurements
  - consider induction of labour for obstetric or medical indications, not as routine

Midwifery Management and Care

- Detailed booking history to refer at-risk couples to a specialist clinic
- Multi-disciplinary management, including obstetrician, haematologist, anaesthetist, haemoglobinopathy specialist nurse and midwife
- Continue antibiotics and increase folic acid to 5 mg daily
- Give nutritional advice to enhance the management of chronic anaemia
- Encourage the woman to keep well hydrated, avoid both cold environments and excessive physical exertion
- Advise reporting of infection or crises for prompt medical treatment

Labour Issues

At risk of:
- Premature birth
- Pre-eclampsia[7]
- Placental abruption
- Sickle cell crises precipitated by immobilisation
- Blood loss hypoxia during labour and birth
- Hypertension
- Dehydration
- Infection
- Transfusion reactions

Medical Management and Care

- Blood taken for FBC, group and save
- Refer to anaesthetist – discuss epidural analgesia as recommended for pain relief
- Keep warm and well hydrated – warmed intravenous fluids are essential
- Ensure optimal oxygenation
- Avoid prolonged labour with early recourse to caesarean section for slow progress
- Graduated compression stockings

Midwifery Management and Care

- Minimise stress in labour and provide one to one support
- Encourage alternative positions during labour and childbirth
- Maintain basic hygiene needs, adequate oxygen, hydration, pain relief and continuous monitoring of fetal heart rate[10]
- Cord blood taken at birth for haemoglobin electrophoresis
- Avoid opiates such as pethidine
- Maintain fluid balance with strict records of input and output[10]

Postpartum issues

Mother is at risk of:
- Postpartum haemorrhage
- Dehydration
- Tissue hypoxia
- Infections
- Thrombo-embolism
- Sickle cell crises

Recurrent pregnancies increase frequency of crises[8]. Intrauterine contraceptive devices (IUCD) are relatively contraindicated[7] due to risk of infections but maternal compliance with contraception is essential.
  The baby requires:
- Universal screening of newborn
- Repeat electrophoresis at six weeks of age
- Prophylactic antibiotic therapy from three months of age is advised[5]

Medical Management and Care

- Vigilant follow-up due to increased risk of sickle cell crisis
- Refer to paediatrician for results of neonatal screening and follow-up arrangements prior to discharge
- Prescribe antibiotics and thrombo-prophylaxis
- Early treatment of suspected endometritis

Midwifery Management and Care

- Early ambulation[10], good hydration and oxygenation encouraged in first 24 hours postpartum
- Four hourly TPR observations[7]
- Use of thrombo-embolic deterrent stockings and daily subcutaneous heparin, because thrombo-embolic prophylaxis is recommended until fully mobile
- Discuss family planning options to space pregnancies[7]; includes progesterone only preparations, but ensure the choice is acceptable to the woman to ensure compliance
- Arrange relevant maternal and neonatal follow-up appointments[10]

14.5 Thrombocytopenia in Pregnancy

Incidence
Gestational: 5–8% of pregnancies[1]
Immune: 0.1% of pregnancies[1,2]

Risk for Childbearing
High Risk

EXPLANATION OF CONDITION

Thrombocytopenia is a reduced platelet (thrombocyte) count which can lead to bleeding in the skin, called **purpura**, and can result in spontaneous bruising and post-injury bleeding[3]. Up to 50% of women with pre-eclampsia will also develop thrombocytopenia[4]. There are several categories, of which the midwife is likely to encounter two.

Gestational Thrombocytopenia

Gestational thrombocytopenia is also known as incidental thrombocytopenia of pregnancy[4]. It is exclusive to pregnancy and presents in the late second or third trimesters. The decreased platelet count is associated with haemodilution, and with increased platelet 'trapping,' and with destruction in the placenta[1]. Usually asymptomatic, diagnosis often arises from a routine antenatal FBC[5] or can be retrospective, after delivery[4]. The platelet levels gradually fall reaching $50–150 \times 10^9/l$ by term. It is considered a benign condition[6] and does not affect the fetus[1]. The platelet count usually returns to normal by six weeks postpartum[4].

Immune Thrombocytopenic Purpura

Immune thrombocytopenic purpura (ITP) was formerly called idiopathic thrombocytopenic purpura. It can have an acute presentation, often occurring in children, and may follow a viral infection[6]. Alternatively, it can be chronic and mainly affects young to middle-aged women, with the incidence increasing with age[8]. It is this version the midwife may encounter in the pre-conception period. It may also present for the first time in pregnancy.

ITP results from the body producing IgG autoantibodies that act against the woman's own platelets[9], reducing their lifespan from ten days to a few hours. As the bone marrow cannot keep pace with replacement, the count drops[9] from a normal value of $150–400 \times 10^9/l$ to $10–140 \times 10^9/l$, with the risk of purpura and haemorrhage. Most cases are idiopathic (unknown cause) but some are secondary to drugs, HIV infection and connective tissue disorders[4].

Diagnosis is difficult as it is based on excluding other illnesses, such as SLE or von Willebrand's disease[5], and side effects of drugs that cause a low platelet count. Additionally, 30% of patients do not have antibodies detected on laboratory investigation.

If thrombocytopenia presents for the first time in pregnancy, diagnosis is complex, as pregnancy symptoms 'overlap'[1], and it is difficult to differentiate between gestational and immune thrombocytopenia. For this reason gestational thrombocytopenia may be considered a high-risk condition as well as ITP. The small IgG antibodies cross the placental barrier sometimes initiating neonatal thrombocytopenia[4].

HELLP syndrome[1] can be an associated condition.

COMPLICATIONS

- Impaired haemostasis[4]
- Bleeding from nose and gums[7]
- Bruising[7]
- Menorrhagia[7] and secondary anaemia
- Splenomegaly is rare in isolated thrombocytopenia[7]
- Major haemorrhage is rare[7]
- Side effects of steroids, e.g. diabetes, hypertension

NON-PREGNANCY TREATMENT AND CARE

- Corticosteroids, e.g. prednisone, to reduce the production of autoantibodies and the removal of antibody-coated platelets; complete response in 20% of cases and no further treatment necessary[7]
- IV gammaglobulin is given to prolong the clearance time of antibody-coated platelets[5]
- Immunosuppressant drugs, e.g. azathioprine, ciclosporine, vincristine, danazol (see Appendix 11)
- Consideration of platelet transfusion in life-threatening situations or immediately before surgery under the advice of a haematologist; only a short-term effect as transfused platelets also have short life-span[5]
- Splenectomy if medical management has failed. Removal of the spleen improves condition in 90% of cases[7] because the spleen is the principal site for production of IgG autoantibodies, as well as being the location for sequestration of antibody-coated platelets[5]. This operation is not recommended for children[7] or HIV-positive adults[10], because of a subsequent risk of pneumococcal infection.

PRE-CONCEPTION ISSUES AND CARE

- Former advice to avoid pregnancy, or deliver by caesarean section, no longer applies due to modern management[11]
- When a woman had ITP in a previous pregnancy the course of the disease and the effect on the fetus is likely to be similar in future pregnancies
- If the woman is still on treatment, she should be referred back to the haematologist for a risk–benefit analysis to maintain or alter drug therapy
- The woman might be investigated for other immune conditions, such as pernicious anaemia
- Usual pre-conception care is given, with additional consideration of:
  - prophylactic antibiotics if post-splenectomy
  - encourage a healthy diet that is rich in iron and folates
  - advising the mother *not* to discontinue her maintenance therapy once she suspects she is pregnant, without prior discussion with the haematologist

Pregnancy Issues

- In immune thrombocytopenia the IgG autoantibodies can cross the placental barrier, causing fetal, and later neonatal, thrombocytopenia[4,13]
- The only reliable predictor of neonatal outcome is a prior affected pregnancy[13]
- There is a risk of severe thrombocytopenia in approximately 1% of neonates[11]
- Splenectomy in pregnancy can precipitate pre-term labour[13]
- Therapy for pregnant women is similar to that of non-pregnant women[11]
- Little correlation exists between maternal and fetal platelet counts, so it is not possible to predict fetal outcome from non-invasive tests[3]
- Thrombocytopenia can arise secondary to pre-eclampsia and HELLP syndrome[12]

Medical Management and Care

- Regular FBC for platelet count, frequency dependent upon the severity of the condition
- Adjust steroids in ITP (usually prednisolone) in relation to platelet count
- Intravenous immunoglobulins (IVIG) if required[11]
- Prophylactic antibiotics if a previous splenectomy[6]
- Splenectomy is best avoided, but if necessary should be performed in the second trimester[16,1]; alternatively it might be combined with caesarean section in third trimester[17] in very rare situations
- Maternal platelet transfusion only if severely compromised
- Avoid cordocentesis if possible[11,15]
- IV Anti D is an experimental treatment used in specialist centres only
- Aim to optimise third trimester platelet count to maximise the prospect of a vaginal delivery near term

Midwifery Management and Care

- Book for hospital confinement and for antenatal care by the multidisciplinary team at a combined obstetric/haematology clinic
- Discuss with the mother a realistic care and birth plan, with consultation with haematologist and obstetrician
- Encourage healthy diet and lifestyle
- Iron and folate tablets throughout pregnancy
- Aim to keep pregnancy otherwise as normal as possible

Labour Issues

- Risk of intrapartum haemorrhage[1], especially from a surgical incision
- Higher chance of pre-term delivery[12]
- Theoretical risk of epidural haematoma[1], however, epidural is considered safe if the platelet count $>80–100 \times 10^9/l$[14]
- There is a small risk of fetal intracranial haemorrhage[11], with chance of fetal bruising and significant cephalhaematoma

Medical Management and Care

- Maintain iv access during labour
- Take blood for FBC and platelets, group and save
- Caesarean section only for obstetric reasons[11,14]
- Avoid ventouse and forceps delivery[14]
- Avoid fetal blood sampling[2,11,15]
- Risk–benefit analysis for epidural if platelet count $<80 \times 10^9/l$
- The anaesthetist may prefer a spinal anaesthetic to an epidural[1]
- Avoid im injections if platelet count $<40 \times 10^9/l$

Midwifery Management and Care

- Inspect iv cannulation site regularly for signs of bleeding
- Aim for normal vaginal delivery if all is otherwise well
- Leave adequate length of umbilical cord, below the cord clamp, to allow blood samples to be taken
- Active management of third stage of labour; consider use of iv Syntocinon if im injections are contraindicated (see above)
- All perineal trauma to be sutured promptly[14] and expertly
- Take placental cord blood for neonatal platelet count, and ascertain if other samples are required[14]
- Confirm with paediatrician if the neonatal vitamin K can be given im
- Neonatal assessment by paediatrician, and possible transfer to the neonatal unit for concerns about bleeding or general condition

Postpartum Issues

- Risk of postpartum haemorrhage if platelet count is low[12]
- ITP secondary to pre-eclampsia or HELLP syndrome often deteriorates immediately post delivery
- The risk of thrombocytopenia in the neonate cannot be predicted from clinical or laboratory test results in the mother[15]
- 6% risk of the neonate having severe thrombocytopenia with a limited risk of intracranial haemorrhage[13]

Medical Management and Care

- Avoid maternal non-steroidal drugs if platelet count $<100 \times 10^9/l$[15]
- Review platelet count post delivery[14] and repeat regularly if pre-eclamptic

Midwifery Management and Care

- The neonate is not for early discharge if daily platelet counts, from umbilical cord stump, are required[1,5]
- Vigilant postnatal examination to ascertain if vaginal loss is excessive and to ascertain if effective uterine involution is occurring
- Vigilant daily examination of the newborn to look for signs of bleeding from cord stump and other areas
- Be alert for intracranial bleeding symptoms such as seizures, bulging fontanelle or altered responses, especially if paediatric advice is that there is a risk of haemorrhage

14.6 Von Willebrand's Disease and Other Bleeding Disorders

Incidence
1% of the UK population have low von Willebrand Factor[1]
7–20% of women with menorrhagia have von Willebrand's Disease[2]

Risk for Childbearing
VWD Type 1 and 2 – Variable Risk
VWD Type 3 – High Risk

EXPLANATION OF CONDITION

A familial haematological disorder, characterised by bleeding, was described in 1926 by von Willebrand in Finland[3], hence the term *von Willebrand's disease* (VWD). This is a condition in which there is either a defect, or deficiency, of the von Willebrand factor (VWF), a carrier protein for clotting factor VIII[4]. There are three[5] basic types:

1. **Type 1** – 75% of cases[4]; partial quantitative deficiency of normal VWF[1,5]
2. **Type 2** – 20% of cases[4]; qualitative deficiencies of VWF of which there are four variations[1]
3. **Type 3 (Severe)** – 5% of cases[4]; almost complete deficiency of VWF and reduced factor VIII[1,5]

VWD is the most common inherited bleeding disorder in pregnancy[6], and is inherited as an autosomal dominant condition. Hence, children of either gender may inherit the clotting deficiency[7]. However, women are more likely to present with symptomatic VWD due to menstruation and childbearing[4]. There are no ethnic differences[8].

Non-pregnant patients usually present as young adults with excess bleeding, in the form of:

*   Epistaxis (nosebleeds)[1,5]
*   Menorrhagia (heavy and prolonged periods)[1,2,5,9]
*   Bleeding after dental extraction or surgery[1,5]
*   Bruising[1,5]

Screening tests[8] entail:

*   Full blood count (FBC) – usually normal but a mild thrombocytopenia may occur in Type 2 patients[8]
*   Serum ferritin
*   Clotting screen – prothrombin time is normal, but the activated partial thromboplastin time may be prolonged
*   Bleeding time – usually prolonged, but may be normal in mild forms of VWD[8]
*   Platelet aggregation test – measures platelet efficiency[8]
*   Von Willebrand factor antigen, and factor VIII

Other Bleeding Disorders

*   **Factor XI deficiency** – similar problems to VWD Type 3
*   **Haemophilia A and B** – female carriers can have low levels, and an associated bleeding risk
    –   Bleeding history and non-pregnant levels of factor VIII or IX should be identified

COMPLICATIONS

*   Haemorrhage (severity varies from VWD Type 1 to 3)
*   Joint bleeding and pain (in VWD Type 3)
*   Anaemia and fatigue
*   Pregnancy problems

NON-PREGNANCY TREATMENT AND CARE

Common Treatments

*   Combined oral contraceptive pill (COCP) – to increase levels of factor VIII and von Willebrand factor, reduce menstrual blood volume, and prevent pregnancy[8]
*   Iron supplementation – if clinical condition necessitates
*   Vaccination against hepatitis A and B[5]
*   Tranexamic acid (to inhibit bleeding) – slows the breakdown of blood clots; tablet form, or syrup for children[1]
*   Desmopressin – a synthetic hormone (not a blood product) that enables VWF to be released into the blood circulation
    –   given iv at specialist centres[1]
    –   nasal spray is available
*   Clotting factor concentrate – derived from human plasma, and used to treat severe cases of VWD[1]

Advice[1]

*   **Avoid aspirin**
*   Carry 'green card' from haemophilia centre at all times in case of accident or emergency
*   For children, parents should inform the school
*   Caution with certain holiday destinations, and a 'travel pack' of drugs may have to be issued
*   Encourage exercise, but discourage contact sports
*   Maintain a healthy lifestyle with an iron-rich diet

PRE-CONCEPTION ISSUES AND CARE

Women with a history of heavy menstrual bleeding since menarche, and a family history suggestive of a coagulation disorder, should be screened for coagulation disorders[10].

Von Willebrand's Disease

*   There is no evidence that fertility is impaired[4]
*   Pre-conception care aims to optimise maternal health
*   The risk of a mother with Type 1 transmitting the condition to her child is 50% but only 33% of these will be clinically affected[7]
*   Opportunity for prenatal diagnosis for women with Type 3, whose genetic mutation is identifiable[7]
*   If parents already have a child with Type 3, the chance of each subsequent child being affected is 25%[7]

Haemophilia

*   Women with relevant family histories are assessed for carrier status and counselled over reproductive options[7]

Factor XI Deficiency

*   Prenatal diagnosis should be discussed if the woman's condition is severe[7]

Pregnancy Issues

There is considerable variability of the haemostatic response of VWD to pregnancy.[7]

Both factor VIII and VWF levels rise in second and third trimesters[2] which may lead to a 'normalisation' of these levels with improvement in minor bleeding problems[8] but makes diagnosis of VWD difficult[8]. However, the first trimester retains a risk of bleeding. In severe VWD, levels remain low throughout[8].

VWD miscarriage risk is not significantly different from that of the general population[2].

Desmopressin is used with caution in pregnancy due to concerns over inducing contractions, placental insufficiency, hyponatraemia, and its antidiuretic effect[8]. It can be used once based on a risk–benefit assessment. It should not be used in the presence of pre-eclampsia[7].

Co-existing thrombocytopenia can worsen[8].

Medical Management and Care

- Pregnancy in women with VWD or other clotting disorders should be managed by a multi-disciplinary team comprising obstetrician, haematologist, senior anaesthetist[7], specialist nurse or midwife
- Counsel about prenatal diagnosis and options arising
- Chorionic villus sampling for fetal DNA analysis might be performed

Von Willebrand's disease
- Check factor levels including VWF:Ag, VWF:AC and FVIII:C at booking, 28 and 34 weeks and prior to invasive procedures[7]
- Aim for factor VIII level ≥50% to cover delivery and postpartum[8]
- Prophylactic treatment when factor levels are <50 IU/dl to cover invasive procedures and delivery[7]
- Platelet count is monitored regularly with VWD Type 2b[7]
- Monitor clinically, advising the laboratory of haemorrhage potential[8]
- If desmopressin is used, advise to restrict fluid intake[8] and observe closely for water retention[7]
- Avoid external cephalic version for malpresentation

Midwifery Management and Care

- Ensure the mother is booked for antenatal care at a specialist haematological/obstetric clinic and delivery at a consultant unit
- Be aware 'booking bloods' will be augmented by the doctor to include FBC, bleeding time or platelet closure time[8]; these are repeated prior to invasive procedures[8]
- Report abnormal blood test results promptly, especially platelets
- Encourage parent-craft attendance, but advise that an epidural *might* be contraindicated and discuss alternative pain relief options

Labour Issues

Delivery is a significant haemostatic challenge[8], hence staff should be alert for intrapartum and postpartum haemorrhage.

Von Willebrand's disease
- Epidurals can be sited by a senior anaesthetist for VWD Type 1 where VWF >50 IU/dl[7,8], but its use is debatable for Type 2[8], and contraindicated for Type 3[7]
- Prompt removal of epidural catheter reduces risk of bleeding[8]
- Effort should be made to ensure a prompt third stage with complete placenta[11]

Haemophilia carriers: for most haemophilia carriers labour and anaesthesia carry normal risk, but those with low factor levels should be identified and a plan agreed.

Medical Management and Care

- In advance agree a delivery/anaesthetic plan, seek haematological advice, ascertain laboratory facilities, and order clotting factors[8]
- IVI, FBC, coagulation screen and group and save in labour[8]
- Avoid fetal blood sampling
- Avoid ventouse and mid-cavity rotational forceps delivery[7]
- Tranexamic acid can be used in the treatment of PPH, after obstetric causes have been treated[7]
- Avoid prolonged labour; early recourse to caesarean section should be considered[7] ensuring surgical haemostasis[8]

Midwifery Management and Care

- Avoid fetal scalp electrodes for continuous fetal monitoring
- Active management of third stage of labour is essential[7]
- If needed, give desmopressin *after* clamping of the umbilical cord[2]
- Ask the doctor if im injections, including Syntometrine, can be given
- Prompt and expert suturing of all perineal trauma
- Ascertain if cord bloods should be taken for fetal VWF[7]
- Prompt administration to the neonate of *oral* vitamin K[7]

Postpartum Issues

- Levels of factor VIII and VWF fall markedly 24 hours postpartum[8], putting mothers of all three types of VWD[2] at:
  - 22% risk of primary PPH[8]
  - 25% risk of secondary PPH[8], which can occur up to *five weeks* postpartum[2]
- The safety of desmopressin in breast-feeding has not been studied[8]
- Neonates who inherit VWD Type 3 are at risk of intracranial haemorrhage, cephalhaematoma from labour[7] and umbilical stump bleeding postpartum

Medical Management and Care

- Check VWF level if there was a low pre-pregnancy baseline[7]
- Desmopressin can be used immediately postpartum[8]

Midwifery Management and Care

- This mother is not for early discharge
- Vigilant postnatal maternal observations, being alert for PPH[8]
- If desmopressin is used, confer with paediatrician over breast-feeding
- Vigilant daily neonatal examinations being alert for intracranial bleeding or umbilical cord stump bleeding
- Advise the parents that circumcision, or other invasive procedures, of the baby must be delayed until the haematologist is in agreement[7]
- When *heel prick* (Guthrie) tests are performed, apply local pressure for a full five minutes and report excess bleeding or bruising[7]

14.7 Disseminated Intravascular Coagulation

Incidence	Risk for Childbearing
Rare, less than 1:1000 pregnancies[1]	High Risk

EXPLANATION OF CONDITION

Disseminated intravascular coagulation (DIC), also known as consumptive coagulopathy, is an acquired disorder of haemostasis, which often heralds the onset of multi-organ failure.[2]
Underlying causes[3]:

- **Infection** – especially *Escherichia coli, Neisseria meningitidis, Streptococcus pneumoniae* and malaria
- **Cancer** – especially lungs, pancreas[3], gynaecological[4]
- **Trauma, burns, surgery** and **snake bite**[5]
- **Pregnancy** – especially:
  - placental abruption
  - major haemorrhage
  - pre-eclampsia
  - retained dead fetus or placenta
  - amniotic fluid embolism[3]

Endothelial damage arising from one of the above results in thromboplastins being released from the damaged cells[6], *triggering* the extrinsic pathway to initiate a coagulation cascade[3]. With DIC, the tissue damage is so severe that blood clotting occurs at the original site *and* throughout the vascular tree. Hence the term *disseminated* intravascular coagulation. This process consumes large quantities of fibrinogen, thrombocytes (platelets) and clotting factors V and VIII[3]. The micro-thrombi produced occlude some small blood vessels, resulting in ischaemic damage (dead tissue) to body organs[6]. The damaged tissue releases more thromboplastins and a vicious cycle develops[6].

Eventually all the clotting factors and platelets are consumed and bleeding results[5]. The patient is in the ironic situation of having both widespread blood clotting *and* a clotting deficiency. Bleeding occurs, petechiae develop in the skin and, if untreated, **major haemorrhage** can result.

DIC can be subclinical, only detected on laboratory investigations, or may present with massive haemorrhage[9]. Bleeding is observed at vascular access points, GI tract, nose, genitourinary tract, iv cannulation sites and wounds. Investigations[2] reveal:

- Increase in prothrombin time
- Increase in partial thromboplastin time
- Increase in fibrin degradation products
- Decrease in platelets
- Decrease in fibrinogen

COMPLICATIONS

- **Damaged kidneys** – renal failure and anuria[6]
- **Damaged liver** – liver failure and jaundice[6]
- **Damaged lungs** – dyspnoea and cyanosis[6]
- **Brain damage** – convulsions or coma[6]
- **Retinal damage** – damaged sight or blindness[6]
- **Pituitary damage** – Sheehan's syndrome[6]
- **Major haemorrhage** – hypovolaemia then death

NON-PREGNANCY TREATMENT AND CARE

- DIC is essentially a clinical diagnosis; laboratory tests confirm the diagnosis and guide replacement of blood component[7]
- Coagulation screen comprising:
  - whole blood film
  - FBC, especially platelet count[8]
  - fibrinogen degradation products/D-dimers[5,8,9]
  - prothrombin time (normal 10–14 seconds)[8]
  - thrombin time (normal 1–15 seconds)[8]
  - partial thromboplastin time (normal 35–45 seconds)
  - fibrinogen levels (normal 2.5–4 g/l)[8]
- Insert indwelling urinary catheter, ideally with a measuring chamber, and monitor urinary output
- Strict monitoring and recording of fluid balance
- Repeat the coagulation screen as clinically indicated
- Central venous pressure (CVP) monitoring[10]
- IVI fresh frozen plasma[2], which contains all the clotting factors[11]
- IVI platelets[6]
- IVI packed cells (blood)[6,11]
- Identify and treat the underlying cause if possible[2]
- Institute high dependency care, transfer if necessary
- Respiratory support if indicated[12]
- IV antibiotics for suspected septicaemia[2]
- Correct exacerbating factors, especially:
  - dehydration
  - acidosis
  - renal failure
  - hypoxia[2]
- Analgesia[12]
- Anticoagulation with heparin rarely used and requires supervision by a haematologist[5,9]
- Concentrates of blood factors (antithrombins and/or protein C) are effective in the non-pregnant state
- Recombinant activated protein C is used for sepsis in non-pregnant patients[9]
- Steroids may be used for precipitating factors

PRE-CONCEPTION ISSUES AND CARE

If a woman had DIC in a previous pregnancy, the recurrence risk will be that of the precipitating cause. Follow-up and de-briefing of any woman who had acute DIC is essential.

Women with chronic DIC may be at high risk of pregnancy complications and need to be assessed and advised by a haematologist before cessation of contraception.

Pregnancy Issues

The activated coagulation system in pregnancy reduces the threshold for DIC[13], putting the mother at risk.

Associated with DIC in pregnancy
- Miscarriage, particularly septic
- Septic, illegal termination[14,4]
- Hydatidiform mole[10]
- Placenta accrete and PPH[10]
- Retained dead fetus[7,10]
- Acute fatty liver of pregnancy[10]
- Placental abruption – most common cause
- Placenta praevia[4,10]
- Pre-eclampsia[4,10]
- HELLP syndrome[4]
- Amniotic fluid embolism[7,10]
- Mismatched blood transfusion[7,10]
- Breast/ovarian/uterine cancer[4]

Possible clinical presentations
- One of the above trigger factors
- Haemorrhage
- Ecchymoses (discoloured skin patches)
- Haematuria
- Shock
- Thrombotic complications in the brain, kidneys or lungs
- Acute pulmonary hypertension if the trigger was amniotic fluid embolism[13]

Maternal mortality associated with DIC
- Placental abruption = 1%[10]
- Infection/shock = 50–80%[10]

Accurate record keeping is of paramount importance.

Medical Management and Care

General
- All women with an associated condition (see opposite) should have a full blood count and coagulation screen[13]
- Before attributing a platelet count of $\leq 100 \times 10^9/l$ to gestational thrombocytopenia, other causes of a reduced platelet count should be excluded[13], especially DIC

If DIC presents acutely with haemorrhage
- Multi-disciplinary team approach, so call haematologist and anaesthetist
- Precipitating factor must be identified and treated immediately[13]
- Investigations – as for non-pregnancy (previous page)
- Blood samples for group and cross-match are especially important as operative delivery may be imminent
- Treatment – as for non-pregnancy (previous page)
- If haemorrhage commences, implement the institution's **major obstetric haemorrhage protocol**

Midwifery Management and Care

- Be aware that DIC can present chronically or acutely, the latter leading to major obstetric haemorrhage (a life-threatening event) and that the midwife might be the first to recognise the problem

If DIC presents acutely with haemorrhage
- Remain with the mother, giving reassurance and oxygen, whilst preparing for an acute emergency
- **Send for medical aid**
- Initiate observations of vital signs, including measurement of blood loss and retaining blood-soaked items for inspection later
- Summon an assistant to prepare an IVI with blood giving set, and venepuncture equipment for the above blood samples
- Summon an assistant to attend the baby if the mother has delivered
- Insert indwelling urinary catheter and monitor fluid balance strictly
- Once medical aid arrives the midwife's role is to assist the medical team and to care for the mother and baby
- If there is a fetus or placental tissue *in utero*, the mother is likely to be transferred to obstetric theatre, otherwise, the mother should be transferred to high-dependency care area, which may well be delivery suite

Labour Issues

Labour and delivery needs to be planned and attended by senior obstetric and anaesthetic staff. If vaginal delivery can be achieved within a reasonable time frame this should be attempted. This will depend upon feto-maternal wellbeing.

Epidural and spinal anaesthesia are generally contraindicated. Hence, general anaesthetic (GA) is likely for operative delivery.

Medical Management and Care

- Caesarean section may be required[13]
- Evacuation of the uterus if there are retained feto-placental products
- Close liaison with haematologist and blood bank

Midwifery Management and Care

- Prepare for, and assist with, an emergency delivery
- Keep mother nil by mouth in case of GA
- If a vaginal delivery – active management of the third stage and all perineal trauma must be sutured promptly
- Vigilant examination of the placenta and ascertain if it, or cord blood samples, need to be sent to the laboratory
- Accurate estimation of blood loss, observe for clotting and possibly retain for inspection by the medical team

Postpartum Issues

- The coagulation imbalance usually resolves 24–48 hours post delivery, and the low platelet count (thrombocytopenia) within a week[11]
- The baby may have been admitted to NNU

Medical Management and Care

- Obstetric postnatal review – debrief; advice for future pregnancies

Midwifery Management and Care

- Careful post-operative care paying particular attention to wound and cannulation sites for signs of bleeding
- Post-operative observations might be continued longer than usual
- Assist the mother to visit her baby on NNU

14 Haematological Disorders

PATIENT ORGANISATIONS

Idiopathic Thrombocytopenia Support Association
Synehurst
Kimbolton Road
Bolnhurst
Bedfordshire MK44 2EW
http://www.itpsupport.org.uk

Women Bleed Too Project (The Haemophilia Society)
http://www.haemophilia.org.uk/uploads/guidetolivingvonwill.pdf

Hospital Information Services
(for Jehovah's Witnesses)
IBSA House
The Ridgeway
London NW7 1RN
his@wtbts.org.uk

SHOT – Serious Hazards of Transfusion (www.shotuk.org)

Dietary information sheets (normal diet, Traditional Asian diet, Asian vegetarian diet) from:
Leicestershire Nutrition and Dietetic Service
Units 11 & 12 Warren Park Way
Enderby
Leicestershire LE19 4SA

UK Thalassaemia Society
19 The Broadway
Southgate Circus,
London N14 6PH
E-mail: office@ukts.org

NHS Sickle cell/Thalassaemia Screening Programme,
Kings College London
Dept. Public Health Sciences
Capital House,
42 Weston Street,
London SE1 5QD
http://www.kcl-phs.org.uk/haemscreening/

Sickle Cell Society
54 Station Road
London NW10 4UA
www.sickecellsociety.org

Sickle Cell and Thalassaemia Centre
Haematology Department
Sandwell and West Birmingham NHS Trust
Lyndon
West Bromwich B71 4HJ
E-mail: Jayne.Swingler:swbh.nhs.uk

UK Forum on Haemoglobin Disorders
http://www.haemoglobin.org.uk

ESSENTIAL READING

Anionwu, E.N. and Atkin, K. (2001) **The Politics of Sickle Cell and Thalassaemia**. UK; Open University Press.

Anon (2001) **A Guide for Women Living with Von Willebrand's Disease.** London; Haemophilia Society. http://www.haemophilia.org.uk/uploads/guidetolivingvonwill.pdf

Billington, M. and Stevenson, M. (2006) **Critical Care in Childbearing for Midwives**. Oxford; Blackwell.

British Committee for Standards in Haematology General Haematology Task Force (2003). Guidelines for the investigation and management of idiopathic thrombocytopenic purpura in adults, children and pregnancy. **British Journal of Haematology, 120**, 570–596.

Chi, C., Shiltagh, N., Kingman, C.E.C. *et al.* (2006) Identification and management of women with inherited bleeding disorders: a survey of obstetricians and gynaecologists in the United Kingdom. **Haemophilia, 12**(4): 405–412.

Clarke, P. and Greer, I.A. (2006) Chapters 3 and 9. **Practical Obstetric Haematology**. London; Taylor & Francis.

Contreras, M. (1998) **ABC of Blood Transfusion**, 3rd Edn. Oxford; BMJ Books/Blackwell.

Dyson, S.M. (2005) **Ethnicity and Screening for Sickle Cell/Thalassaemia. Lessons for Practice from the Voices of Experience**. Oxford; Churchill Livingstone.

Green, D. and Ludham, C.A. (2006) **Fast Facts: Bleeding Disorders**, pp. 90–92. Oxford; Health Press.

Lee, C.A., Chi, C. and Pavord, S. *et al.* (2006) The obstetrical and gynaecological management of women with inherited bleeding disorders – review with guidelines produced by a taskforce of UK Haemophilia Centre Doctors' Organisation. **Haemophilia, 12**, 311–336.

Okpala, I. (2004) **Practical Management of Haemoglobinopathies**. Oxford; Blackwell Publishing.

Strong, J. (2006) Von Willebrand disease and pregnancy. **Current Obstetrics and Gynaecology, 16**, 1–5.

THROMBO-EMBOLIC DISORDERS 15

Daksha Elliott and Sue Pavord

15.1 Deep Vein Thrombosis

Incidence	Risk for Childbearing
1 in 1000 in pregnancy[1]	High Risk

EXPLANATION OF CONDITION

Deep vein thrombosis (DVT) is the formation of a blood clot or thrombus in a deep vein, partially or completely occluding the flow of blood. It commonly affects the leg veins but can occur elsewhere. In pregnant women, 85% of DVT occurs in the left leg[2] due in part to compression of the left iliac vein by the right iliac artery as they cross[3]. Virchow described the factors that promote venous thrombosis:

- Reduction of blood flow (stasis)
- Alteration of the constituents of the blood (hypercoagulability)
- Abnormalities/damage to the vessel wall

All three elements of this triad are affected by pregnancy. Pressure of the gravid uterus on the inferior vena cava and pelvic veins, an increase in coagulation factors and reduction in natural inhibitors to anticoagulation and decreased venous tone all predispose to venous thrombo-embolism (VTE).

Symptoms of DVT

- Pain in area of clot
- Unilateral and occasionally bilateral swelling
- Redness or discolouration
- Difficulty weight bearing on the affected leg
- Low grade pyrexia
- Lower abdominal pain if the pelvic veins are affected

COMPLICATIONS

Pulmonary Embolus (PE)

This occurs when a fragment of thrombus breaks away, travels through the right side of the heart and lodges in the pulmonary arterial circulation. Approximately 25% of DVT will be complicated by PE if left untreated. The risk is higher with femoral or ileofemoral thrombus than for more distal DVT.

Post-Thrombotic (or Post-Phlebitic) Syndrome

This long-term complication of DVT arises due to damage of venous valves, resulting in incompetence with reflux and backflow of blood. This increases hydrostatic pressure below the damaged area and causes disruption of the more distal valves, which in turn become incompetent. The venous hypertension leads to oedema and hypoxia of the tissues.

Symptoms range from mild to severe and include:

- Pain
- Oedema
- Eczematous dermatitis
- Pruritus
- Hyperpigmentation
- Skin ulceration
- Cellulitis

Post-thrombotic syndrome occurs in 50% of patients following a DVT[4,5,6,7], with onset of symptoms often several months or even years after the initial event.

NON-PREGNANCY TREATMENT AND CARE

Prompt treatment is necessary to reduce the risk of extension and propagation of the thrombus and to minimise the risk of post-thrombotic syndrome. Urgent referral is therefore required for all patients with a suspected DVT to confirm the diagnosis objectively. Diagnosis is made from a combination of clinical probability score and radiological imaging. Non-invasive techniques, such as Doppler ultrasound, should be used where possible.

Negative D-dimers associated with a low clinical probability score reliably excludes VTE[8]. D-dimers are breakdown products of cross-linked fibrin and are raised in inflammatory, infective or malignant conditions. They should not be used to aid positive diagnosis of venous thrombosis but have a high negative predictive value in patients whose clinical probability of VTE is low as assessed by a formal scoring system, e.g. Wells (see Appendix 15.1).

Heparin is the initial treatment of choice, because of its fast onset of anticoagulation and evidence for reduced risk of further thrombo-embolic events[8]. Low-molecular-weight heparin has a number of advantages over unfractionated heparin, including predictable dose-response and longer half-life enabling once daily administration. In patients with moderate to high clinical probability scores, heparin should be commenced immediately and continued until the diagnosis is excluded by diagnostic imaging[9].

Once a DVT has been confirmed, oral anticoagulation is initiated, in non-pregnant patients, and should be overlapped with heparin therapy until the International Normalized Ratio is greater than 2.0 on two consecutive days[9].

The recommended duration of anticoagulation following a first episode of DVT is 3–6 months[8], but this needs to be continued depending upon on-going presence of risk factors.

PRE-CONCEPTION ISSUES AND CARE

Pregnancy increases the risk of VTE ten-fold, which increases to 25–fold in the puerperium[10]. Undetected proximal venous thrombosis can increase the risk of premature labour and abruption. Therefore, where possible, women should be encouraged to optimise health prior to undertaking a pregnancy:

- If overweight, advise on diet and exercise
- Stop smoking
- Reduce caffeine and alcohol intake

Warfarin is contraindicated in pregnancy, other than in exceptional circumstances, and women who are on long-term warfarin should be made aware of the teratogenic risks if taken at 6–12 weeks gestation.

Pregnancy Issues

The risk of thrombosis is present from the first trimester until at least six weeks postpartum.

All pregnant women should have thrombotic risk assessment at booking, taking into account their personal and family history, the presence of acquired risk factors and any known thrombophilia (see Appendix 15.2). This should be repeated if circumstances change, such as excessive weight gain, immobility or vomiting with dehydration.

Women should be given advice on ways to reduce thrombotic risk:

- Keep hydrated
- Remain as active as possible
- Avoid standing for long periods
- Elevate feet when sitting
- Leg care (massage legs gently with oil or cream)
- Avoid unnecessary, long journeys by aeroplane, bus or car

Women with a past history of venous thrombo-embolic disease must be booked for antenatal care and delivery at a consultant unit.

If a DVT arises for the first time during pregnancy, the care and place of delivery must be transferred to a consultant unit, if not already done so.

An objective confirmation of diagnosis in pregnancy is crucial, as appropriate treatment reduces morbidity and mortality[11], but a false diagnosis has implications for:

- The current pregnancy
- Subsequent pregnancies
- Contraceptive choices
- HRT decisions
- Family members

D-dimers are less likely to be helpful in excluding the diagnosis because levels increase as pregnancy advances. Where DVT is suspected, non-invasive testing by ultrasound should be performed.

In addition to warfarin embryopathy during the first trimester, the risks continue throughout pregnancy, with neurological complications in later stages and the risk of fetal intracranial haemorrhage during delivery[1,12,13]. Heparin is therefore the treatment of choice for DVT in pregnancy.

Medical Management and Care

- If a DVT is suspected full anticoagulation should be initiated until thrombo-embolic disease is excluded[14]
- If a Doppler ultrasound is negative but there is a high clinical suspicion of DVT and symptoms persist, the investigations should be repeated after seven days

Venography confers a small radiation risk to the fetus and should be avoided if possible. However, if on balance of risk it is felt that venography is necessary to obtain a diagnosis, then the fetus should be shielded from radiation.

In the absence of contraindications treatment is with low-molecular-weight heparin (LMWH)[15]:

- Heparin does not cross the placenta and therefore does not affect the fetus
- LMWH is given subcutaneously and can be self administered, allowing out-patient management
- LMWH has a more predictable dose response allowing the doses to be based upon patient weight
- For treatment of DVT, LMWH should be given 12 hourly to minimise peaks and troughs
- Aim for antiXa levels of $0.4–1.0\,\mu/ml$; may be variable between laboratories and depends on the type of LMWH used
- Heparin-induced thrombocytopenia (HIT) is rare in pregnancy but the platelet count should be checked 5–7 days after starting therapy[16]
- A small proportion of patients develop cutaneous allergy and may require changing to a different LMWH
  - a degree of cross-reactivity exists[17] and alternative anticoagulants such as fondaparinux (Arixtra®) may be required
- Anticoagulation should continue for at least six months but some experts prefer to reduce to prophylactic doses after 3–4 weeks if symptoms have resolved

Midwifery Management and Care

- The mother should be taught correct self-injection technique
- Ensure that she is given a sharps bin and knows how to dispose of sharps safely
- The side effects of heparin should be discussed:
  - osteoporosis
  - HIT
  - cutaneous allergy
- Reinforce general antithrombotic advice regarding hydration, mobility, leg care and avoidance of unnecessary long journeys
- Ensure that compression stockings have been prescribed, are a good fit and encourage compliance
- Graduated elastic compression stockings should be worn on the affected leg following proximal DVT for at least two years, to reduce the incidence of severe post-thrombotic syndrome[7,6,18]
- Ensure that the woman is seen by an anaesthetist prior to delivery
- Be aware of, and report any signs and symptoms of complications of this condition
- In particular be aware of the risk of a DVT causing pulmonary embolism

Labour Issues

The intrapartum period is associated with an increase in both thrombotic and bleeding risks, and a careful assessment of these risks needs to be undertaken when planning safe management for the patient.

Ideally women should be allowed to labour spontaneously, as this reduces the need for obstetric intervention. However, depending on staffing levels, some centres may prefer a planned delivery.

Regional anaesthesia carries a possible risk of significant spinal bleeding and should be avoided within 12 hours of a prophylactic dose of LMWH and within 24 hours of a treatment dose.

General anaesthesia is associated with a higher thrombotic risk due to immobility, but may have to be considered for a caesarean section if temporary interruption of heparin is not thought suitable.

Prolonged labour and dehydration increase thrombotic risk.

Medical Management and Care

An intrapartum care plan must be worked out on an individual basis with each patient, involving the consultant obstetrician, consultant haematologist and consultant anaesthetist.

Women who are admitted in spontaneous labour or for a planned delivery will have been advised to omit their LMWH injection at the onset of contractions. This should avoid the problem of having an anticoagulant effect at the time of delivery and facilitate the use of epidural anaesthesia.

Women who are considered to be at high risk of further venothrombotic events may need to be converted to intravenous unfractionated heparin. This allows more flexibility in controlling anticoagulation and minimises time with trough levels. The heparin would need to be interrupted temporarily for the second and third stages of labour. These women **should not** be given intramuscular injections or NSAIDs.

Midwifery Management and Care

- TED stockings
- Encourage mobility by changes of position in labour
- Passive leg exercises if mother has an epidural
- Ensure that the woman remains hydrated, and consider iv fluids if necessary
- Avoid prolonged use of lithotomy position
- Active management of third stage after vaginal delivery, including the use of intravenous oxytocin
- Early suturing of perineal tears/episiotomy

Postpartum Issues

The risk of thrombosis increases 25-fold in the puerperium[10], therefore particular vigilance should be given to:

- Leg care
- Hydration
- Mobility
- Use of compression stockings
- Consideration to the most suitable form for continued anticoagulation
- Length of time that treatment should be continued for postnatally

Breast-feeding is safe on heparin or warfarin treatment and should be promoted[19].

Reliable contraception should be advised, however the combined oral contraceptive pill should be avoided in women with a history of thrombo-embolism.

- Depo-provera, the progesterone only pill (mini-pill) and condoms (with the addition of a spermicide) may be considered. Intrauterine devices, including intrauterine progestogen-only devices, are also suitable although are unlikely to be inserted in the immediate postpartum period
- There is interaction between warfarin and oral contraception. Note that oestrogen and progesterone antagonise the anticoagulant effect

Medical Management and Care

- A follow-up plan must be documented in the notes
- LMWH should be restarted four hours after removal of epidural catheter or two hours after vaginal delivery with no epidural, unless there are complications such as bleeding or the need for surgery
- Anticoagulation should always be continued until at least six weeks postpartum, when the coagulation status returns to pre-pregnancy levels
- If treatment is to be continued for longer than this, in order to complete six months anticoagulation for those with acute thrombosis, the woman may need to convert to warfarin

Midwifery Management and Care

- If converting to warfarin, counsel regarding safety issues with warfarin therapy, drug and food interactions
- Discuss contraception choices before discharge
- Make sure that follow-up appointments have been made including thrombophilia testing for those with acute VTE
- If further pregnancy is planned, ensure information is given regarding teratogenicity of warfarin therapy

15.2 Pulmonary Embolism

Incidence
60–70/100,000 of the general population
Risk increases to 0.5–3/1000 pregnancies

Risk for Childbearing
High Risk and Life Threatening
Pulmonary embolism is the leading cause of direct
maternal death in the UK[2]

EXPLANATION OF CONDITION

Pulmonary embolism (PE) is an occlusion of the pulmonary arterial circulation, usually occurring when a thrombus breaks free from a distant site, often the deep veins in the leg. More rarely they may originate in the pelvic or renal veins or upper extremities or in the right heart chambers.

Typical symptoms of pulmonary embolism include:

- Severe sudden onset of shortness of breath
- Sharp chest pain which is worse on inspiration (pleuritic pain)
- Cough with blood (haemoptysis)

Risk factors for venous thrombo-embolism include:

- Age (over 35 years)
- Increased body mass index (>30 kg/m^2)
- Immobility
- Surgery
- Pregnancy and particularly the puerperium
- Combined oral contraceptive pill
- Hormone replacement therapy
- A past history of venous thrombo-embolism
- A strong family history of venous thrombo-embolism
- An inherited clotting tendency (thrombophilia)
- An acquired clotting tendency, e.g. antiphospholipid syndrome or acquired activated protein C resistance
- Dehydration
- Myeloproliferative disorders
- Drugs such as Tamoxifen
- Nephrotic syndrome

COMPLICATIONS

Large clots may lodge in the pulmonary artery or lobar branches and cause haemodynamic compromise including:

- Cardiac arrest and sudden death
- Heart failure or shock
- Severe breathing difficulty
- Arrhythmias
- Pleural effusion

Smaller clots continue travelling distally to occlude smaller vessels in the lung periphery. These are more likely to produce pleuritic chest pain by initiating an inflammatory response involving the pleura.

Chronic thrombo-embolic disease with recurrent pulmonary embolism and pulmonary hypertension is more unusual.

Untreated, there is a mortality of 30%[1].

NON-PREGNANCY TREATMENT AND CARE

Pulmonary embolus is potentially fatal and urgent referral is necessary for all women with a suspected PE to confirm the diagnosis objectively. Diagnosis is made from a combination of clinical probability score and radiological imaging.

A negative D-dimer test reliably excludes PE in patients with low clinical probability; such patients do not require imaging for VTE. Patients with raised D-dimers and/or moderate or high clinical probability score should have either a ventilation perfusion (VQ) scan or computed tomographic pulmonary angiography (CTPA) performed. CTPA provides a more definitive diagnosis and will detect any additional lung pathology, but is not available in all centres.

Heparin, usually low-molecular-weight heparin, should be commenced at presentation. Once a PE has been confirmed, oral anticoagulation is initiated in non-pregnant patients and should be overlapped with heparin therapy until the International Normalized Ratio (INR) is within therapeutic range (usually 2–3) on two consecutive tests. Anticoagulation should be continued for 3–6 months, but a longer duration may be necessary depending on the presence of on-going risk factors.

Massive or sub-massive PE associated with cardiac compromise, require thrombolytics in addition to heparin. Resuscitative measures include oxygenation and supporting cardiac output.

PRE-CONCEPTION ISSUES AND CARE

Pregnancy increases the risk of PE ten-fold, which is further increased in the postpartum period[3]. Women should be encouraged to minimise their acquired risk factors and improve fitness prior to undertaking a pregnancy.

Women who are on long-term warfarin therapy should be made aware of the teratogenic risks. The risk is greatest when the daily warfarin dose exceeds 5 mg. If taken at 6–12 weeks' gestation, the risk of warfarin embryopathy is around 5% including:

- Chondrodysplasia punctata
- Nasal hypoplasia
- Growth restriction
- Short proximal limbs

Women should keep a diary of their menstrual cycle and seek immediate medical advice once pregnancy is suspected so that warfarin can be replaced by heparin within two weeks of the first missed menstrual period.

Pregnancy issues

All pregnant women should have thrombotic risk assessment at booking and again if circumstances, such as excessive weight gain, immobility or vomiting with dehydration, change[4]. Women should be given advice on ways to reduce thrombotic risk.

Additional risk factors
- Hyperemesis
- Parity >4
- Caesarean section, particularly if emergency
- Operative vaginal delivery
- Pre-eclampsia
- Ovarian hyperstimulation

Rare causes of PE
- Amniotic fluid embolism, caused by entry of amniotic fluid and fetal antigen into the maternal circulation, invoking an anaphylactic reaction; associated with 80% mortality
- Air embolism caused by intrauterine manipulation or neck vein cannulation

Diagnosis of PE is much more problematic in pregnant patients, mainly due to the fears of the effects of harmful radiation on the fetus. However, the potential risks associated with the radiological tests used are minimal when compared with the consequences of inaccurate diagnosis.

Diagnostic difficulties are compounded by the relative frequency of chest pain and shortness of breath in pregnant patients and the rise with D-dimers as pregnancy advances, rendering them less useful for diagnostic exclusion in low-probability cases. As a consequence, only 10% of patients investigated for a suspected pulmonary embolism are confirmed thromboses.

Medical Management and Care

Objective confirmation of thrombo-embolism is crucial because of implications for the current pregnancy, subsequent pregnancies, contraceptive choices and HRT decisions. In addition, it is well established that treatment reduces morbidity and mortality[5].

Clinical suspicion of PE warrants a chest X-ray and Doppler ultrasound of the legs. If there is confirmation of DVT, lung scanning is not required, as the diagnosis of PE can be presumed.

A pulmonary ventilation/perfusion scan (VQ scan) is a sequenced nuclear scan test that uses inhaled and injected material to measure breathing (ventilation) and circulation (perfusion). Acute pulmonary embolism results in perfusion defects which are not matched by ventilation defects. VQ carries a slight increased risk of childhood cancer (1:280,000)[6].

Computed tomography pulmonary angiogram (CTPA) involves multiple X-rays being passed through the lungs. This produces cross-sectional images, or 'slices', on a cathode-ray tube, to construct a three-dimensional image of the lungs. Intravenous iodine is used to highlight the structure of the lungs. The advantages are a more definitive result and identification of other lung pathology. However, it is associated with a life-time risk of breast cancer of 13.6%[7]. Women should be given full information where possible and consent obtained.

Low-molecular-weight heparin is the preferred option for use as it has clear advantages over unfractionated heparin. Reduced binding to non-specific plasma proteins provides a predictable dose-response effect, allowing doses to be based on patient weight, without the need for intense monitoring. The long half-life facilitates self-administration on an out-patient basis.

Anticoagulation should be the same as treatment for DVT.

Midwifery Management and Care

If a woman presents with the signs and symptoms of PE, she should be referred immediately to hospital. After diagnosis she should be informed of the result and the need to be treated with heparin.
- The woman should be taught correct self-injection technique
- Ensure that the woman is given a sharps bin and knows how to dispose of sharps safely
- The side effects of heparin should be discussed:
  - osteoporosis
  - heparin-induced thrombocytopenia
  - cutaneous allergy
- Reinforce general antithrombotic advice regarding hydration, mobility and leg care
- Ensure that compression stockings have been prescribed, are a good fit and encourage compliance
- Ensure that the woman is seen by an anaesthetist prior to delivery
- Be aware of and report any signs and symptoms of complications

Labour Issues

Labour and delivery are associated with a further increase in hypercoagulability as well as risks of uterine haemorrhage and bleeding from surgical sites. The balance between these risks needs to be carefully assessed and managed, to ensure safety of the patient during this unstable period.

Both thrombotic and bleeding risks are further increased by:

- Prolonged labour
- Interventional vaginal delivery
- Caesarean section, particularly when undertaken as an emergency

Ideally, patients on prophylactic or therapeutic anticoagulation should be allowed to labour spontaneously, as this reduces the need for intervention.

Inferior vena caval filters are rarely needed but may be required if anticoagulation is contraindicated and the risk of PE is felt to be significant. However, whilst the PE rate is reduced, the DVT risk is increased and only retrievable filters should be used.

Epidural should be timed to avoid bleeding complications[8] and general anaesthesia may have to be considered for caesarean section in women on full anticoagulation.

Medical Management and Care

An intrapartum care plan must be worked out on an individual basis with each patient, involving the consultant obstetrician, consultant haematologist and consultant anaesthetist.

Women who are admitted in spontaneous labour or for a planned delivery will have been advised to omit their LMWH injection at the onset of contractions. This should avoid the problem of having an anticoagulant affect at the time of delivery and facilitate the use of epidural anaesthesia.

Women who are considered to be at high risk of further veno-thrombotic events may need to be converted to intravenous unfractionated heparin, as this allows more flexibility in controlling anticoagulation and minimises time with trough levels. The heparin would need to be temporarily interrupted for the second and third stages of labour. These women should *not* be given intramuscular injections or NSAIDs.

Midwifery Management and Care

- Encourage mobility with regular changes of position
- TED stockings
- Passive leg exercises if epidural given
- Attention to hydration and consideration to iv fluids if necessary
- Regular observations in labour
- Active management of third stage after vaginal delivery, including the use of intravenous oxytocin
- Early suturing of perineal tears/episiotomy

Postpartum Issues

The risk of thrombosis increases 25-fold in the puerperium[8]. Signs of PE, e.g. chest pain or breathlessness, need to be taken seriously and regarded as an emergency.

Particular vigilance should be given to:

- Leg care
- Hydration
- Mobility
- Use of compression stockings
- Most suitable form of continued anticoagulation
- Length of time that treatment should be continued postnatally

The mother should be informed of the safety of breast-feeding whilst on heparin or warfarin treatment[9].

Reliable contraception should be advised:

- The combined oral contraceptive pill is relatively contraindicated with a history of thrombo-embolism
- Depo-Provera, the progesterone only pill (mini-pill) and condoms (with the addition of a spermicide) may be considered. Intrauterine devices, including intrauterine progestogen-only devices, are also suitable although are unlikely to be inserted in the immediate postpartum period
- There is interaction between warfarin and oral contraception. Note that oestrogen and progesterone antagonise the anticoagulant effect

Medical Management and Care

- A follow-up plan must be documented in the case notes
- LMWH should be restarted four hours after removal of epidural catheter or two hours after vaginal delivery with no epidural unless there are complications such as bleeding or need for surgery
- Anticoagulation should always be continued until at least six weeks postpartum
- If treatment is to be continued for longer than this, in order to complete six months anticoagulation, then the woman may need to convert to warfarin

Midwifery Management and Care

- If converting treatment to warfarin, counsel the mother regarding safety issues with warfarin therapy
- Before discharge make sure that follow-up appointments have been made, including thrombophilia testing for those with an acute VTE
- Discuss contraception choices before discharge
- If further pregnancy is planned, ensure information is given regarding teratogenicity of warfarin
- Pay attention to postnatal observations, including pulse, respiration and leg swelling
- Be aware that PE can present suddenly in the puerperium, necessitating emergency re-admission

15.3 Thrombophilia and Inherited Clotting Disorders

Incidence	Risk for Childbearing
Approximately 10% of the general population have an inherited thrombophilia	Variable or High Risk – depending upon type of disorder

EXPLANATION OF CONDITION

The term thrombophilia refers to disorders of the haemostatic system that result in an increased risk of thrombosis. It includes inherited and acquired risk factors.

Inherited

- Factor V Leiden (FVL)
- Prothrombin 20210
- Protein C deficiency
- Protein S deficiency
- Antithrombin deficiency

Acquired

- Antiphospholipid syndrome (see Section 11.4)

Complex

- Raised factor VIII levels
- Hyperhomocysteinaemia

COMPLICATIONS

- The relative risk of VTE varies with the nature of the thrombophilia but is greatest for antithrombin deficiency and antiphospholipid syndrome
- Thrombophilias existing in combination act synergistically, with a resulting risk greater than would be expected for the sum of the individual factors
- There is increased risk for gestational venous thrombosis, recurrent miscarriage and late pregnancy complications

NON-PREGNANCY TREATMENT AND CARE

Women with a previous history of thrombosis should be screened for thrombophilia prior to pregnancy.

Other indications for testing include:

- Individuals with a first-degree family history of VTE or known thrombophilia who are planning pregnancy or intending to undergo a procedure or course of treatment that would greatly increase their risk of thrombosis:
  - orthopaedic surgery
  - hormone replacement therapy
  - combined oral contraceptive pill
  - invasive vascular procedures
- Unexplained or unusually-sited thrombosis
- Children or young adults with thrombosis
- Women with a history of unexpected pregnancy complications should be tested for antiphospholipid antibodies (see section 11.4):
  - three or more early miscarriages
  - late fetal loss
  - stillbirth
  - early or severe pre-eclampsia
  - placental abruption
  - poor fetal growth
- Young patients with unexplained arterial thrombosis should be investigated for antiphospholipid antibodies

PRE-CONCEPTION ISSUES AND CARE

For potential childbearing there are:

- Increased thrombotic risks
- Potential associations with:
  - recurrent miscarriage
  - fetal loss
  - placental abruption
  - pre-eclampsia
  - poor fetal growth

Women with thrombophilia should be informed of their diagnosis and its implications. Counselling should be reinforced by written patient information where possible.

- Advise against using the combined oral contraceptive pill, which acts in synergy with FVL and other thrombophilia to greatly enhance thrombotic risk
- Precautions for travel should be highlighted and the importance of additional thromboprophylaxis for high-risk situations such as surgery, prolonged immobility and plaster casts should be emphasised
- Plans for pregnancy should be discussed before conception and should include thromboprophylactic measures and any need for heparin
- Ideally patients should be placed on a database and issued with a registration card bearing details of their condition and phone numbers for contact
- Women with previous thrombosis and who are on long-term warfarin should be made aware of the teratogenic risks. They should keep a diary of their menstrual cycle and seek immediate medical advice if they suspect that they are pregnant
- Anticoagulation should not be interrupted but provision made to ensure that warfarin is stopped and replaced with heparin no later than six weeks gestation

Pregnancy Issues

Thrombosis is usually a *multi-hit phenomenon*, with cumulative risk factors triggering a clinical event.

Pregnancy significantly increases the risk for patients with underlying thrombophilia, due to a combination of various physiological changes including:

- A further increase in hypercoagulability as pregnancy advances
- Decreased venous return secondary to compression of the pelvic veins by the gravid uterus
- Reduced vessel tone with venous pooling

Of those women with previous VTE, those with underlying thrombophilia are more at risk of recurrent thrombosis than those without. The relative risk varies according to the nature of the thrombophilia, with antithrombin deficiency and antiphospholipid syndrome being the highest.

Antiphospholipid syndrome is characterised by the presence of persistent antiphospholipid antibodies (lupus anticoagulant and anticardiolipin antibodies) in association with clinical complications. In addition to venous and arterial thrombotic events, it is associated with recurrent miscarriages and late fetal loss, as well as complications in advanced pregnancy including pre-eclampsia, stillbirth and intrauterine growth retardation (IUGR) (see Section 11.4). There is also recent focus on the association of inherited thrombophilia with poor pregnancy outcome.

Pregnant women with acquired thrombophilia, and those with inherited thrombophilia and a complex obstetric or thrombosis history, should be managed by a multi-disciplinary team which includes a consultant obstetrician and consultant haematologist. Ideally, the women would be seen in a joint obstetric haematology clinic.

Medical Management and Care

All women should undergo an assessment of thrombotic risk in early pregnancy, taking into account their personal and family histories, the nature of their thrombophilia and any additional acquired risk factors, such as age and obesity. Repeat assessments should be made in the second and third trimesters and each time the circumstances and risk factors change. The risks for VTE, thromboprophylaxis and management for the pregnancy should be discussed with the mother.

Thrombophilia and a history of VTE – these mothers should be offered thromboprophylaxis with antenatal LMWH, and also for at least six weeks postpartum[1].

Antiphospholipid (Hughes) syndrome – this is associated with a recurrent thrombotic risk of up to 70%[2] and therefore women with antiphospholipid syndrome and previous venous thrombosis should receive heparin from the onset of pregnancy until six weeks postpartum. If the condition was diagnosed because of recurrent miscarriages, treatment may not be required in the postpartum period. The addition of aspirin has been shown to improve pregnancy outcome in antiphospholipid syndrome patients with a prior history of obstetric complications[3,4] (see Section 11.4).

Asymptomatic inherited or acquired thrombophilia – these women may require antenatal or postnatal thromboprophylaxis depending on the specific thrombophilia. Antithrombin deficiency carries a 30% increased risk of thrombosis in pregnancy and these women should always receive heparin in high prophylactic or treatment doses from the onset of pregnancy. Other thrombophilias requiring antenatal prophylaxis include combined defects and homozygous states. Women with protein C and protein S deficiency may need to start heparin antenatally.

Absent thrombophilia but previous VTE – these women should be offered postpartum prophylaxis with LMWH. It may be reasonable not to use antenatal prophylaxis with heparin for a previous single VTE associated with a temporary risk factor that has now resolved[1]. However, thromboprophylaxis has been advocated if the previous VTE was related to the combined oral contraceptive pill or if additional acquired risk factors are present[5]. Also, if there is a positive first-degree family history of VTE, recurrent VTE or a history of thrombosis affecting an unusual site LMWH should be offered antenatally and for at least six weeks postnatally[1].

Midwifery Management and Care

- The midwife should be a point of contact so that the woman can inform her regarding the onset of pregnancy. This contact should be continued throughout the pregnancy to report any concerns or changes in circumstances which increase the thrombotic risk
- The woman should be taught correct self-injection technique and educated regarding safe disposal of 'sharps'
- Potential side effects of heparin should be discussed:
  - osteoporosis
  - HIT
  - cutaneous allergy
- Reinforce general antithrombotic advice regarding hydration, mobility, travel and leg care
- Ensure that TED stockings have been provided, are a good fit and encourage compliance
- Ensure use of compression stockings where necessary
- Be aware of and report any signs and symptoms of complications
- Effective communication with the community midwife and other members of the multi-disciplinary team

Labour Issues – as for DVT and PE

Management and Care – as for DVT and PE

Postpartum Issues – as for DVT and PE

Management and Care – as for DVT and PE

15 Thrombo-embolic Disorders

PATIENT ORGANISATIONS

Hughes Syndrome Foundation
Louise Coote Lupus Unit
Gassiot House
St. Thomas's Hospital
London SE1 7EH
http://www.hughes-syndrome.org

Thrombosis Research Institute
Emmanuel Kaye Building
Manresa Road
London SW3 6LR
http://www.tri-london.ac.uk

Lifeblood: The Thrombosis Charity
PO Box 1050
Spalding PE12 6YF
http://www.thrombosis-charity.org.uk

Electronic Quality Information for Patients:
Blood and Circulation Disorders
http://www.equip.nhs.uk/topics/blood.html

ESSENTIAL READING

Boyle, M. (2004) *Thromboembolism in pregnancy.* In: **Emergencies Around Childbirth**. Oxford; Radcliffe Medical Press.

De Swiet, M. (Ed) (2002) *Thromboembolism; Antiphospholipid syndrome, systemic lupus erythematosus and other connective tissue disease.* In: **Medical Disorders in Obstetric Practice.** Oxford; Blackwell Scientific.

Dike, P. (2007) *Haematological disorders* part 2. In: **Critical Care in Childbearing for Midwives** (Eds M. Billington and M. Stevenson), pp. 83–8. Oxford; Blackwell Publishing.

Lifeblood: The Thrombosis Charity, Fact Sheet: **Thrombosis and Pregnancy**.
www.thrombosis-charity.org.uk/Thrombosis_and_pregnancy_factsheet.pdf

Nelson-Piercy, C. (2002) *Thromboembolic disease.* In: **Handbook of Obstetric Medicine**, 2nd Edn. London; Martin Dunitz.

NICE (2007) **Clinical Guideline 46**. Venous Thromboembolism. http://guidance.nice.org.uk/CG46/quickrefguide/pdf/English

RCOG (2004) **Clinical Green Top Guidelines No. 37 Thromboprophylaxis during pregnancy, labour and after vaginal delivery.** London; Royal College of Obstetricians and Gynaecologists.
http://www.rcog.org.uk/index.asp?PageID=535

RCOG (2007) **Clinical Green Top Guidelines No. 28 Thromboembolic Disease in Pregnancy and the puerperium: Acute Management**. London; Royal College of Obstetricians and Gynaecologists.
http://www.rcog.org.uk/resources/Public/pdf/green_top_28_thromboembolic_minorrevision.pdf

16

ADDICTIVE DISORDERS

Miranda Hayer and Tanu Singhal

16.1 Alcohol Addiction

Incidence	Risk for Childbearing
Exact incidence of alcohol addiction is unknown 0.33–1.9 per 1000 births have fetal alcohol syndrome (FAS)	Variable Risk – related to quantity and frequency of maternal alcohol consumption

EXPLANATION OF CONDITION

Alcohol abuse, also known as alcohol dependence, is a disease. Alcoholics will continue to drink despite serious family, health or legal problems[1,2]. The risk of developing alcohol addiction is influenced by genetic and lifestyle factors. Alcohol addiction is known to 'run in families' but does not mean that a child of an alcoholic parent will automatically become an alcoholic as well. Some develop alcoholism even though no one in their family has a drinking problem[2,3,4,5].

Alcohol tolerance is the need for increased amounts of alcohol to achieve intoxication or a diminished effect with continued use of the same amount of alcohol[1]. Alcohol withdrawal symptoms are two or more of the following developing within several hours to a few days of reduction in heavy or prolonged alcohol use:

- Sweating or rapid pulse
- Increased hand tremor
- Insomnia
- Nausea and vomiting
- Physical agitation
- Anxiety
- Transient visual, tactile or auditory hallucinations
- Grand mal seizures[1,2,4,5,6,7]

The Food Standards Agency (FSA) recommends no more than one or two units of alcohol once or twice per week[8]. One unit of alcohol approximates to:

- Half a pint of ordinary-strength beer, lager, or cider
- A quarter of a pint of strong beer or lager
- One small glass of wine
- One single measure of spirits
- One small glass of sherry

COMPLICATIONS

Moderate alcohol use, up to two units per day, is not considered harmful for most adults. However, consequences of alcohol misuse are serious and can be life threatening[9,10,11,12]. Heavy drinking increases the risk of developing cancer of the liver, oesophagus, throat and larynx.

Alcohol consumption can also cause:

- Subfertility
- Liver cirrhosis
- Immune system problems
- Brain damage
- Harm to the fetus during pregnancy

Furthermore, it increases the risk of death from automobile crashes as well as recreational and occupational injuries[9,10,11].

According to the most current UK government information, both homicides and suicides are more likely to be committed by persons who have been drinking alcohol[10,12].

Fetal Alcohol Syndrome (FAS)

Women who drink over six units of alcohol per day are at greatest risk of having a child with fetal alcohol syndrome (FAS)[9]. This results in growth restriction, hand and facial deformities and intellectual impairment (see next page).

Fetal Alcohol Effect

Children of women who drank more than two 'glasses' of alcohol a day throughout their pregnancy were found to have more problems with learning speech, language, attention span and hyperactivity than babies of women who did not drink[9] (assume a 'glass' ≥one unit of alcohol). This collection of characteristics is known as fetal alcohol effects (FAE). Although less severe than FAS, the effects of FAE are still harmful[9].

NON-PREGNANCY TREATMENT AND CARE

- Detoxification for alcohol and many drugs must be done under medical supervision to ensure this process is completed as safely and painlessly as possible
- Detoxification is the medical withdrawal of an alcohol-dependent patient from the drug
- It should be conducted in an inpatient setting and under medical supervision
- It can be completed in pregnancy when it should include collaboration with an obstetrician to ensure:
  - close observation and monitoring of maternal alcohol withdrawal status
  - continual monitoring of fetal wellbeing[11]
- Information leaflets about detoxification programmes should be available
- Ensure access to specialist substance-abuse services and treatment options, with pharmacy support
- Offer holistic support to partner and family to make lifestyle changes to sustain long-term compliance

PRE-CONCEPTION ISSUES AND CARE

Prospective parents should be made aware of the risks of continued alcohol use. Alcohol is teratogenic *and* feto-toxic.

While the safe acceptable level of alcohol intake is controversial, the DoH and RCOG suggest limiting intake to 1–2 units not more than once or twice a week, while the Medical Council on Alcohol suggest abstinence in the first trimester then limiting intake to 1–2 units once or twice a week[3,4,6]. Assess for risk of STD – prevention advice and/or screening should be made available. Women should be strongly advised against binge drinking.

Counselling for women who already have a child with FAS helps prevent a recurrence. Women most likely to have an affected child are those who are sexually active whilst 'drinking heavily' and not intending to conceive.

Pregnancy issues

Drinking alcohol during pregnancy is not advisable as there is no evidence to support a safe level of maternal drinking for the fetus. Binge drinking in early pregnancy is particularly harmful[8].

Alcohol consumption during pregnancy can cause fetal alcohol syndrome, which includes one or more of:

- IUGR and post-birth growth restriction, which is dose/consumption dependent
- Neurological abnormalities
- Developmental delays
- Behavioural dysfunction
- Intellectual impairment
- Skull or brain malformations
- Characteristic facial features:
  - skin folds at eye corner
  - small head circumference
  - small eye opening
  - thin upper lip
  - indistinct nasal philtrum
- Major structural anomalies are seen with alcohol consumption of >35 g/day[4,8,9,10,11]
- Cognitive impairment endures with age and features become more apparent as the child develops[9]

Medical Management and Care

Where alcohol use is confirmed:

- Consultant-led care with a specialist team
- Detailed anomaly scan
- Serial sonography to assess fetal growth
- Multi-disciplinary care with neonatologists, anaesthetists and detoxification teams if required
- Screening for other substance abuse and STD if suspected
- Serial liver function tests if a heavy alcohol intake is suspected

Midwifery Management and Care

- Assess pregnant women where episodic binge or regular heavy alcohol use may be an issue
- Consider the woman's social support and emotional wellbeing in relation to the alcohol abuse. These should be re-visited postpartum:
  - domestic violence
  - homelessness
  - self-harm or self-neglect
  - poor appetite/anorexia and sub-nutrition
  - mental health, stability and psychological issues
  - environmental issues
  - potential parenting capability
  - preparation for the baby
- Information should be available on effects of alcohol abuse
- There should be easy access to specialist midwifery services, counselling, detoxification programmes and support agencies
- Ascertain related health issues, such as oesophageal varices and blood-borne infections
- Assessment for any child-protection issues

Labour Issues

There is no indication to induce labour if there is normal fetal growth. Induction of labour should follow standard obstetric indications.

If the mother is intoxicated, issues of competence and consent should be considered prior to investigations and procedures.

Medical Management and Care

- Liver function tests and clotting test if indicated by level of drinking
- Early involvement of anaesthetic team for pain-relief strategy
- Senior input with any operative intervention especially if concerns arise regarding maternal competence to giving of consent

Midwifery Management and Care

- An initial assessment of fetal wellbeing, with auscultation of fetal heart and cardiotocograph (CTG), should be performed
- Continual electronic fetal monitoring when in labour
- Assessment of analgesic needs as determined by level of intoxication
- Apart from the above, labour can be managed normally by the midwife

Postpartum Issues

The risk of sudden infant death syndrome (SIDS) and sudden unexpected death in infancy (SUDI) increase with alcohol consumption (see Appendix 16.1). In particular, safe sleeping practices must be discussed.

Involve paediatricians in the neonatal examination to assess for FAS or FAE, with explanation and support regarding long-term implications.

Medical Management and Care

- Appropriate follow-up for any medical problems detected, e.g. abnormal liver function, STD, etc.
- Ongoing support arrangements for detoxification

Midwifery Management and Care

Prior to discharge from hospital the following should be ascertained, with finding referred to the multi-disciplinary team:

- Parenting capability
- Mental health, stability and psychological issues
- Environmental issues
- Preparation for the baby
- Child-protection issues, including risk assessment
- Observe for features of FAS or FAE
- Paediatrician, rather than a midwife, to conduct the neonatal examination
- Community midwife should reinforce safe sleeping practices and liaise with the multi-disciplinary team

16.2 Cannabis Use

Incidence
British Crime Surveys 2001–2006 indicate:
44% of 16–29 year olds *tried* cannabis in 2000
8.7% of 16–59 year olds *used* cannabis in 2005–2006

Risk for Childbearing
Low Risk – for fetal compromise
Variable Risk – for adverse maternal mental health and SIDS

EXPLANATION OF CONDITION

Cannabis is the most widely-used illegal drug in Britain[1]. It is a naturally-occurring drug made from parts of the cannabis plant. The dried leaves and flower are used as a source of marijuana, bhang, pot and the resinous part as hashish. It is a mild hallucinogen, often giving sedative-like effects making some people feel relaxed and others nauseated. Cannabis is usually smoked but can be inhaled through a *bong*, cooked and eaten in food. It is inexpensive and widely available.

In the UK cannabis is a class C drug that is illegal and harmful. The maximum sentence for possessing cannabis is two years in prison and an unlimited fine. The maximum penalty for supplying cannabis is 14 years in prison and an unlimited fine[2]. Cannabis has been used medically to treat chronic pain and conditions such as myalgic encephalomyelitis (ME), also known as chronic fatigue syndrome. However, this is not recommended during pregnancy.

COMPLICATIONS

Smoking cannabis is associated with illnesses such as bronchitis, emphysema and cancer. Heavy, frequent cannabis use is associated with increased susceptibility to respiratory disorders, dependency, precipitation or exacerbation of mental health problems in vulnerable people and cognitive impairment. The UK is just beginning to recognise the health care needs of cannabis users[3,4,5,6,7].

Some people experience unpleasant effects, such as anxiety, panic attacks or paranoia, when they use cannabis. It can affect memory. Usually these symptoms stop once the cannabis has *'worn off'*. Some cannabis users feel tense or agitated after smoking pot. Some have uncontrolled thoughts or become confused *'after a joint'*[7,8,9,10].

If there is a family history of mental conditions, cannabis can trigger serious conditions, such as schizophrenia. There is also concern that people who use cannabis liberally when they are young may be vulnerable to mental health problems later in life[7,8,9,10]. If a user already has a mental health problem, cannabis will probably exacerbate their symptoms[7].

NON-PREGNANCY TREATMENT AND CARE

Care should focus on:

- Offering holistic support to partners and family to prevent relapse
- Marijuana use is strongly associated with use of tobacco and alcohol, both of which also need addressing[6,7,8]
- Provision of information leaflets and contact details of organisations that can help with reducing cannabis use

PRE-CONCEPTION ISSUES AND CARE

Ascertain Level of Cannabis Use

- Some users become dependent on cannabis in a similar way to other drugs
- Using cannabis *'most days'* can result in psychological dependency

Explore Personal Issues

Make positive changes:

- Financial concerns – one of the most common problems associated with cannabis use is the financial expenditure and finding a source of 'cash'
- Difficult relationships
- Conflict with family or friends
- Struggling to meet work or study commitments
- Ill-health, especially respiratory problems
- Mental health problems (anxiety, depression, schizophrenia)
- Liaise with the GP about any psychological or mental health issues
- Cannabis use can affect relationships and sexual activity
- Cannabis use can affect motivation and ability to parent effectively

Advice for the Prospective Mother

- Consider stopping or cutting down
- Contact support groups or specialist substance abuse service
- Promote health benefits of reducing or stopping cannabis use
- Provide information on the short- and long-term problems of cannabis use, which comprise:
  - anxiety and paranoia
  - memory and concentration problems
  - increased risk of accidents
  - bizarre thoughts, extreme paranoia and hallucinations
  - increased risk of throat and lung disease
  - dependence
  - financial problems
  - social isolation
  - less motivation
  - existing mental health problems made worse
  - possibility of premature birth
  - babies may suffer from temporary tremor and distress

Pregnancy Issues

Fetus

There is no conclusive evidence that cannabis is teratogenic. However, it is known to affect fetal growth by reducing the oxygen-carrying capacity of red blood cells, and by impairing oxygen exchange at tissue level[5,6].

Mother

Wellbeing – maternal diet and general health can be compromised[5,6].

Dependency – during the last few years it has become clear that cannabis use can result in dependency and lead to problems.

The symptoms of maternal dependence are:

- Using more cannabis or using for longer periods with a constant desire to use
- Trying to '*give it up*' and failing
- Spending excess time getting supplies, '*using*' and taking longer to recover
- Spending less time on important activities, or giving them up altogether
- Continue '*using*', despite knowledge of the harm this entails
- Tolerance (needing more of the drug to get the same effect)
- '*Withdrawal*' (unpleasant symptoms upon cessation)

Medical Management and Care
- Multi-disciplinary approach to care
- Fetal growth assessment
- Scans as necessary
- If mental health problems are identified, liaise with psychiatric services
- Provide supportive, non-judgemental care

Midwifery Management and Care
- Conduct the booking history with tact, and ensure the mother is booked for antenatal care at a specialist clinic, especially if there is also other drug use, alcohol or social problems
- Book for delivery at a consultant unit with a neonatal care unit
- Use of observational skills and history taking to ascertain amount of cannabis use and level of dependency
- Provide advice on short- and long-term effects of cannabis use
- Ensure regular antenatal care and reinforce any medical advice or treatment given
- Assessment of need to refer to social care if lifestyle chaotic or adversely affected by dependency on cannabis
- Referral to specialist substance abuse services if indicated
- Assess mental health and refer to the medical staff if concerned
- Be aware of signs of cannabis withdrawal:
  - anxiety and/or depression
  - anger, confusion or irritability
  - urge or craving to smoke
  - sleep problems and night sweats
  - restlessness
  - loss of appetite
  - tremors
  - diarrhoea

Labour Issues
- Maternal hypertension and tachycardia may occur, resulting in reduced blood flow to the placental site[5,6,8]
- Cannabis use affects concentration, and can create feelings of paranoia and anxiety
- Lack of concentration or drowsiness may affect the way labour is perceived, and have implications for informed consent if fetal compromise requires medical intervention

Medical Management and care
- Careful review of maternal condition to detect hypertension or tachycardia, and act promptly once identified

Midwifery Management and Care
- Provide non-judgemental, supportive environment
- Perform regular observations of maternal blood pressure and pulse
- Assess level of concentration and ability to give informed consent
- Be aware that some withdrawal (as above) may occur in labour

Postpartum Issues
- Both mother and baby are at risk of withdrawal symptoms
- In the neonate the symptoms are tremors and signs of distress
- There is an increased risk of sudden infant death syndrome (SIDS) and sudden infant deaths in infancy (SUDI), and this has been related to co-sleeping (see Appendix 16.1)

Medical Management and care
- Continued support for giving up cannabis and associated substances of abuse
- Support and treatment for mental health problems

Midwifery Management and Care
- Observe for signs of withdrawal in mother and baby
- Provide supportive environment to enable adjustment to motherhood and parenting
- Provide general advice on effects of cannabis withdrawal on the baby and mother
- Refer to paediatrician if the baby shows signs of withdrawal
- Promote positive parenting
- Advise to avoid co-sleeping with baby
- Provide information on SIDS
- Support breast-feeding
- Encourage the provision of a smoke-free environment for the baby

16.3 Cocaine Addiction

Incidence	Risk for Childbearing
5.9% of 16–24 year olds have reported cocaine use in the British Crime Survey 2005–2006	Variable to High Risk for the mother Moderate Risk for the fetus

EXPLANATION OF CONDITION

Cocaine is a short-acting central nervous system stimulant, with an effect that is said to be intense, immensely pleasurable but relatively brief. Onset of action is within ten minutes, with a half-life of 20–90 minutes, depending on the route of administration[1].

Powder cocaine, cocaine hydrochloride (HCl) is extracted from the leaves of the coca plant: it is water soluble and usually snorted, sniffed rubbed into gums or injected.

'Freebase' and 'crack' cocaine are colourless and odourless. They are insoluble in water but soluble in alcohol, ether and acetone. Heating converts them into a stable substance which can be inhaled. Freebase is a flammable compound because ether is used in its extraction; hence users risk facial and tracheal burns.

Crack cocaine is produced by heating cocaine HCl with sodium bicarbonate, making 'rocks' or crystals. These crackle when heated but are a stable mixture without risk of flammability. Cocaine may also be injected, combined with heroin, when it is known as speedball[2,3,4,5,6].

COMPLICATIONS

Cocaine acts on the peripheral sympathetic nerve system, affecting nerve conduction, as well as the central nervous system. It causes intense euphoria, heightened energy, enhanced alertness and increased self-confidence. However, it also increases a risk of:

- Tachycardia
- Hypertension
- Uterine contractility
- Myocardial infarction
- Stroke
- Intracranial haemorrhage
- Seizures
- Other motor or visual abnormalities
- Smoking crack cocaine also leads to respiratory diseases[2,3,4,5,6]

The associated problems include:

- Sexually transmitted diseases (STD) are higher in these women, due to high-risk sexual behaviour
- Anorexia is common, causing a suboptimal nutritional state

After the intense stimulation comes the crashing low that brings with it anxiety, tension, mood swings, paranoia and depression, reinforcing the need for more stimulation. Although cocaine is not highly addictive, its use can cause psychological dependence. Physical symptoms of a 'crash' or 'low' include:

- Tachycardia
- Tachypnoea
- Sweating
- Shaking
- Agitation
- Nausea
- Altered mood

Prolonged use can lead to:

- Insomnia
- Loss of appetite
- Stress
- Skin problems
- Impaired immune system
- Hyperthermia
- Hallucinations
- Liver damage
- Hypertension
- Myocardial infarction
- Stroke[3,4,5,6]

NON-PREGNANCY TREATMENT AND CARE

Lifestyle issues need to be explored to help the user understand their drug habit so that changes can be made to reduce or stop cocaine use. A holistic approach to support is needed to address psychological dependency alongside issues of housing needs, debt management, education and skills acquisition as well as exercise, social activities and nutrition.

Crack cocaine and cocaine use can affect the user's sexual function, causing impotence in men and amenorrhea and infertility in women.

PRE-CONCEPTION ISSUES AND CARE

- Access to health care may be delayed due to amenorrhoea and result in a late diagnosis of pregnancy
- Assess the level of crack cocaine and/or cocaine use
- Assess the affects of cocaine use on lifestyle; encourage the user to abstain, because there is no substitute drug to relieve symptoms
- Education, support and information are crucial in making positive choices
- Explore sexual history and offer screening for STD if high-risk sexual behaviour is identified
- Provide holistic support to address issues of housing, debt management; may include exploration of social issues such as prostitution and/or criminal activity to support the cocaine habit
- Lifestyle issues may need to be addressed to assist relapse prevention
- Explore the willingness of the user to want to stop using crack cocaine or cocaine
- Multi-drug usage is common as is alcohol intake and they need addressing together
- Refer to appropriate specialist substance misuse service and specialist services that are discreet and maintain anonymity if requested
- Discuss the detrimental effects of cocaine addiction on pregnancy, emphasising that these are worsened further by consumption of alcohol and cigarette smoking
- During pregnancy, metabolism of cocaine to inactive compounds is reduced, and metabolism to active compound norcaine is increased; it rapidly crosses the placenta and the fetus is exposed to a high concentration of cocaine
- Child-protection assessment may be necessary, especially if lifestyle is chaotic and there is an unwillingness to address cocaine use prior to conception

Pregnancy Issues

Cocaine use in pregnancy *might* cause:
- Miscarriage
- Low birth weight
- Pre-term birth
- Increased perinatal morbidity
- Disturbed behaviour in newborn babies

Several studies report increased incidence of cranial abnormalities, limb reduction defects, urogenital defects and intestinal abnormalities[7]. Many of these are due to associated compounding factors, such as multi-drug use, alcohol and smoking and malnutrition etc.[7,8,9]

Studies suggest cocaine use may increase uterine contractility. Placental abruption may result from vasoconstriction and transient hypertension due to the vasoconstrictor properties of the drug[11].

Intrauterine growth retardation and low birth weight are the most frequent adverse effects reported. Reduced utero-placental flow impairs transfer of nutrients and oxygen[4,9]. Maternal appetite is also suppressed[12].

Pregnant cocaine users require effective medical and midwifery attention, and to look after themselves throughout the pregnancy. Avoiding proper medical care, poor nutrition, smoking cigarettes and drinking alcohol can all have major effects upon the health of the baby[7,8,9,10,11,12].

Medical Management and Care

The myths surrounding cocaine often arise from lack of knowledge and poor communication, which can undermine the effectiveness of treatment. Issues affecting treatment and care are:
- Access to treatment
- Lifestyle issues
- Relationships with drug workers
- Ongoing treatment

Effective care
- Multi-disciplinary care, led by a consultant obstetrician with expertise in substance misuse
- Neonatologist, anaesthetist, pharmacist, specialist midwife and social worker involvement and teamwork, highlighting child-protection issues
- Toxicology and STD screening with consent
- Detailed anomaly and serial growth ultrasound scans
- Supportive, non-judgemental care

Midwifery Management and Care

- Good history taking to assess level of cocaine use and willingness to stop using
- Early treatment experiences of the user will make a difference to the user's later commitment to treatment; previous bad experience can affect the user's willingness to engage in treatment options during pregnancy
- Use of a non-judgemental approach to users with an appreciation of how cocaine fits into their lifestyles
- Refer to appropriate specialist substance abuse service
- Encourage attendance at antenatal clinics and classes
- Establish whether there are child-protection concerns, and a necessity for Social Services referral

Labour Issues

CTG changes, due to cocaine's transfer across placental and fetal blood–brain barrier, present as:
- Fetal tachycardia
- Reduced beat to beat variability
- Lack of accelerations

Maternal hypertension leads to *in utero* cerebral infarction. There is increased risk of placental insufficiency, intrapartum hypoxia and meconium-stained liquor.

Use of opiate-based analgesia in labour should be avoided. There is a risk of thrombocytopenia, and a risk of developing an epidural haematoma. Adrenaline/epinephrine may not be effective in treating hypotension.

Medical Management and Care

- Inform anaesthetist and neonatal services to ensure appropriate pain relief and neonatal assessment
- Intervention only for obstetric indications
- Increased risk of operative delivery due to CTG complications, so plan to deliver on consultant-led unit

Midwifery Management and Care

- Continuous electronic fetal monitoring in labour
- Individualised, non-judgemental care
- Avoid use of opiate-based analgesia, because pain relief receptors may already be saturated; might also encourage a relapse if the mother has been drug free in recent times
- Discuss the feasibility of an epidural with the anaesthetist, and discuss pain relief options with the mother taking anaesthetic risks into account

Postpartum Issues

Ensure all relevant professionals know about the delivery and any concerns identified.

Cocaine, whilst not physically addictive, can cause severe withdrawal effects in neonates exposed to both cocaine and opiods. Due to the delay in the effects of some drugs, babies should stay in hospital for a minimum of 4–5 days. Symptoms include poor sucking, feeding problems, irritability, hypertonia, yawning and sneezing[9,10,13].

Mothers require support in caring for babies with minor symptoms that do not require treatment.

Cocaine can be passed on to the child through breast milk. Hence, the decision to breast-feed should be individualised taking into account lifestyle and any contraindications[13].

Medical and Midwifery Management and Care

- Normal baby care should be commenced with regular assessments and transfer to NNU if condition deteriorates
- Liaison with substance abuse service/drug liaison midwife
- Provide support in parenting as even babies *not requiring* medical treatment may still be irritable, unsettled and have difficulties feeding
- Make the mother aware that cocaine passes into breast milk with associated risks
- Assess the potential sequelae to the baby if the mother chooses to breast-feed whilst using cocaine
- Ensure a paediatrician performs the neonatal examination and is informed of baby's condition daily until discharge
- Recommend immunisation to reduce acquisition of infection
- Inform relevant professionals of delivery and postnatal care details
- Address any child-protection issues

16.4 Heroin Addiction

Incidence	Risk for Childbearing
No reliable data	Maternal: Moderate to High Risk
0.2% of 16–24 year olds report having used heroin in the last year in the British Crime Survey 2005–2006	Fetal: Moderate Risk

EXPLANATION OF CONDITION

Heroin is a class A drug, derived from morphine, which is obtained from the opium poppy. It is known colloquially as *boy, brown, china white, dragon, gear, H, horse, junk, skag* and *smack*.

It is sold as a powder, which comes in different colours, from white, if it is pure, to dark brown if it has been mixed with other substances. It can be smoked, sniffed or made into a solution for injection.

Heroin takes effect quickly and can last several hours, depending on how much is taken and whether it is smoked, sniffed or injected. It produces a feeling of warmth, relaxation and detachment with a lessening of anxiety[1].

COMPLICATIONS

Heroin use can cause nausea and vomiting but these effects stop with regular use. An overdose can produce stupor and coma, sometimes leading to death from respiratory failure[2].

Giving up heroin after regular use causes aches, tremor, sweating, chills and muscular spasms. Physical long-term effects include chronic constipation, irregular periods for women, occasionally pneumonia and decreased resistance to infection, thrombophlebitis and bacterial endocarditis[1,2].

These problems may be made worse by self-neglect. Heroin addicts tend to focus on their next 'fix' and are unable to maintain employment, become homeless and resort to crime as a means of obtaining money for drug purchase[1,2].

NON-PREGNANCY TREATMENT AND CARE

There are several schools of thought on treatment for heroin dependency, ranging from abstinence to maintenance. The National Treatment Agency (NTA) formulates policy for treatment in England. As part of the national drug strategy their target is to double the numbers in treatment by 2008[3,4,5,6].

Methadone is the leading drug for substitute prescribing and can be used to maintain or detoxify. It has a reputation among users as being more difficult to detoxify from compared to heroin[3].

From April 2001 buprenorphine has been prescribed by general practitioners (GPs). This is marketed under the trade name Subutex and may be useful when methadone is not the best choice, for example when a person is in the early stages of dependency[4,5].

Naltrexone implants can be used to block the effects of heroin as part of a treatment programme. They are not yet licensed in the UK but are available from private practitioners[3].

There is support for the idea that doctors should return to prescribing heroin as they did in the 1960s rather than methadone. This is because users prefer it and by prescribing heroin the controversial view is that the illicit market would be undercut.

Heroin use can affect the user's sexual function, causing impotence in men and amenorrhea and infertility in women.

PRE-CONCEPTION ISSUES AND CARE

- Access to health care may be delayed due to amenorrhoea and result in a late diagnosis of pregnancy
- Discuss options available, health-related issues and support systems in place
- Offer referral for substitution therapy/detoxification under specialist supervision
- Advantages of methadone for substitution include continued contact with medical services, purity of preparation and 24-hour duration of action, preventing fluctuations in blood levels; available as oral linctus
- Discuss harmful effects of heroin to self and a future baby
- Dependency can affect co-ordination, concentration and thus parenting
- Risk of hepatitis B and C infections as well as HIV with iv drug abuse, therefore essential to offer screening for blood-borne infections after full counselling[7,8]
- Advise the prospective mother to explore financial issues prior to considering a family
- Address any other multi-drug use, alcohol intake and smoking
- Increased risk of prematurity, low birth weight, neonatal withdrawal and sudden infant death syndrome (SIDS)
- Promote folic acid supplementation and standard pre-conception care as outlined at the beginning of Chapter 1

Pregnancy issues

Heroin is not teratogenic. It is associated with:

- Pre-term delivery
- Fetal growth restriction
- Antepartum haemorrhage
- Multiple pregnancy

Pregnant women who are addicted to heroin are advised to switch to methadone. This is administered at regular intervals and keeps the levels of the drug in the bloodstream relatively stable, causing fewer problems for both mother and fetus. With expert professional help, a woman may be able to reduce the amount she takes. Women are not advised to try to quit the drug when they are pregnant as this can cause distress and withdrawal symptoms in the developing baby which could be very harmful[9].

It is vital that mothers with a heroin problem seek expert help so that the best care can be given to them and their babies before and after the birth[10,11,12,13,14].

The short half-life of heroin causes repeated withdrawals, resulting in smooth muscle spasms which cause:

- Uterine contractions and pre-term delivery
- Placental vasospasm and fetal compromise
- Fetal gut spasm, releasing meconium
- Fetal distress

Medical Management and Care

- Consultant with expertise in substance abuse should lead care
- Multi-disciplinary care with neonatologists, anaesthetists, substance abuse team and a specialist midwife
- Serial ultrasound scans for fetal growth
- Assess for multiple pregnancy
- Document plan for intrapartum pain relief antenatally
- Address any related health issues – STD, etc.
- Identify and document any child care/protection issues

Midwifery Management and Care

- Encourage engagement with specialist substance misuse services for treatment
- Encourage regular antenatal care and refer to consultant care
- Normalise midwifery care as much as possible
- Recognise the social, medical and emotional impacts of heroin use
- Provide honest and accurate information regarding the risks to mother and baby
- Ensure regular communication with multi-professional team, including liaison with social care for pre-birth risk assessment
- Discuss effects of drug abusing lifestyle and develop a care plan that minimises harm and stabilises lifestyle
- Arrange pre-birth visit to the neonatal unit
- Discuss options for pain relief
- Document multi-agency care plan to ensure all professionals involved in the care are aware of needs in labour and post birth

Labour Issues

The main issues are:

- Analgesia in labour
- Increased risk of fetal distress

Use naloxone with extreme care for reversal, as it can precipitate severe fetal distress or shock in the neonate[10,11].

Medical Management and Care

- Continuous fetal monitoring
- Intervention for obstetric indications only
- Continue ongoing prescription for methadone

Midwifery Management and Care

- Inform the neonatologist of labour
- Continuous fetal monitoring in labour
- If prescribed methadone, epidural should be offered as the preferred choice of pain relief
- Avoid the use of opiates, e.g. diamorphine, pethidine, especially if the woman is drug free, as this increases risk of reintroducing craving for heroin

Postpartum Issues

Babies exposed to heroin or methadone before birth also suffer extreme symptoms of withdrawal after delivery, needing treatment which may last for weeks. Symptoms include:

- Irritability
- Restlessness
- Feeding and breathing difficulties
- General distress

The baby will need expert care to overcome these symptoms[10,11,12,13].

Withdrawal from heroin is usually observed within 24 hours of delivery, whilst methadone symptoms may be delayed for 48 hours[12,13,14].

Medical Management and Care

- Ongoing care plan for all health care issues identified in pregnancy

Midwifery Management and Care

- **Do not use naloxone** (Narcan) for babies of women who are using opiates (including methadone)
- Normal baby care with observation for neonatal abstinence syndrome (NAS) for 3–5 days
- Breast-feeding can be encouraged if drug use is stable, unless mother is using high doses of benzodiazepines or is HIV positive
- Provide parenting education and support
- Inform social worker, health visitor and specialist substance misuse services of delivery and the need for postnatal support
- Offer hepatitis B and BCG vaccination if required
- Arrange a follow-up appointment for babies of women who are HIV, hepatitis C or B positive

16.5 Amphetamine Addiction

Incidence	Risk for Childbearing
No reliable data	Maternal: Low Risk
3.3% of 16–24 year olds reported use in the British Crime Survey 2005–2006, a reduction from 11.6% reported in 1996	Fetal: Moderate Risk – related to cardiovascular anomalies

EXPLANATION OF CONDITION

Amphetamine is not a naturally-occurring compound, but a synthetic molecule first synthesised in Germany in 1887. It is structurally similar to ephedrine, a natural stimulant found in some plants. Like ephedrine, amphetamine dilates the bronchial sacs of the lungs. Medical use of amphetamine began in the 1930s, with the introduction of the Benzedrine inhaler[1,2,3].

Speed is the street name for amphetamine, and it is also known as *amphetamine sulphate, phet, billy, whizz, sulph, base, amphetamine, paste, dexamphetamine, dexies, dexedrine.*

It is Britain's least pure illegal drug. It is often taken along with *ecstasy* (methylenedioxymethamphetamine). It can be swallowed, smoked, snorted or injected[3,4].

- Amphetamine makes people feel wide awake, excited and chatty
- It may be impossible to sit still or sleep
- It makes some people panicky
- Sniffing a lot in a short space of time may cause hallucinations
- Amphetamine can be addictive; the more is taken the greater chance a person will need to take more to get the same effect, known colloquially as a *'buzz'*
- The effects begin after about half an hour if ingested but much quicker if injected or smoked (methamphetamine) and can last for up to six hours. The high is followed by a long, slow comedown

COMPLICATIONS

- Amphetamine users have died from overdose[3,4]
- Amphetamine use can lead to anxiety, depression, irritability and aggression
- Amphetamine use can lead to mental illnesses such as psychosis and paranoid feelings; can lead to delusions and suicidal ideation
- Short-term physiological effects include decreased appetite, increased stamina and physical energy[5]
- Long-term abuse or overdose effects can include tremor, restlessness, changed sleep patterns, and weakened immune system[6]
- Injecting any drug can cause vein damage, ulcers and gangrene
- Dirty or shared needles and injecting works can help the spread of hepatitis and HIV[7,8,9]
- Unstable lifestyle, poor nutrition and mixing with other drugs of abuse contribute to harmful effects[10,11]

NON-PREGNANCY TREATMENT AND CARE

- Provide information and leaflets on effects of amphetamine and ecstasy use
- Ensure access to specialist substance abuse services and treatment options
- Benefits of substitution therapy are controversial; dexamphetamine substitute is prescribed both orally and intravenously as part of a programme to reduce and stop amphetamine use. A small retrospective study found over half those injecting stopped, and more than a third did so within two months of commencing treatment[12]
- Offer holistic support to partner and family to make lifestyle changes to enable user to stop

PRE-CONCEPTION ISSUES AND CARE

- It is essential that prospective parents are aware of the risks of continued use of amphetamines and ecstasy during pregnancy
- Ensure access to specialist substance abuse services
- Pregnancy can be a good motivator to cease amphetamine use
- Discuss adverse effects on parenting skills with continued use
- There are no specific effects associated with intermittent or recreational use in pregnancy
- High dose continual use causes harmful effects with added effects of unstable lifestyle, poor nutrition and multiple drug usage[11]
- Some, but not all, studies suggest that amphetamines may cause an increased risk of birth defects, including cleft palate, and heart and limb defects[6]
- Use also appears to contribute to pregnancy complications, including maternal high blood pressure which can cause slow fetal growth, premature delivery and post-partum haemorrhage
- Advise parents that babies exposed to amphetamines undergo withdrawal-like symptoms after birth, including jitteriness, drowsiness and breathing problems[13,14], and usually require admittance to a neonatal unit.

The use of ecstasy has increased dramatically in recent years. To date there have been few studies on how the drug may affect pregnancy. One small study found a possible increase in congenital heart defects and, in females only, of the skeletal defect *clubfoot*. Babies exposed to ecstasy before birth may face similar risks as babies exposed to other types of amphetamine[9].

Pregnancy issues

Fetal

There is a higher than expected occurrence of:

- Growth retardation/restriction
- Pre-term delivery
- Heart defects
- Central nervous system defects
- Talipes (especially with ecstasy)
- Cleft lip and palate[5,6]

None of the above studies involved the use of amphetamines alone, but amphetamines and sympathomimetics (cough and cold remedies), ecstasy and multiple drug use. Though the published data is conflicting as regards the fetal effects, the National Teratology Information System (NTIS) for Newcastle-upon-Tyne's prospective data collection suggests an overall malformation rate of 17.7%. Overall incidence of cardiovascular defects was 65/1000 pregnancies compared to the expected 5–10/1000[5,6,7,8,9,10].

Maternal

Because of their anorectic impact, amphetamines may severely affect maternal nutrition prior to and during pregnancy. There is further risk of:

- Hypertension
- Postpartum haemorrhage

Medical Management and Care

- Consultant with expertise in substance abuse should lead care
- Detailed anomaly and fetal cardiac scan
- Serial growth scans
- Counsel regarding risk of pre-term delivery
- Paediatric input as indicated

Midwifery Management and Care

- Accurate history taking to ascertain level of amphetamine use
- Book for antenatal care at a maternal medicine clinic with delivery booked at consultant unit with a neonatal unit
- Assess if amphetamine use is associated with other drug or alcohol abuse
- Provide holistic approach to care
- Ensure access to specialist substance abuse services
- Assess willingness to stop taking amphetamines
- Assess whether there are any child protection/parenting concerns
- Refer to appropriate social services for support

Labour Issues

Amphetamine use in pregnancy has been correlated with:
- Reduced birth weight
- Prematurity
- Postpartum haemorrhage
- Retained placenta

It can result in maternal and fetal tachycardia affecting fetal heart rate monitoring.

Medical Management and care

- IVI, full blood count and blood group and save in labour

Midwifery Management and care

- Ensure appropriate analgesia and give supportive care
- Care of IVI and accurate recording of fluid balance
- Be aware of the risk of postpartum haemorrhage and retained placenta
- Active management of third stage of labour
- Ensure paediatrician aware of possible fetal abnormalities and low birth weight
- Continuous electronic fetal heart monitoring

Postpartum Issues

- It is important to provide care and support if any fetal abnormality is present
- There may be issues about feeding if a baby has a cleft palate
- Amphetamines can cause restlessness, irritability and poor sleep patterns for mother, interfering with safe parenting
- Increased risk of SIDS
- Impaired lactation in regular amphetamine users

Medical Management and Care

- Continued efforts to support giving up drug

Midwifery Management and Care

Babies born to amphetamine users can show an increase in jitteriness, drowsiness and respiratory distress, suggesting an amphetamine withdrawal syndrome. Hence, the following care should be implemented:

- Regular observations for signs of withdrawal
- Paediatrician to perform neonatal examination
- Documentation of neonatal observations
- Information on SIDS should be given to the parents
- Careful consideration should be given to breast-feeding as lactation may be impaired in regular amphetamine users[15]

16 Addictive Disorders

PATIENT ORGANISATIONS

ADDACTION UK – Charity working solely in the field of drug and alcohol treatment
www.addaction.org.uk 0207 251-5860

ADFAM
Charity supporting families affected by drugs/alcohol
www.adfam.org.uk 0207 928-8898

BARNARDO'S UK – Charity supporting vulnerable children and their families
www.barnardos.org.uk 0208 550-8822

FRANK – a confidential, anonymous and discreet service for advice, information + support on drugs
www.talktofrank.com 0800 776600

PHOENIX HOUSE – Charity providing specialist treatment for drug and alcohol users across the UK
www.phoenixhouse.org.uk

TURNING POINT
Social care charity across England and Wales
www.turningpoint.co.uk

ALCOHOL CONCERN
National agency for alcohol misuse
www.alcoholconcern.org.uk

BABY CENTRE: UK Team – www.bwbycentre.co.uk

NARCONON – www.drugrehab.co.uk

Know Cannabis
www.knowcannabis.org.uk

National Treatment Agency www.nta.nhs.uk

Amphetamine (PIM 934) www.inchem.org

Amphetamine use and Pregnancy www.obfocus.com

DRUGSCOPE UK – Centre of expertise for drugs conducting research on drug-related issues
www.drugscope.org.uk 0207 928-1211

HIT Drug cards and leaflets for clubbers, plus 'holiday protection' booklet. www.hit.org.uk 0870 990-9702

LIFELINE Leaflets on Drug Myths and Facts for parents
www.lifeline.org.uk 0161 839-2075

QUIT Charity offering advice to help smokers to stop
www.stopsmoking@quit.org.uk 0800 002200

Drinkline – 0800 917-8282

NHS Smoking Helpline 0800 169-0169
AL-ANON/ALATEEN Range of publications on living with an alcoholic partner or parent
www.al-anonuk.org.uk

ESSENTIAL READING

COCA (Conference on Cocaine and Crack) www.coca.org.uk

Criminal Policy Research Unit South Bank University (2003) **On the rocks: a follow-up study of crack users in London.**

Cross-Government Website for Professionals
www.drugs.gov.uk

Department Of Health (2002) **Tackling Crack Cocaine – A National Plan**. London.

Home Office (2004) **Drug use among vulnerable groups of young people: findings from the Crime and Justice Survey (2003)**. London; The Stationery Office.

Howell, E., Heiser, N. and Harrington, M. (1999) A review of recent findings on substance abuse treatment for pregnant women. **Journal of Substance Abuse Treatment, 16**:195–219.

Kaltenbach, K. and Finnegan, L. (1997) Children of maternal substance misusers. **Current Opinion in Psychiatry, 10**: 220–224.

PM's Strategy Unit (2003) **Alcohol Harm Reduction Strategy for England.** www.strategy.gov.uk

RCOG (1999) **Clinical Green Top Guideline No.9: Alcohol consumption in pregnancy.** http://www.rcog.org.uk/index.asp?PageID=509

Siney, C. (2001) **The Pregnant Drug Addict**, 2nd Edn. Books for Midwives Press.

Strang, J. and Gossop, M. (1994) **Heroin Addiction and Drug Policy: The British System**. Oxford; Oxford University Press.

Thompson, M. and Kingree, J. (1998) The frequency and impact of violent trauma among pregnant substance abusers. **Addictive Behaviours**. 23:257–262.

Various Authors (1999) Maternal and obstetric effects of prenatal drug exposure, pp. 75–86; Interpreting research on prenatal substance exposure in the context of multiple confounding factors, pp. 39–54; Perinatal effects of prenatal drug exposure. Neonatal aspects, pp. 87–106; Early development of infants exposed to drugs prenatally, pp. 107–150. **Clinics in Perinatology, 26.**

Winyard, R. (2005) **Substance Misuse in Primary Care: a multidisciplinary approach**. Oxford; Radcliffe.

PSYCHIATRIC DISORDERS

17

Kathryn Gutteridge and Renuka Lazarus

17.1 Antenatal Psychiatric Disorders

Incidence	Risk for Childbearing
10–15%	Moderate Risk Increased risk if past or family history of severe mental illness Increased risk with social problems

EXPLANATION OF CONDITION

There is a socio-cultural expectation that pregnancy and childbirth are times of happiness and wellbeing. This makes it difficult for women to seek help for mental health problems during the perinatal period[1]. Pregnancy was previously considered to be protective against mental illness[2]. However, mental health problems during pregnancy are at least as common as they are postnatally and are increasingly recognised as important forerunners of postnatal illness[3,4].

Some degree of emotional lability and anxiety during pregnancy is normal. Sleep deprivation is common. However this needs to be differentiated from depressive and anxiety disorders occurring during this period[5].

Although any psychiatric disorder may present in pregnancy, the clinical issues to note are:

- Most first-onset conditions are mild depressive and anxiety disorders, and the cause is commonly psychosocial[6]
- Relapses and recurrences of previous mental illness may occur both during pregnancy and in the postnatal period[6]
- Relapses of the following disorders may occur:
  – depressive and anxiety disorders
  – obsessive compulsive disorder
  – schizophrenia
  – bipolar disorder
  – substance misuse
- Antidepressants and antipsychotics should not automatically be discontinued once the woman becomes pregnant[7] as this is a frequent cause of relapse
- Mild to moderate disorders may be managed in primary care
- Past or current severe illness should be referred to specialist psychiatric services, preferably to a perinatal psychiatric service[7,8]
- Good communication between all health professionals both in primary and secondary services is crucial[4]

Common psychosocial factors associated with mild antenatal depressive and anxiety symptoms are[9]:

- Previous infertility or obstetric loss
- Lack of support; relationship problems
- Unplanned pregnancy or ambivalence towards it
- Financial problems
- Teenage pregnancy
- Pregnancy-related medical problems
- Domestic violence
- Poor experience of own mothering
- Past sexual abuse
- Bereavement

COMPLICATIONS

Antenatal psychiatric disorders may be associated with[9,10,11,12]:

- Poor attendance at antenatal clinic
- Low birth weight
- Prematurity
- Smoking and substance misuse
- Poor general health and nutrition
- Deliberate self-harm and suicide
- Safeguarding children issues
- Maternal–infant attachment dysfunction

Any depression or anxiety during pregnancy that is unrecognised and untreated increases the risk of suicide during the last trimester[4].

NON-PREGNANCY TREATMENT AND CARE

Mild to moderate mental illness may be managed in primary care. Management includes:

- Advice on lifestyle, exercise and coping with stress
- Talking therapies
- Psychotropic medication

Severe mental illness is usually managed by psychiatric services either in the community or in a psychiatric unit.

PRE-CONCEPTION ISSUES AND CARE

Women with previous mental illness should receive advice about the following issues in a manner that is socially and culturally sensitive:

- Contraception
- Risk of recurrence of mental illness in perinatal period
- Risks and benefits of medication in pregnancy
- Counselling regarding risk of mental illness in offspring

Good communication between professionals is important. Advice may be given by primary care services; liaison with specialist psychiatric services is needed for women with past or current mental illness.

Pregnancy Issues

Persistent anxiety and depressive symptoms affect the woman's general health and satisfaction with pregnancy. The increased production of maternal and fetal cortisol in these patients may also be associated with increased uterine artery resistance which may result in[11,12]:

- Fetal growth retardation
- Low birth weight
- Prematurity
- Long-term behavioural and cognitive deficits in the child

Some women may adopt maladaptive ways of coping with stress, and these could also indirectly affect the pregnancy. These include:

- Smoking
- Alcohol and substance misuse
- Poor dietary habits
- Lack of exercise
- Self-harming behaviour

Management and Care

Early detection of perinatal mental illness by all health professionals is crucial. Care pathways should be clearly defined and good communication between professionals is important. Psychiatric management should be detailed in the woman's care plan including risk assessment and child protection issues.

Medical Care

- Mild to moderate depressive and anxiety symptoms are the most frequent psychiatric problems in pregnancy and may be managed in primary care
- Psychological therapies such as self-help strategies, non-directive counselling and other brief therapies may be indicated
- Advice may be sought from specialist psychiatric services if needed, regarding commencing or continuing medication
- All women with severe mental illness (past or current) should be referred to specialist services, preferably to a specialist perinatal psychiatry team[7]
- The risk–benefit ratio of psychotropic medication is assessed and decisions regarding medication during pregnancy are made after discussions with the woman and her partner

Midwifery Care

- At the booking visit, the midwife will screen for past or present severe mental illness in the woman and her family and refer to appropriate services if necessary
- She should establish a trusting relationship with the woman that is socially and culturally sensitive
- Advice regarding smoking cessation, diet and exercise, breast-feeding, birth preparation and support services

Labour Issues

- There are no physical reasons why the birth should be managed differently
- Anxiety management techniques may be useful in anxious women
- Specialist perinatal psychiatric team may need to be contacted for advice or assessment
- Neonatologists should be contacted if the mother is on psychotropic medication

Medical Management and Care

- Advice regarding psychotropic medication during labour should be entered in the pre-birth care plan
- Drugs should be used judiciously in view of possible effects on the baby

Midwifery Management and Care

- Labour should be managed from a normal perspective
- Discuss methods of support for labour pain to reduce anxiety
- Support throughout labour is important
- Consent should be obtained throughout labour

Postpartum Issues

The main risk is an escalation of antenatal psychiatric symptoms after delivery, or a recurrence of previous mental illness. These may manifest as:

- Increased anxiety and agitation
- Low mood, excessive tearfulness or apathy
- Poor handling or attachment to baby
- Bizarre or unusual behaviour
- Delusions and hallucinations
- Thoughts, or acts, of harming herself or the baby
- Breast-feeding may be possible with planned medication management

Medical Management and Care

- Specialist perinatal psychiatry team should be contacted if symptoms are severe
- Many psychotropic drugs are safe in breast-feeding and need not be discontinued
- Transfer to a specialist psychiatric Mother and Baby Unit may be indicated if the patient is too ill to be discharged home

Midwifery Management and Care

- Observe mother and baby interaction
- Discuss rest, diet and self-care
- Assess how mother is coping
- Reassure if mood change is due to postnatal blues
- Observe baby if breast-feeding mother is on psychotropic medication
- Communicate with specialist services and refer if needed

17.2 Postnatal Psychiatric Disorders

Incidence
Depression: 10–15%[1,2]
Puerperal psychosis: 0.2%[3]

Risk for Childbearing
Moderate Risk for depression
High Risk for psychosis

EXPLANATION OF CONDITIONS

Psychiatric disorders following childbirth are common, and include both new episodes specific to the postpartum period, as well as recurrences of previous illnesses. Depression and puerperal psychosis will be described here.

Depression

The term 'postnatal depression' is often used inappropriately to describe all postnatal psychiatric disorders, and is best avoided[4]. The presentation and manifestation of symptoms of depression occurring in the postnatal period do not differ from depression outside of childbirth[5].

Normal emotional changes following childbirth may mask or be mistaken for depressive symptoms. **'Postnatal blues'** are experienced by 50–80% of women, are transient and occur 3–10 days after delivery[6,7]. They are characterised by irritability, tearfulness, low mood, euphoria and sleep disturbance. They resolve spontaneously and the woman and her family need reassurance and support.

Depression in the postnatal period may range from mild to severe. Prediction and early detection are important. The key features include a two-week history of the following symptoms[4]:

- Low mood, loss of interest and enjoyment and reduced energy
- Associated symptoms such as:
  – reduced concentration and self-esteem
  – ideas of guilt
  – hopelessness
  – thoughts or acts of self-harm or suicide
  – sleep and appetite disturbance

At the booking visit and at all subsequent visits the midwife should ask the following questions to detect depression[8]:

- During the past month, have you often felt low, depressed or hopeless?
- During the past month, have you had little interest or pleasure in doing things?

Puerperal Psychosis

This illness is relatively rare and is a psychiatric emergency requiring urgent hospital admission. Mothers with a positive past history or family history of bipolar disorder are particularly at risk[9]. There is also an association with primiparity and obstetric complications[10]. The clinical picture includes:

- Mood changes: elation, depression or irritability
- Perplexity and confusion
- Agitation and abnormal behaviour
- Delusions and hallucinations
- Thoughts or acts of harm to self or others
- Difficulty in caring for self and baby

COMPLICATIONS

Complications depend on the duration and the severity of the illness. They include:

- Self-harm and suicide[3]
- Neglect of baby and infanticide[9]
- Dysfunction of mother–infant attachment and interaction[9,11]
- Long-term emotional, behavioural and cognitive problems in the child[10]
- Relationship problems and family breakdown[4]
- Social, occupational and financial complications[6]
- Depression in the partner[8]

NON-PREGNANCY TREATMENT AND CARE

Depression in the non-pregnant population is managed in primary care if it is mild to moderate, and referred to the psychiatric services if it is severe[12]. The following management options are available:

- Advice on lifestyle, exercise and coping with stress
- Talking therapies, e.g. cognitive behaviour therapy
- Antidepressant medication
- Mood stabilisers, e.g. lithium

PRE-CONCEPTION ISSUES AND CARE

Women with a past history of severe depression or puerperal psychosis should be counselled regarding relapse rates (about 50%) in future pregnancies. Medication should not be abruptly discontinued. Many antidepressants are safe in pregnancy; mood stabilisers may cause fetal defects, but again the risk–benefit ratio should be assessed to decide whether discontinuation is indicated.

Other issues that may be associated with depression and require advice and support are[12]:

- Poor diet and nutritional status
- Smoking
- Substance/alcohol abuse
- Self-harming behaviour
- Relationship breakdown

Pregnancy issues

Psychosocial risk factors play a role in causing mild to moderate depression. However, in severe depression and in puerperal psychosis, biological factors are more important.

Women with the following history need to be supported and advised regarding the possible risk of developing postnatal psychiatric illness:

- Past or family history of severe depression
- Past or family history of bipolar disorder[10]
- Antenatal depression
- Severe postnatal blues
- Social problems and lack of social support
- Recent negative life events
- Long-standing difficulties in coping
- Sexual abuse and/or rape

Medical Management and Care

- Antenatal depression may be treated either with talking therapies or antidepressants
- Psychotropic medication need not be discontinued
- Women at risk should have access to a specialist perinatal psychiatry service for advice or assessment if needed

Midwifery Management and Care

- At the booking visit, the midwife will screen for past or present severe mental illness in the woman and her family and refer to appropriate services if necessary[8]
- Communication with other professionals is vital if the woman is at risk of developing postnatal psychiatric illness
- The care plan should include psychiatric management and should be recorded in all versions of the maternity notes[8]
- A trusting relationship should be established with the woman that is socially and culturally sensitive
- Advice should be given regarding smoking cessation, diet and exercise, breast-feeding, birth preparation and support services
- Safeguarding children principles should be observed

Labour Issues

- There are no physical reasons why the birth should be managed differently
- Obstetric complications may increase the risk for developing postnatal psychiatric disorders
- Specialist perinatal psychiatric team may need to be contacted for advice or assessment
- Neonatologists should be contacted if the mother is on psychotropic medication

Medical Management and Care

- Psychotropic medication may be indicated in women with past or present psychiatric illness
- Drugs should be used judiciously in view of possible effects on the baby

Midwifery Management and Care

- Discuss all care fully with the woman and birth partner
- Ensure that any plan has the woman's full consent
- Psychological and physical support is important throughout labour
- Avoid unnecessary interventions
- Encourage skin-to-skin contact between mother and baby
- Breast-feeding to be encouraged if not pharmacologically contraindicated

Postpartum Issues

- Postnatal blues and normal emotional changes should be distinguished from depression
- Depression usually presents within the first 12 weeks postpartum; one-third to one-half of these are severe and tend to present early, usually by 4–6 weeks postpartum
- Puerperal psychosis presents acutely, usually 3–7 days postpartum
- Severe depression and puerperal psychosis need referral to specialist perinatal psychiatric services
- Suicide is the foremost cause of maternal mortality; it can be prevented by early detection and treatment

Medical Management and Care

- Specialist perinatal psychiatry team should be contacted if symptoms are severe
- Risk assessment and child-protection issues are important
- Psychotropic medication may be indicated and may be safe in breast-feeding
- Admission to a specialist psychiatric Mother and Baby Unit may be indicated if the patient is severely ill

Midwifery Management and Care

- Observe mother and baby interaction
- Discuss rest, diet and self-care, and how the mother is coping
- Reassure if mood change is due to postnatal blues
- Observe baby if breast-feeding mother using medication
- Ask screening questions for depression; scales such as the EPDS may be used, but only as part of an assessment[1]
- Communicate with specialist services and refer if needed
- Refer to Social Services if *safeguarding of children* concerns are raised

17 Psychiatric Disorders

PATIENT ORGANISATIONS

PNI-UK
http://www.pni-uk.com/pniuk.html

ForParentsbyParents
http://www.depression-in-pregnancy.org.uk/

Meet a Mum Association
http://www.mama.co.uk/default.asp?nc=4104&id=1
0845 120 3746

Mind
www.mind.org.uk
Tel: 08457 660 163

National Childbirth Trust (NCT)
www.nctpregnancyandbabycare.com
Tel: 0870 444 8707

Association for Postnatal Illness
www.apni.org
Tel: 020 7386 0868

Perinatal Illness UK
www.pni-uk.com

Action on Puerperal Psychosis
www.bham.ac.uk/app

Birth Trauma Association
www.birthtraumaassociation.org

PaNDa
www.vicnet.net.au/-panda

Royal College of Psychiatrists
Perinatal Special Interest Group
www.rcpsych.ac.uk/college/sig/peri.htm

CRY-SIS
www.cry-sis.com
Tel: 0207 404-5011

ESSENTIAL READING

POLICY AND GUIDELINES
NICE (2007) Clinical Guideline 45: **Antenatal and Post-natal Mental Health** http://guidance.nice.org.uk/CG45/niceguidance/

The Scottish Intercollegiate Guidelines Network (SIGN) (2002) **Guidelines: Postnatal depression and puerperal psychosis** (includes screening, diagnosis, management for a multi-disciplinary team).
http://www.sign.ac.uk/guidelines/fulltext/60/index.html

WHO UK Collaborating Centre (2005) **Introduction to Post-natal Disorders**.
http://www.libraries.nelh.nhs.uk/mentalhealth

EVIDENCE AND BEST PRACTICE
The Cochrane Library has systematic reviews on: **Antide-pressant prevention of postnatal depression**
http://dx.doi.org/10.1002/14651858.CD004363.pub2

Dennis, C-L and Creedy, D. (2004) **Psychosocial and psychological interventions for preventing postpartum depression**. Cochrane Database
http://dx.doi.org/10.1002/14651858.CD001134.pub2

MIDIRS Informed Choice Leaflet 20: **Postnatal depression**.
http://www.clinicalevidence.com/ceweb/conditions/pac/1407/1407.jsp

BOOKS
Dalton, K. (2001) **Depression after Childbirth: How to Recognize, Treat, and Prevent Postnatal Depression**, 4th edn. Oxford; Oxford University Press.

Gutteridge, K.E.A. and Waheed, W. (2007) **Maternal Mental Health: Working in Partnership in Essential Midwifery Practice:** Public Health (Eds S. Byrom and G. Edwards). Oxford; Blackwell Publishing.

Hanzak, E. (2005) **Eyes without Sparkle: A Journey through Postnatal Illness**. Oxford; Radcliffe.

Littlewood, J. and McHugh, N. (1997) **Maternal Distress And Postnatal Depression**. Basingstoke; Macmillan.

Price, S. (Ed) (2007) **Mental Health in Pregnancy and Childbirth**. Oxford; Blackwell Publishing.

Raphael-Leff, J. (1991) **Psychological Processes of Child-bearing**. London; Chapman and Hall.

Shaw, F. (2001) **Out of Me**. London; Virago Press.

NEOPLASIA 18

Julie Goddard, Jo Matharu and
S. Elizabeth Robson

18.1 Breast Cancer

Incidence	**Risk for Childbearing**
1:9 lifetime risk[1]	Variable Risk
3:10,000 risk of diagnosis in pregnancy[2]	

EXPLANATION OF CONDITION[1,3,4]

Breast cancer is most commonly associated with post-menopausal women but is increasingly affecting women of child-bearing age. The classic presentation is with a painless, slow growing and palpable mass. Other symptoms include nipple discharge and breast skin changes.

Risk factors include:

- Increased age
- Nulliparity
- Family history
- Early menarche
- Late menopause
- HRT use

Breast cancer once diagnosed is attributed a 'stage' in order to guide treatment decisions.

- **Stage 0** – non-invasive breast cancer with no invasion of surrounding tissue
- **Stage I** – invasive breast cancer in which the tumour measures <2 cm and there is no lymph node involvement
- **Stage II** – the tumour measures at least 2 cm but <5 cm **or** cancer has spread to the lymph nodes in the axilla on the same side as the affected breast
- **Stage IIIA** – tumour size is >5 cm **or** there is significant lymph node involvement, where the nodes stick to one another or surrounding tissue
- **Stage IIIB** – tumour has spread to the breast skin, chest wall or internal mammary lymph nodes; includes inflammatory breast cancer
- **Stage IV** – tumour has spread beyond the breast, axilla and internal mammary nodes and may have spread to lymph nodes at neck base, lungs, liver, brain or bone

COMPLICATIONS[1,3]

- Metastasis (secondaries)
- Anaemia
- Anorexia
- Fatigue
- Secondary infection
- Depression
- Side effects of treatment:
  - **radiotherapy**: lethargy, anorexia, localised skin reactions
  - **chemotherapy**: (it is of note that cytotoxic drugs used currently have significantly less severe side effects than previously) nausea, vomiting, hair loss, fatigue, infections, mouth sores and irregular menstruation
  - **hormone therapy**: mood swings, depression, weight gain, hot flushes, bloating and early menopause

NON-PREGNANCY TREATMENT AND CARE[1,4]

Prompt Referral and Diagnosis

Diagnosis is by a combination of examination, mammography, ultrasound and fine-needle aspiration cytology.

Surgery

Surgery may include:

- lumpectomy
- mastectomy
- lymphadenectomy
- reconstructive surgery, where appropriate

Chemotherapy

Chemotherapy treats the entire system by disrupting the ability of cancer cells to divide and grow. A combination of drugs is often used, as different drugs attack cancer cells at different stages of their growth. Drugs are usually administered every 2–4 weeks for 4–6 months to allow for a recovery period from side effects of treatment.

Radiotherapy

Radiotherapy involves the use of high-energy X-rays to destroy the cancer cells. This painless administration of X-rays is usually given over a period of time to optimise the effect of destroying the cancer cells whilst avoiding damage to normal cells. Radiotherapy may reduce the risk of recurrence by 50–60%.

Hormone Therapy

Oestrogen-sensitive cancers comprise 50–75% of breast cancers. Commonly-used hormone drugs include anti-oestrogens (e.g. tamoxifen), LHRH agonists (e.g. Zoladex) and aromatase inhibitors.

Psychological Support

As many as 30% of women diagnosed with breast cancer will develop a depressive illness within a year of diagnosis. The psychological impact of a diagnosis of breast cancer merits the input of the multi-disciplinary team to support the woman and her family.

PRE-CONCEPTION ISSUES AND CARE

Women with a previous history of breast cancer who are contemplating pregnancy should seek advice from their obstetrician, breast surgeon and oncologist.

In general, a delay of two years post cancer treatment is recommended to allow for early recurrences to be detected[5]. Younger women (<33 years) may be advised to wait three years before conception as they have a higher relapse rate[6]. Women with a poor prognosis may be advised to avoid further pregnancy. Pregnancy does not appear to affect long term survival after breast cancer, but women with a poor prognosis are likely to die while they have young children.

Women with previous early stage breast cancer and no signs of recurrence have a good prognosis following subsequent pregnancy, with survival rates of 71–90%[7].

Pregnancy Issues

Breast cancer is the most common cancer found in pregnancy and accounts for 3% of all breast cancers[7].

Pregnancy following breast cancer
Pregnancy after treatment for breast cancer appears to be associated with a higher rate of miscarriage[8]. Current literature shows no evidence of previous use of cytotoxic drugs causing any adverse fetal or neonatal development effects. Consequently women with a previous history of breast cancer should be managed with regard to their pregnancy as normal.

Breast cancer diagnosed during pregnancy
Prognosis may be worse in pregnancy, as diagnosis may be delayed due to normal physiological changes which may mask symptoms/signs of cancer. However, recent studies indicate that survival is unaffected in pregnant women with breast cancer when compared with non-pregnant women with the same stage of disease[9,10].

Surgical intervention is the preferred management[7], ideally performed after the first trimester in order to reduce risk of miscarriage. It may involve modified radical mastectomy or lumpectomy and axillary clearance with deferred reconstruction.

Chemotherapy is associated with risk of congenital malformations in the first trimester, with critical susceptible period of 5–10 weeks[11]. Chemotherapy in the second and third trimesters appears safe although there may be a link with IUGR and low birth weight[12].

Radiotherapy and tamoxifen are usually avoided until post delivery. If radiotherapy is indicated, early delivery may be required to commence treatment as soon as possible[12].

Medical Management and Care

For women with a previous history of breast cancer
- Manage pregnancy as normal
- Encourage surveillance for any signs of recurrence

For women diagnosed in pregnancy
- Diagnosis is as for non-pregnancy, but mammography is less useful due to pregnancy-induced changes in breast tissue[13]
- Discussion regarding continuation of pregnancy if diagnosis in first trimester[14]
- Whilst termination of pregnancy has not been shown to have any beneficial effect on outcomes it may require discussion if the treatment required is limited by continued pregnancy and/or for emotional and social reasons[15]
- Planned multi-disciplinary care including obstetricians, midwives, oncologists, anaesthetists, paediatricians and Macmillan nurses
- Negotiation about optimum time and mode of delivery depending upon need for treatment in pregnancy
- Steroid administration for fetal lung maturation and liaising with paediatricians if premature delivery is required

Midwifery Management and Care

For women with a previous history of breast cancer
- Encourage careful breast self-examination
- Educate about the normal physiological breast changes in pregnancy, but be alert to how these may mask symptoms
- Immediate referral to specialist obstetrician and oncology team if suspicious about these changes
- Provide psychological and emotional support for pregnant women who have experienced breast cancer; fears regarding future recurrence and issues around mortality may be heightened during pregnancy and impending parenthood

For women diagnosed in pregnancy
- Importance of maternal wishes are paramount; act as advocate and provide information for the woman and her family
- Extra vigilance regarding fetal growth, regular antenatal appointments and 'small for dates' recordings
- Advise about fetal movements
- Direct women to appropriate support networks (see Essential Reading)
- Basic nursing care may be required, especially if the mother has had recent surgery and requires wound care
- 'Parent-craft' education may have to be given on a one-to-one basis and include advice on lifting the baby if arm movement is impaired

Labour Issues

If mastectomy is required in the third trimester this could be combined with caesarean section, depending on gestation. The placenta requires histology, and the pathologist should examine for evidence of placental metastases.

Medical Management and Care
- Delivery may be expedited early to allow radiotherapy or tamoxifen treatment to begin

Midwifery Management and Care
- Prepare for a potential pre-term delivery with a mother who might be physically 'run down' and anxious, and possibly post-operative
- Care with positioning of CTG monitor belts, and when assisting the mother to move; she may have weak arm movement if post surgery
- Send placenta to histology with detailed clinical history

Postpartum Issues
- Breast-feeding is contraindicated during chemotherapy and radiotherapy[7]
- Lactation might fail to occur as a consequence of radiation therapy

Medical Management and Care
- Discuss contraception: the COCP is contraindicated after a diagnosis of breast cancer

Midwifery Management and Care
- Teach partner parenting skills
- Psychological and physical support; advise how to hold the baby
- Encourage breast-feeding if possible, or advise on formula feeds

18.2 Malignant Melanoma

Incidence[1]	Risk for Childbearing
8,000 cases per annum in UK	Variable Risk
1,800 deaths per year in UK	

EXPLANATION OF CONDITION

Malignant melanoma is a tumour originating from the normal melanocytes within the skin which proliferate and transform into aggressive tumours. It is thought that genetic predisposition and exposure to ultraviolet radiation are the primary contributors to the development of the disease[2].

Malignant melanomas may begin as an existing mole/nevus or arise *de novo*. Generally they present as dark pigmented skin lesions, expanding in size, but they may be amelanotic and thus red or pale in colour. The lesions may be painful, itch, bleed or ulcerate. Any suspicious skin changes necessitate investigation.

Risk factors for malignant melanoma include fair skin, history of childhood sun exposure, episodic sunburn, living in a hot country, multiple nevi (moles) and family history.

There are four main types of melanoma[3]:

1. **Superficial spreading melanoma:** most common, accounting for 70% of melanomas. These are common in the middle-aged population. They grow laterally and then vertically and are often found to arise from pre-existing benign nevi.
2. **Nodular melanoma:** accounting for 25% of melanomas, these are more common in men, develop quickly and usually arise *de novo*. The tumour invades vertically and is typically deep at presentation. This type of melanoma presents as an elevated nodule and is more likely to ulcerate or bleed. Nodular melanoma has the worst prognosis of the four types.
3. **Lentigo malignant melanoma:** accounts for 10% of melanomas and is most common in the elderly population. It is usually found on sun-exposed areas of the body (e.g. face). This melanoma is less likely to metastasise and has the best prognosis.
4. **Acral lentiginous melanoma:** most commonly found on the palms of hands, soles of feet and under nails. These tumours grow vertically and are characterised by a flat pigmented area around the focus of the melanoma. Tumours around the nailbed are the most difficult to diagnose and have the poorest prognosis.

Malignant melanomas are attributed a **stage** by combining the score for the depth of the tumour (Breslow scale) along with the Tumour-Nodes-Metastases staging system. Broadly speaking, the stages are categorised as follows[4]:

- **Stage I** – <1 mm thick
- **Stage II** – >1 mm thick
- **Stage III** – spread to local lymph nodes
- **Stage IV** – distant metastases

Malignant melanoma is almost completely curable if detected early. Five year survival rates are 96% for local lesions, 60% if regional spread and 14% if distant metastases[5]. The overall survival rate for women is 85%.

NON-PREGNANCY TREATMENT AND CARE

Any person with a lesion suspicious of melanoma should be referred promptly by the primary care team for further assessment. Excision of a suspicious lesion is performed as a full-thickness skin biopsy with a 2–5 mm clinical margin of normal skin laterally and with a cuff of sub-dermal fat. This allows diagnosis and decisions regarding further treatment[4].

Following diagnosis a thorough physical examination is required to look for the presence of other possible melanomas and to assess the clinical stage of the disease.

Most malignant melanomas are treated entirely with surgical removal. Early stage disease is treated with wide local excision with margins of normal tissue of 1–3 cm[4]. More advanced disease is difficult to treat and some treatments are intended to be palliative rather than curative. Possible treatments include lymph node dissection, chemotherapy, radiotherapy and interferon therapy[6].

Management of patients with malignant melanoma requires a multi-disciplinary team approach including primary care, dermatology, surgery, oncology, histopathology and clinical nurse specialists.

PRE-CONCEPTION ISSUES AND CARE

Current opinion is that conception should be delayed for 2–3 years following treatment for malignant melanoma[7]. Whilst no evidence suggests that pregnancy affects the cancer or the chance of it recurring, recurrence rates are significantly higher in the two years following diagnosis. Women who have had an early-stage melanoma completely excised and have had no recurrence within 2–3 years are likely to be cured.

Women with metastatic or recurrent disease should be advised to avoid pregnancy due to poor prognosis and difficult treatment decisions during pregnancy.

Pregnancy issues

The incidence of malignant melanoma is rising. It accounts for one-third of all new cancers in the 15–39 year age group[6]. Thirty-five percent of women with melanoma are of child-bearing age and the co-existence of melanoma and pregnancy although still rare is increasing[8].

There is no evidence that pregnancy affects the prognosis of malignant melanoma. The outcome of pregnancies associated with stage I melanoma is generally excellent[9]. Termination of pregnancy does not affect the prognosis and should not be routinely offered.

Diagnosis and treatment should not be delayed due to pregnancy. Management of early-stage disease is identical to the non-pregnant patient.

Advanced-stage disease in pregnancy requires an individualised treatment plan with multi-disciplinary team input. Palliative chemotherapy to slow tumour growth and control symptoms is relatively safe for the fetus in the second and third trimesters (see Section 18.1).

Melanoma can, rarely, metastasise to the placenta. It is the commonest tumour to do so, accounting for up to a third of all reported cases[10].

Medical Management and Care

- Do not delay referral for suspicious lesions in pregnancy
- Surgical removal of tumour should not be delayed due to pregnancy; preferably performed under local anaesthetic, but general anaesthesia need not be avoided in pregnancy
- Termination is not indicated for early-stage disease
- In the case of metastatic disease, mean survival is six months[8] therefore termination may need discussion, although prognosis is unaffected
- Management decisions regarding metastatic disease in pregnancy are difficult and are based on symptoms, maternal wishes, likely length of survival and potential fetal outcome; involvement of the multi-disciplinary team is vital and maternal wishes are paramount

Midwifery Management and Care

General issues

- Encourage vigilant observation of pre-existing moles/nevi
- Discourage any use of sun beds
- Advocate 'sensible sunlight exposure' to gain vitamin D without getting sunburnt (see Appendix 1.3)
- Immediate referral to a specialist if pregnant woman reports suspicious skin changes

For women with melanoma in pregnancy

- Psychological support
- Offer contact details of support groups and sources of further information
- Support for partner and family members
- Encourage a healthy lifestyle, with a vitamin- and iron-rich diet, and avoidance of smoking and alcohol

Labour Issues

Labour and delivery can be managed as normal for any women with a previous history of melanoma.

In the rare circumstance of advanced melanoma during pregnancy, delivery depends on the clinical situation and is likely to be pre-term and by caesarean section.

Medical Management and Care

- Anticipate normal labour for women with early-stage or previous disease

Midwifery Management and Care

- Normal midwifery care in labour
- Care not to damage any skin area that has received treatment; protective dressing might be required
- For women with current melanoma send the placenta for histological examination with detailed history for the pathologist (to examine for placental metastasis)

Postpartum Issues

In the rare circumstance of advanced melanoma with metastasis to the placenta there is a risk of spread to the fetus, therefore the baby needs careful follow-up to exclude disease. Melanoma in the neonate has a high mortality rate[11].

Medical Management and Care

- Normal postpartum care
- Follow-up with skin cancer specialists

Midwifery Management and Care

- Normal postpartum care
- Encourage breast-feeding unless the mother is currently undergoing chemotherapy or radiotherapy. If the latter applies, then advice on formula feeds is necessary and instruction should be given about the sterilisation of infant feeding equipment
- Arrange any necessary follow-up appointments for both mother and baby

18.3 Hodgkin's Lymphoma

Incidence	Risk for Childbearing
1500 cases a year in UK[1] 1:20,000 pregnancies are affected [2]	Variable Risk

EXPLANATION OF CONDITION [3,4]

Hodgkin's lymphoma (HL) is a rare malignancy of the lymphatic system. A specific type of cell called Reed Steinberg cells are characteristic of this condition and they are thought to arise from B-lymphocytes.

- **Presentation** is usually with a painless, slow-growing, enlarged lymph node in the neck, axilla or groin. In 30% of patients there are associated symptoms of night sweats, fever and weight loss. Other variable symptoms include fatigue, anorexia, pruritus and rarely alcohol-induced pain in the affected lymph nodes
- **Peak incidence** is in the third decade and it is commoner in men (ratio 1.3:1)
- **Risk factors** include family history, immunosuppression and infection with Epstein Barr virus
- **Histological types** of Hodgkin's lymphoma are divided into classical HL (95%) and nodular lymphocyte predominant HL (5%). Classical HL is further divided into 4 subtypes:
  - nodular sclerosing HL (70%)
  - lymphocyte-rich HL (5%)
  - mixed cellularity HL (25%)
  - lymphocyte-depleted HL (rare)
- **Diagnosis** is by:
  - lymph-node biopsy
  - abnormal blood parameters associated with HL include normocytic anaemia, raised ESR, raised LDH and abnormal LFT
- **Staging** is important as it guides treatment and affects prognosis. It involves physical examination, blood tests, chest X-ray and CT scan +/− positron-emission tomography (PET) scan. There are four stages:
  - Stage I – single lymph node group affected
  - Stage II – two lymph node groups affected on same side of diaphragm
  - Stage III – lymph nodes affected on both sides of diaphragm
  - Stage IV – disseminated disease
- **Classification:**
  - **A** refers to absence of systemic symptoms
  - **B** refers to presence of systemic symptoms
  - **X** refers to bulky disease
- **Prognosis** for Hodgkin's lymphoma is good, with a five-year survival rate of 75–80%. Most recurrences occur within three years. Survival rate decreases with:
  - advanced stage of disease
  - presence of B symptoms
  - bulky disease
  - abnormal blood parameters
  - increasing patient age

NON-PREGNANCY TREATMENT AND CARE

Prompt referral is required if there is a suspicion of lymphoma. Current guidelines suggest referral for investigation within two weeks in the following situations[5]:

- Lymphadenopathy persisting >6 weeks in the absence of infection
- Constellation of symptoms such as night sweats, fever, weight loss, fatigue and pruritus

Diagnosis is as detailed earlier.

Treatment depends on the stage and histological type of the disease and consists of radiotherapy, chemotherapy or a combination of both. Decisions regarding treatment are made in a multi-disciplinary team setting in conjunction with the patient.

For early-stage disease, until recently the treatment of choice was radiotherapy. Although this resulted in high cure rates there were concerns regarding the risk of relapse and the side effects of radiotherapy on surrounding healthy tissue. Treatment for early-stage disease now usually consists of short-term chemotherapy with involved field radiotherapy[6]. This type of radiotherapy is directed at the group of lymph nodes affected and minimises damage to surrounding tissue.

For advanced disease, the treatment of choice is combination chemotherapy over 6–8 months[6]. Various combinations can be used with equal efficacy but the preferred regimen in the UK comprises: Adriamycin, bleomycin, vinblastine and dacarbazine, as this regimen minimises side effects.

Psychological support is an important aspect of treatment which must not be neglected.

PRE-CONCEPTION ISSUES AND CARE

General advice is to delay conception until 2–3 years following treatment for Hodgkin's lymphoma, as the majority of recurrences occur during this time.

There is no evidence that pregnancy increases the chance of recurrence.

Previous chemotherapy does not increase the risk of congenital malformation.

Some women will have reduced fertility or early menopause following radiotherapy or chemotherapy. These women may need referral for fertility treatment if required[1].

Pregnancy Issues

Hodgkin's lymphoma occurring during pregnancy is rare and there is limited data available to guide management. Pregnancy does not appear to adversely affect prognosis in existing Hodgkin's lymphoma, and pregnancy outcome is generally good[2].

There is no evidence that offering termination in an affected pregnancy affects the disease course or prognosis.

If staging is required in pregnancy, MRI and ultrasound should be considered as an alternative to CT scanning to reduce the radiation load to the fetus[7].

Treatment in pregnancy should be individualised to take account of the mother's wishes, gestation at diagnosis, the stage and growth velocity of the tumour and the effect of treatment on the fetus:

- Radiotherapy is avoided if possible during pregnancy but, if required, supradiaphragmatic radiotherapy with shielding of the fetus has been shown to be relatively safe[8]
- Chemotherapy should be avoided in the first trimester but is relatively safe in the second and third trimesters[7] (see Section 18.1)

Medical Management and Care

- Pregnancy in women with a previous history of Hodgkin's lymphoma should be managed as low risk
- Any symptoms of recurrence should merit immediate referral for investigation
- Termination of pregnancy should not routinely be offered for women with HL in pregnancy but may require discussion in some cases
- Good communication between the members of the multi-disciplinary team is essential
- If treatment is commenced in pregnancy, regular ultrasound for fetal wellbeing and growth is appropriate
- Cancer is a risk factor for thrombosis, therefore consider need for thromboprophylaxis if other risk factors present (see Section 15.2)

Midwifery Management and Care

- Accurate booking history is essential, and it may be necessary to obtain case notes from outside the area
- Ascertain if a management plan had been made pre-conception
- The mother may be eligible for 'low-risk' care if her condition is well controlled, but this decision should be made by the doctors concerned (see above) as such decisions are outside the scope of midwifery practice
- The mother needs to understand that if her condition deteriorates she will need re-referral to her existing physician to receive 'high-risk' obstetric treatment
- Tactfully ascertain what information has been understood by the mother and husband/partner in relation to her long-term prognosis
- Complex, emotive family issues may arise as child care is considered
- Effective multi-disciplinary teamwork is important, especially if future care arrangements for the baby might have to be made
- Care should be supportive and tailored to individual needs
- Be alert for disease recurrence (previous page) and refer promptly
- Be alert for signs of infection and, if necessary, take relevant swabs or MSU, for culture and sensitivity and refer promptly to a doctor

Labour Issues

Some women with Hodgkin's lymphoma diagnosed after the second trimester will opt to delay treatment until after pregnancy, therefore these women are likely to be delivered early by caesarean section. Some women will undergo early induction of labour for the same reason if successful induction is likely.

Lymphoma is extremely unlikely to metastasise to the placenta.

Medical Management and Care

- If delivery requires expediting early, prescribe steroids as required to optimise fetal lung function, ensure delivery in a hospital with appropriate neonatal facilities and involve the paediatricians in planning delivery
- Mode of delivery is decided depending on factors such as gestation, parity, fetal wellbeing and maternal wishes

Midwifery Management and Care

- Administer any prescribed steroids, as above
- The midwife will be able to manage labour normally in many cases
- Alternatively, the midwife may have to prepare for an operative and/or pre-term birth (see Chapter 1)

Postpartum Issues

- If treatment has been delayed until after pregnancy, it can commence immediately following delivery
- Breast-feeding is not recommended during concurrent treatment with chemotherapy or radiotherapy (see Section 18.1)

Medical Management and Care

- Normal postpartum care
- Consider need for thrombo-prophylaxis (see Section 15.2)

Midwifery Management and Care

- Normal, supportive postnatal care
- Additional attention to thrombo-prophylaxis
- Encourage and support breast-feeding, unless the mother is receiving treatment, when advice on formula feeds and sterilisation of feeding equipment will have to be given to the mother and any others who are likely to be involved in the care of the baby
- Additional support may be required at home, and involvement of social services may be necessary

18.4 Gestational Trophoblastic Disease

Incidence	Risk for Childbearing
1 per 714 live births in UK[1]	Previous GTD – Low Risk
1200 cases per year in UK[2]	Current Choriocarcinoma – High Risk

EXPLANATION OF CONDITION

Gestational trophoblastic disease (GTD) encompasses several related tumours arising from placental tissue.

- **Complete hydatidiform mole** – in this condition the conceptus is diploid and androgenetic in origin. It arises after duplication of the haploid sperm following fertilisation of an empty ovum. There is usually no fetal tissue present.
- **Partial hydatidiform mole** – this is triploid in origin and results from dispermic fertilisation of the ovum. There is often a fetus present.
- **Choriocarcinoma** – this tumour is diagnosed histologically after uterine evacuation. It has the potential to metastasise widely, commonly to the lung and brain.
- **Placental site trophoblastic tumours** – this extremely rare type of tumour (0.23% of all GTD)[3] has a variable prognosis.

GTD most commonly presents with vaginal bleeding in the first trimester, associated with typical ultrasound findings. Historically, the presenting symptoms were: severe early onset pre-eclampsia, large-for-dates uterus, hyperthyroidism or hyperemesis but these presentations are now rare with the availability of first trimester high quality ultrasound[4].

GTD can, rarely, present after an ectopic pregnancy, miscarriage or full-term pregnancy. The usual presenting symptom in these cases is irregular vaginal bleeding[2].

Complete moles are usually diagnosed by ultrasound findings of an anembryonic pregnancy, associated with typical placental appearances. Partial moles can be more difficult to diagnose ultrasonographically[5].

TREATMENT AND CARE

Treatment starts with evacuation of the uterus, which should be surgical in the case of a complete mole[6]. Oxytocic agents should be avoided due to the theoretical risk of causing disseminated trophoblastic disease. The products of conception must be sent for histological confirmation. In view of the difficulty in diagnosing partial moles, it is recommended that tissue for histology is sent following surgical or medical evacuations for all non-viable first trimester pregnancies[7]. Most molar pregnancies remit spontaneously following evacuation of the uterus. In rare circumstances a second uterine evacuation is required[8].

All women with GTD must be registered with the UK Trophoblastic Disease Registration and Surveillance scheme (or other national equivalent) which has been running since 1973. Follow up in the UK is undertaken at three centres, Dundee, Sheffield and London. Women are followed up with serial serum and urinary bHCG levels to allow diagnosis and treatment of persistent trophoblastic disease.

Persistent Trophoblastic Disease

The need for further treatment following a molar pregnancy is identified by evidence of persistent disease activity which is thought unlikely to resolve spontaneously. Persistent trophoblastic disease occurs following 8% of complete moles and 0.5% of partial moles[2].

Chemotherapy is the treatment of choice and this is carried out in Sheffield or London. There are stringent criteria used to identify women needing chemotherapy. These include bHCG level >20,000 after evacuation of retained products of conception (ERPC), static or rising bHCG levels after ERPC, persistent bHCG six months after ERPC or evidence of metastasis[9]. A diagnosis of choriocarcinoma always requires chemotherapy. Prognosis is variable depending on factors including:

- Age
- Length of time following previous pregnancy
- Pre-treatment bHCG level
- Size of tumour
- Site and number of metastases
- Previous failed chemotherapy[9]

Cure rates are high, with an overall survival rate of 94% over 15 years[2]. The highest mortality rate (21%) occurs in women who have developed choriocarcinoma after a normal full-term delivery[10].

Follow up and monitoring of bHCG levels is important to exclude recurrence of disease. At the Sheffield centre, women with a complete mole are followed up for two years and those with a partial mole for one year. Women who have required chemotherapy are followed up for five years.

Diagnosis can have a profound effect on the woman[11], and when discussing clinical findings it is important to acknowledge this as a pregnancy loss[12].

PRE-CONCEPTION ISSUES AND CARE

Women who have had a molar pregnancy have a 1 in 76 chance of having another molar pregnancy. If this occurs it is usually of the same histological type[2].

Women who have had a molar pregnancy are advised not to conceive until six months after their bHCG levels have normalised[5]. The combined oral contraceptive pill (COCP) should be avoided until bHCG levels are normal, and intrauterine contraceptive devices and systems (IUCD, IUS) are best avoided due to bleeding risk. Advise on barrier method contraception, or refer to a family planning clinic.

Women who have required chemotherapy are advised not to conceive for 12 months following completion of treatment due to the theoretical risk of teratogenicity. The risk of recurrent GTD is also highest in the first 12 months following treatment[9]. The above contraceptive advice applies.

Women can be reassured that fertility is generally not affected following chemotherapy and 90% of those who wish to conceive will do so. There is no evidence of increased risk of fetal abnormality[2].

Pregnancy Issues

Women with previous GTD have a 98% chance of having a normal pregnancy[5]. A normal dating scan at 12 weeks gestation should reassure women that their pregnancy is likely to be normal.

A rare situation occasionally arises with a twin pregnancy where one is viable and the other is molar. In this situation, pregnancy can be allowed to continue if the mother wishes as there is no increased risk of developing persistent trophoblastic disease, and the outcome after chemotherapy, if required, is unaffected. These pregnancies are high risk, with increased rates of early miscarriage, second trimester loss and pre-eclampsia. The chance of a successful pregnancy with a live baby is 40%[13].

Medical Management and Care

- Most pregnancies following a molar pregnancy can be managed as low risk with community midwife based care
- If a woman conceives within 12 months of chemotherapy, joint assessment involving obstetrician, oncologist and fetal medicine specialist is required to ascertain the risk of teratogenicity
- In the case of an affected twin pregnancy, regular monitoring for signs of pre-eclampsia is essential; regular scans for growth and fetal wellbeing are indicated

Midwifery Management and Care

- If a midwife identifies a mother in early pregnancy with vaginal discharge/ bleeding, a *large for dates* uterus and possibly hyperemesis, then the mother should be referred to a consultant unit for assessment
- Care should be taken not to alarm the mother, as these symptoms could also be related to a multiple pregnancy

GTD presenting in pregnancy
- The management is as described on the previous page
- In the UK the mother is likely to be admitted to a gynaecological unit and be cared for by nurses; however the midwife may be involved with pre-operative preparation and psychological support
- If the mother is rhesus negative, anti-D is indicated
- In certain circumstances, midwives might be involved with aftercare, and should be alert for haemorrhage; if abnormal bleeding or a 'boggy uterus' present, re-refer to the relevant gynaecological unit

Pregnancy following a molar pregnancy
- Encourage early booking, and take a thorough case history and if necessary obtain former hospital records
- Arrange a dating scan and reassure of the low risk of recurrence
- Ensure that the screening centre where the molar pregnancy was registered is aware that the woman is pregnant to ensure appropriate postnatal follow-up
- In the case of an affected twin pregnancy, provide psychological support and be vigilant for signs of pre-eclampsia

Labour Issues

- Following a previous molar pregnancy, anticipate normal labour
- The mode of delivery for an affected twin pregnancy depends on obstetric factors such as gestation, previous obstetric history and pregnancy complications

Medical Management and Care

- No medical input is required for women with an uncomplicated pregnancy following a molar pregnancy

Midwifery Management and Care

Pregnancy following a molar pregnancy
- Normal midwifery care in labour
- Placental samples are not usually required, but it might be advisable to check with the obstetric team

Postpartum issues

The screening centre for trophoblastic disease where the woman is registered will request postnatal urine bHCG samples to identify recurrent disease.

In rare cases women with no history of molar pregnancy can develop gestational trophoblastic disease following a normal pregnancy. This possibility needs to be considered in women with irregular vaginal bleeding postpartum, a positive bHCG and no evidence of an intra- or extrauterine pregnancy. Prognosis tends to be worse in these women, partly due to delayed diagnosis[10].

Medical Management and Care

- Liaise with appropriate trophoblastic screening centre if any suspicion of recurrent or *de novo* gestational trophoblastic disease
- Advise against the COCP until the bHCG level is within normal levels

Midwifery Management and Care

Pregnancy following a molar pregnancy
- Ensure arrangements have been made for follow-up care; otherwise normal postnatal care is given
- Explain that an HCG urine sample is needed in six weeks, and advise upon practical arrangements
- Be aware that whilst grief over the former pregnancy loss usually resolves by about four months, this can persist in some mothers[12] and might 're-surface' postpartum
- The midwife might have to give advice on barrier methods of contraception if the combined oral contraceptive pill is contraindicated due to high HCG levels[14] (see Pre-conception Care)

18 Neoplasia

PATIENT ORGANISATIONS

Hydatidiform Mole & Choriocarcinoma Support Service
www.hmole-chorio.org.uk

The Miscarriage Association
c/o Clayton Hospital
Northgate, Wakefield
West Yorkshire WF1 3JS
www.miscarriageassociation.org.uk

Lymphoma Association
PO Box 386
Aylesbury
Buckinghamshire HP20 2GA
www.lymphoma.org.uk
www.lifesite.info

Gynae C (Gynaecological cancer)
1 Bolingbroke Road
Swindon
Wiltshire SN2 2LB
www.communigate.co.uk/wilts/gynaec

Cancer Research UK
PO Box 123
Lincoln's Inn Fields
London WC2A 3PX
www.cancerresearchuk.org

CancerHelp UK (aligned to Cancer Research UK)
www.cancerhelp.org.uk

Breast Cancer Care
Kiln House
210 New Kings Road
London SW6 4NZ
www.breastcancercare.org.uk

Marie Curie Cancer Care
89 Albert Embankment
London SE1 7TP
www.mariecurie.org.uk

Macmillan Cancer Support
89 Albert Embankment
London SE1 7UP
www.macmillan.org.uk

Cancerbackup
3 Bath Place
Rivington Street
London EC2A 3JR
www.cancerbackup.org.uk

ESSENTIAL READING

Breast Cancer Care (2005) **Factsheet: Breast cancer during pregnancy**.
www.breastcancercare.org.uk

Grosser, L. (2004) Breast cancer during pregnancy. **British Journal of Midwifery, 12**(5):299–304.

Hatton, C., Collins, G. and Sweetenham, J. (2007) **Fast Facts – Lymphoma**. Oxford; Health Press.

James, D.K., Steer, P.J., Weiner, C.P. and Gonik, B. (2006) Malignant disease. In: **High Risk Pregnancy: Management Options**, 3rd Edn. USA; Elsevier.

Kal, H.B. and Struikmans, H. (2005) Radiotherapy during pregnancy: fact and fiction. **The Lancet, 6,** 328–333.

Karim, S.A. and Shafi, M.I. (2005) Malignancy in pregnancy. **Current Obstetrics and Gynaecology, 15,** 414–416.

McEwan, A. (2002) Cancer in pregnancy. **Current Obstetrics and Gynaecology, 12,** 307–313.

Paterson, G. (2004) Cancer in the pregnant woman. **British Journal of Midwifery, 12**(8):496–501.

RCOG (2004) **Guideline No. 12: Pregnancy and Breast Cancer.** January. London; Royal College of Obstetricians and Gynaecologists.

RCOG (2004) **Guideline No. 38: The Management of Gestational Neoplasia.** February. London; Royal College of Obstetricians and Gynaecologists.

Smith, J.R. and Barron, B.A. (1999) **Fast Facts – Gynaecological Oncology**. Oxford; Health Press.

Thorstensen, K. A. (2000) Midwifery management of first trimester bleeding and early pregnancy loss. **Journal of Midwifery and Women's Health, 45**(6):481–497.

APPENDICES

Appendix 1.1 UK Maternal Deaths – Causes and Risk Factors

Number of deaths from consecutive UK confidential enquiries into maternal mortality[1]

Type of Cause of Death	Triennial Report			
	1994–96	1997–99	2000–02	2003–05
DIRECT CAUSES (up to 42 days postpartum)				
Thrombosis and thrombo-embolism	48	35	30	41
Hypertensive disease of pregnancy	20	15	14	18
Haemorrhage	12	7	17	14
Amniotic fluid embolism	17	8	5	17
Ectopic pregnancy	12	13	11	10
Spontaneous miscarriage	2	2	1	1
Legal termination of pregnancy	1	2	3	2
Other early pregnancy deaths	0	0	0	1
Genital tract sepsis	14	14	11	18
Genital tract trauma	5	2	1	3
Fatty liver	2	4	3	1
Anaesthetic	1	3	6	6
Other direct causes	0	1	4	0
Total number of direct deaths	**134**	**106**	**106**	**132**
INDIRECT CAUSES (up to 42 days postpartum)				
Cardiac	39	35	44	48
Psychiatric	9	15	16	18
Other indirect causes	86	75	90	87
Indirect malignancies	N/A	11	5	10
Total number of indirect deaths	**134**	**136**	**155**	**163**
COINCIDENTAL DEATHS	**36**	**29**	**36**	**55**
LATE DEATHS (42–365 days postpartum)				
Direct causes	4	7	4	11
Indirect causes	32	39	45	71
Coincidental	36	61	45	–
Total number of late deaths	**72**	**107**	**94**	**82**
Total of all deaths	**376**	**378**	**391**	**432**

Risk factors for maternal deaths from CEMACH 'Why Mothers Die 2000–2002' Report[2]

Factor	Risk
Social disadvantage	20 times more likely to die
Poor communities	45% higher death rate
Minority ethnic groups	3 times more likely to die
Black African women (especially newly arrived and asylum seekers)	7 times more likely to die
Late booking or poor attendance	20% of direct and indirect maternal deaths
Obesity	35% of the women who died in 2000–02*
Substance abuse	8% of the women who died in 2000–02**
Domestic violence	14% of the women who died in 2000–02***

* This table is not repeated in the 2003–05 report, where over 50% of the women who died were either overweight or obese, with 15% being morbidly obese having a BMI of 35 or above.
** 11% had problems with substance abuse, again showing an increase[3].
*** The incidence remained static at 14% for domestic violence.
Reproduced from the sixth[1,2] and seventh[3] reports of the Confidential Enquiries into Maternal Death, with the permission of the Royal College of Obstetricians and Gynaecologists, and from CEMACH.

Appendix 1.2 UK Maternal Deaths by Type of Antenatal Care and Place of Delivery

Maternal death by type of antenatal care, United Kingdom 2003–05[1]

Type of Antenatal Care	Classification of Death					
	Direct n	Indirect n	Direct & Indirect n ~ %	Coincidental n	Late n	TOTAL n ~ %
Team-based or 'shared' care	54	60	114 ~ 39%	17	6	137 ~ 33%
Consultant-led unit only	15	39	54 ~ 18%	9	1	64 ~ 15%
Midwife only	11	16	27 ~ 9%	8	0	35 ~ 8%
Midwife and GP	5	4	9 ~ 3%	6	6	18 ~ 4%
Death before booking or after miscarriage or ToP	22	9	31 ~ 11%	5	0	36 ~ 9%
Unaware of pregnancy	5	1	6 ~ 2%	1	0	7 ~ 2%
Suboptimal antenatal care: • Concealed pregnancy • No antenatal care • Late booking/poor attender	3 4 11	2 6 24	5 ~ 2% 10 ~ 3% 35 ~ 12%	0 4 5	0 0 1	5 ~ 1% 14 ~ 3% 41 ~ 10%
Not stated	2	2	4 ~ 1%	55	0	59 ~ 14%
Total	132	163	295 ~ 100%	110	14	416 ~ 100%

Source: Table 1.4 from the CEMACH Report 'Saving Mothers' Lives' 2003-05

Maternal death by place of delivery, United Kingdom 1994–2005

Venue	Triennial Report			
	1994–96	1997–99	2000–02	2003–05
Consultant-led Obstetric Unit	152	132	152	202
Stand alone GP/midwife-led birth centre	1	3	1	2
Accident and Emergency Department	12	11	15	14
Intensive Care Unit	2	2	1	4
Hospital other	0	3	3	5
Home	2	4	3	3
Total	169	155	175	230

Source: Table 22.9 from the CEMACH Report 'Why Mothers Die 2000–2002'[2]
Table 1.6 from the CEMACH Report 'Saving Mothers' Lives 2003–05'[3]

Adapted and reproduced from the sixth and seventh[3] reports of the Confidential Enquiries into Maternal Death, with the permission of the Royal College of Obstetricians and Gynaecologists, and from CEMACH.

Appendix 1.3 Daily Vitamin and Mineral Dietary Intake for Pregnancy and Lactation

Vitamin[1,2]	RDA (Recommended Daily Dietary Amount/Allowance)*	Sources[1,2]	Overdose[2]	Notes
A Retinol	Pregnancy 2700–8000 IU[3] Lactation 3–4000 IU[3,4]	Liver, fish liver oil, green leafy vegetables, carrots, yellow fruits, egg yolks, enriched margarine, milk products	A fat soluble vitamin which accumulates in the body[2]. Overdose in pregnancy can be dangerous[3]. 8000 IU is the maximum dose. High doses may be teratogenic[3].	Pregnant women should not take supplements, and should avoid eating liver[3].
B₁ Thiamine	Pregnancy 1.5 mg[3] Lactation 1.6 mg[3]	Yeast products, liver, rice, wholemeal products, peanuts, pork, milk	A water-soluble vitamin that is excreted in urine, so overdose unlikely[2].	Destroyed by alcohol[2].
B₂ Riboflavin	Pregnancy 1.6 mg[3] Lactation 1.8 mg[3]	Yeast products, milk, liver, fish, cheese, green leafy vegetables	A water-soluble vitamin that is excreted in urine, so no danger of overdose.	Destroyed by alcohol[2].
B₆ Pyridoxine	Pregnancy 2.2 mg[3] Lactation 2.1 mg[3]	Fish, bananas, chicken, pork, wholegrains, dried beans	May cause nerve problems in large doses. Conflicting evidence about maximum safe dose.	Destroyed by alcohol and the contraceptive pill[2].
B₁₂ Cobalamin	Pregnancy 2.2 µg[3] Lactation 2.6 µg[3]	Fish, liver, beef, pork, milk and cheese	A water-soluble vitamin that is excreted in urine, so no danger of overdose.	
C Ascorbic Acid	Pregnancy 70 mg[3] Lactation 95 mg[3]	Citrus fruits, berries, tomatoes, cauliflower, green leafy vegetables, peppers	Large doses can cause diarrhoea. Excessive doses, ≥1000 mg, *might* damage DNA.	
D	Pregnancy 400 IU[3] Lactation 400 IU[3]	80% from sunlight 20% from cod liver oil, sardines, herrings, salmon, tuna, and milk products	A fat-soluble vitamin which accumulates in the body[2]. High doses are teratogenic in animals[3].	Australia advocates daily sunlight exposure 15 min to prevent deficiency[5]; no data for the UK.
E Tocopherol	Pregnancy 10 mg[3] Lactation 12 mg[3]	Eggs, nuts, soya, wholemeal products, beans, vegetable oil, broccoli, sprouts, spinach	A fat-soluble vitamin with a slight risk of overdose.	
Folic Acid	Pre-conception 0.4 mg[3] Pregnancy 0.4 mg[3] Lactation 0.28 mg[3] NB: Higher doses are given for folate deficiency[3].	Liver, yeast products, egg yolk, carrots, melon, apricots, avocado, beans, whole wheat, green leafy vegetables	A water-soluble vitamin that is excreted in urine, so no danger of overdose.	Essential for production of erythrocytes and other body cells. Use in periconception period reduces risk of neural tube defects.
Mineral	**RDA**	**Sources[1,2]**	**Overdose[2]**	**Notes**
Calcium	Pregnancy 1000 mg[4] Lactation 1000 mg[4]	Dairy products and green leafy vegetables	High doses lead to hypertension, headaches, renal or gall bladder stones[2].	
Iron	Pregnancy 27mg[4**] Lactation 9 mg[4]	Red meat, oily fish, egg yolk, green leafy vegetables, dried apricots, nuts, wholegrain foods	Iron accumulates in the body. High doses lead to nausea and constipation and can be fatal.	Deficiency leads to anaemia. Best taken with folic acid to aid absorption.
Magnesium	Pregnancy 350 mg[4] Lactation 310 mg[4]	Green leafy vegetables, wholegrain foods, nuts	High dose causes diarrhoea.	
Zinc	Pregnancy 11 mg[4] Lactation 12 mg[4]	Meat, shellfish, milk, brown rice and wholegrain foods	High dose results in nausea and vomiting.	

* RDA figures are based on the USA National Academy of Sciences Recommendations[3,4].

** This figure is lower in the UK, and the exact dosage is debated in the midwifery press.

Appendix 2 Dermatoses Specific to Pregnancy

Any blistering rash in pregnancy requires urgent referral for a medical opinion.

Intrahepatic cholestasis of pregnancy (see Chapter 10)

- Onset is usually in the third trimester
- Initially pruritus may be localised, e.g. palms and soles, but later more generalised
- There are no skin lesions just excoriations
- The condition resolves after delivery
- Obstetric cholestasis (OC) occurs occasionally in some patients postpartum if given the combined oral contraceptive pill

Treatment: emollients and topical antipruritic agents, such as 0.5% menthol in aqueous cream. Further management of OC is discussed in Chapter 10.

Polymorphic eruption of pregnancy

(Pruritic urticarial papules and plaques of pregnancy) (PUPP)

- Occurs in 1:200 pregnancies, is the commonest rash peculiar to pregnancy and is of unknown course
- It usually occurs in the third trimester in the abdominal striae and spares the umbilicus
- A variety of lesions occur:
  - urticarial papules
  - plaques
  - polycyclic lesions, sometimes with small vesicles
- The rash is itchy and usually spreads but rarely involves the palms, soles or face
- It disappears one week after delivery and there is no risk for mother or baby
- Recurrence with subsequent pregnancies is unusual

Treatment: symptomatic, with emollients, topical steroid creams and, if severe, oral prednisolone.

Pemphigoid gestationis

This is a rare autoimmune blistering disease occurring in 1:50,000 pregnancies. It starts in the second or third trimester (occasionally postpartum) with pruritic urticarial-like lesions, often around the umbilicus.

- May progress to become more generalised and bullous
- Involvement of the palms, soles of the feet and face may occur

- Occasionally improves in late pregnancy or 'flares' after delivery
- In some cases the rash recurs with menstruation or the combined OCP
- Occasionally there are transient bullous lesions in the baby
- Referral to the dermatology department is necessary for a skin biopsy to confirm the diagnosis and for further management

Treatment: high dose steroids or, if steroid resistant, ciclosporin and/or plasmapheresis may be necessary.

Prurigo of pregnancy

- This can occur during any trimester and its cause is unknown
- There is an increased risk if the woman has a history of atopy
- The rash consists of itchy papules and nodules on the extensor surfaces of the limbs and sometimes on the abdomen
- There is no adverse effect for the mother or baby

Treatment: symptomatic with medium potency steroid creams, oral antihistamines and protective bandages.

Pruritic folliculitis of pregnancy

This occurs from 16–40 weeks of pregnancy with follicular papules and sterile pustules which are widely distributed. The cause is unknown and it will resolve within three weeks postpartum. There is no risk to mother or baby.

Treatment: topical steroids, benzoyl peroxide, UVB phototherapy.

Impetigo herpetiformis

This is a rare skin condition and some dermatologists regard it as pustular psoriasis in pregnancy.

- There are erythematous patches with sterile pustules at the edges
- The patients are unwell, with fever, malaise and diarrhoea and vomiting
- There is significant risk to the mother of tetany, seizures and hepatic and renal impairment
- There is also a high risk of stillbirth
- **These patients require urgent dermatology referral for diagnosis**

Treatment: high dose steroids and early-timed delivery.

Appendix 3.1 British Hypertension Society's Blood Pressure Measurement Recommendations

WITH MERCURY BLOOD PRESSURE MONITORS[1]

- The patient should be seated for at least five minutes, relaxed and not moving or speaking
- The arm must be supported at the level of the heart
- Ensure no tight clothing constricts the arm
- Place the cuff on neatly, with the centre of the bladder over the brachial artery
- The bladder should encircle at least 80% of the arm (but not more than 100%)
- The column of mercury must be vertical, and at observer's eye level
- Estimate the systolic pressure beforehand:
  - palpate the brachial artery
  - inflate cuff until pulsation disappears
  - deflate cuff
  - estimate systolic pressure
- Then inflate to 30 mmHg above the estimated systolic level needed to occlude the pulse
- Place the stethoscope diaphragm over the brachial artery and deflate at a rate of 2–3 mm/sec until you hear regular tapping sounds
- Measure systolic (first sound) and diastolic (disappearance) to the nearest 2 mmHg

Cuff Sizes	Width (cm)	Length (cm)	Bladder width and length (cm)	Arm circumference (cm)
Small adult/child	10–12	18–24	12 × 18	<23
Standard adult	12–13	23–35	12 × 26	<33
Large adult	12–16	35–40	12 × 40	<50
Adult thigh cuff	20	42		<53

Points to Note

- The date of next servicing should be clearly marked on the sphygmomanometer (six monthly)
- All maintenance necessitating handling of mercury should be conducted by the manufacturer or specialised service units
- Aneroid manometers tend to deteriorate and need regular checking
- In many instances aneroid monitors cannot be corrected accurately, therefore they should not be used as a substitute for mercury sphygmomanometers

WITH ELECTRONIC BLOOD PRESSURE MONITORS[2]

- The patient should be seated for at least 5 minutes, relaxed and not moving or speaking
- The arm must be supported at the level of the heart
- Ensure no tight clothing constricts the arm
- Place the cuff on neatly, with the centre of the bladder over the brachial artery
- The bladder should encircle at least 80% of the arm (but not more than 100%)
- Most monitors allow manual blood pressure setting selection where you chose the appropriate setting; other monitors will automatically inflate and re-inflate to the next setting if required
- Repeat three times and record measurement as displayed
- Initially test blood pressure in both arms, and use arm with highest reading for subsequent measurement

Cuff Sizes	Width (cm)	Length (cm)	Bladder width and length (cm)	Arm circumference (cm)
Small adult/child	10–12	18–24	12 × 18	<23
Standard adult	12–13	23–35	12 × 26	<33
Large adult	12–16	35–40	12 × 40	<50
Adult thigh cuff	20	42		<53

Points to Note

- If checking against a mercury sphygmomanometer the blood pressure may differ slightly between devices
- It is good practice to occasionally check the monitor against a mercury sphygmomanometer or another validated device
- It is important to have a monitor calibrated according to the manufacturer's instructions

NB: A4-size colour posters of both of these columns can be downloaded from the BHS website as www.bhsoc/bp_monitors/BLOOD_PRESSURE_1784a.pdf www.bhsoc/bp_monitors/BLOOD_PRESSURE_1784b.pdf

Reproduced with kind permission of the British Hypertension Society.

Appendix 3.2 Blood Pressure Devices for Use in Pregnancy and Obesity

This section outlines blood pressure measuring devices that have been tested according to the revised BHS protocol (1993) and/or the International Protocol and/or the AAMI Protocol, that have met the British Hypertension Society's criteria and that are currently available in the UK[1]. To meet these criteria, devices must achieve a minimum B grade for both systolic and diastolic measurements for the revised BHS protocol or pass the accepted criteria of the International Protocol or the AAMI Protocol[1]. The references for each of these protocols can be found on the Publications page of the British Hypertension Society's website, www.bhsoc.org/Blood_pressure_Publications.stm.

Further details, including links to distributors, can be found on www.bhsoc.org/bp_monitors/special.stm.

Pregnancy and Pre-eclampsia

Device
Microlife 3BTO-A (2)[2]
Arm monitor

Grade
Validated for use in pregnancy and pre-eclampsia
BHS A/B

Cuff Sizes
Standard Adult – 22–32 cm
Large adult – 32–42 cm
These cuffs are included for accurate blood pressure measurement in pregnancy as weight and arm circumference increase

Weight
430 g

Dimensions
$180 \times 114 \times 75$ mm

Batteries
Uses $4 \times$ AA batteries
Mains adaptor also available

Obese Adults and the Elderly

Device
Omron 637-IT[3]
Wrist monitor

Grade
Validated for use in obese adults and the elderly
International protocol

Cuff Size
Fits 13.5–21.5 cm

Weight
165 g

Dimensions
$79 \times 66.5 \times 38$ cm

Batteries
$2 \times$ AAA alkaline batteries

Reproduced with kind permission of the British Hypertension Society.

Appendix 4.1 Glossary of Cardiac Terms

Afterload: the amount of resistance to ejection of blood from a ventricle.

Anuria: urine output of less than 50 ml per 24 hours.

Atrial fibrillation: the normal regular rhythm of the heartbeat is lost and replaced by an irregular rhythm which may be episodic (paroxysmal atrial fibrillation) or persistent. The loss of normal atrial contraction produces a risk of clot formation in the atria. Anticoagulation and drugs to slow the heart rate are required.

Cardiac failure: heart failure; cardiac output insufficient to meet the demands of the body resulting in shortness of breath, pulmonary oedema, peripheral oedema and tiredness.

Cardiac output (CO): the amount of blood pumped out of the heart in one minute.

Cardioversion: the procedure of applying electrical shock to the chest to change an abnormal heartbeat into a normal one.

Compliance: the elasticity or amount of 'give' when blood enters the ventricle.

Congestive heart failure (CHF): a fluid overload condition (congestion) that may or may not be caused by HF; often an acute presentation of HF with increased amount of fluid in the blood vessels.

Contractility: the force of ventricular contraction; related to the number and state of myocardial cells.

Diastolic heart failure: the inability of the heart to pump sufficiently because of an alteration in the ability of the heart to fill; current term used to describe a type of HF.

Dyspnoea on exertion (DOE): shortness of breath that occurs with exertion.

Ejection fraction (EF): percent of blood volume in the ventricles at the end of diastole that is ejected during systole; a measurement of contractility.

Electrical cardioversion: used to shock the heart back into normal rhythm. If this procedure is necessary, it is carried out under general anaesthesia.

Heart failure (HF): the inability of the heart to pump sufficient blood to meet the needs of the tissues for oxygen and nutrients; signs and symptoms of pulmonary and systemic congestion may or may not be present.

Ischaemia: inability to supply adequate oxygen leading to tissue damage or death.

Left-sided heart failure (left ventricular failure): inability of the left ventricle to fill or pump (empty) sufficient blood to meet the needs of the tissues for oxygen and nutrients; traditional term used to describe patient's HF symptoms.

Oliguria: diminished urine output; less than 400 ml per 24 hours.

Orthopnoea: shortness of breath when lying flat.

Paroxysmal nocturnal dyspnoea (PND): shortness of breath that occurs suddenly during sleep.

Pericardiocentesis: procedure that involves surgically entering the pericardial sac, usually with a needle.

Pericardiotomy: surgically-created opening of the pericardium.

Pre-load: the amount of myocardial stretch just before systole caused by the pressure created by the volume of blood within a ventricle.

Pulmonary hypertension: elevated blood pressure in the pulmonary arteries from constriction; causes problems with the blood flow in the lungs, and makes the heart work harder. If left untreated, this can lead to heart failure.

Pulmonary oedema: abnormal accumulation of fluid occurring in the interstitial spaces or in the alveoli of the lungs.

Pulseless electrical activity (PEA): condition in which electrical activity is present but there is not an adequate pulse or blood pressure because of ineffective cardiac contraction or circulating blood volume.

Pulsus paradoxus: systolic blood pressure that is more than 10 mmHg higher during exhalation than during inspiration; difference is normally less than 10 mmHg.

Right-sided heart failure (right ventricular failure): inability of the right ventricle to fill or pump (empty) sufficient blood to the pulmonary circulation.

Stroke volume (SV): amount of blood pumped out of the ventricle with each contraction.

Systolic heart failure: inability of the heart to pump sufficiently because of an alteration in the ability of the heart to contract; current term used to describe a type of heart failure (HF).

Thermo-dilution: method of determining cardiac output that involves injecting fluid into the pulmonary artery catheter. A thermistor measures the difference between the temperature of the fluid and the temperature of the blood ejected from the ventricle. Cardiac output is calculated from the change in temperature.

Thrombolytic therapy: Treatment to break up blood clots in the circulatory system.

Ventricular ejection fraction: (see ejection fraction).

NB: Cardiac abbreviations are to be found within the glossary of abbreviations at the beginning of this book.

Appendix 4.2 New York Heart Association 1994 Classification of Heart Disease

Classification of Functional Capacity and Objective Assessment

In 1928 the New York Heart Association published a classification of patients with cardiac disease based on clinical severity and prognosis. This classification has been updated in seven subsequent editions of *Nomenclature and Criteria for Diagnosis of Diseases of the Heart and Great Vessels* (Little, Brown & Co.). The ninth edition, revised by the Criteria Committee of the American Heart Association, New York City Affiliate, was released on 4th March 1994. The new classifications are summarised below[1].

Functional Capacity

Class	Description
I	Patients with cardiac disease but without resulting limitation of physical activity. Ordinary physical activity does not cause undue fatigue, palpitation, dyspnoea or anginal pain.
II	Patients with cardiac disease resulting in slight limitation of physical activity. They are comfortable at rest. Ordinary physical activity results in fatigue, palpitation, dyspnoea or anginal pain.
III	Patients with cardiac disease resulting in marked limitation of physical activity. They are comfortable at rest. Less than ordinary activity causes fatigue, palpitation, dyspnoea or anginal pain.
IV	Patients with cardiac disease resulting in inability to carry on any physical activity without discomfort. Symptoms of heart failure or the anginal syndrome may be present even at rest. If any physical activity is undertaken, discomfort increases.

Objective Assessment

A. No objective evidence of cardiovascular disease
B. Objective evidence of minimal cardiovascular disease
C. Objective evidence of moderately severe cardiovascular disease
D. Objective evidence of severe cardiovascular disease

Examples

- A patient with minimal or no symptoms but a large pressure gradient across the aortic valve or severe obstruction of the left main coronary artery is classified:
  Function Capacity I, Objective Assessment D
- A patient with severe anginal syndrome but angiographically normal coronary arteries is classified:
  Functional Capacity IV, Objective Assessment A

Reproduced with kind permission of the American Heart Association.

Appendix 4.3 Drugs for Cardiac Disease – An Overview for Midwives

This table is to give the midwife an **overview** of cardiac drug use and the implications for pregnancy. These drugs are prescribed, by a doctor, if the expected benefit to the mother outweighs any effect upon the fetus (see legend).

Type of Drug	Name	Risk		Notes
		Pregnancy[1]	Breast-feeding	
Diuretics to reduce fluid retention	Amiloride	B	Probably compatible[1]	
	Bumetanide	C	Probably compatible[1]	Used for prompt diuresis[3]
	Chlorothiazide	C	Compatible[1]	
	Frusemide/Furosemide	C	Probably compatible[1]	
	Spironolactone	C	Probably compatible[1]	
ACE inhibitors to lower BP and treat heart failure	Captopril	C	Compatible[1]	Teratogenic risk in first trimester (animal studies) and fetal renal toxicity in second and third trimesters (human data)[1,3,5]. Most cardiologists stop ACE inhibitors promptly pre-conception and restart them post delivery.
	Enalapril	C	Probably compatible[1]	
	Lisinopril	C	Probably compatible[1]	
	Losartan	C	Probably compatible[1]	
	Ramipril	C	Probably compatible[1]	
	Valsartan	C	Probably compatible[1]	
Beta-blockers to reduce frequency/force of the heartbeat, treat heart failure, lower BP	Atenolol	D	Potential toxicity[1]	All may cause minor growth restriction[1,3,5] in second and third trimesters, but this is rarely of clinical significance. Some are excreted to a lesser extent than others in breast milk, hence a prescriber should seek individual drug details.
	Carvedilol	C	Potential toxicity[1]	
	Metoprolol	C	Potential toxicity[1]	
	Nadolol	C	Potential toxicity[1]	
	Propranolol	C	Potential toxicity[1]	
	Sotalol	B	Potential toxicity[1]	
Nitrates to dilate coronary arteries	Glyceryl trinitrate/ nitroglycerin	B	Probably compatible[1]	
	Isosorbide mono-/dinitrate	C	Probably compatible[1]	
Anti-arrhythmics to steady an irregular heartbeat	Adenosine	C	Probably compatible[1]	Maternal benefit >> fetal risk[1]
	Amiodarone	**D**	**Contraindicated**[1]	Pregnancy risk
	Bretylium	C	Hold breast-feeding[1]	No pregnancy data[1]
	Digoxin/digitalis	C	Compatible[1]	
	Disopyramide	C	Probably compatible[1]	Risk in 3rd trimester[1]
	Flecainide	C	Probably compatible[1]	Moderate risk[1]
	Verapamil	C	Probably compatible[1]	
Anticoagulants	Aspirin – low dose	Safe[2]	Safe[2]	See NSAID in Appendix 11
	Aspirin – standard	C	Use with caution[1]	
	Heparin	C	Compatible[1]	Does not pass to placenta or breast[1]
	Dalteparin	B	Compatible[1]	Low molecular weight heparins
	Enoxiparin	B		
	Warfarin	**D or X**	Compatible[1]	One manufacturer rates X[1] Contraindicated in first trimester[1]
Antihypertensives to lower blood pressure	Doxazocin	C	Potential toxicity[1]	
	Methyldopa	B	Probably compatible[1]	
	Nifedipine	C	Probably compatible[1]	See vasodilators in Appendix 11
	Nicardipine	C	Probably compatible[1]	
Others to treat pulmonary hypertension	Prostacycline/epoprostenol	B	Probably compatible[1]	
	Sildenafil (Viagra; Revatio)	No data	No data	
	Bosentan	X	**Contraindicated**[5]	Contraindicated pregnancy/lactation[3,5]

Key: Pregnancy risk factors[1]: **A** = Little or no risk (human studies)[1]; **B** = Little risk (animal studies)[1]; **C** = Some adverse effects (animal studies); used if benefit outweighs risk[1]; **D** = Positive evidence of risk (human studies); used with serious conditions[1]; **X** = Risk outweighs possible benefits, contraindicated in pregnancy[1]

Midwives: Mothers should be advised to continue with existing medication until a doctor with experience of prescribing such medications in pregnancy has been consulted, because sudden cessation of any medication without careful thought for substitution can be associated with adverse feto-maternal outcome.

Doctors: This simple table cannot address factors for prescribing, and a more authoritative source **must** be used, e.g. **British National Formulary**, latest issue from the BMA, or on-line www.bnf.org.; Briggs, G.G., Freeman, R.K. and Yaffe, S.J. (2005) **Drugs in Pregnancy and Lactation**, 7th Ed. USA; Lippincott.

Appendix 5 Asthma in Pregnancy: An Information Leaflet for Pregnant Women

Congratulations on your pregnancy!
The maternal medicine clinic aims to make your pregnancy as problem-free as possible. We try to ensure that you receive the best possible care for your pregnancy and asthma in one location, and to reduce the stress of appointments in several different places. Occasionally we may need to refer you to see a chest consultant.

Naturally you may be a little worried about how your asthma may affect your unborn baby. We hope to dispel some of your common concerns with this leaflet. If this leaflet does not answer all your questions, please ask us and we will try to find out for you.

Asthma is a common condition. Approximately 5% of pregnant women suffer from asthma. We know that approximately one third will see no change in their condition during pregnancy, one third will improve and one third may get worse. It is difficult to predict which category you will fall into.

Will my asthma affect my unborn baby?
It is important that your asthma is well controlled. As you will know, your baby relies on you for his/her supply of oxygen. You are 'breathing for two'. If you are unwell with asthma, your baby may not receive sufficient oxygen and your baby's growth may be affected.

Is it safe to take my asthma medications during pregnancy?
Yes. One of the common concerns of pregnant women with asthma is whether the medication they take for their asthma will affect their baby. There are no known harmful effects from inhaled relievers (e.g. Ventolin, Serevent and Bricanyl) or inhaled steroids (Becotide, Pulmicort or Flixotide). It is therefore safe to take them.

If you need oral steroids (prednisolone) regularly to control your asthma, then you should take them. The benefits of well-controlled asthma outweigh any risk. There is known to be minimal effect with using them. Some of the newer drugs, such as Singular, are untested in pregnancy. However, it is far more harmful to have poorly controlled asthma. Your medications are designed to help you. By keeping you well, they help your baby to develop normally.

What can I safely use for pain relief in labour?
Most drugs are safe to use in labour for most women, but discuss what is on offer and make an informed decision.

You may like to talk to one of our consultant anaesthetists, particularly if your asthma is difficult to control. They will discuss the options with you. They will also discuss your options should the need for a caesarean section arise. An epidural or spinal anaesthetic is generally the safest option for all women, but especially for women with breathing problems.

Will my asthma become worse in labour?
This is rare, but please do not forget to bring **all** your normal medication in with you when you come to hospital. It may help to keep a reliever (blue inhaler) packed in your suitcase ready for coming in.

Can I labour in a *Home from Home* room?
This will depend upon how bad your asthma is. It also depends on how well controlled it is during your pregnancy and at time of labour. Discuss this with your midwife, but remember, nothing is *written in stone* and circumstances or decisions can change. Obviously if you are unwell at the time of labour we will need to monitor the condition of you and your baby closely – and then Home from Home would not be an option.

Will it be safe to breast-feed my baby?
Breast-feeding is the recommended method of feeding for all women, particularly if you suffer from allergies. Recent research shows that children who are breast-fed for the first four months of life are less likely to wheeze at six years of age. The amounts of inhaled drugs and even oral steroids that enter breast milk are extremely small. If you are taking **theophylline** it may be better if you take it **after** feeding your baby, to minimise side effects.

What advice should I seek from a professional?
We aim to see all women with moderate or severe asthma in the maternal medicine clinic at booking, then at 28 and 36 weeks of pregnancy. We would also see any asthmatic woman whose condition worsened during pregnancy. Examples of circumstances when you should seek advice include any **one** of the following:

- **Worsening symptoms where you use your reliever more than four times a day**
- **Your reliever is not working, or it works for less than four hours**
- **Being awakened at night by asthma symptoms**
- **Shortness of breath on exertion**
- **Persistent cough**
- **Peak flow below 60% of your normal best**

Who should I contact?
Speak to your community midwife, practice nurse or GP. Ask them to refer you to the maternal medicine clinic, or telephone the clinic directly and ask to speak to a midwife.
Important telephone numbers are …………..

Finally
Don't forget that smoking is harmful to you and your inborn baby, so we advise you to stop. For advice please telephone
………………………..

On the whole your pregnancy should be uneventful. We will work together to make sure it stays that way, but please contact us if you have any concerns.
The Maternal Medicine Team

Appendix 6 Replacement of Renal Function by Dialysis

In medicine, dialysis is a method of replacing renal function that has been lost due to either acute or chronic renal failure. Dialysis works on the principle of diffusion of low molecular weight solutes down a concentration gradient across a semi-permeable membrane. Fluid can be removed by exerting a hydrostatic or osmotic gradient across the membrane. Blood is present on one side of the semi-permeable membrane and dialysis fluid on the other.

The concentration of undesired solutes, such as potassium, in the dialysis fluid is low and a buffer is also present to facilitate the removal of metabolic acid. There are two types of dialysis.

HAEMODIALYSIS (HD)

During haemodialysis the patient's blood is pumped by machine through a filter (dialyser) containing a semi-permeable membrane with a large surface area. A physiological dialysis fluid (dialysate), is pumped on the other side of the semi-permeable membrane in the opposite direction. Excess water and metabolic waste products are cleared from the blood by the processes of diffusion, convection and ultrafiltration.

To prevent the blood from clotting whilst circulating through the machine, a low dose of heparin is infused into the blood tubing.

Normally a patient will receive haemodialysis three times per week, for approximately four hours at a time. Some dialysis patients pass no urine at all, and fluid intake is usually restricted to only 500 ml per day (equivalent to daily insensible losses through breathing, sweating, etc.), plus the amount of the previous days urinary output. Otherwise, in between dialyses this fluid will accumulate in the body causing 'overload', hypertension and pulmonary oedema.

There are other dietary restrictions such as potassium, which if elevated will cause cardiac arrhythmias, and phosphate which can accumulate and lead to renal bone disease and extravascular calcification.

Access to the vascular system is required for haemodialysis by:

- Insertion of a dual lumen catheter (VasCath) into a major vein
- Arterio-venous fistula: surgical procedure to join together an artery and a vein, usually at the wrist; blood from the artery then flows directly into the vein, the increased pressure causes the vein to thicken and dilate
- Arterio-venous graft (synthetic such as Gore-Tex®), again between the artery and a vein, just beneath the skin

It is very important not to cannulate, or take blood, or blood pressure on the arm with the graft or the fistula, as this may cause unnecessary damage to it.

PERITONEAL DIALYSIS (PD)

With PD, the peritoneal membrane serves as a semi-permeable membrane and its blood supply provides blood flow. After the insertion of a soft plastic tube into the peritoneal cavity, dialysis fluid (usually ~2 l), is infused. The fluid is left to dwell in the peritoneal cavity, dialysis occurs and the fluid is then drained out and discarded. Fresh fluid is instilled back into the peritoneal cavity and the cycle is repeated.

Most commonly patients perform four exchanges per day, at breakfast, lunch, teatime, and bedtime, and the fluid remains in the abdomen for approximately four hours between exchanges. This is called continuous ambulatory peritoneal dialysis (CAPD). Another alternative is to use a machine that automatically cycles the fluid exchanges in and out of the peritoneal cavity continuously overnight whilst the patient sleeps. This is called automated peritoneal dialysis (APD).

The composition of the dialysis fluid is similar to that used for haemodialysis. The major difference is that PD fluid contains high concentrations of glucose to enable the removal of fluid from the patient by osmosis. Therefore, for example, a patient may instil in 2 l of fluid and then later drain out 2.5 l of fluid.

The PD fluid is prepared with different glucose concentrations so that the amount of fluid removal can, to some degree, be tailored to individual patient requirements. Because this fluid is warm and sugary, there is a high chance of infection. This may result in PD peritonitis, a painful and potentially serious complication of treatment. Scrupulous hygiene is therefore required when changing the bags.

Dietary restrictions are less rigorous for PD patients because dialysis is occurring constantly. Patients must avoid constipation, as this will restrict the draining out of the dialysis fluid.

Appendix 7 Diabetes Mellitus

CRITERIA FOR THE DIAGNOSIS OF DIABETES MELLITUS

The 1999 WHO Revised Criteria for Glucose Intolerance:

- Diabetes mellitus requires symptoms of hyperglycaemia and a fasting venous plasma glucose concentration ≥7.0 mmol/l and/or random venous plasma glucose ≥11.1 mmol/l
- Otherwise an oral glucose tolerance test is required:

75 g Oral Glucose Tolerance Test		Venous Plasma Glucose Concentration (mmol/l)
Diabetes mellitus	Fasting	≥7.0
	2 hr	≥11.1
Impaired glucose tolerance	Fasting	<7.0
	2 hr	≥7.8 and <11.1
Increased fasting glucose	Fasting	≥6.1 and <7.0
	2 hr	<7.8

SUGGESTED REGIMEN FOR MANAGEMENT OF DIABETES DURING LABOUR

The target capillary blood glucose should be within the range of 4–8mmol/l.
Once the woman is in established labour insert an iv cannula and infuse:

- Line 1: 5% D-glucose + 10 mmol potassium chloride 500 ml at 100 ml/hour
- Line 2: 0.9% sodium chloride 49.5 ml + human soluble insulin (50 IU) via a syringe driver
- Titrate the rate of infusion against capillary blood glucose level according to the scale below
- Give parallel infusions through a Y-connector; avoid 3-way taps
- Monitor glucose hourly during labour
- All results to be charted by the midwife

Capillary Blood Glucose Concentration (mmol/L)	Insulin Infusion Rate (IU/h)
<3.5	• Stop infusion and recheck blood glucose in 20 minutes • Inform doctor
3.5–4	0.5
4.1–7	1.0
7.1–11	2.0
11.1–14	3.0
14.1–17	4.0
>17	8.0 • Check urine for ketones and inform doctor

- After delivery continue infusion until woman is able to eat and drink
- Subcutaneous insulin must be given 30 minutes before the infusion is stopped

FEATURES OF THE METABOLIC SYNDROME

Abnormal glucose tolerance (type 2 diabetes or IGT) plus two or more of the following:

- Insulin resistance
- Central obesity
  - body mass index >30 kg/m^2
  - waist:hip ratio >0.85 (females)
- Hypertension: BP >160/90 mmHg
- Dyslipidaemia
  - fasting triglycerides >1.7 mmol/l
  - HDL-cholesterol <1.0 mmol/l (females)
- Microalbuminuria
- Albumin:creatinine ratio >3.5 (females)

Appendix 8.1 Drugs Used for Neurological Conditions

Drug Name	Possible Side Effects	Potential Effects on Fetus	Rate of Major Congenital Malformation (MCM) (%)
Carbamazepine	Acne, hirsutism, dizziness, double vision, headaches, decreased appetite, aplastic anaemia, thrombocytopenia, erythrocytopenia, leucocytopenia, hypotension, vitamin K deficiency and folate deficiency	• Neural tube defects • Craniofacial defects • Digital defects • Cardiac malformations • Developmental delay	2.2[1]
Phenytoin	Slurred speech, ataxia, insomnia, twitching, nausea, vomiting, constipation, rash with fever, gingival hyperplasia, megaloblastic anaemia, vitamin K deficiency, hypocalcaemia, folate deficiency and systemic lupus erythematosus	• Craniofacial, limb and digital abnormalities • Hernias • IUGR • Development delay • Congenital heart defects • Orofacial clefts	3.7[1]
Sodium valproate	Ataxia, tremors, sedation, increased weight gain, gastric irritation, liver dysfunction, pancreatitis, rash, hair loss, thrombocytopenia, folate deficiency, and vitamin K deficiency	• Fetal valproate syndrome, facial dysmorphia, impaired psychomotor development • Neural tube defects • Digital defects • Urogenital defects	6.2[1]
Lamotrigine	Rashes, fever, malaise, drowsiness, hepatic dysfunction, dizziness		3.2[1]
Benzodiazepine	–	–	
Topiramate	–	–	7.1[1]
Gabapentin	–	–	3.2[1]
Levetiracetam	Drowsiness, asthenia, dizziness	–	Insufficient data
Primidone	Extreme sedation, vitamins D and K deficiencies	• Dysmorphic face • Digital abnormalities • Hypoplastic fingernails	Insufficient data

Midwives: Mothers should be advised to continue with existing medication until a doctor with experience of prescribing such medications in pregnancy has been consulted, because sudden cessation of any medication without careful thought for substitution can be associated with a poor pregnancy outcome.

Doctors: This simple table cannot address factors for prescribing, and a more authoritative source **must** be used, e.g.:
Briggs, G.G., Freeman, R.K. and Yaffe, S.J. (2005) **Drugs in Pregnancy and Lactation**, 7th Ed. USA; Lippincott.

Morrow, J., Russell, A., Guthrie, E. *et al.* (2006) Malformation risks of epileptic drugs in pregnancy: a prospective study from the UK Epilepsy and Pregnancy Register. **Journal of Neurology, Neurosurgery and Psychiatry**, 77, 193–8.

Appendix 8.2 Advice for Epileptic Women with Babies

Advice for epileptic women with babies, if the seizures are not well controlled:

- Avoid excessive tiredness; share care of baby at night to avoid becoming fatigued
- When feeding the baby, ensure you are sitting safely with a back rest
- Consider feeding on the floor
- Use high chair in lowest setting in safe surroundings, making sure it cannot be knocked over
- Dress and change baby on floor to prevent falling
- Use a buggy/pram with brakes preferably that initiate when you release the handle
- Bath the baby when support is available[1]
- Bath baby in shallow water
- Use safety gates[2]

Appendix 9.1 Pain Therapy Ladder for Pregnancy

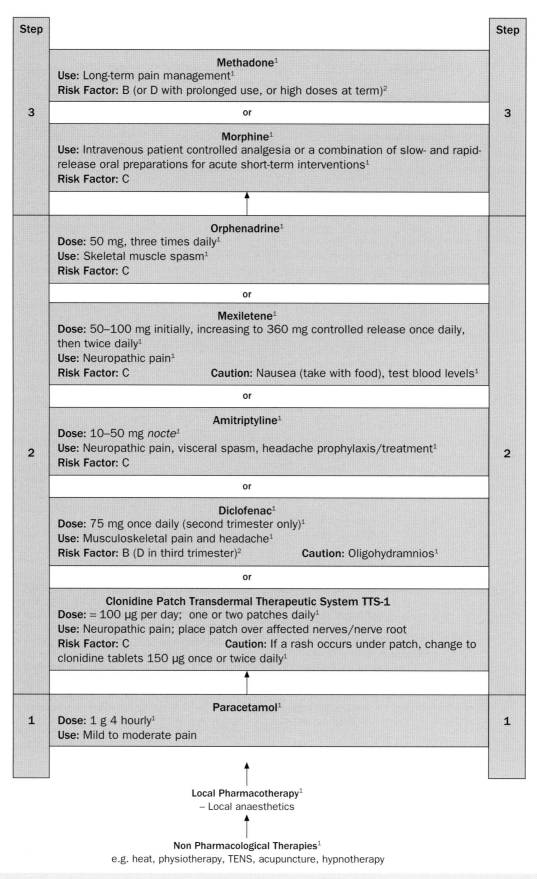

Step 3

Methadone[1]
Use: Long-term pain management[1]
Risk Factor: B (or D with prolonged use, or high doses at term)[2]

or

Morphine[1]
Use: Intravenous patient controlled analgesia or a combination of slow- and rapid-release oral preparations for acute short-term interventions[1]
Risk Factor: C

Step 2

Orphenadrine[1]
Dose: 50 mg, three times daily[1]
Use: Skeletal muscle spasm[1]
Risk Factor: C

or

Mexiletene[1]
Dose: 50–100 mg initially, increasing to 360 mg controlled release once daily, then twice daily[1]
Use: Neuropathic pain[1]
Risk Factor: C   Caution: Nausea (take with food), test blood levels[1]

or

Amitriptyline[1]
Dose: 10–50 mg *nocte*[1]
Use: Neuropathic pain, visceral spasm, headache prophylaxis/treatment[1]
Risk Factor: C

or

Diclofenac[1]
Dose: 75 mg once daily (second trimester only)[1]
Use: Musculoskeletal pain and headache[1]
Risk Factor: B (D in third trimester)[2]   Caution: Oligohydramnios[1]

or

Clonidine Patch Transdermal Therapeutic System TTS-1
Dose: = 100 µg per day; one or two patches daily[1]
Use: Neuropathic pain; place patch over affected nerves/nerve root
Risk Factor: C   Caution: If a rash occurs under patch, change to clonidine tablets 150 µg once or twice daily[1]

Step 1

Paracetamol[1]
Dose: 1 g 4 hourly[1]
Use: Mild to moderate pain

Local Pharmacotherapy[1]
– Local anaesthetics

Non Pharmacological Therapies[1]
e.g. heat, physiotherapy, TENS, acupuncture, hypnotherapy

Risk to Fetus Key: A = little or no risk (human studies)[2]; **B** = little risk (animal studies)[2]; **C** = some adverse effects (animal studies); used if benefit outweighs risk[2]; **D** = positive evidence of risk (human studies); used with serious conditions[2]; **X** = risk outweighs possible benefits, contraindicated in pregnancy[2]

Appendix 9.2 Biochemical Changes in Hypovitaminosis D

The diagnosis of vitamin D deficiency is relatively easily made by biochemical tests that should be available from most laboratories. The diagnosis of osteomalacia is traditionally made on bone biopsy but this is very rarely necessary now as calcidiol and related biochemical measures (see below) are widely available.

The biochemical measures used and changes seen in low vitamin D are:

- *Serum calcidiol (25-(OH) Vit D):* vitamin D deficient <25 nmol/l, insufficient <50 nmol/l
- *Serum total adjusted calcium* (corrected for variation in serum albumin level): normal range 2.10–2.60 mmol/l; newborn up to 2.90 mmol/l; serum calcium may often be normal but if low, parenthesise may occur and in neonates significant risk of fits remain
- *Serum phosphate (PO_4):* adult normal range 0.80–1.40; up to 4 weeks 3.1 mmol/l; neonates and infants 0.80–2.40 mmol/l; characteristically low but may be normal
- *Total serum alkaline phosphatase:* will be raised and indicates deficiency of some severity. The normal range of alkaline phosphates varies in different health localities and this needs to be checked from each laboratory and should be provided on the result form. The placenta also produces alkaline phosphatase, which would be detectable in the mother's blood in the third trimester of pregnancy and for a few days after delivery
  - for assessment of vitamin D deficiency and osteomalacia a bone-specific alkaline phosphatase measurement may be needed
  - in moderate and severe vitamin D deficiency the bone alkaline phosphatase would typically be raised and indicates vitamin D deficiency of some severity and duration
  - non-pregnant adult range 40–130 IU/l; up to 4 weeks 400 IU/l; up to 12 years 350 IU/l
- *Serum parathyroid hormone level (PTH): see* your institution's own laboratory reference range. Our range is 1.6–7.5 pmol/l; raised parathyroid hormone level in the presence of vitamin D deficiency is very supportive of a diagnosis

- The earliest changes would be low 25-(OH) Vit D level followed by a raised PTH and in advanced cases other biochemical changes follow

These normal ranges quoted are from our local laboratory. Each locality should check its own normal ranges.

Appendix 10.1 Reflux Treatment Guidelines for Over-the-Counter Medications[1]

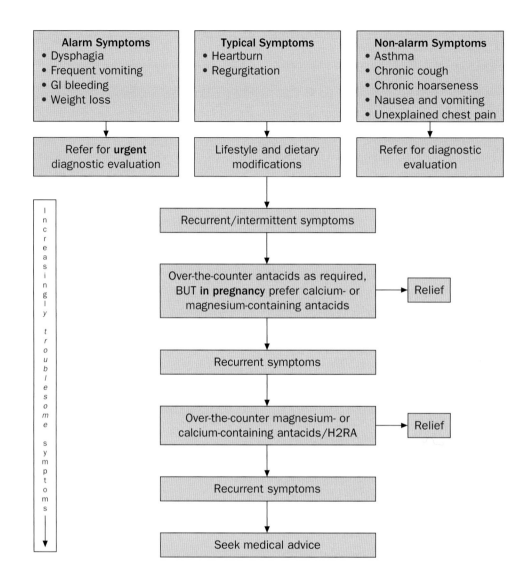

Source:
Tytgat, G.N., Heading, R.C., Muller-Lissner, S. *et al.* (2003) Contemporary understanding and management of reflux and constipation in the general population and pregnancy: a consensus meeting. **Alimentary Pharmacology and Therapeutics**, **18**:291–301. Reproduced with permission of Blackwell Publishing.

Appendix 10.2 Reflux Treatment Guidelines for Prescribed Medications in Non-pregnancy[1]

If a woman becomes pregnant whilst on this regimen the midwife should refer her to a doctor so that a risk–benefit analysis can be made for continuation or alteration of treatment.

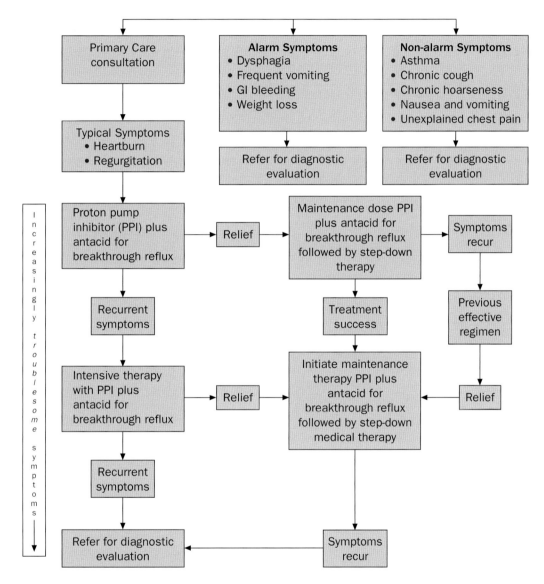

Source:
Tytgat, G.N., Heading, R.C., Muller-Lissner, S. *et al.* (2003) Contemporary understanding and management of reflux and constipation in the general population and pregnancy: a consensus meeting. **Alimentary Pharmacology and Therapeutics, 18:**291–301. Reproduced with permission of Blackwell Publishing.

Appendix 10.3 Rome II Diagnostic Criteria for Irritable Bowel Syndrome[1]

The Rome II diagnostic criteria for irritable bowel syndrome were developed by the Committee on Functional Bowel Disorders and Functional Abdominal Pain, Multinational Working Teams to Develop Diagnostic Criteria for Functional Gastrointestinal Disorders (Rome II). The four-year collaboration arrived at an international consensus for symptom-based diagnostic standards[1].

Diagnostic Criteria for Irritable Bowel Syndrome
Twelve weeks or more, not necessarily consecutive, in the past twelve months of abdominal discomfort or pain that has two out of three features:
1   Relieved with defecation
2   Onset associated with a change in frequency of stool
3   Onset associated with a change in form (appearance) of stool
NB: There is an absence of structural or metabolic abnormalities to explain the symptoms

Symptoms that Cumulatively Support the Diagnosis of Irritable Bowel Syndrome
• Abnormal stool frequency (>3 bowel movements per day or <3 bowel movements per week)
• Abnormal stool form (lumpy/hard or loose/watery stool) more than one quarter of defecations
• Abnormal stool passage (straining, urgency or feeling of incomplete evacuation) more than one quarter of defecations
• Passage of mucus more than one quarter of defecations
• Bloating or feeling of abdominal distension more than one quarter of days

Source:
Thompson, W.G., Longstreth, G.F., Drossman, M., Heaton, K.W., Irvine, E.J. and Muller-Lissner, S.A. (1999) Functional bowel disorders and functional abdominal pain. **GUT**, 45, supplement II ii43–ii47. Adapted and used with permission of the BMJ Publishing Group.

Appendix 11 Drugs for Autoimmune Disease – An Overview for Midwives

This table is to give the midwife an **overview** of autoimmune drug use at different pregnancy stages. These drugs are prescribed, by a doctor, in pregnancy, if the expected benefit to the mother outweighs any effect upon the fetus.

Type of Drug	Name	RISK		Notes
		Pregnancy	Breast-feeding	
NSAIDs Non-steroidal Anti-inflammatory Drugs to control symptoms	Aspirin – low dose	Safe[1]	Safe[1]	Aspirin does not cross the placenta, and single use is considered safe in breast-feeding[1,2,3,4,5]
	Aspirin – standard	C	Potential toxicity Use with caution[2]	Regular use with children is associated with Reye's syndrome[3,6]
	Ibruprofen (*Brufen, Nurofen*)	B	Compatible[2]	*Regular* NSAID use in third trimester is associated with fetal:
	Naproxen (*Naprosyn*)	B	Probably compatible[2]	– ductus arteriosus constriction[1]
	Indomethacin (*Indomod*)	B	Probably compatible[2]	– impaired renal function[1]
	Phenylacetic acid (*Diclofenac*)	B	Probably compatible[2]	Breast-feeding *prior* to a maternal dose minimises infant exposure[1]
	Ketocid (*Ketoprofen*)	B	Probably compatible[2]	
DMARDs Disease-modifying Anti-rheumatic Drugs to modify disease	Azathioprine (*Imuran*)	D	Potential toxicity[2] Human/animal data suggest risk[2]	Transplant patients continue use[3] Pregnancy dosage ≤2 mg/kg/day[1] Evidence is emerging for breast-feeding use based on a risk–benefit analysis[6,7]
	Ciclosporin (*Neoral*)	C	Potential toxicity[2] Limited risk data[2]	Use in pregnancy to be supervised by specialist clinic Present in breast milk[1,3]
	Gold (*Myocrisin, Ridaura*)	C	Probably compatible[2]	Prolonged elimination time in breast milk[2]
	Hydroxychloroquine (Plaquenil)	C	Compatible[2]	Use in pregnancy to be supervised by specialist clinic[3]
	Leflunomide (Arava)	X	Potential toxicity[2] Contraindicated[2]	Pregnancy should not be attempted until plasma level ≤0.02 mg[3,4,5]
	Methotrexate (*Maxtrex*)	X	Toxicity reported[2] Contraindicated[2]	Avoid pregnancy for ≥3 months after ceasing treatment[3] Folate supplements required throughout pregnancy[1]
	Penicillamine (*Distamine*)	D	Potential toxicity[2] Limited risk data[2]	Fetal anomalies found in rodents[4] Continue use in second and third trimesters with Wilson's disease[2,4]
	Sulfasalazine (*Salazopyrin*)	B	Limited data[2] Use with caution[2]	Theoretical risk of neonatal haemolysis, so folate supplements are required[1,3,4,5]
TNF Tumour Necrosis Factor to inhibit immune response	Etanercept (*Enbrel*)	B	Limited data[2] Probably compatible[2]	Limited data so most advise avoidance or caution with use in pregnancy
	Infliximab (*Remicade*)	C	Limited data[2] Contraindicated[2]	Avoid pregnancy for ≥6 months after ceasing treatment[1,3,4,5] Manufacturer advises against use in breast-feeding[2]
Steroids to reduce inflammation	Prednisolone (*Deltacortril*)	C	Compatible[2]	Neonate unaffected if maternal dose ≤40 mg daily Benefit usually outweighs risk[1]
Vasodilators	Nifedipine (*Adalat*)	C	Limited data[2] Probably compatible[2]	Modified release version is preferred in pregnancy[8] Antenatal exposure is *not* grounds for invasive prenatal screening[9]

Key: A = little or no risk (human studies)[2]; **B** = little risk (animal studies)[2]; **C** = some adverse effects (animal studies); used if benefit outweighs risk[2]; **D** = positive evidence of risk (human studies); used with serious conditions[2]; **X** = risk outweighs possible benefits, contraindicated in pregnancy[2]

Midwives: Mothers should be advised to continue with existing medication until a doctor with experience of prescribing such medications in pregnancy has been consulted, because sudden cessation of any medication without careful thought for substitution can be associated with a poor pregnancy outcome. This especially applies to mothers with renal transplants, and also sudden cessation of DMARDs resulting in lupus 'flare' and pregnancy loss.

Doctors: This simple table cannot address factors for prescribing, and a more authoritative source **must** be used, e.g.: Briggs, G.G., Freeman, R.K. and Yaffe, S.J. (2005) **Drugs in Pregnancy and Lactation,** 7th Ed. USA; Lippincott;
Ostensen, M., Khamashta, M., Lockshin, M. *et al.* (2006) Anti-inflammatory and immunosuppressive drugs and reproduction. **Arthritis Research and Therapy**, 8, 209–28. http://arthritis–research.com/content/8/3/209.

Appendix 12.1 The ABC of Hepatitis[1]

	Hepatitis A (HAV)	Hepatitis B (HBV)	Hepatitis C (HCV)	Hepatitis D (HDV)	Hepatitis E (HEV)
What is it?	HAV is a virus that causes inflammation of the liver. It does not lead to chronic disease.	HBV is a virus that causes inflammation of the liver. It can cause liver cell damage, leading to cirrhosis and cancer.	HCV is a virus that causes inflammation of the liver. It can cause liver cell damage, leading to cirrhosis and cancer.	HDV is a virus that causes inflammation of the liver. It only infects those persons with HBV.	HEV is a virus that causes inflammation of the liver. It is rare in the US. There is no chronic state.
Incubation Period	2–7 weeks Average 4 weeks	6–23 weeks Average 17 weeks	2–25 weeks Average 7–9 wks	2–8 weeks	2–9 weeks Average 40 days
How is it Spread?	Transmitted by faecal/oral (anal/oral sex) route, close person to person contact or ingestion of contaminated food and water. Hand to mouth after contact with faeces, such as changing diapers.	Contact with infected blood, seminal fluid, vaginal secretions, contaminated needles, including tattoo and body-piercing tools. Infected mother to newborn. Human bite. Sexual contact.	Contact with infected blood, contaminated iv needles, razors and tattoo and body-piercing tools. Infected mother to newborn. Not easily spread through sex.	Contact with infected blood, contaminated needles. Sexual contact with HDV infected person.	Transmitted through faecal/oral route. Outbreaks associated with contaminated water supply in other countries.
Symptoms	Children may have none. Adults usually have light stools, dark urine, fatigue, fever, nausea, vomiting, abdominal pain and jaundice.	May have none. Some persons have mild flu-like symptoms, dark urine, light stools, jaundice, fatigue and fever.	Same as HBV	Same as HBV	Same as HEV
Treatment of Chronic Disease	Not applicable	Interferon, entecavir, lamivudine, telbivudine, and adefovir dipivoxil control replication of the virus with varying success.	Pegylated interferon with ribavirin with varying success.	Interferon with varying success.	Not applicable
Vaccine	Two doses of vaccine to anyone over one year of age.	Three doses may be given to persons of any age.	None	HBV vaccine prevents HDV infection.	None
Who is at Risk?	Household or sexual contact with an infected person or living in an area with HAV outbreak. Travellers to developing countries, persons engaging in anal/oral sex and injection drug users.	Infants born to infected mother, having sex with an infected person or multiple partners, injection drug users, emergency responders, healthcare workers, persons engaging in anal/oral sex, and haemodialysis patients.	Blood transfusion recipients before 1992, healthcare workers, injection drug users, haemodialysis patients, infants born to infected mother, multiple sex partners.	Injection drug users, persons engaging in anal/oral sex and those having sex with an HDV infected patient.	Travellers to developing countries, especially pregnant women.
Prevention	Vaccination. Immune globulin within two weeks of exposure. Washing hands with soap and water after going to the toilet. Use household bleach (10 parts water to 1 part bleach) on surfaces contaminated with faeces, such as changing tables. Safer sex.	Vaccination provides protection for 20 plus years. Hepatitis B immune globulin within one week of exposure. Clean up infected blood with household bleach and wear protective gloves. Do not share razors, toothbrushes, or needles. Safer sex.	Clean up spilled blood with household bleach. Wear gloves when touching blood. Do not share razors, toothbrushes, or needles with anyone. Safer sex.	Hepatitis B vaccine to prevent HBV /HDV infection. Safer sex.	Avoid drinking or using potentially contaminated water.

Grid 2007

HEPATITIS FOUNDATION INTERNATIONAL
504 Blick drive, Silver Spring, Maryland 20904
Tel: 1-800-891-0707 Fax: 301-622-4702
Website: www.hepatitisfoundation.org
Reproduced with kind permission

Appendix 12.2 Other Infectious Viral Diseases

General Details	Symptoms and Signs	Fetal Risks	Trimester of Risk	Management
Rubella RNA togavirus known as *German measles* Most UK women are vaccinated, hence protected from infection IP – up to 21 days (typically 7–10 days) Infective from seven days before rash to seven days after rash	May be symptomless May present with: • Macular rash (spreads from ears and face) • Mild febrile illness • Pharyngitis • Lymphadenopathy • Arthralgia	Congenital defects: • Ocular defects (e.g. cataracts) • Sensorineural hearing impairment • Cardiac abnormalities (e.g. patent ductus arteriosus) • Hepatosplenomegaly • Jaundice • Thrombocytopenic purpura • Low birth weight • Mental retardation	First trimester mainly: nearly all pregnancies are affected if acquired in the first 10 weeks 13–16 weeks: Less risk, mainly sensorineural deafness	Ensure women are immune pre–pregnancy If not immune, immunise after delivery If infected in first 16 weeks refer for multi-disciplinary counselling to plan for further management Termination of pregnancy should be discussed
Human parvovirus B19 DNA virus Causes *erythema infectiosum,* also known as *fifth disease* or *slapped cheek syndrome* IP – 4–20 days Infective mainly before symptoms arise Infection gives life-long immunity; 50–60% adults immune Outbreaks occur and can last for several months	Often symptomless In children: • Febrile illness • Maculopapular rash (causing flushing of cheeks) Adult women are particularly likely to complain of arthralgia or arthritis which may last a couple of weeks and predominantly affects the peripheral joints	Fetal infection is usually benign and self-limiting Asymptomatic infection occurs in approximately 50% following maternal infection[1] • Miscarriage, risk increased by approx 10%[2] • Fetal anaemia • Hydrops fetalis, approximately 3% risk[2] • Fetal death There is no risk of congenital abnormality[2]	Risk to fetus is in the first 20 weeks only The interval between infection and development of hydrops fetalis is 2–7 weeks, with an average of 5 weeks[2]	Serological testing to confirm diagnosis Monitoring of fetus post maternal infection is by ultrasound assessment at 1–2 weekly intervals for up to 12 weeks If evidence of hydrops fetalis: fetal blood sampling and intrauterine blood transfusion when appropriate
Cytomegalovirus (CMV) DNA virus; member of the herpes family Reactivation and reinfection are common The virus can be transmitted: • transplacentally intrapartum (by exposure to virus in cervix) • postnatally (in breast milk) • Cross infection (especially from other babies in nurseries)	Often symptomless May take the form of a glandular-fever-like illness with: • Fever • Hepatitis • Lymphocytosis (but no pharyngitis) It may cause hepatitis or other abnormal liver function It causes a more severe and widespread disease in immunosuppressed patients	Most commonly asymptomatic infection with no long-term sequelae Associations include: • Mental retardation • Microcephaly • Hepatosplenomegaly • Jaundice • Thrombocytopenic purpura • Low birth weight • Chorioretinitis	All trimesters Most infected fetuses not affected About 5–10% of infected newborns are symptomatic at birth	Diagnosis can be made from viral culture from urine, nasopharynx or blood, or by serological tests Discuss invasive testing to establish fetal infection Consider termination of pregnancy if early gestation and fetal infection confirmed Ultrasound surveillance of the infected or at *risk* fetus; arrange paediatric follow-up of infected neonates
Measles RNA virus; paramyxovirus IP – 10–14 days Immunity life long Well-established vaccination programme NB: Vaccine contraindicated in pregnancy	Usually a self-limiting illness in children with: • Fever • Rash • Cough More severe illness in adults with possible complications of: • Pneumonia • Hepatitis • Encephalitis	Not associated with congenital abnormalities Newborn delivered to a woman with active disease may develop severe neonatal measles Maternal pyrexia may precipitate premature delivery	Throughout pregnancy	Treat pyrexia aggressively, e.g. with paracetamol and cold sponging, and be alert for signs of pre-term labour

IP = incubation period

Appendix 12.3 Other Infectious Bacterial Diseases

General Details	Symptoms and Signs	Fetal Risks	Management
Syphilis Caused by the spirochaete *Treponema pallidum* Incubation period 10–90 days Classified as congenital or acquired	Characterised by stage: Primary syphilis • Primary anogenital chancre (ulcer) • Lymphadenopathy Secondary syphilis • Widespread maculopapular rash • Lymphadenopathy • Mucocutaneous lesions • Condylomata lata (wart-like genital lesions) Late syphilis • Gummatous lesions which may affect respiratory tract, skin, bones, joints • Possible cardiac and CNS (*neurosyphilis*) complications	70–100% of fetuses will be infected if the woman has untreated primary syphilis in pregnancy; one third of these fetuses will die *in utero* Congenital syphilis *Early features* include skin lesions, e.g. rash, raised moist mucocutaneous lesions, 'snuffles', periostitis, hepatosplenomegaly, lymphadenopathy, osteochondritis. *Late features* include interstitial keratitis, deafness and characteristic facial features, e.g. Hutchinson's incisor, mulberry molars, frontal bossing, short maxilla, saddlenose deformity and protuberance of the mandible.	All pregnant women should be screened for syphilis at the initial antenatal visit. Those that screen positive should be managed by genitourinary physicians, obstetricians and midwives and treatment needs to be commenced promptly. First line treatment: im procaine penicillin G for 10 days[3] (erythromycin or azithromycin if penicillin allergy – treatment of baby needed if either of these are used). All babies of women treated for syphilis, either in pregnancy or in the past, should have paediatric follow-up for evidence of congenital syphilis, and serology performed[3].
Tuberculosis Caused by *Mycobacterium tuberculosis* and, rarely, *Mycobacterium bovis* Transmission is by respiratory droplets, however *M. bovis* is acquired by ingestion of contaminated milk Seen as acid-alcohol fast bacilli in a Ziehl-Neelsen stain	Infection often subclinical. Approximately 5% of newly-infected people develop clinically-active disease. This is more likely if immunosuppressed or at the extremes of life. HIV is a significant risk factor for TB and complicates management. Active TB normally manifests as pulmonary TB. The symptoms and signs include malaise, night-sweats, productive cough and haemoptysis, however it may be asymptomatic. Miliary TB occurs when the bacilli invade blood vessels and disseminate to multiple organs. This is rare but more common if immunosuppressed.	There is no increase in congenital malformations or fetal damage when rifampicin, isoniazid, ethambutol and pyrazinamide are used. Streptomycin, however, has been shown to cause fetal sensorineural deafness when used at any stage in pregnancy and must therefore be avoided. Congenital TB is rare however it is more common if the woman has miliary TB and is associated with increased neonatal mortality. Delays in diagnosis can result in an increase in prematurity, low birth weight and perinatal mortality[4]. If the woman is diagnosed and treated early the outcome is good[4].	Clinical infection is diagnosed by detecting acid-fast bacilli in sputum or evidence on chest X-ray. Any woman with symptoms suggestive of TB should be screened or if there has been prolonged close contact with newly-diagnosed infectious TB. Aim to diagnose and treat women prior to pregnancy. If detected in pregnancy treatment should be started without delay and coordinated by the local TB specialist and is likely to require six months of treatment[4]. It is rarely necessary to separate the neonate at delivery. If the infant has been exposed to infectious TB then it will require treatment. The neonatologist and TB specialist should be involved.
Group B Streptococcus (GBS) Lancefield Group B *Streptococcus* Gram-positive coccus	Normal commensal of female genital tract – carried in up to about 25% of mothers in the lower genital tract or rectum. Can be associated with septic abortion, puerperal or gynaecological sepsis. May cause infection in elderly or immunosuppressed patients.	Vast majority of babies born to mothers who carry GBS are not infected. Pre-term babies however are more at risk. *If affected, may have:* Early onset GBS infection Occurs within the first seven days of life and affects approximately one baby per 2000 live births. Symptoms include temperature instability, poor feeding, irritability, and respiratory distress. Late onset GBS infection Less common than early onset GBS disease, typically presents with fever and meningitis and occurs after days seven from delivery but within the first few months of life. GBS is not associated with congenital abnormalities.	Routine screening for GBS carrier state is not recommended in the UK at present[5]. If GBS is detected in pregnancy, antenatal treatment is not recommended, however consideration for intrapartum antibiotics should be given[5]. Risk factors for neonatal GBS include prematurity, prolonged ruptured membranes (>18 hrs) and intrapartum fever. Intrapartum antibiotics should be offered to all women with a previous baby affected by GBS[5]. If GBS is detected in urine then the woman should be treated antenatally and intrapartum antibiotics should be offered. The antibiotic of choice is intravenous penicillin and clindamycin if allergic to penicillin[5]. Any baby showing signs of GBS disease should be treated promptly with appropriate antibiotics.

Appendix 13 Body Mass Index

WORLD HEALTH ORGANISATION – BODY MASS INDEX[1]

The Body Mass Index (BMI) is assessed by calculating the woman's weight in kilograms divided by the square of her height in metres (kg/m^2).

Body Mass Index Range	Classification	Risk of Associated Comorbidities[1]
<18.5	Underweight	Low risk, but at increased risk of other medical problems
18.5–24.9	Normal weight	Average
25.0–29.9	Overweight	Mildly increased
30.0–39.9	Obesity	High
40.0	Extreme Obesity	Very high

Appendix 14.1 Blood and Blood Products for Midwives

MIDWIFERY RESPONSIBILITY

Midwives are responsible for the administration and recording of a number of blood products. It is essential to locate and review local policies and practice guidelines, and also be aware of national policies for this practice.

The risk of transmitting infective agents via blood products cannot be excluded, therefore blood products and blood transfusion are only used when absolutely necessary and all other options, such as intravenous iron, have been tried. Hence, the old-fashioned practice of 'postpartum top-up transfusions' is inappropriate unless there is cardiac compromise or risk of serious bleeding.

Women should, where feasible, be given verbal and written information about blood products, and this should include when anti-D is advocated. Counselling about options and risk should be given by a health professional with knowledge and experience in this field. This ensures every effort has been made to help mothers and their partners make a balanced and informed decision, knowing the relative risks and benefits. This counselling and giving of information should be recorded in the case notes.[1]
See http//:www.blood.co.uk/pages/e34patnt.html

The counselling can be reinforced with additional information in the form of patient information leaflets. Mothers can be made aware of credible websites and reputable self-help groups.

Some women may decline products or blood transfusion, and this important issue is addressed in Chapter one. Appendix 14.2 also has a care plan for women who are Jehovah's witnesses and wish to decline blood products or blood transfusion.

Midwives should also ensure they know how adverse reactions may present, who to inform and how they are managed. This information is collected and published by SHOT – Serious Hazards of Transfusion (www.shotuk.org). The most common incidents include errors at the bedside[2].

A midwife should have a sound understanding of the blood products on which she is giving advice, and which she might administer.

The common blood products a midwife is likely to encounter are described below.

BLOOD PRODUCTS

The following are blood and blood products for administration which a midwife is likely to encounter. Other products may be given in the care of a pregnant woman with a specific condition. If unfamiliar, the midwife should ask for further information about this product and its administration from the prescriber.

All blood-derived products are organised and supplied by the blood transfusion services who can give expert and detailed advice.

Red Blood Cells

Packed red cells
This is the form of blood cell most commonly administered in obstetrics. Each unit is prepared from whole blood collected into an anticoagulant solution. Each unit is about 250 ml and has a haematocrit of 55–80% (normal haematocrit 35–50%).

- All units produced in the UK are *leucocyte depleted* as this has been shown to reduce viral and possibly prion transmission
- Red cells may be irradiated (for immunodeficient women) or CMV (cytomegalovirus) negative for immunosuppressed women and neonates
- Packed cells are indicated for women with symptomatic anaemia who require rapid alleviation of symptoms or women with Hb <7 g/dl in whom blood loss is a significant risk
- Also given for major blood loss when initial measures including volume expansion and cell salvage have been used
- Adverse reactions include:
  - raised temperature
  - rigors
  - allergic reaction (rashes, reduced BP)
  - haemolysis
- More severe, rarer, reactions include:
  - transfusion related acute lung injury (TRALI)
  - graft versus host disease (GVH)
- In the longer term RBC antibody formation and viral infection (hepatitis, CMV, HIV, CJD) may occur

Whole blood
Whole blood is now rarely used, but may be available in specific circumstances for resuscitation.

- Administration would be in conjunction with blood bank and the haematology services
- Red blood cell preparations such as these have a shelf life of approximately 35 days stored at the appropriate temperature
- Transfusion must be started within 30 minutes of removal from the fridge and completed within four hours
- Blood can be requested in different forms depending upon urgency:
  - uncrossmatched O negative
  - group specific (~30 minutes)
  - full cross-match (45–60 minutes)

Platelets

In obstetrics, platelet transfusion is most likely to be seen either in the acute situation of haemorrhage, disseminated intravascular coagulopathy (DIC) or in a woman with ITP and evidence of impaired haemostasis. Also given prophylactically in a woman with a platelet count of less than 10,000 at risk of bleeding.

- Most of the platelet units used in maternity care will be concentrates from whole blood
- Can be stored for up to 5 days at room temperature but must be continually agitated to prevent clumping
- It is usual to use ABO and Rh compatible platelets
- Side effects include:
  - temperature and rigors in 1% (rising to 30% in those who have had multiple platelet transfusions)

- risk of viral transmission (higher than for red cells because platelets are pooled from a number of donors)
    - allergic reaction
- Pay close attention to surgical and obstetric causes of bleeding as part of the decision to transfuse platelets

Plasma Products

Intravenous immunoglobulin (IVIg)

This may be given to women with a falling platelet count in immune thrombocytopenic purpura (ITP), prevention of fetal bleeding in feto-maternal alloimmune thrombocytopenia (FMAIT) and other immunologically based disorders. The dose is weight- and condition-based and is usually given once per week or two weeks. Infusion takes several hours.

- This is again a pooled plasma product associated with a small risk of infection transmission
- Headache and malaise are also reported
- Alternatives should be carefully considered before the use of IVIg because of monetary and convenience costs and side effects, as well as the risks of blood products

Cryoprecipitate

The main use of cryoprecipitates in obstetrics is replacement of fibrinogen and factors XII and VIII in massive haemorrhage,

to complement transfusion of more than eight units of blood (red cell transfusion is poor in clotting factors), and as part of the management of DIC.

- It is prepared from a single rather than a multiple donation and is 20–40 ml/unit
- It is stored at −30 C° for up to 12 months and must be thawed to body temperature before use
- ABO compatible units should be used

Fresh frozen plasma (FFP)

This again is produced from a single donation. It is also used as an adjunct to massive transfusion and in the management of DIC. Each bag contains all the clotting factors, albumin and gamma globulin. It must be used immediately after thawing, and in maternity care should be Rhesus compatible.

Anti-D

Anti-D is a pooled plasma product, which is usually used for prevention of formation of anti-D antibodies. While there are no recorded cases of infection or prion transmission it must be remembered, and patients told, that it is a blood product.

Appendix 14.2 Hospital Information Services for Jehovah's Witnesses Care Plan for Women in Labour Refusing a Blood Transfusion

A pregnant woman who is a Jehovah's Witness might present this care plan to a midwife or doctor at an antenatal visit, and also when admitted to delivery suite, and ask for one copy to be kept in her obstetric notes.

This care plan **must** be discussed with the most senior clinician on duty.

In addition, midwives and other clinicians should refer to the policies of their own institution in relation to mothers who refused blood products and blood transfusion.

CARE PLAN FOR WOMEN IN LABOUR REFUSING A BLOOD TRANSFUSION[#]

As referred to in the *RCOG News* (October 2000) and the MOET course manual 2003 of the Royal College of Obstetricians and Gynaecologists

This document has been prepared as an aid for medical staff and midwives who are managing a Jehovah's Witness or other patient who refuses a blood transfusion and is at risk of, or experiencing, postpartum haemorrhage. We urge clinicians to plan in advance for blood loss, which includes correction of antenatal anaemia (see: 'Management of postpartum anaemia,' second bullet point, italicised note). This should be discussed with the patient in keeping with her wishes that blood or blood products will not be used. Readiness to act promptly to prevent or stop bleeding is paramount.

- Consider booking high-risk patients into a unit with facilities such as interventional radiology, cell salvage and surgical expertise[1]
- Please ensure that the **consultant obstetrician and anaesthetist are aware a Jehovah's Witness has been admitted in labour**
- All such patients should have the **third stage of labour actively managed with oxytocic drugs** together with early cord clamping and controlled cord traction after placental separation
- Do not leave the patient alone for the first hour after delivery

Risk Factors Predisposing to Postpartum Haemorrhage

If the patient has any of the risk factors below, an iv infusion of **oxytocin (Syntocinon)** should be considered after delivery of the baby:

- Previous history of bleeding, ante- or postpartum haemorrhage
- Prolonged labour (especially when augmented with oxytocin)
- Abnormal placentation
- Large baby (>3.5 kg) and/or polyhydramnios
- Increased maternal age (>40 years)
- Fibroids/myomyectomy scars
- More than 3 children

- Maternal obesity
- Multiple pregnancy

Management of Active Haemorrhage

First steps:

- Involve **obstetric, anaesthetic** and **haematology consultants**
- Establish iv colloid infusion, e.g. **Gelofusine**
- Give **oxytocic drugs first, then exclude retained products of conception or trauma** (this could save time)
- Proceed with **bimanual uterine compression**
- Give oxygen
- Catheterise and monitor urine output
- Consider CVP line
- **Aortic compression** against the spine, using a fist just above the umbilicus, may buy time in an emergency[2]
- Slow but persistent blood loss requires action
- Anticipate coagulation problems
- Keep patient fully informed

Proceed with following strategies if bleeding continues:

- **Ergometrine** with **oxytocin (Syntometrine)** marginally more effective than oxytocin alone. If patient is hypertensive, use **oxytocin** 10 U (not 5 U) by slow iv injection (in PPH, benefits of the higher dose outweigh the risks)[3,4].
- **Carboprost (Hemabate)** 250 μg/ml im, can be repeated after 15 minutes. Direct intra-myometrial injection is faster (less hazardous at open operation). If not available use 1–2 **Gemeprost** pessaries in the uterus[5].
- **Oral misoprostol (Cytotec** 200 μg tablets**)** (prostaglandin E_1 analogue), **600** μg (3 tablets). Use when unresponsive to oxytocin and ergometrine[6]. **Intrauterine misoprostol** 800 μg (4 tablets), has been successfully used when refractory to oxytocin, ergometrine and also to carboprost[7,8]. **Rectal misoprostol** 800 or 1000 μg (5 tablets), rapid absorption and control of haemorrhage reported when unresponsive to oxytocin and ergometrine; avoids problems associated with oral administration[9,10]. Misoprostol does not cause hypertension.
- **Recombinant factor VIIa (rFVIIa; NovoSeven)** 90 μg/kg, provides site-specific thrombin generation. Increasingly used to treat uncontrollable haemorrhage successfully, for example: in placenta accreta/percreta, ruptured uterus, uterine atony and HELLP syndrome[11-17] (in seven of these cases bleeding was controlled even in the presence of DIC, despite the failure of all conventional therapies, including packing of pelvis, arterial ligation and hysterectomy[12-16]). Expert advice on this drug will be available from the local Haemophilia Comprehensive Care Centre or Novo Nordisk 24-hour medical advice line (0845 600 5055; emergency UK-wide delivery available). *Some hospitals now hold a small stock of factor VIIa to avoid delivery delay.*
- **Aprotinin (Trasylol),** 2,000,000 U followed by 500,000 U/h or **tranexamic acid (Cyklokapron),** 1 g iv tds; both are anti-fibrinolytic agents, well established for controlling haemorrhage[18-20]. Additionally, consider iv **vitamin K.**

- **Intrauterine balloon tamponade:** stomach balloon of a Sengstaken-Blakemore tube used to control PPH in 14 of 16 cases, including bleeding from an atonic uterus in nine cases[21,22]. Rüsch urological balloon catheter also used[23]. *Consider having a purpose-designed 500 ml tamponade balloon available* (J-SOS-100500-Bakri. Cook [UK] Ltd. tel. 01462 473100)[24]. Balloon tamponade is able to indicate if bleeding will stop (as measured via catheter drainage shaft; the 'tamponade test'), thus avoiding unnecessary surgery[21]. Systematic **uterine packing** also an option[25].
- **B-Lynch brace suture**[26,27]. Simple suture technique to control massive haemorrhage. Can be combined with intrauterine balloon catheter if bleeding persists[28]. (NB: **prophylactic insertion of this suture** has been used in high-risk caesarean section[29].)
- **Embolisation/ligation of internal iliac arteries, or embolisation/bilateral mass ligation of uterine vessels**[27,30].
- **Blood salvage** may be life-saving if substantial blood-loss anticipated[1,31]. Check if acceptable to patient. Used at caesarean section in at least 400 reported cases, without complications of amniotic fluid embolism or coagulopathy[32]. A **cell saver with leucocyte depletion filter** together with **separate suction** (one for amniotic fluid and one for blood salvage) minimises amniotic fluid contamination[32,33].
- **Hysterectomy:** subtotal hysterectomy can be just as effective, also quicker and safer[34]. Clamp uterine arteries as early as possible.

Management of Postpartum Anaemia

- For severe anaemia give oxygen and use **recombinant human erythropoietin (rHuEPO, NeoRecormon or Eprex)** 300 IU/kg (not 50 U) × 3 weekly subcutaneously or iv **without delay,** for accelerated haemoglobin recovery[5,36,37]. Augment with **iron, vitamin B$_{12}$ and folic acid.**
- Iron supplementation essential with EPO. *Oral iron is too slow and unreliable,* use iv **iron sucrose** (Venofer) by drip infusion or slow iv bolus (200 mg × 3 weekly)[35,36]. This drug is *rarely associated with anaphylaxis.* (**NB: *Optimisation of antenatal haemoglobin essential.** When unresponsive to oral iron,* **iron sucrose** *can be efficacious in reversing iron deficiency*[38,39]. *The addition of* **EPO** *[which does not cross the placenta and is reportedly safely used in pregnancy] enhances the response*[29,31,39,40]. *Suggested dosages of EPO and iv iron as above, but × 2 weekly*[39].)
- Consider elective **ventilation** in the ICU. Use **microsampling** techniques (such as HemoCue haemoglobin analyser).
- **Hyperbaric oxygen therapy** is an option in life-threatening anaemia due to PPH[41] – tel 0151 648 8000 (24-hrs) for available centres.

This document reflects current clinical and scientific knowledge and is subject to change. The strategies are not intended as an exclusive guide to treatment. Good clinical judgement, taking into account individual circumstances, may require adjustments.

#Reviewed by consultants in obstetrics and gynaecology, anaesthesia and haematology (including experts in haemostasis).

Recommendation to Mothers: You have two copies of this document, one of which should be placed in your obstetric notes (usually a folder in which your antenatal workup records are kept). It should be discussed with the most senior clinician at the antenatal visit. The other copy should be presented to the obstetrician on admission to the maternity/labour ward for delivery of the baby.

Produced by the Hospital Information Services for Jehovah's Witnesses 0208 906 2211 (24-hour); his@wtbts.org.uk **Sept 2005**

Appendix 14.3 Protocol for Community Management of Anaemia in Pregnancy*

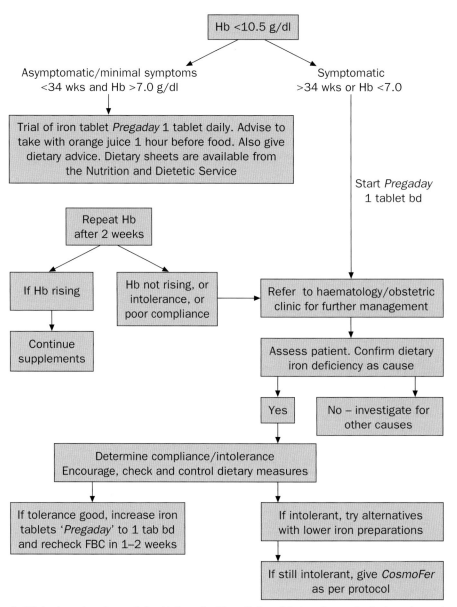

Hb <10.5 g/dl

Asymptomatic/minimal symptoms
<34 wks and Hb >7.0 g/dl

Symptomatic
>34 wks or Hb <7.0

Trial of iron tablet *Pregaday* 1 tablet daily. Advise to take with orange juice 1 hour before food. Also give dietary advice. Dietary sheets are available from the Nutrition and Dietetic Service

Start *Pregaday*
1 tablet bd

Repeat Hb
after 2 weeks

If Hb rising

Hb not rising, or intolerance, or poor compliance

Refer to haematology/obstetric clinic for further management

Continue supplements

Assess patient. Confirm dietary iron deficiency as cause

Yes

No – investigate for other causes

Determine compliance/intolerance
Encourage, check and control dietary measures

If tolerance good, increase iron tablets 'Pregaday' to 1 tab bd and recheck FBC in 1–2 weeks

If intolerant, try alternatives with lower iron preparations

If still intolerant, give *CosmoFer* as per protocol

* Clinical protocol used for University Hospitals of Leicester, adapted and used with permission

Appendix 14.4 Management Plan for Sickle Cell Crisis – A Worked Example

PATIENT DETAILS:
Mrs. YYYY XXXXX
Unit Number: 11111

DIAGNOSIS: Sickle β thalassaemia
Pregnant
Gestational diabetes

BACKGROUND:
4 crises requiring treatment in hospital
2001 severe crisis and chest syndrome following dehydration. Required exchange transfusion.
2004 postpartum splenic sequestration and widespread splenic infarction.
NB: Sibling died with sickle crisis.

BASELINE RESULTS: Hb 8.7 g/dl
Hb El Hb F +A +S Hb F 19% Hb S 68%
Blood Group B Positive   No atypical antibodies
Husband's Hb El normal

MANAGEMENT PLAN FOR SICKLE CRISIS

- Admit to haematology ward if <26/40 pregnant
- Admit to delivery suite if >26/40
- Make sure both haematology and obstetric teams are informed

ANALGESIA   Diclofenac 50 mg orally stat, then tds for a maximum of 2 days
Regular paracetamol
For moderate to severe pain:
1. Loading dose 100μg/kg iv/im morphine sulphate
2. Followed by 50 μg/kg im after 15 minutes if pain is not controlled

WARNING Risk of opiate toxicity – monitor respiratory rate and state of consciousness every 15–30 min

IV FLUIDS   500 ml 4-hourly (fluids may need to be warmed through a blood warmer)
Careful monitoring of fluid balance

BLOOD TESTS   FBC
U&E
Group and Save

Consider exchange transfusion:
- If chest syndrome, pre-eclampsia or severe crisis
- Discuss with consultant haematologist first
- Ensure that blood products, if used, are Rhesus genotyped, Kell neg and sickle neg

MICROBIOLOGY   Blood cultures, throat swab, MSU, sputum cultures if available

OTHER INVESTIGATIONS   Chest X-ray only if there is a suspicion of chest syndrome

OTHER MEDICATIONS
- Continue penicillin prophylaxis
- Add amoxicillin 500 mg tds if febrile
- Continue folic acid 5 mg once daily

REASSESS
- Investigations
- Response to pain relief
- Evidence of infection

MONITOR FOR
- Evidence of chest/girdle syndrome (severe pain unrelieved by analgesia, hypoxia)
- Shadowing on chest X-ray
- Evidence of splenic/hepatic sequestration – precipitate fall in Hb, circulatory failure
- Evidence of pre-eclampsia – hypertension, proteinuria, oedema

NB: If these conditions arise, the woman needs urgent exchange transfusion and consider transfer to ITU

Contact:
- Lead Haematologist
- Obstetrician for Obstetric Haematology
- Lead for Haemoglobinopathies

Clinical protocol used for University Hospitals of Leicester, adapted and used with permission

Appendix 15.1 Wells Prediction Rule for Clinical Assessment of Deep Vein Thrombosis[1]

Clinical Feature	Score
Active cancer (patient receiving treatment for cancer within the previous six months or currently receiving palliative treatment)	1
Paralysis, paresis or recent plaster immobilisation of the lower extremities	1
Recently bedridden for three days or more or major surgery within the previous four weeks	1
Localised tenderness along the distribution of the deep venous system	1
Entire leg swollen	1
Calf swelling – circumference at least 3 cm larger than that on the asymptomatic side when measured 10 cm below tibial tuberosity	1
Pitting oedema confined to the symptomatic leg	1
Collateral superficial veins (non-varicose)	1
Alternative diagnosis at least as likely as deep vein thrombosis	–2
Total Score	
Scoring: Add all the scores to get the total. In patients with symptoms in both legs, use the scores for the more symptomatic leg.	

Interpretation of Total Score	
Probability of DVT is low	<1
Probability of DVT is moderate	1 or 2
Probability of DVT is high	>2

Reproduced with permission of the Lancet.

Appendix 15.2 Risk Factors[a] for Venous Thrombo-embolism in Pregnancy and the Puerperium[1]

Pre-existing

Previous VTE

Congenital Thrombophilia

     Antithrombin deficiency

     Protein C deficiency

     Protein S deficiency

     Factor V Leiden

     Prothrombin gene variant

Antiphospholipid syndrome

Age over 35 years

Obesity (BMI >30 kg/m^2) either pre-pregnancy or pregnancy

Parity >4

Gross varicose veins

Paraplegia

Sickle cell disease

Inflammatory disorders, e.g. inflammatory bowel disease

Some medical disorders, e.g. nephrotic syndrome, certain cardiac diseases

Myeloproliferative disorders, e.g. essential thrombocythaemia, polycythaemia vera

New onset or transient[b]

Surgical procedure in pregnancy or puerperium, e.g. evacuation of retained products of conception, postpartum sterilisation

Hyperemesis

Dehydration

Ovarian hyperstimulation syndrome

Severe infection, e.g. pyelonephritis

Immobility (>4 days bed rest)

Pre-eclampsia

Excessive blood loss

Long-haul travel

Prolonged labour

Midcavity instrumental delivery

Immobility after delivery

Legend

a – Although these are all accepted as thrombo-embolic risk factors, with many of them there are few data to support the degree of increased risk.

b – These risk factors are potentially reversible and may develop or resolve at later stages in gestation than the initial risk assessment. Therefore ongoing individual risk assessment is important.

Appendix 16.1 Sudden Unexpected Deaths in Infancy 1993–1996: Contributory Factors Involving Carers[1]

Below is a result of analysis in five English health regions of all post perinatal deaths (7–365 days of life)

Area of Concern	Instances			
	SIDS		Explained Deaths	
	n = 346	%	n = 71	%
Personal Situation (total)	26	7.5	6	8.5
Maternal depression	6	1.7	1	1.4
Other illness in mother	2	0.6	0	0
Poor hygiene	4	1.2	0	0
Poor bonding	3	0.9	0	0
Lack of support	5	1.4	1	1.4
Immaturity of mother	1	0.3	1	1.4
Learning difficulties of mother	1	0.3	0	0
Violence of the father	0	0	1	1.4
Mendacity (untruthfulness)	1	0.3	0	0
Prostitution	1	0.3	0	0
Poor command of English	0	0	1	1.4
Mother absent from home	0	0	1	1.4
Mother abused in childhood	2	0.6	0	0
Social Circumstances (total)	21	6.1	3	4.2
Poverty	8	2.3	2	2.8
Disorganised household	10	2.9	0	0
Travelling family	1	0.3	1	1.4
Mother in prison	1	0.3	0	0
Father in prison	1	0.3	0	0
Substance Abuse (total)	137	39.6	14	19.7
Cigarettes	100	28.9	8	11.3
Alcohol	13	3.8	4	5.6
Illegal drugs	24	6.9	2	2.8
Infant Care (total)	45	13.0	7	9.9
Incorrect feeding	7	2.0	2	2.8
Inadequate supervision of baby	7	2.0	4	5.6
Suspected abuse	8	2.3	0	0
Carer under the influence of alcohol	13	3.8	0	0
Generally poor standards	10	2.9	1	1.4
Sleeping arrangements (total)	137	39.6	6	8.5
Inappropriate place	12	3.5	0	0
Use of unsafe cot or bunk bed	0	0	3	4.2
Settee shared with adult	6	1.7	0	0
Bed-sharing under influence of alcohol	13	3.8	0	0
Other bed-sharing	19	5.5	1	1.4
Use of soft pillow	5	1.4	0	0
Placing baby prone	31	9.0	1	1.4
Over-wrapping	29	8.4	0	0
Keeping baby too warm	16	4.6	1	1.4
Use of electric blanket	1	0.3	0	0
Leaving fire burning near baby all night	4	1.2	0	0
Not keeping baby warm enough	1	0.3	0	0
Use of services (total)	31	9.0	15	21.1
Late booking at antenatal clinic	5	1.4	2	2.8
Refusal to use services or accept advice	15	4.3	2	2.8
Failure to give medication/other treatment	2	0.6	1	1.4
Failure to recognise illness or seek advice	8	2.3	7	9.9
Refusal of hospital for baby	0	0	1	1.4
Taking baby out of hospital against advice	0	0	1	1.4
Incorrect resuscitation	1	0.3	1	1.4

The shaded areas pertain directly to subjects discussed in this book.

Appendix 16.2 Neonatal Abstinence Syndrome

Neonatal abstinence syndrome (NAS) is a condition that results from antenatal exposure to opiates, and presents post-delivery when the exposure ceases.

OPIATE EXPOSURE

Opioid receptors are found throughout the central nervous system and other peripheral sites, where they mediate analgesia and have a range of other functions.

Long-term exposure to opiates results in CNS adaptation to the presence of the drug, leading to the development of tolerance. Increased amounts of the drug are required to achieve the same physical effects. In acute opiate withdrawal, such as following childbirth, specific physical symptoms are experienced that involve the central nervous system, respiratory system, gastrointestinal system and vasomotor system. These are mainly due to the decrease in the production of endogenous opioids and a rebound increase in noradrenergic activity.

OPIATE WITHDRAWAL

Opiate withdrawal is characterised by a generalised hyperactive state with symptoms of anxiety, enhanced startle and altered sleep pattern.

Signs and Symptoms of Opiate Withdrawal

Central Nervous System
- Hyperactivity
- Hyper-irritability – excessive crying, high-pitched cry
- Increased muscle tone
- Exaggerated reflexes
- Tremors
- Sneezing
- Hiccoughs
- Yawning
- Short, restless sleep pattern
- Pyrexia

Respiratory System
- Tachypnoea
- Excess secretions
- Stuffy nose

Gastrointestinal
- Disorganised, vigorous sucking
- Vomiting, posseting
- Sensitive gag
- Hyperphagia
- Diarrhoea
- Abdominal cramps
- Drooling

Vasomotor
- Flushing
- Sweating
- Sudden pallor

Withdrawal symptoms vary greatly from one baby to another. Symptoms depend on:

- The type of drug used
- Amount of drug used
- The route of administration
- When the last dose was taken by the mother
- Whether other drugs were used in conjunction with the main drug of choice

Withdrawal symptoms usually occur within 24–48 hours after birth. Methadone has a longer half-life and withdrawal symptoms may not present until 72 hours. Symptoms may be further delayed with polydrug use, especially benzodiazepine use.

MANAGEMENT OF MINOR SYMPTOMS

It is important to ensure other medical causes are considered in the assessment of symptoms that are causing concern, e.g. raised temperature may be due to infection.

- Encourage parents to cuddle/gently rock baby
- Kangaroo care, skin to skin (if appropriate) can be soothing
- Prevent overheating
- Maintain calm atmosphere, with dim lighting and keep noise to a minimum
- Breast-feeding may assist with minimising withdrawal symptoms
- The use of a dummy may help comfort the baby

INDICATIONS FOR PHARMACOLOGICAL MANAGEMENT

Pharmacological management is indicated if the baby is unable to feed and sleep sufficiently with the above supportive measures.

If the baby develops diarrhoea and/or vomiting resulting in dehydration or unacceptable weight loss, or develops seizures, then pharmacological treatment should be commenced promptly.

Appendix 17 Treatment Guidance for Antenatal and Postnatal Psychiatric Disorders

MANAGEMENT OF DEPRESSION

When choosing an antidepressant for pregnant or breast-feeding women, prescribers should, while bearing in mind that the safety of these drugs is not well understood, take into account that[1]:

- Tricyclic antidepressants, such as amitriptyline, imipramine and nortriptyline, have lower known risks during pregnancy than other antidepressants
- Most tricyclic antidepressants have a higher fatal toxicity index than selective serotonin reuptake inhibitors (SSRI)
- Fluoxetine is the SSRI with the lowest known risk during pregnancy
- Imipramine, nortriptyline and sertraline are present in breast milk at relatively low levels
- Citalopram and fluoxetine are present in breast milk at relatively high levels
- SSRI taken after 20 weeks' gestation may be associated with an increased risk of persistent pulmonary hypertension in the neonate
- Paroxetine taken in the first trimester may be associated with fetal heart defects
- Venlafaxine may be associated with increased risk of high blood pressure at high doses, higher toxicity in overdose than SSRI and some tricyclic antidepressants, and increased difficulty in withdrawal
- All antidepressants carry the risk of withdrawal or toxicity in neonates; in most cases the effects are mild and self-limiting

For a woman who develops mild or moderate depression during pregnancy or the postnatal period, the following should be considered[1]:

- Self-help strategies (guided self-help, computerised cognitive behavioural therapy or exercise)
- Non-directive counselling delivered at home (listening visits)
- Brief cognitive behavioural therapy or interpersonal psychotherapy

Appendix 18 Advice to Patients on Coping with Cancer Symptoms and Side Effects

The following is an excerpt from the Cancerbackup website, www.cancerbackup.org.uk, accessed May 2007. Health professionals are advised to direct patients and relatives to this reliable source of credible information.

FATIGUE

Fatigue means feeling excessively tired or exhausted all or most of the time. The tiredness is not relieved by rest and can affect you physically, psychologically and emotionally. People who have fatigue have no energy and find it difficult to do simple, everyday things that people usually take for granted. Coping with fatigue can be addressed by:

Diet

- Keep a diary of what and when you eat daily
- Try to take advantage of the times when your appetite is best
- Drink plenty of liquids
- If your taste changes, try new foods, or eat the foods that taste best to you
- Ask for any leaflets that are available which give dietary advice
- You can also ask your doctor to refer you to a dietitian, who can give you helpful ideas

Exercise

It is important to try and exercise a little if you can, even when you are unwell. Research has found that exercise may actually help the symptoms of fatigue. The problem is that while too much exercise might make you tired, so can too little, so it's important to find your own level. A good balance between being active and getting plenty of rest is best. The physiotherapist at the hospital may be able to advise you about what would suit you. General rules are:

- Regular, light exercise such as walking has been shown to reduce fatigue as well as nausea and vomiting, and can help some people to sleep better
- Plan some activity or light exercise into your day
- If exercise is impossible try to stay active in your daily routine
- Pay attention to how your body reacts to exercise: How did you sleep? How did you feel the next day?
- Drink plenty of fluids before, during and after exercise
- Perhaps keep a record of your activities to share with your doctor or nurse, so they can help monitor your progress
- It is important to find a balance between activity and rest, and exercise in a way that allows the muscles to recover after activity

Sleep

It's very important to try and keep a normal sleeping routine when you are ill, even though your fatigue may make you feel like sleeping all the time. The following might be a useful guide:

1. *Sleep just long enough* Sleep as much as you need to feel refreshed and healthy during the following day, but not more than necessary. Limiting time in bed seems to produce better-quality sleep. Too much time in bed can lead to disturbed/shallow sleep.
2. *Wake up at the same time every day* A regular wake-up time in the morning seems to strengthen most people's sleep routine and lead eventually to regular times of going to sleep.
3. *Exercise regularly if you can* A steady daily amount of exercise may help to deepen sleep over the long term.
4. *Reduce noise* Occasional loud noises, such as aircraft flying overhead, disturb sleep, even if you don't remember the disturbance later. If your bedroom is noisy, you could mask some of the noise using a small electric fan, or you could use ear-plugs.
5. *Keep a steady temperature in your bedroom* Although a very warm room disturbs sleep, so does a very cold one. Room temperature should be comfortably warm.
6. *Have a bedtime snack* Hunger may disturb sleep. A light bedtime snack or a hot drink can help some to sleep better.
7. *Avoid stimulants* Many people who have problems sleeping are very sensitive to stimulants. It is best to avoid cola drinks, coffee, strong tea and chocolate for a few hours before bedtime.
8. *Know how naps affect you* Some people find that day-time naps help them sleep better at night, while others sleep less well after them. Find out what suits you best.
9. *Limit your intake of alcohol* Alcohol can help tense people to fall asleep more quickly, but the sleep tends to be broken. So avoid large amounts of alcohol near bedtime.
10. *Know when to say 'enough'* Rather than lying in bed tossing and turning you could get up and watch television or read a book. Wait until you feel tired again and then go back to bed. Audio tapes with stories can help you to sleep, and are stocked in most bookshops and libraries.

Lymphoedema

Lymphoedema can occur in the arm after breast cancer treatment to the armpit, or in the leg if cancer or its treatment affects nodes in the groin area or the pelvis.

The affected arm or leg may become swollen, stiff, uncomfortable and awkward to move, making daily activities, such as dressing or washing, difficult. Lymphoedema can develop weeks, months or even years after cancer treatment and it is difficult to know who will be affected or how bad the lymphoedema will be.

It is not possible to replace lymph nodes that have been removed or lymphatic vessels that have been damaged. Once lymphoedema has developed it cannot be cured permanently. However, it can usually be reduced and controlled.

Lymphoedema may cause the following symptoms in the affected area:

- A feeling of fullness or heaviness
- Tightness and stretching of the skin swelling
- Reduced movement of the joints
- Thickening and dryness of the skin
- Discomfort and/or pain

You may first realise you have swelling because clothing, shoes or jewellery (such as rings or watches) feel tighter than usual.

Occasionally, in more severe lymphoedema, the skin may become broken and the colourless lymph fluid can leak out onto the surface. This is known as *lymphorrhoea* (pronounced 'lim-for-ria'). This happens when too much fluid builds up in the tissues or when the skin is damaged. However, it is important to remember that most people with lymphoedema only have mild symptoms.

ASCITES

Inside the abdomen is a membrane called the peritoneum, which has two layers. One layer lines the abdominal wall and the other layer covers the organs inside the abdominal cavity. The peritoneum produces a fluid that acts as a lubricant and allows the abdominal organs to glide smoothly over one another. Sometimes too much of this fluid can build up between the two layers and this is called ascites.

The symptoms of ascites can be very distressing. The abdomen becomes very swollen and distended, which can be uncomfortable or painful. It can also cause difficulty in getting comfortable, sitting up or walking. It can make you feel very tired (lethargic) and breathless. It may cause feelings of sickness (nausea) or make you sick (vomiting). You may also suffer indigestion and a reduced appetite.

In order to relieve symptoms, the treatment of ascites involves slowing the build-up of the fluid and putting a tube into the abdomen to drain it (known as paracentesis). Ascites can build up again and drainage may need to be carried out more than once.

PAIN

Not everyone with cancer has pain, but approximately 3 in 10 people with cancer who are having treatment will have pain. When the cancer is advanced, around 7 in 10 people will have pain.

Physical Causes

Pain may occur for a number of reasons:

- A cancer may press on the tissues around it, or on a nerve.
- Infection can cause pain, by creating inflammation in the affected part of the body.
- Damage to tissues following surgery or radiotherapy may lead to pain.
- A cancer may spread from its original (*primary*) place in the body to form other tumours (*secondaries* or *metastases*). These may cause pain, especially in the bones.
- Sometimes, pain can seem to occur in parts of the body far away from the cancer that is causing it. This is called *referred pain*.

Understandably, someone with cancer may assume that a new ache or pain means that their cancer has come back, or is getting worse, or that the cancer has spread, but this is not always the case.

Emotions and Pain

Emotions such as fear, anxiety, depression and tiredness can make your pain worse. This does not mean that cancer pain is 'all in the mind'.

Social Effects on Pain

Sometimes pain can be made worse by other social or work related things happening in your life which cause you stress (for example, friends avoiding you).

Treatment for Pain

International guidelines set out the types of painkillers that are most effective for different levels of pain. This is known as the *analgesic* ladder:

1. **Mild pain** – mild painkillers or anti-inflammatory drugs (e.g. paracetamol or ibuprofen)
2. **Moderate pain** – weak opioid painkillers (e.g. codeine)
3. **Severe pain** – strong opioid painkillers (e.g. morphine)

Often, painkillers from two different groups will be used at the same time, as they work in different ways. Other drugs that help to control pain, such as bisphosphonates and steroids, can also be used alongside the painkillers.

ALOPECIA

Cancer treatments such as chemotherapy and radiotherapy can make your hair fall out. There are many ways of dealing with this. You may not mind your bald head, but if you do want to cover up there are many types of wigs or hairpieces, hats, turbans or scarves that you can use.

FERTILITY PROBLEMS

Protecting Your Fertility

Many women who are concerned that their cancer treatment may cause infertility are advised to store either embryos (fertilised eggs) or eggs, before their treatment starts. Embryos and unfertilised eggs are usually frozen for up to ten years, although in some situations this can be extended until the woman reaches 55.

Your doctor or nurse can discuss the possibility of infertility and the collection and storage of eggs or embryos with you and can refer you to a fertility clinic. Sometimes the NHS will pay for storage of the eggs or embryos, but some health authorities will not.

Collection and Storage of Eggs

The whole process takes 3–4 weeks and involves stimulating the ovaries to produce more eggs than normal. This is done by giving doses of the hormones GnRH, FSH and LH. A fourth hormone, called human chorionic gonadotrophin (HCG), is also used. Usually at least six eggs are collected, which will increase the chances of achieving a pregnancy.

Eggs are collected in one of two ways. Either an ultrasound-guided needle is passed through the wall of the vagina, or a small cut is made in the abdominal skin below the navel and a fine needle is inserted to remove the eggs. These procedures can be uncomfortable and painkilling drugs may be needed. A general anaesthetic may be used.

Some women need to start their cancer treatment straight away and it may not be possible to delay it in order to have the ovarian stimulation.

There is a risk with some cancers, such as breast cancer, that the hormones used in ovarian stimulation may also stimulate the cancer to grow. It therefore may not be advisable to have ovarian stimulation. Your doctors will be able to discuss this with you. It may be possible to collect one or two eggs without ovarian stimulation, although this reduces the chances of a successful pregnancy.

Using collected eggs

Once the eggs have been collected, they can either be frozen and stored, or fertilised using *in vitro* fertilisation (IVF) and then frozen. IVF involves putting the eggs and sperm together in a test tube in a laboratory for fertilisation to occur.

In order to fertilise the eggs to form an embryo, sperm from a partner will be needed. Both the woman and the man will need to sign a consent form and neither can use the embryos to start a pregnancy without the other's permission. If a woman has no partner, sperm from an anonymous sperm donor can be used. When the embryos are needed, they are thawed and placed in the womb. Pregnancy rates are much lower, however, than from fresh embryo transfer. Freezing more embryos than are needed usually improves a woman's chance of becoming pregnant.

Freezing Unfertilised Eggs

This is a newer process, which is much less successful. This method is still largely experimental at the moment. When the eggs are thawed they are fertilised by injecting a sperm into the egg. This is known as *intra-cytoplasmic sperm injection* (ICSI). The fertilised egg is then placed in the womb. ICSI is done to improve the chance of a pregnancy.

Ovarian Tissue Freezing

A newer technique is to take some ovarian tissue for freezing. It is thought that the ovarian tissue can be put back into the body at a later date and eggs can then be collected. This type of infertility treatment is still very experimental at the moment.

There are no guarantees of pregnancy with these treatments, as you will learn when discussing them at the fertility clinic. If you have not been able to store any eggs or embryos, or if you do not become pregnant by the above methods, it may be possible for you to become pregnant using eggs from another woman (donor eggs). If treatment has made you infertile but you manage to become pregnant by one of the above methods, it is likely that you will need to be given hormones to maintain the pregnancy. The hormones are usually given by injection.

Used with kind permission of Cancerbackup.

Cancerbackup is the UK's leading cancer information charity, offering information, support and understanding to all those affected by cancer, through a comprehensive range of information available free direct to patients and families, as well as online at www.cancerbackup.org.uk, and via a freephone helpline, staffed by experienced cancer nurses: 0808 800 1234 (Mon–Fri, 9 am–8 pm).

Appendices References

Appendix 1.1 UK Maternal Deaths: Causes and Risk Factors

1. Lewis G and Drife J (Eds):2004 **Why Mothers Die 2000–2002, 6th Report. Confidential Enquiries into Maternal and Child Health.** RCOG Press Table 1.4
2. Lewis G and Drife J (Eds):2004 *Midwifery summary* in **Why Mothers Die 2000–2002 6th Report. Confidential Enquiries into Maternal and Child Health.** London, RCOG Press 2
3. Lewis G (Ed):2007 **Saving Mothers' Lives: Reviewing Maternal Deaths to Make Motherhood Safer. 7th Report of the Confidential Enquiries into Maternal and Child Health.** London; CEMACH

Appendix 1.2 UK Maternal Deaths by Type of Antenatal Care and Place of Delivery

1. Lewis G and Drife J 2004 **Why Mothers Die 2000–2002 6th Report. Confidential Enquiries into Maternal and Child Health.** RCOG Press Table 22.9
2. Lewis G and Drife J 2004 **Why Mothers Die 2000–2002 6th Report. Confidential Enquiries into Maternal and Child Health.** RCOG Press. Source: Table 1.7
3. Lewis G (Ed):2007 **Saving Mothers' Lives: Reviewing Maternal Deaths to Make Motherhood Safer. 7th Report of the Confidential Enquiries into Maternal and Child Health.** London; CEMACH

Appendix 1.3 Daily Vitamin and Mineral Dietary Intake for Pregnancy and Lactation

1. Food Standards Agency (UK):website www.eatwell.gov.uk/ healthydiet/nutritionessentials/vitaminsandminerals/folicacid/ [accessed 04–06–2007]
2. Rutherford D 2007 **Vitamins and Minerals – What Do They Do?** www.netdoctor.co.uk/health_advice/facts/vitamins_which.htm [accessed 4–6–2007]
3. Briggs GG, Freeman RK and Yaffe SJ 2005 **Drugs in Pregnancy and Lactation**, 7th Ed. Philadelphia; Lippincott
4. National Academy of Sciences (USA):2004 **Dietary Reference Intakes** www.iom.edu/Object.File/Master/21/372/DRI%20Tables%20af ter%20electrolytes%20plus%20micro–macroEAR_2.pdf [accessed 04–06–2007]
5. Nowson CA and Margerison C 2002 Vitamin D intake and vitamin D status of Australians. **Medical Journal of Australia**, 177(3): 149–152

Appendix 3.1 BHS Blood Pressure Measurement Recommendations

1. British Hypertension Society 2007 Factsheet: **Blood Pressure Measurement with Mercury Blood Pressure Monitors** www. bhsoc/bp_monitors/BLOOD_PRESSURE_1784a.pdf [accessed 08–06–2007]
2. British Hypertension Society 2007 Factsheet: **Blood Pressure Measurement with Electronic Blood Pressure Monitors** www. bhsoc/bp_monitors/BLOOD_PRESSURE_1784b.pdf [accessed 08–06–2007]

Appendix 3.2 Blood Pressure Devices for Use in Pregnancy and Obesity

1. British Hypertension Society 2007 www.bhsoc.org/bp_monitors/ special.stm [accessed 08–06–2007]
2. Reinders A, Cuckson AC, Lee JTM and Shennan AH 2005 An accurate automated blood pressure device for use in pregnancy and pre-eclampsia: the Microlife 3BTO–A. **British Journal of Obstetrics and Gynaecology**, 112:1–6
3. Altunkan S, Oztas K and Altunkan E 2006 Validation of the Omron 637IT wrist blood pressure measuring device with a position sensor according to the International Protocol in adults and obese adults. **Blood Pressure Monitoring**, 11(2):79–85

Appendix 4.2 New York Heart Association 1994 Classification of Heart Disease

1. American Heart Association 2007 **Classification of Functional Capacity and Objective Assessment** www.americanheart.org/ presenter.jhtml?identifier=4569

Appendix 4.3 Drugs for Cardiac Disease – an Overview for Midwives

1. Briggs GG, Freeman RK and Yaffe SJ 2005 **Drugs in Pregnancy and Lactation**, 7th Ed. USA; Lippincott
2. Ostensen M, Khamashta M, Lockshin M, *et al.* 2006 Anti-inflammatory and immunosuppressive drugs and reproduction. **Arthritis Research and Therapy**, 8:209–228 http://arthritis–research.com/content/8/3/209
3. MIMS 2007 **Monthly Index of Medical Specialities,** May. London; Haymarket Medical Publications
4. Steer PJ, Gatzoulis MA and Barker P (Eds) 2006 **Heart Disease and Pregnancy**. London; RCOG Press
5. British National Formulary 2007 No. 54 online www.bnf.org [accessed 04-09-2007]

Appendix 5 Asthma in Pregnancy – an Information Leaflet for Pregnant Women

1. Smith J 2007 **Asthma in Pregnancy: An Information Leaflet for Pregnant Women**. Leicester; University Hospitals of Leicester NHS Trust

Appendix 8.1 Drugs Used for Neurological Conditions

1. Morrow J, Russell A, Guthrie E, Parsons L, Robertson I, Waddell R, Irwin B, McGivern R, Morrison P and Craig J 2006 Malformation risks of epileptic drugs in pregnancy: a prospective study from the UK Epilepsy and Pregnancy Register. **Journal of Neurology, Neurosurgery and Psychiatry**, 77:193–198

Appendix 8.2 Advice for Epileptic Women with Babies

1. Cornelissen M, Steegers-Theunissen R, Kollee L, Eskes T, Vogels-Mentink G, Motohara K, De Abreu R and Monnens L 1993 Increased incidence of neonatal vitamin K deficiency resulting from maternal anticonvulsant therapy. **American Journal of Obstetrics and Gynaecology**, 168(3):923–928
2. Epilepsy Action 2005 **Mothers in Mind** http://www.epilepsy. org.uk/downloads/pdf/epilepsyaction_mothersinmind.pdf

Appendix 9.1: Pain Therapy Ladder for Pregnancy

1. Roche S and Hughes EW 1999 Pain problems associated with pregnancy and their management. **Pain Reviews**, 6:239–261
2. Briggs GG, Freeman RK and Yaffe SJ 2005 **Drugs in Pregnancy and Lactation**, 7th Ed. USA; Lippincott

Appendix 10.1 Reflux Treatment Guidelines for Over-The-Counter Medicines

1. Tytgat GN, Heading RC, Muller-Lissner S, *et al.* 2003 Contemporary understanding and management of reflux and constipation in the general population and pregnancy: a consensus meeting. **Alimentary Pharmacology and Therapeutics**, 18:291–301 Figure 2

Appendix 10.2 Reflux Treatment Guidelines for Prescribed Medicines in Non-Pregnancy

1. Tytgat GN, Heading RC, Muller-Lissner S, *et al.* 2003 Contemporary understanding and management of reflux and constipation in the general population and pregnancy: a consensus meeting. **Alimentary Pharmacology and Therapeutics**, 18:291–301 Figure 3

Appendix 10.3 Rome II Diagnostic Criteria for Irritable Bowel Syndrome

1. Thompson WG, Longstreth GF, Drossman M, Heaton KW, Irvine EJ and Muller-Lissner SA 1999 Functional bowel disorders and functional abdominal pain. **Gut**, 45(suppl. II):ii43–ii47

Appendix 11: Drugs for Autoimmune Disease – an Overview for Midwives

1. Ostensen M, Khamashta M, Lockshin M, *et al.* 2006 Anti-inflammatory and immunosuppressive drugs and reproduction. **Arthritis Research and Therapy**, 8:209–228 http://arthritis–research.com/content/8/3/209
2. Briggs GG, Freeman RK and Yaffe SJ 2005 **Drugs in Pregnancy and Lactation,** 7th Ed. Philadelphia, USA; Lippincott
3. BNF 2006 **British National Formulary**. Issue 51 http://www.bnf.org/bnf/ [accessed 23-11-2006]
4. Weiner CP and Buhimschi C 2004 **Drugs for Pregnant and Lactating Women**. London; Churchill Livingstone
5. MIMS 2006 **Monthly Index of Medical Specialities** (November). London; Haymarket Medical Publications
6. Khare M, Lott J and Howarth E 2003 Is it safe to continue azathioprine in breast feeding mothers? **Journal of Obstetrics and Gynaecology**, 23(Suppl. 1):S53
7. Sau A, Clarke S, Bass J, *et al.* 2007 Azathioprine and breastfeeding – is it safe? **British Journal of Obstetrics and Gynaecology**, 114:498–501
8. Prodigy 2006 www.prodigy.nhs.uk/pk.uk/raynauds_phenomenon/extended_information/management_issues [accessed 16–05–2006]
9. NTIS 2006 **Exposure to Nifedipine during Pregnancy**. National Teratology Information Service, Regional Drug and Therapeutics Centre

Appendix 12.1 The ABC of Hepatitis

1. Hepatitis Foundation International 2007 ABC of Hepatitis www.hepatitisfoundation.org [accessed 02–07–2007]

Appendices 12.2 and 12.3 Other Bacterial and Viral Infections

1. Koch WC, Harger JH, Barnstein B, *et al.* 1998 Serological and virologic evidence for frequent intrauterine transmission of human parvovirus B19 with a primary maternal infection during pregnancy. **Journal of Pediatric Infectious Disease,** 17:489–494
2. Miller E, Fairley CK, Cohen BJ, *et al.* 1998 Immediate and long term outcome of human parvovirus B19 infection in pregnancy. **British Journal of Obstetrics and Gynaecology,** 105:174–178
3. Clinical Effectiveness Group 2002 **UK National Guidelines on the Management of Early Syphilis**. www.bashh.org/guidelines
4. Health Protection Agency 2006 Pregnancy and Tuberculosis www.hpa.org.uk/infections/topics_az/tb/menu.htm
5. RCOG 2003 **Clinical Guideline 36 – Prevention of Early Onset Neonatal Group B Streptococcal Disease**. London; Royal College of Obstetricians and Gynaecologists

Appendix 13 Body Mass Index

1. DH 2006 **Care Pathways for the Management of Overweight and Obesity** www.dh.gov.uk

Appendix 14.1 Blood and Blood Products

1. NPSA 2006 **Safer Practice Notice 14 – Right Patient, Right Blood**
2. SHOT – Serious Hazards of Transfusion www.shotuk.org/Summary%202005.pdf [accessed 18–05–2007]

Appendix 14.2 Hospital Information Services for Jehovah's Witnesses

1. Hall MH 2006 Chap. 4 *Haemorrhage* in **Why Mothers Die 2000–2002. Confidential enquiry into maternal and child deaths.** www.cemach.org.uk/publications/WMD2000_2002/wmd–04.htm [accessed 24–08–2005]
2. Riley DP, Burgess RW 1994 External abdominal aortic compression: A study of a resuscitation manoeuvre for postpartum haemorrhage. **Anaesthesia and Intensive Care,** 22: 571–575
3. Scottish Obstetric Guidelines and Audit Project (SOGAP). The management of postpartum haemorrhage. **Section 2.4.6 Arresting the Bleeding**. www.sign.ac.uk/guidelines/sogap/sogap4.html [accessed 18.08.2005]
4. Choy CMY, Lau WC, Tam WH and Yuen PM 2002 A randomised controlled trial of intramuscular Syntometrine and intravenous oxytocin in the management of the third stage of labour. **British Journal of Obstetrics and Gynaecology,** 109:173–177
5. Barrington JW and Roberts A 1993 The use of gemeprost pessaries to arrest postpartum haemorrhage. **British Journal of Obstetrics and Gynaecology,** 100:691–692
6. El-Refaey H, O'Brien P, Morafa W, Walder J and Rodeck C 1997 Use of oral misoprostol in the prevention of postpartum haemorrhage. **British Journal of Obstetrics and Gynaecology,** 104: 336–339
7. Oboro VO, Tabowei TO and Bosah JO 2003 Intrauterine misoprostol for refractory postpartum hemorrhage. **International Journal of Gynecology and Obstetrics,** 80:67–68
8. Adekanmi OA, Purmessur S, Edwards G and Barrington JW 2001 Intrauterine misoprostol for the treatment of severe recurrent atonic secondary postpartum haemorrhage. **British Journal of Obstetrics and Gynaecology,** 108:541–542
9. Lokugamage AU, Sullivan KR, Niculescu I, Tigere P, Onyangunga F, El Refaey H, Moodley J and Rodeck CH 2001 A randomized study comparing rectally administered misoprostol versus Syntometrine combined with an oxytocin infusion for the cessation of primary post partum hemorrhage. **Acta Obstetrica et Gynecologica Scandinavica,** 80:835–839
10. O'Brien P, El-Refaey H, Gordon A, Geary M and Rodeck CH 1998 Rectally administered misoprostol for the treatment of postpartum hemorrhage unresponsive to oxytocin and ergometrine: A descriptive study. **Obstetrics and Gynaecology,** 92:212–214
11. Branch DW and Rodgers GM 2003 Recombinant activated factor VII: A new weapon in the fight against hemorrhage. **Obstetrics and Gynaecology,** 101:1155–1156
12. Moscardó F, Pérez F, de la Rubia J, Balerdi B, Lorenzo JI, Senent ML, Aznar I, Carceller S and Sanz MA 2001 Successful treatment

of severe intra-abdominal bleeding associated with disseminated intravascular coagulation using recombinant activated factor VII. **British Journal of Haematology**, 114:174–176

13. Zupančić Šalek S, Sokolić V, Visković T, Šanjug J, Šimić M and Kaštelan M 2002 Successful use of recombinant factor VIIa for massive bleeding after caesarean section due to HELLP syndrome. **Acta Haematologica**, 108:162–163Š

14. Bouwmeester FW, Jonkhoff AR, Verheijen RHM, van Geijn HP 2003 Successful treatment of life-threatening postpartum hemorrhage with recombinant activated factor VII. **Obstetrics and Gynaecology**, 101:1174–1176

15. Segal S, Shemesh IY, Blumenthal R, Yoffe B, Laufer N, Ezra Y, Levy I, Mazor M and Martinowitz U 2003 Treatment of obstetric hemorrhage with recombinant activated factor VII(rFVIIa). **Archives of Gynecology and Obstetrics**, 268:266–267

16. Price G, Kaplan J and Skowronski G 2004 Use of recombinant factor VIIa to treat life-threatening non-surgical bleeding in a post-partum patient. **British Journal of Anaesthesia**, 93: 298–300

17. Ahonen J, Jokela R 2005 Recombinant factor VIIa for life-threatening post-partum haemorrhage. **British Journal of Anaesthesia** 94:592–595

18. Valentine S, Williamson P and Sutton D 1993 Reduction of acute haemorrhage with aprotinin. **Anaesthesia**, 48:405–406

19. Gai M-Y, Wu L-F, Su Q-F and Tatsumoto K 2004 Clinical observation of blood loss reduced by tranexamic acid during and after caesarian section: A multi-centre, randomized trial. **European Journal of Obstetrics, Gynaecology and Reproductive Biology**, 112: 154–157

20. As AK, Hagen P and Webb JB 1996 Tranexamic acid in the management of postpartum haemorrhage. **British Journal of Obstetrics and Gynaecology**, 103:1250–1251

21. Condous GS, Arulkumaran S, Symonds I, Chapman R, Sinha A and Razvi K 2003 The 'tamponade test' in the management of massive postpartum hemorrhage. **Obstetrics and Gynaecology**, 101:767–772

22. Katesmark M, Brown R and Raju KS 1994 Successful use of a Sengstaken-Blakemore tube to control massive postpartum haemorrhage. **British Journal of Obstetrics and Gynaecology**, 101:259–260

23. Johanson R, Kumar M, Obhrai M and Young P 2001 Management of massive postpartum haemorrhage: use of a hydrostatic balloon catheter to avoid laparotomy. **British Journal of Obstetrics and Gynaecology**, 108:420–422

24. Bakri YN, Amri A and Abdul Jabbar F 2001 Tamponade-balloon for obstetrical bleeding. **International Journal of Gynaecology and Obstetrics**, 74:139–142

25. Maier RC 1993 Control of postpartum hemorrhage with uterine packing. **American Journal of Obstetrics and Gynecology**, 169(2 pt 1):317–323

26. Lynch C, Coker A, Lawal AH, Abu J and Cowen MJ 1997 The B–Lynch surgical technique for the control of massive postpartum haemorrhage: an alternative to hysterectomy? Five cases reported. **British Journal of Obstetrics and Gynaecology**, 104: 372–375

27. Dildy III GA 2002 Postpartum hemorrhage: New management options. **Clinical Obstetrics and Gynecology,** 45:330–344

28. Danso D and Reginald P 2002 Combined B–Lynch suture with intrauterine balloon catheter triumphs over massive postpartum haemorrhage. **British Journal of Obstetrics and Gynaecology**, 109:963

29. Kalu E, Wayne C, Croucher C, Findley I and Manyonda I 2002 Triplet pregnancy in a Jehovah's Witness: recombinant human erythropoietin and iron supplementation for minimising the risks of excessive blood loss. **British Journal of Obstetrics and Gynaecology**, 109:723–725

30. Drife J 1997 Management of primary postpartum haemorrhage. **British Journal of Obstetrics and Gynaecology**, 104:275–277

31. de Souza A, Permezel M, Anderson M, Ross A, McMillan J and Walker S 2003 Antenatal erythropoietin and intra-operative cell salvage in a Jehovah's Witness with placenta praevia. **British Journal of Obstetrics and Gynaecology**, 110: 524–526

32. Catling S and Joels L 2005 Cell salvage in obstetrics: the time has come. **British Journal of Obstetrics and Gynaecology**, 112:131–132

33. Waters JH, Biscotti C, Potter PS and Phillipson E 2000 Amniotic fluid removal during cell salvage in the caesarean section patient. **Anesthesiology**, 92:1531–1536

34. Johanson R, Cox C, Grady K and Howell C 2003 **Managing Obstetric Emergencies and Trauma – The MOET Course Manual**. RCOG Press 246

35. Busuttil D and Copplestone A 1995 Management of blood loss in Jehovah's Witnesses. Recombinant human erythropoietin helps but is expensive. **British Medical Journal**, 311:1115–1116

36. Breymann C, Richter C, Hüttner C, Huch R and Huch A 2000 Effectiveness of recombinant erythropoietin and iron sucrose vs. iron therapy only, in patients with postpartum anaemia and blunted erythropoiesis. **European Journal of Clinical Investigation**, 30:154–161

37. Rizzo JD, Lichtin AE, Woolf SH, Seidenfeld J, Bennett CL, Cella D, *et al.* 2002 Use of epoetin in patients with cancer: evidence-based clinical practice guidelines of the American Society of Clinical Oncology and the American Society of Hematology. **Blood**, 100:2303–2320

38. Perewusnyk G, Huch R, Huch A, Breymann C 2002 Parenteral iron therapy in obstetrics: 8 years experience with iron-sucrose complex. **British Journal of Nutrition**, 88:3–10

39. Breymann C, Visca E, Huch R and Huch A 2001 Efficacy and safety of intravenously administered iron sucrose with and without adjuvant recombinant human erythropoietin for the treatment of resistant iron-deficiency anemia during pregnancy. **American Journal of Obstetrics and Gynecology**, 184:662–667

40. Sifakis S, Angelakis E, Vardaki E, Koumantaki Y, Matalliotakis I and Koumantakis E 2001 Erythropoietin in the treatment of iron deficiency anemia during pregnancy. **Gynecologic and Obstetric Investigations**, 51:150–156

41. McLoughlin PL, Cope TM and Harrison JC 1999 Hyperbaric oxygen therapy in the management of severe acute anaemia in a Jehovah's Witness. **Anaesthesia**, 54:891–895

Appendix 15.1   Wells Prediction Rule for Clinical Assessment of Deep Vein Thrombosis

1. Wells PS, Anderson DR, Bormanis J, *et al.* 1997 Value of assessment of pre-test probability of deep-vein thrombosis in clinical management. **The Lancet**, 350(9094):1795–1798

Appendix 15.2   Risk Factors for Venous Thromboembolism in Pregnancy and the Puerperium

1. RCOG 2004 **Clinical Guideline 37 – Thromboprophylaxis during Pregnancy, Labour and After Vaginal Delivery**. London; Royal College of Obstetricians and Gynaecologists

Appendix 16.1   Sudden Unexpected Deaths in Infancy – Contributory Factors Involving Carers

1. Fleming P, Blair P, Bacon C and Berry J 2000 **Sudden Unexpected Deaths in Infancy: The CESDI SUDI Studies 1993–1996**. London; The Stationery Office

Appendix 17   Treatment Guidance for Antenatal and Postnatal Psychiatric Disorders

1. NICE 2007 **Clinical Guideline 45 – Antenatal and Postnatal Mental Health**. London; National Institute for Clinical Excellence 8–9 http://guidance.nice.org.uk/CG45/niceguidance/pdf/English/download.dspx

Appendix 18   Advice to Patients on Coping with Cancer Symptoms and Side Effects

1. www.cancerbackup.org.uk/Aboutcancer [accessed July 2007]

Chapter References

Preface

1. RCM 2002 Guidance Paper 26 – Refocusing the role of the midwife. **Midwives** 5(4):128–129
2. Freeman-Wang T and Beski S 2002 The older obstetric patient. **Current Obstetrics and Gynaecology**, 12:41–46
3. Karnad D and Guntupalli MD 2004 Critical Illness and pregnancy: Review of a global problem. **Critical Care Clinics**, 20(4): 555–576
4. Kaaja R and Greer I 2005 Manifestations of chronic disease during pregnancy. **Journal of the American Medical Association** 294(21):2751–2757
5. Lewis G and Drife J 2002 **CEMACH 6th report: Why Mothers Die 2000–2002 Confidential Enquiries into Maternal and Child Health.** Section 1 part 2. London; RCOG Press
6. NMC 2007 NMC Consultation 'Review of pre-registration midwifery education' – decisions. London; Nursing and Midwifery Council online www.nmc–uk.org/aFrameDisplay.aspx? DocumentID=2271 [accessed 9–7–2007]
7. Frazer D 1996 Pre-registration midwifery programmes: a case study evaluation of the non-midwifery placement. **Midwifery**, 12(1):16–22
8. Lee-Colereidge H 2003 Information technology in midwifery. **Midwives**, 6(10):444–445
9. Mashiach R, Seidman G, and Seidman D 2002 Use of mifepristone as an example of conflicting and misleading medical information on the internet. **British Journal of Obstetrics and Gynaecology**, 109:437–442
10. Wilson J and Symon A 2002 **Clinical Risk Management in Pregnancy: The Right to a Perfect Baby.** Oxford; Books for Midwives Press 56–65
11. UKCC 2001 **Fitness for Practice and Purpose.** London; United Kingdom Central Council for Nursing, Midwifery and Health Visiting 4.10 and 5.14
12. O'Sullivan S 2005 Healthcare watchdog reports to Parliament. **Midwives**, 8(9):392
13. Enkin M, Keirse MJNC, Neilson J, Crowther C, Duley L, Hodnett E and Hofmeyr J 2000 Chap.7 *Risk scoring* in **A Guide to Effective care in Pregnancy and Childbirth.** Oxford; Oxford University Press 49–52
14. EU second midwifery directive 80/155/EEC Article 4 in NMC **2004 Midwives Rules and Standards.** London; Nursing and Midwifery Council 36

Chapter 1 Midwifery Care and Medical Disorders

1. Schrander-Stumpel C 1999 Pre-conception care: challenge of the new millennium? **American Journal of Medical Genetics**, (89):58–61
2. Treacy A, Byrne P, Collins C and Geary M 2006 Pregnancy outcome in immigrant women. **Irish Medical Journal**, 99(1):22–23
3. Nelson-Piercy C 2002 **Handbook of Obstetric Medicine.** London; Martin Dunitz
4. Heyes T, Long S and Mathers N 2002 Preconception care – practice and beliefs of primary care workers. **Family Practice**, 21(1):22–27
5. Burden B and Jones T 2004 Chap.10 *Preconception care.* In Henderson C and Mcdonald S (Eds) **Mayes' Midwifery: A Textbook for Midwives**, 13th Ed. London; Baillière Tindall 143–155
6. Chan KL and Kean LH 2004 Routine antenatal management at the booking clinic. **Current Obstetrics and Gynaecology**, 14:79–85

7. Glenville M 2007 **Health Professional's Guide To Pre-Conception Care** (booklet) Bognor; Foresight www.foresight–preconception.org.uk/booklet_healthproguide.htm
8. Enkin M, Keirse MJNC, Neilson J, Crowther C, Duley L, Hodnett E and Hofmeyr J 2000 **A Guide to Effective care in Pregnancy and Childbirth.** Oxford; Oxford University Press Chapters 3 and 18
9. NICE 2003 **Clinical Guideline: Antenatal care.** London; National Institute for Clinical Excellence www.nice.org.uk/guidance/ CG6 [under review]
10. NMC 2005 **Guidelines for Records and Record Keeping.** London; Nursing and Midwifery Council
11. Shepherd J, Rowan C and Powell E 2004 Chap.16 *Confirming pregnancy and care of the pregnant woman* in Henderson C and Mcdonald S (Eds) **Mayes' Midwifery: A textbook for midwives**, 13th Ed. London; Baillière Tindall 235–259
12. Chan KL and Kean LH 2004 Routine antenatal management in later pregnancy. **Current Obstetrics and Gynaecology**, 14:86–91
13. Janssen B and Wiegers T 2006 Strengths and weaknesses of midwifery care from the perspective of women. **Evidence Based Midwifery**, 4(2):53–59
14. Alfirevic Z 2006 **RCOG/RCM Joint Statement No.1: Immersion in Water during Labour and Birth.** London; Royal College of Obstetricians and Gynaecologists and Royal College of Midwives www.rcm.org.uk/info/docs/RCOG_RCM_Birth_ in_Water_FINAL_COPY_1.pdf
15. Harris T 2004 Chap.30 *Care in the third stage of labour* in Henderson C and Mcdonald S (Eds) **Mayes' Midwifery: A textbook for midwives**, 13th Ed. London; Baillière Tindall 507–523
16. Speidel B, Fleming P, Henderson J, Leaf A, Marlow N, Russell G and Dunn P 1998 Chap.4 *Routine care of the newborn infant* in **A Neonatal Vade-mecum**, 3rd Ed. London; Arnold 47–53
17. NMC **2004 Midwives Rules and Standards** *Rule 9: Records.* London; Nursing and Midwifery Council
18. MacArthur 1999 What does postnatal care do for women's health? **The Lancet**, 353(9150):343–344
19. NICE 2006 **Clinical Guideline No. 37: Routine postnatal care of women and their babies.** London; National Institute for Clinical Excellence http://www.nice.org.uk/CG037
20. NMC **2004 Midwives Rules and Standards** *Rule 2: Interpretation.* London; Nursing and Midwifery Council
21. NMC **2004 Midwives Rules and Standards** *Rule 6: Responsibility and sphere of practice.* London; Nursing and Midwifery Council
22. Tiran D 2006 Complementary therapies in pregnancy: midwives' and obstetricians' appreciation of risk. **Complementary Therapies in Clinical Practice**, 12(2):126–131
23. Anderson F and Johnson C 2005 Complementary and alternative medicine in obstetrics. **International Journal of Gynaecology and Obstetrics**, 91(2):116–124
24. NMC **2004 Midwives Rules and Standards** *Rule 7: Administration of Medicines.* London; Nursing and Midwifery Council
25. Young F 2001 Using over the counter medication in pregnancy. **British Journal of Midwifery**, 9(10):613–616
26. Briggs GG, Freeman RK and Yaffe SJ 2005 **Drugs in Pregnancy and Lactation**, 7th Ed. Philadelphia, USA; Lippincott
27. Lewis G and Drife J 2004 **Why Mothers Die 2000–2002 6th Report. Confidential Enquiries into Maternal and Child Health.** London; RCOG Press
28. RCM 1997 **Position Paper 17 Conscientious Objection.** London; Royal College of Midwives
29. Simpson C 2004 Chap.34 *The pre-term baby and the small baby* in Henderson C and Mcdonald S (Eds) **Mayes' Midwifery: A Textbook for Midwives**, 13th Ed. London; Baillière Tindall 637

30. Hospital Liaison Committee Network for Jehovah's Witnesses Leaflet – An information and Referral Service, London; HIS www.his@wtbs.org.uk

31. RCM 2006 **Position Paper 26 Refocusing the Role of the Midwife**. London; Royal College of Midwives

32. NMC **2004 Midwives Rules and Standards** *EU Activities of a Midwife*. London; Nursing and Midwifery Council 36

33. Edwards G 2007 Chap.16 *Midwifery* in Lewis G (Ed) **Saving Mothers' Lives: Reviewing Maternal Deaths to Make Motherhood Safer. 7th Report of the Confidential Enquiries into Maternal and Child Health**. London; CEMACH 199–212

34. Whitty JE 2002 Maternal cardiac arrest in pregnancy. **Clinical Obstetrics and Gynaecology**, 45(2):377–392

35. Germain S, Wyncollb D and Nelson-Piercy C 2006 Management of the critically ill obstetric patient. **Current Obstetrics and Gynaecology**, 16:125–133

36. De Sweit M 2002 **Medical Disorders in Obstetric Practice**. Oxford; Blackwell Scientific 135

37. Boyle M (Ed) 2002 **Emergencies Around Childbirth: A Handbook For Midwives**. UK; Radcliffe Medical Press

38. Resuscitation Council (UK) 2005 **In Hospital Resuscitation** www.resus.org

39. Jevon P and Raby M 2001 **Resuscitation in Pregnancy**. Oxford; Books for Midwives Press

Chapter 2 Skin Disorders

2.1 Eczema

1. Diepgen TL 2000 *Is the prevalence of atopic dermatitis increasing?* in Williams HC (Ed) **Atopic Dermatitis**. Cambridge; Cambridge University Press

2. Kroumpouzos G and Cohen L M 2001 Dermatoses of pregnancy. **Journal of the American Academy of Dermatology** 45:1–19

3. Snijders BE, Thijs C, Kummeling I, Penders J and van den Brandt PA 2007 Breastfeeding and infant eczema in the first year of life in the KOALA birth cohort study: a risk period-specific analysis. **Pediatrics**, Jan; 119(1):e137–41

4. Reed BR 1997 Dermatological drug use during pregnancy and lactation. **Dermatologic Clinics**, 15:197–206

2.2 Psoriasis

1. Krueger GG, Bergstresser PR, Lowe NJ, *et al.* 1984 Psoriasis. **Journal of the American Academy of Dermatology**, 11:937–974

2. Murase J, Chan K, Garite T, Cooper D and Weinstein G 2005 Hormonal effect on psoriasis in pregnancy and post partum. **Archives of Dermatology**, 141(5):601–606

3. Rees JL and Farr PM 1997 Psoriasis. **Journal of the Royal College of Physicians of London**, 31(3):238–240

4. BNF 2006 **British National Formulary No:52** London; BMA and RPSGB as http://www.bnf.org/bnf/ [accessed May 2007]

5. McHugh NJ and Laurent MR 1989 The effect of pregnancy on the onset of psoriatic arthritis. **British Journal of Rheumatology**, 28:50–52

6. Tauscher AE, Fleischer AB Jr, Phelps KC and Feldman SR 2002 Psoriasis and pregnancy. **Journal of Cutaneous Medicine and Surgery**, 6:561–570

Chapter 3 Hypertensive Disorders

3.1 Chronic Hypertension

1. Chesley LC 1978 **Hypertensive disorders in pregnancy**. New York; Appleton-Century-Crofts 478

2. Butler NR and Bonham DG 1963 **Perinatal Mortality**. Edinburgh; E & S Livingstone 87–100

3. Williams MA, Lieberman E, Mittendirf R, Monson RR and Schoenbaum SC 1991 Risk factors for abruptio placentae. **American Journal of Epidemiology**, 134:965–972

4. Williams B, Poulter NR, Brown MJ, *et al.* 2004 British Hypertension Society guidelines for hypertension management (BHS–IV) summary. **British Medical Journal**, 328:634–640

5. Milne F, Redman C, Walker J, *et al.* 2005 The pre-eclampsia community guideline. PRECOG: how to screen for and detect onset of pre-eclampsia in the community. **British Medical Journal**, 330:576–580

6. Tuffnell DJ, Shennan AH, Waugh JJS and Walker JJ 2006 **RCOG Guideline 10(A):The Management of Severe preeclampsia/eclampsia**. London; Royal College of Obstetricians and Gynaecologists

7. RCOG 2001 Evidence Based Clinical Guideline No 8. **The Use of Electronic Fetal Monitoring**. London; RCOG Press

3.2 Pre-eclampsia

1. Shennan AH and Waugh JJS 2003 **Pre-eclampsia**. London; RCOG Press

2. Duckitt K, Harrington D 2005 Risk factors for pre-eclampsia at antenatal booking: systematic review of controlled studies. **British Medical Journal**, 330:565–567

3. Duley L, Henderson Smart DJ, Knight M, *et al.* 2003 Antiplatelet agents for preventing pre-eclampsia and its complications. **Cochrane Database of Systematic Reviews** Issue 4. Article CD004659 DOI:10.1002/14651858.CD004659

4. Hoffmeyer GJ, Atallah AN, Duley L 2006 Calcium supplementation during pregnancy for preventing hypertensive disorders and related problems. **Cochrane Database of Systematic Reviews** Issue 3 Article CD001059. DOI:10.1002 /14651858.CD001059.pub2

5. NICE 2003 **Clinical Guideline: Antenatal care**. London; National Institute for Clinical Excellence http://www.nice.org.uk/guidance/CG6

6. Shennan AH, Gupta M, Halligan A, *et al.* 1996 Lack of reproducibility in pregnancy of Korotkoff phase IV as measured by mercury sphygmomanometry. **Lancet**, 347:139–142

7. Waugh JJS, Bell SC, Kilby MD, *et al.* 2005 Optimal bedside urinalysis for the detection of proteinuria in hypertensive pregnancy: a study of diagnostic accuracy. **British Journal of Obstetrics and Gynaecology**, 112:412–417

8. Tuffnell DJ, Shennan AH, Waugh JJS and Walker JJ 2006 **RCOG Guideline No. 10(A):The Management of Severe preeclampsia/eclampsia**. London; Royal College of Obstetricians and Gynaecologists

3.3 Severe pre-eclampsia/HELLP/Eclampsia

1. Tuffnell DJ, Shennan AH, Waugh JJS, Walker JJ 2006 **RCOG Guideline 10(A) The Management of Severe preeclampsia/eclampsia**. London; Royal College of Obstetricians and Gynaecologists

Chapter 4 Heart Disease

4.1 Mild Structural Heart Disease

1. Walker F 2006 Chap.5 *Antenatal care of women with cardiac disease: a cardiologist's perspective* in Steer PJ, Gatzoulis M and Baker P (Eds) **Heart Disease in Pregnancy**. London; RCOG Press 55–66

2. Wren C and O'Sullivan JJ 2001 Survival with congenital heart disease and need to follow up in adult life. **Heart**, 85:438–443

3. Vause S, Thorne S and Clarke B 2006 Chap.1 *Preconceptual counselling for women with cardiac disease* in Steer PJ, Gatzoulis M and Baker P (Eds) **Heart Disease in Pregnancy**. London; RCOG Press 3–8

4. Stout K 2005 Pregnancy in women with congenital heart disease: the importance of evaluation and counselling. **Heart**, 91:713–714

5. Macpherson G 2004 **Black's Student Medical Dictionary**. London; A and C Black Publishers

6. Shinebourne EA, Babu-Narayan SV and Carvalho JS 2006 Tetralogy of Fallot: from fetus to adult. **Heart**, 92:1353–1359

7. Perloff J and Warnes C 2001 Challenges posed by adults with repaired congenital heart disease. **Circulation**, 103:2637

8. Neumayer U, Stone S and Somerville J 1998 Small ventricular septal defects in adults. **European Heart Journal**, 19:1573–1582

9. Siu SC and Colman J 2001 Heart disease in pregnancy. **Heart**, 710–715

10. Hyett J, Perdu M, Sharland G, Snijders R and Nicolaides KH 1999 Using fetal nuchal translucency to screen for major congenital cardiac defects at 10–14 weeks of gestation: population based cohort study. **British Medical Journal**, 318:81–85

11. Zuber M, Gautschi N and Oechslin E 1999 Outcome of pregnancy with congenital shunt lesions. **Heart**, 81:271–275

12. Pitkin RM, Perloff JK, Kos BJ and Beall MH 1990 Pregnancy and congenital heart disease. **Annals of Internal Medicine**, 112:445–454

13. Thorne SA 2004 Pregnancy in heart disease. **Heart**, 90:450–456

14. Nelson-Piercy C 2007 Chap.9 *Cardiac Disease* in Lewis G (Ed) 2007 **Saving Mothers' Lives: Reviewing Maternal Deaths to Make Motherhood Safer. 7th Report of the Confidential Enquiries into Maternal and Child Health**. London; CEMACH 117–130

15. Tomlinson M 2006 Chap.37 *Cardiac disease* in James DK, Steer PJ, Weiner CP and Gonik B (Eds) 2006 **High Risk Pregnancy: Management Options**, 3rd Ed. London; Elsevier 790–827

16. Thorne S 2006 Chap.13 *Mitral and aortic stenosis* in Steer PJ, Gatzoulis M and Baker P (Eds) **Heart Disease in Pregnancy**. London; RCOG Press 183–190

17. Khairy P, Quyang DW and Fernandes S 2006 Pregnancy outcomes in women with congenital heart disease. **Circulation**, 113:1564–1571

18. Gelson E, Johnson M, Gatzoulis M and Uebing A 2007 Cardiac disease in pregnancy. Part 1: congenital heart disease. **The Obstetrician and Gynaecologist**, 9:15–20

4.2 Moderate Structural Heart Disease

1. Swan L 2006 *Aortopathies including Marfan's syndrome and coarctation* in Steer PJ, Gatzoulis M and Baker P (Eds) **Heart Disease in Pregnancy**. London; RCOG Press

2. Warnes C 2005 The Adult with Congenital Heart Disease – Born to be Bad? **Journal of the American College of Cardiology**, 46:1–8

3. Celermajer D and Greaves K 2002 Survivors of coarctation repair: fixed but not cured. **Heart**, 88:113–114

4. Cohen M, Fuster V, Steele PM, Driscoll D and McGoon DC 1989 Coarctation of the aorta. Long-term follow-up and prediction of outcome after surgical correction. **Circulation**, 80(4):840–845

5. Raja SG and Basu D 2005 Pulmonary hypertension in congenital heart disease. **Nursing Standard**, 19(50):41–49

6. Presbitero P, Somerville J, Rabajoli F, *et al.* 1995 Corrected transposition of the great arteries without associated defects in adult patients: clinical profile and follow-up. **British Heart Journal**, 74:57–59

7. Shah S and Calderon D 2005 **Aortic Coarctation**. www. emedicine.com/med/topic154.htm [accessed 30/08/2007]

8. Serfontein SJ and Kron IL 2002 Complications of coarctation repair. **Seminars in Thoracic and Cardiovascular Surgery: Pediatric Cardiac Surgery Annual**, 5:206–211

9. Gatzoulis MA, Balaji S, Webber SA, *et al.* 2000 Risk factors for arrhythmia and sudden cardiac death late after repair of tetralogy of Fallot: a multicentre study. **The Lancet**, 356:975–981

10. Connolly HM, Grogan M and Warnes CA 1999 Pregnancy among women with congenitally corrected transposition of great arteries. **Journal of the American College of Cardiology**, 33(6): 1692–1695(4)

11. Adamson D, Dhanjal C, Nelson-Piercy C and Collis R 2007 *Cardiac disease in pregnancy* in Geer I, Nelson-Piercy C and Walters B (Eds) **Maternal Medicine – Medical Problems in Pregnancy**. Edinburgh; Churchill/Elsevier

12. Nelson-Piercy C 2007 Chap.9 *Cardiac Disease* in Lewis G (Ed) 2007 **Saving Mothers' Lives: Reviewing Maternal Deaths to Make Motherhood Safer. 7th Report of the Confidential Enquiries into Maternal and Child Health**. London; CEMACH 117–130

13. Thorne SA 2004 Pregnancy in heart disease. **Heart**, 90:450–456

14. Siu SC, Sermer M, Colman JM, *et al.* 2001 Prospective multicentre study of pregnancy outcomes in women with heart disease. **Circulation**, 104:515–521

15. Guedes A, Mercier L, Leduc L, Berube L and Marcotte F 2004 Impact of pregnancy on the systemic right ventricle after a Mustard operation for transposition of the great arteries. **American College of Cardiology**, 21:44(2):433–437

4.3 Severe Structural Heart Disease

1. Abbas AE, Lester SJ and Connolly H 2005 Pregnancy and the cardiovascular system. **International Journal of Cardiology**, 98:179–189

2. Gatzoulis MA, Webb GD and Daubeny PEF (Eds) 2003 **Diagnosis and management of adult congenital heart disease**. London; Churchill Livingstone/Elsevier 136

3. Siu SC, Sermer M, Colman JM, *et al.* 2001 Prospective multicentre study of pregnancy outcomes in women with heart disease. **Circulation**, 104:515–521

4. Presbitero P, Somerville J, Sone S, *et al.* 1994 Pregnancy in cyanotic congenital heart disease – outcome of mother and fetus. **Circulation**, 89:2673–2676

5. Tomlinson M 2006 Chap.37 *Cardiac disease* in James DK, Steer PJ, Weiner CP and Gonik B (Eds) 2006 **High Risk Pregnancy: Management Options**, 3rd Ed. London; Elsevier 790–827

6. Thorne SA 2004 Pregnancy in heart disease. **Heart**, 90:450–456

7. Gilbert ES 2007 Chap.11 *Cardiac disease* in **High Risk Pregnancy and Delivery**, 4th Ed. London; Mosby/Elsevier 270–285

4.4 Valvular Heart Disease

1. Braunwald E 2001 *Valvular heart disease* in Braunwald E and Zipes DP (Eds) **Heart Disease: A Textbook of Cardiovascular Medicine**, 6th Ed. London; Saunders/Elsevier

2. Tomlinson M 2006 Chap.37 *Cardiac disease* in James DK, Steer PJ, Weiner CP and Gonik B (Eds) 2006 **High Risk Pregnancy** (3rd Ed). London; Elsevier 790–827

3. Bayer AS, Bolger A F, Taubert KA, *et al.* 1998 Diagnosis and management of infective endocarditis and its complications. **Circulation**, 98:2936–2948

4. Stuart 2006 Chap.19 *Maternal endocarditis* in Steer PJ, Gatzoulis M and Baker P (Eds) **Heart Disease in Pregnancy**. London; RCOG Press 267–284

5. Elkayam U 2005 Valvular heart disease and pregnancy part 11 prosthetic valves. **Journal of the American College of Cardiology**, 46(3):403–410

6. Reimold S and Rutherford J 2003 Valvular heart disease in pregnancy. **New England Journal of Medicine**, 349(1):52–59

7. Prasad A and Ventura H 2001 Valvular heart disease and pregnancy. **Post Graduate Medicine**, 110(2):69–88

8. Nelson-Piercy C 2007 Chap.9 *Cardiac disease* in Lewis G (Ed) 2007 **Saving Mothers' Lives: Reviewing Maternal Deaths to Make Motherhood Safer. 7th Report of the Confidential Enquiries into Maternal and Child Health**. London; CEMACH 117–130

9. Nelson-Piercy C 2006 **Handbook of Obstetric Medicine**, 3rd Ed. Abingdon; Informa Health Care 23–43

10. Silversides CK, Coleman JM, Sermer M and Siu SC 2003 Cardiac risk in pregnant women with rheumatic mitral stenosis. **American Journal of Cardiology**, 91:182–185

11. Ray P, Murphy GJ and Shutt, LE 2004 Recognition and management of maternal cardiac disease in pregnancy. **British Journal of Anaesthesia**, 93:428–439

12. Hameed A, Karaalp I, Tummala P, *et al.* 2001 The effect of valvular heart disease on maternal and fetal outcome of pregnancy. **Journal of the American College of Cardiology**, 37(3): 893–899

13. Tucker D, Liu D and Ramoutar P 1996 Myocardial infarction at term – a case report to consider management options. **Journal of Obstetrics and Gynaecology**, 16:522–524

14. Niwa K and Tateno S 2006 Chap.18 *Maternal cardiac arrhythmias* in Steer PJ, Gatzoulis M and Baker P (Eds) **Heart Disease in Pregnancy**. London; RCOG Press 251–265

15. Chan WS, Anand S and Ginsberg JS 2000 Anticoagulation of pregnant women with mechanical heart valves a systematic review of the literature. **Archives of Internal Medicine**, 160: 191–196

16. Gilbert ES 2007 Chap.11 *Cardiac disease* in Gilbert ES **High Risk Pregnancy and Delivery**; 4th Ed. London; Mosby/Elsevier 270–285

17. Breast Feeding Network 2007 www.breastfeedingnetwork.org.uk/ supporterline/medication.php [accessed 17-6-2007]

4.5 Marfan's syndrome

1. Lalchandani S and Wingfield M 2003 Pregnancy in women with Marfan's syndrome. **European Journal of Obstetrics Gynaecology and Reproductive Biology**, 110(2):125–130
2. Rubenstein D, Wayne D and Bradley J 2003 **Lecture Notes on Clinical Medicine**, 6th Ed. Oxford; Blackwell/Wiley 280–281
3. Marfan's Association 2007 Factsheet online marfan.org.uk/content/view/14/31/ [accessed 02-09-2007]
4. De Swiet M 2002 **Medical Disorders in Obstetric Practice**, 4th Ed. Oxford; Blackwell/Wiley 149–150
5. Chen H 2006 Marfan's Syndrome www.emedicine.com/ped/topic1372.htm [accessed 30-06-2007]
6. Pyeritz R 2000 The Marfan's syndrome. **Annual Review of Medicine**, 51:481–510
7. Kumar P and Clarke M 2002 **Clinical Medicine**, 5th Ed. London; Saunders/Elsevier 803–804
8. Swan L 2006 *Aortopathies including Marfan's syndrome and coarctation* in Steer P, Gatzoulis M and Baker P (Eds) **Heart Disease in Pregnancy**. London; RCOG Press
9. Stuart AG and Williams A 2007 Marfan's syndrome and the heart. **Archives of Disease in Childhood**, 92(4):351–356
10. Nelson-Piercy C 2002 **Handbook of Obstetric Medicine**, 2nd Ed. London; Martin Dunitz 27–28
11. Ryan-Krause P 2002 Identify and manage Marfan's syndrome in children. **Nurse Practitioner**, 27(10):26–37
12. Oakley GD, McGarry K, Limb DG and Oakley CM 1979 Management of pregnancy in patients with hypertrophic cardiomyopathy. **British Medical Journal**, 1:1749–1750
13. Bonow RO, Carabellow B, de Leon A, Edmunds LH, *et al.* 1998 ACC/AHA guidelines for the management of people with valvular heart disease. A report from the American College of Cardiology/American Heart Association Task Force on Practice Guidelines Committee on Management of Patients with Valvular Heart Disease. **Journal of the American College of Cardiology**, 32:1486–1588
14. Uebing A, Steer PJ, Yentis SM and Gatzoulis MA 2006 Pregnancy and congenital heart disease. **British Medical Journal**, 332: 401–406
15. Elkayam U and Googdwin TM 1995 Adenosine therapy for supraventricular tachycardia during pregnancy. **American Journal of Cardiology**, 75:521–523
16. Meijboom LI, Drenthen W, Pieper PG, *et al.* 2006 Obstetric complications in Marfan's syndrome. **International Journal of Cardiology**, 110(1):53–59
17. Rahman J, Rahman FZ, Rahman W, *et al.* 2003 Obstetric and gynecologic complications in women with Marfan's syndrome. **The Journal of Reproductive Medicine**, 48(9):723–728
18. Oakley C, Child A, Jung B, *et al.* 2003 The task force on the management of cardiovascular disease during pregnancy of the European Society of Cardiology. **European Heart Journal**, 24:761–781
19. Durbridge J, Dresner M, Harding K and Yentis S 2006 Chap.20 *Pregnancy and cardiac disease – peripartum aspects* in Steer P, Gatzoulis M and Baker P (Eds) **Heart Disease in Pregnancy**. London; RCOG Press 285–298
20. Chow SL 1993 Acute aortic dissection in a patient with Marfan's syndrome complicated by gestational hypertension. **Medical Journal of Australia**, 159:760–762
21. Schmaltz A 2002 Pregnancy in maternal congenital heart disease: a review. **Fetal and Maternal Medicine**, 13(1):43–6122
22. Fujitani S and Baldisseri M 2005 Hemodynamic assessment in a pregnant and peripartum patient. **Critical Care Medicine**, 33(Suppl. 10):S354–361
23. Witcher P and Harvey C 2006 Modifying labor routines for the woman with cardiac disease. **Journal of Perinatal and Neonatal Nursing**, 20(4):303–310
24. Thorne S, Nelson-Piercy C, MacGregor A, *et al.* 2006 Pregnancy and contraception in heart disease and pulmonary arterial hypertension. **Journal of Family Planning and Reproductive Health Care**, 32(2):75–81
25. Dhanjal MK 2006 Chap.2 *Contraception in Women with Heart Disease* in Steer P, Gatzoulis M and Baker P (Eds) **Heart Disease in Pregnancy**. London; RCOG Press 9–28

4.6 Functional Heart Disease: Cardiomyopathy

1. Maron BJ 2002 Hypertrophic cardiomyopathy: a systematic review. **Journal of the American Medical Association**, 287:1308–1320
2. Nelson-Piercy C 2006 Chap.16 *Cardiomyopathy* in Steer P, Gatzoulis M and Baker P (Eds) **Heart Disease in Pregnancy**. London; RCOG Press 231–242
3. Tan J 2004 Cardiovascular disease in pregnancy. **Current Obstetrics and Gynaecology**, 14:155–165
4. Valeriano C, Simbre II, Jacob Adams M, *et al.* 2001 Current treatment options. **Cardiovascular Medicine**, 3:493–505
5. Matthews T and Dickinson 2005 Considerations for delivery in pregnancies complicated by maternal hypertrophic obstructive cardiomyopathy. **Australian and New Zealand Journal of Obstetrics and Gynaecology**, 45:526–528
6. Autore C, Conte MR, Piccininno M, *et al.* 2002 Risk associated with pregnancy in hypertrophic cardiomyopathy. **Journal of the American College of Cardiology**, 40:1864–1869
7. Paix B, Cyna A, Belperio P and Simmons S 1999 Epidural analgesia for labour and delivery in a parturient with congenital hypertrophic obstructive cardiomyopathy. **Anaesthesia and Intensive Care**, 27:59–62
8. Macpherson G 2004 **Black's Student Medical Dictionary**. London; A and C Black Publishers
9. Yacoub A and Martel MJ 2002 Pregnancy with primary dilated cardiomyopathy. **Obstetrics and Gynaecology**, 99:928–930
10. Nelson-Piercy C 2007 Chap.9 *Cardiac disease* in Lewis G (Ed) **Saving Mothers' Lives: Reviewing Maternal Deaths to Make Motherhood Safer. 7th Report of the Confidential Enquiries into Maternal and Child Health**. London; CEMACH 117–130
11. Elkayam U 2005 Valvular heart disease and pregnancy part 11: prosthetic valves. **Journal of the American College Cardiology**, 46(3):403–410
12. Murali S and Baldisseri M 2005 Peripartum cardiomyopathy. **Critical Care Medicine**, 33(Suppl.):S340–S346
13. Veille JC 1984 Peripartum cardiomyopathies – a review. **American Journal of Obstetrics and Gynaecology**, 148:805–818
14. Ray P, Murphy GJ and Shutt LE 2004 Recognition and management of maternal cardiac disease in pregnancy. **British Journal of Anaesthesia**, 93:428–439
15. Hendricks CH and Brenner WE 1970 Cardiovascular effects of oxytocic drugs used post partum. **American Journal of Obstetrics and Gynecology**, 108:751–760
16. Durbridge J, Dresner M, Harding K and Yentis S 2006 *Pregnancy and cardiac disease – peripartum aspects* in Steer P, Gatzoulis M and Baker P (Eds) **Heart Disease in Pregnancy**. London; RCOG Press
17. Jordan S 2001 **Pharmacology for Midwives: The Evidence Base**. London; Palgrave Macmillan
18. Ramsay M 2006 *Management of the puerperium in women with heart disease* in Steer P, Gatzoulis M and Baker P (Eds) **Heart Disease in Pregnancy**. London; RCOG Press 299–312
19. Elkayam U, Tummala P and Rao K 2001 Maternal and fetal outcomes of subsequent pregnancies in women with peripartum cardiomyopathy. **New England Journal of Medicine**, 344: 1567–1571
20. Elkayam U 2003 Pregnant again after peripartum cardiomyopathy: to be or not to be. **European Heart Journal**, 23:753–756

4.7 Functional Heart Disease: Arrhythmias

1. Niwa K and Tateno S 2006 Chap.18 *Maternal cardiac arrhythmias* in Steer P, Gatzoulis M and Baker P (Eds) **Heart Disease in Pregnancy**. London; RCOG Press 251–265
2. Macpherson G 2004 **Black's Student Medical Dictionary**. London; A and C Black Publishers
3. Brodsky M, Doria R, Allen B, *et al.* 1992 New-onset ventricular tachycardia during pregnancy. **American Heart Journal**, 123: 933–941
4. Ferrero S, Colombo BM and Ragni N 2004 Maternal arrhythmias in pregnancy. **Archives of Gynecology and Obstetrics**, 269(4): 244–253
5. Trappe H 2006 Acute therapy maternal and fetal arrhythmias during pregnancy. **Journal of Intensive Care Medicine**, 21(5): 305–315

6. Zevitz 2006 Ventricular Fibrillation www.emedicine.com/med/topic2363.htm [accessed 27-6-07]
7. Waldo A 2000 Electrophysiology: treatment of atrial flutter. **Heart**, 84:227
8. Conway D and Yip G 2003 **Atrial Physiology in Cardiac Arrhythmias – A Clinical Approach**. London; Mosby/Elsevier
9. Cox D and Dougall H 2001 Understanding ECGs – bradycardia. **Student BMJ**, 09:443–848 www.studentbmj.com/issues01/12/education/453;php [accessed 12-05-2007]
10. Blomstrom-Lundqvist C, Scheinman MM, Aliot EM, et al. 2003 ACC/AHA/ESC Guidelines for the management of patients with supraventricular arrhythmias – executive summary: a report of the American College of Cardiology/American Heart Association Task Force on Practice Guidelines and the European Society of Cardiology Committee for Practice Guidelines. **Circulation**, 108:1871–1909
11. Rotmensch H, Rotmensch S and Elkayam U 1987 Management of cardiac arrhythmias during pregnancy, current concepts. **Drugs**, 33(6):623–633
12. Bartalena L, Bogazzi F, Braverman LE and Martino E 2001 Effects of amiodarone administration during pregnancy on neonatal thyroid function and subsequent neurodevelopment. **Journal of Endocrinological Investigation**, 1(24):116–130
13. Devendra K, Ching CK, Tan LK, Tan HK and Yu SL 2006 Intrapartum maternal sinus bradycardia with spontaneous resolution following delivery. **Singapore Medical Journal**, 47(11): 971–974
14. Silversides CK, Coleman JM, Sermer M and Siu SC 2003 Cardiac risk in pregnant women with rheumatic mitral stenosis. **American Journal of Cardiology**, 91:182–185
15. Elkayam U, Googdwin TM 1995 Adenosine therapy for supraventricular tachycardia during pregnancy. **American Journal of Cardiology**, 75: 521–523
16. Mark S and Harris L 2002 Arrhythmias in pregnancy in Wilansky S (Ed) **Heart Disease in Women**. Philadelphia; Churchill/Elsevier 497–514
17. Lee S, Chen SA, Wu TJ, et al. 1995 Effects of pregnancy on first onset and symptoms of paroxysmal supraventricular tachycardia. **American Journal of Cardiology**, 76; 675–678
18. Fuster V, Ryden LE, Asinger RW, et al. 2001 ACC/AHA/ESC Guidelines for the management of patients with atrial fibrillation: executive summary – a report of the American College of Cardiology/American Heart Association Task Force on Practice Guidelines. **Circulation**, 104:2118–2150
19. Tomlinson M 2006 Chap.37 Cardiac disease in James D, Steer P, Weiner C and Gonik B (Eds) **High Risk Pregnancy: Management Options**, 3rd Ed. London; Elsevier 790–827
20. Wolbrette D 2005 Arrhythmias during pregnancy a therapeutic challenge – business briefing. **Women's Heath Care**, 51–55
21. Lip G, Hart RG and Conway DSG 2002 ABC of antithrombotic therapy: antithrombotic therapy for atrial fibrillation. **British Medical Journal**, 325(7371):1022–1025
22. Rotmensch H, Rotmensch S and Elkayam U 1987 Management of cardiac arrhythmias during pregnancy, current concepts. **Drugs**, 33(6):623–633

4.8 Ischaemic Heart Disease – Angina and Myocardial Infarction
1. Roos-Hesselink JW 2006 Ischaemic heart disease in Steer P, Gatzoulis M and Baker P (Eds) **Heart Disease in Pregnancy**. London; RCOG Press 243–250
2. Nelson-Piercy C 2007 Chap.9 Cardiac disease in Lewis G (Ed) 2007 **Saving Mothers Lives: Reviewing Maternal Deaths to Make Motherhood Safer. 7th Report of the Confidential Enquiries into Maternal and Child Health**. London; CEMACH 117–130
3. James AH, Abel DE, Brancazio LR 2006 Anticoagulants in pregnancy. **Obstetrical and Gynecological Survey**, 61(1)59–69
4. Anderson C 2007 Pre-eclampsia: exposing future cardiovascular risk in mothers and their children. **Journal of Obstetric, Gynecologic and Neonatal Nursing**, 36:3–8
5. Roth A and Elkayam U 1996 Acute myocardial infarction associated with pregnancy. **Annals of Internal Medicine**, 125(9):751–762

6. James AH, Jamison MG, Biswas MS, Brancazio LR, Swamy JK, Myers ER 2006 Acute myocardial infarction in pregnancy – a United States population based study. **Circulation**, 133(12):1564–1571
7. Tan J 2004 Cardiovascular disease in pregnancy. **Current Obstetrics and Gynaecology**, 14:155–165
8. Ray P, Murphy GJ and Shutt LE 2004 Recognition and management of maternal cardiac disease in pregnancy. **British Journal of Anaesthesia**, 93: 428–439
9. Vinatier D, Viirelizier S and Depret-Mosser S 1994 Pregnancy after myocardial Infarction. **European Journal of Obstetrics, Gynaecology and Reproductive Biology**, 56:89–93
10. Marini J and Wheeler A 2006 **Critical Care Medicine**, 3rd Ed. Philadelphia; Lippincott/Williams and Wilkins
11. Handkins GDV, Wendel GD, Leveno KL and Stoneham J 1985 Myocardial infarction during pregnancy: a review. **Obstetrics and Gynaecology**, 65:139–146
12. Tomlinson M 2006 Chap.37 Cardiac disease in James DK, Steer PJ, Weiner CP and Gonik B (Eds) **High Risk Pregnancy**, 3rd Ed. London; Elsevier 790–827
13. Tsui BC, Stewart B, Fitzmaurice A and Williams R 2001 Cardiac arrest and myocardial infarction induced by post partum intravenous ergonovine administration. **Anaesthesiology**, 94:363–364
14. Shieikh AU and Harper MA 1993 Myocardial infarction during pregnancy management and outcome of two pregnancies. **American Journal of Obstetrics and Gynecology**, 169:279–284
15. McKechnie RS, Patel D, Eitzman DT, Rajagopalan S and Murthy TH 2001 Spontaneous coronary artery dissection in a pregnant woman. **Obstetrics and Gynaecology**, 98:899–902
16. Rubenstein D, Wayne D and Bradley J 2003 **Lecture Notes on Clinical Medicine**, 6th Ed. Oxford; Blackwell 264

4.9 Pulmonary Hypertension and Eisenmenger's Syndrome
1. D'Alonzo GE, Barst RJ, Ayres SM, et al. 1991 Survival in patients with primary pulmonary hypertension: results from a national prospective registry. **Annals of Internal Medicine**, 115:343–349
2. Simon J and Gibbs R 2001 Recommendations on the management of pulmonary hypertension in clinical practice. **Heart**, 86(Suppl. 1):i1–i13
3. Rich S, Dantzker DR, Ayres SM, et al. 1987 Primary pulmonary hypertension. A national perspective study. **Annals of Internal Medicine**, 197:216–223
4. Simonneau G, Galie N, Rubin LJ, Langleben D, Seeger W, et al. 2004 Clinical classification of pulmonary hypertension. **Journal of the American College of Cardiology**, 43(12 supplements): 5s–12s
5. Nichols WC, Koller DL, Slovis B, et al. 1997 Localization of the gene for familial primary pulmonary hypertension to chromosome 2q31–32. **Nature Genetics**, 15(3):277–280
6. Gaille N, Ghofrani HA, Torbicki A, Barst RJ, Rubin LJ, Badesch D, et al. 2005 Sildenafil citrate therapy for pulmonary arterial hypertension. **New England Journal of Medicine**, 353:2148–2157
7. Abenhaim L, Moride Y, Brenot F, et al. 1996 Appetite-suppressant drugs and the risk of primary pulmonary hypertension. International Primary Pulmonary Hypertension Study Group. **New England Journal of Medicine**, 335(9):609–661
8. Kiely D, Elliot C, Webster V and Stewart P 2006 Pregnancy and pulmonary hyper tension: New approaches to management in Steer P, Gatzoulis M and Baker P (Eds) **Heart Disease in Pregnancy**. London; RCOG Press
9. Warnes CA 2004 Pregnancy and pulmonary hypertension. **International Journal of Cardiology**, 97(Suppl. 1):11–3
10. Weiss BM, Zemp L, Seifert B and Hess OM 1998 Outcome of pulmonary vascular disease in pregnancy: a systematic overview from 1978 through to 1996. **Journal of the American College of Cardiology**, 31:1650–1657
11. **Pulmonary Hypertension Association** www.pha–uk.com/ [accessed 17/05/2007]
12. Thorne S, Nelson-Piercy C, MacGregor A, Gibbs S, Crowhurst J, et al. 2006 Pregnancy and contraception in heart disease and pulmonary arterial hypertension. **Journal of Family Planning and Reproductive Health Care**, 32(2):75–81

13. Tomlinson M 2006 Chap.37 *Cardiac disease* in James DK, Steer PJ, Weiner CP and Gonik B (Eds) **High Risk Pregnancy**, 3rd Ed. London; Elsevier 790–827
14. Campbell P and Rudisill P 2006 Psychological needs of the critically ill obstetric patient. **Critical Care Nursing**, 29(1):77–80

Chapter 5 Respiratory Disorders

5.1 The Breathless Pregnant Woman
1. Dilworth JP and Baldwin DR 2002 **Respiratory Medicine Specialist Handbook**. London; Martin Dunitz
2. Hytten FE and Leitch I 1971 *Respiration* in **The Physiology of Human Pregnancy**. Oxford; Blackwell Scientific Publications

5.2 Asthma
1. Nelson-Piercy C 2001 Asthma in pregnancy. **Thorax**, 56:325
2. Rey E and Boulet L-P 2007 Asthma in pregnancy. **British Medical Journal**, 334:582–585
3. British Thoracic Society *et al.* 1990 Guidelines for the management of asthma in adults: 11 – acute severe asthma. **British Medical Journal**, 301:6755:797–800
4. British Thoracic Society/Scottish Intercollegiate Guidelines 2003 Network British guideline on the management of asthma. **Thorax**, 58(Suppl. 10):i1–i94 update www.brit–thoracic.org.uk
5. Price D, Foster J, Scullion J and Freeman D 2004 **Asthma and COPD**. London; Churchill Livingstone
6. Scullion JE 2007 **Fundamental Aspects of Nursing – Respiratory Disorders**. London; Quay Books
7. Tan KS and Thompson NC 2000 Asthma in pregnancy. **American Journal of Medicine**, 109:727
8. WHO 2002 **Infant and Young Child Nutrition – Global Strategy in Infancy And Young Child Feeding**. 55th World assembly. Geneva; World Health Organization

5.3 Pneumonia and Chest Infections
1. Guidelines for the Management of Community Acquired Pneumonia in Adults 2001 **Thorax**, 56(Suppl. IV) 2004 update www.brit–thoracic.org.uk
2. Berkowitz K and Lasala A 1990 Risk factors associated with the increasing prevalence of pneumonia in pregnancy. **American Journal of Obstetrics and Gynecology**, 163:981–985
3. Metlay JP, Kapoor WN and Fine MJ 1997 Does this patient have community-acquired pneumonia? Diagnosing pneumonia by history and physical examination. **Journal of the American Medical Association**, 278:1440

5.4 Tuberculosis
1. NICE 2006 **Guideline CG033: Clinical Diagnosis and Management of Tuberculosis, and Measures for Its Prevention and Control** www.nice.org.uk
2. **Guidelines for the Management of Tuberculosis** www.brit–thoracic.org.uk [accessed March 2007]
3. Omerod P 2001 Tuberculosis in pregnancy and the puerperium. **Thorax**, 56:494
4. de March P 1975 Tuberculosis in pregnancy: Five-in-ten year review of 215 patients in their fertile age. **Chest**, 68:800–880

5.5 Cystic Fibrosis
1. Dilworth JP and Baldwin DR 2002 **Respiratory Medicine Specialist Handbook**. London; Martin Dunitz
2. Gilljam M, Antoniou M, Shin J, Dupuis A, Corey M and Tullis DE 2000 Pregnancy in cystic fibrosis. Fetal and maternal outcome. **Chest**, 118(1):85–91
3. Edenborough FP, Stableforth DE, Webb AK *et al.* 2000 The outcome of 72 pregnancies in 55 women with cystic fibrosis in the UK 1977–1996. **British Journal of Obstetrics and Gynaecology**, 107:254–261

5.6 Sarcoidosis
1. The Diffuse Parenchymal Lung Disease Group of the British Thoracic Society 1999. **Thorax**, 54(Suppl. 1)
2. European Respiratory Monograph 2005. **Sarcoidosis** 32:1–339
3. Baughman RP, Lower EE and du Bois RM 2003 Sarcoidosis. **The Lancet**, 361:1111–1118
4. Selroos O 1990 Sarcoidosis and pregnancy: A review with results of a retrospective survey. **Journal of Internal Medicine**, 227:221

Chapter 6 Renal Disorders

6.1 Urinary Tract Infections
1. NICE 2003 **Clinical Guideline: Antenatal care**. London; National Institute for Clinical Excellence www.nice.org.uk/guidance/CG6
2. Williams D 2006 *Renal disorders* in James DK, Steer PJ, Weiner CP, Gonik B (Eds) **High Risk Pregnancy: Management Options**, 3rd Ed. Philadelphia; W.B. Saunders Company Ltd 50: 1098–1124
3. Lindheimer MD, Grunfeld JP and Davison JM 2000 *Renal disorders* in Baron WM and Lindheimer MD (Eds). **Medical Disorders During Pregnancy**. Chicago, USA; Mosby Inc. 39–70
4. Davison JM 2001 Renal disorders in pregnancy. **Current Opinion in Obstetrics and Gynaecology**, 13:109–114
5. Kincaid-Smith P and Bullen M 1965 Bacteriuria in pregnancy. **The Lancet**, 1:1382–1387
6. Brumfitt W 1975 The effects of bacteriuria in pregnancy on maternal and fetal health. **Kidney International**, 8(Suppl.):S113–119
7. Avorn J, Monane M, Gurwitz JH, Glynn RJ, Choodnovskiy I and Lipsitz LA 1994 Reduction of bacteriuria and pyuria after ingestion of cranberry juice. **Journal of the American Medical Association**, 271:751–754
8. Griffiths P 2003 The role of cranberry juice in the treatment of urinary tract infections (mini-review). **British Journal of Community Nursing**, 8(12):557–561
9. Jepson RG, Milhaljevic L and Craig J 2004 Cranberries for preventing urinary tract infections. **The Cochrane Database of Systematic Reviews** Issue 2. Art. No:CD001321.DOI: 10.1002/14651858.CD001321.
10. RCOG 2003 **Clinical Guideline 36 Prevention of Early Onset Neonatal Group B Streptococcal Disease.** London; Royal College of Obstetricians and Gynaecologists 6
11. Smaill F 2001 Antibiotics for asymptomatic bacteriuria in pregnancy. **The Cochrane Database of Systematic Reviews**. 2. Art. No.: CD000490. DOI: 10.1002/14651858.CD000490
12. British National Formulary 2006 **Issue 51** http:www.bnf.org/bnf/bnf/current/127074.htm [accessed 08-05-2006]
13. Hass DM 2005 Antibiotic treatment for preterm rupture of the membranes. http://www.clinicalevidence.co/ceweb/conditions/pac/1404/1404_13.jsp [accessed 04-05-2006]

6.2 Chronic Kidney Disease
1. www.dh.gov.uk/assetRoot/04/10/26/80/04102680.pdf [accessed 14-09-2006]
2. The Short CKD eGuide, derived from UK CKD Guidelines. 2005 http://www.renal.org/eGFR/eguide.html [accessed 18/05/06]
3. Jones DC and Hayslett JP 1996 Outcome of pregnancy in women with moderate or severe renal insufficiency. **New England Journal of Medicine**, 335:226–226
4. Jungers P and Chaveau D 1997 Pregnancy in renal disease. **Kidney International**, 52:871–885
5. Hou S 1999 Pregnancy in chronic renal insufficiency and end stage renal disease. **American Journal of Kidney Disease**, 33:235–252
6. Davison JM 2001 Renal disorders in pregnancy. **Current Opinion in Obstetrics and Gynaecology**, 13:109–114
7. Branch DW and Porter FF 2006 Chap. 44 *Autoimmune disease* in James DK, Steer PJ, Weiner CP and Gonik B (Eds) **High Risk Pregnancy: Management Options**, 3rd Ed. Philadelphia; W.B. Saunders Company Ltd 949–985
8. Cooper WD, Hernandez Dias S, *et al.* 2006 Major congenital malformations after exposure to ACE inhibitors. **New England Journal of Medicine**, 344(23):2443
9. RCOG 2004 **Clinical Guideline 37 Thromboprophylaxis During Pregnancy, Labour and After Vaginal Delivery**. London; Royal College of Obstetricians and Gynaecologists

6.3 Dialysis in Pregnancy
1. Hou SH 1994 Pregnancy in women on haemodialysis and peritoneal dialysis. **Baillière's Clinical Obstetrics and Gynaecology**, 8:481–500
2. Jungers P and Chaveau D 1997 Pregnancy in renal disease. **Kidney International**, 52:871–885
3. Hussey MJ and Pombar X 1998 Obstetric care for renal allograft recipients or for women treated with haemodialysis or peritoneal dialysis during pregnancy. **Advanced Renal Replacement Therapy**, 5:3–13
4. Hou S 1999 Pregnancy in chronic renal insufficiency and end stage renal disease. **American Journal of Kidney Disease**, 33:235–252

6.4 Renal Transplantation
1. Eardley KS and Lipkin GW 2000 Pregnancy in the renal transplant recipient. **Transplant Topics**, 7:1–6
2. Davison JM 2001 Renal disorders in pregnancy. **Current Opinion in Obstetrics and Gynaecology**, 13:109–114
3. McKay DB and Josephson MA 2006 Pregnancy in recipients of solid organs – effects on mother and child. **New England Journal of Medicine**, 354:1281–1293
4. Hussey MJ and Pombar X 1998 Obstetric care for renal allograft recipients or for women treated with haemodialysis or peritoneal dialysis during pregnancy. **Advanced Renal Replacement Therapy**, 5:3–13

6.5 Nephrotic Syndrome
1. RCOG 2004 **Clinical Guideline 37: Thromboprophylaxis During Pregnancy, Labour and After Vaginal Delivery**. www.rcog.uk/recources/Public/pdf/Thromboprophylaxis_no037.pdf
2. Cooper WD, Hernandez Dias S, *et al.* 2006 Major congenital malformations after exposure to ACE inhibitors. **New England Journal of Medicine**, 344(23):2443
3. Barcelo P, Lopez-Lilo J, Cabero L and Del Rio G 1986 Successful pregnancy in primary glomerular disease. **Kidney International**, 30:914–919
4. Farquharson RG and Grieves M 2006 Chap. 43 *Thromboembolic disease* in James DK, Steer PJ, Weiner CP and Gonik B (Eds) **High Risk Pregnancy: Management Options**, 3rd Ed. Philadelphia; W.B. Saunders Company Ltd 938–948

Chapter 7 Endocrine Disorders

7.1 Hypothyroidism
1. Tonacchera M, Chiovato L and Pinchera A 2002 *Clinical assessment and systemic manifestations of hypothyroidism* in Wass JAM and Shalet SM (Eds) **Oxford Textbook of Endocrinology and Diabetes**. Oxford; Oxford University Press 491–502
2. Girling JC and DeSwiet M 1992 Thyroxine dosage during pregnancy in women with primary hypothyroidism. **British Journal of Obstetrics and Gynaecology**, 99:368–370
3. Girling JC 2003 Thyroid disorders in pregnancy. **Current Obstetrics and Gynaecology**, 13:45–51
4. Franklyn J 2002 *Subclinical hypothyroidism* in Wass JAM and Shalet SM (Eds) **Oxford Textbook of Endocrinology and Diabetes**. Oxford; Oxford University Press 518–522
5. Hershman JM 2002 *Thyroid disease during pregnancy* in Wass JAM and Shalet SM (Eds) **Oxford Textbook of Endocrinology and Diabetes**. Oxford; Oxford University Press 522–524
6. Rennie JM and Roberton NRC 2002 **A Manual Of Neonatal Intensive Care**, 4th Ed. London; Arnold 281–282

7.2 Thyrotoxicosis
1. Orgiazzi J. *Management of Graves' hyperthyroidism* in Wass JAM and Shalet SM (Eds) **Oxford Textbook of Endocrinology and Diabetes**. Oxford; Oxford University Press 453–458
2. Girling JC 2003 Thyroid disorders in pregnancy. **Current Obstetrics and Gynaecology**, 13:45–51
3. Davis LE, Lucas MJ, Hankins GDV, *et al.* 1989 Thyrotoxicosis complicating pregnancy. **American Journal of Obstetrics and Gynecology**, 160:63–70

4. Hershman JM 2002 *Thyroid disease during pregnancy* in Wass JAM and Shalet SM (Eds) **Oxford Textbook of Endocrinology and Diabetes**. Oxford; Oxford University Press 522–524
5. Rennie JM and Roberton NRC 2002 **A Manual of Neonatal Intensive Care**, 4th Ed. London; Arnold 281–282
6. Nelson-Piercy C 2002 **Handbook of Obstetric Medicine**. London; Martin Dunitz 100–105

7.3 Type 1 Diabetes Mellitus
1. CEMACH 2007 **Findings of a National Enquiry: Diabetes in Pregnancy: Are we providing the best care? England, Wales and Northern Ireland**. London; Confidential Enquiry into Maternal and Child Health
2. CEMACH 2005 **Findings of a National Enquiry: Pregnancy In Women With Type 1 And Type 2 Diabetes, England, Wales and Northern Ireland**. London; Confidential Enquiry into Maternal and Child Health
3. Casson IF, Clarke CA, Howard CV, *et al.* 1997 Outcomes of pregnancy in insulin dependent diabetic women: Results of a five year population cohort study. **British Medical Journal**, 315(7103): 275–278
4. Lumley J, Watson L, Watson M and Bower C 2006 Periconceptional supplementation with folate and/or multivitamins for preventing neural tube defects. **Cochrane Pregnancy and Childbirth Group, Cochrane Database of Systematic Reviews**, 3
5. Jackson W 2004 Breastfeeding and Type 1 diabetes mellitus. **British Journal of Midwifery**, 12(3):158–165
6. Howorka K, Pumpral J, Gabriel M, *et al.* 2001 Normalisation of pregnancy outcome in pregestational diabetes through functional insulin treatment and modular out-patient education adapted for pregnancy. **Diabetic Medicine** 18:965–972

7.4 Type 2 Diabetes Mellitus
1. CEMACH 2007 **Findings of a National Enquiry: Diabetes in Pregnancy: Are we providing the best care? England, Wales and Northern Ireland**. London; Confidential Enquiry into Maternal and Child Health
2. CEMACH 2005 **Findings of a National Enquiry: Pregnancy In Women With Type 1 And Type 2 Diabetes, England, Wales and Northern Ireland**. London; Confidential Enquiry into Maternal and Child Health
3. Lumley J, Watson L, Watson M and Bower C 2006 Periconceptional supplementation with folate and/or multivitamins for preventing neural tube defects. **Cochrane Pregnancy and Childbirth Group, Cochrane Database of Systematic Reviews**, 3
4. Casson IF, Clarke CA, Howard CV, *et al.* 1997 Outcomes of pregnancy in insulin dependent diabetic women: Results of a five year population cohort study. **British Medical Journal** 315(7103): 275–278
5. Jackson W 2004 Breastfeeding and Type 1 Diabetes Mellitus. **British Journal of Midwifery**, 12(3):158–165
6. Dunne FP, Brydon P, Smith T, Essex M, Nicholson H and Dunne J 1999 Pre-conception diabetes care in insulin-dependent diabetes mellitus. **Quarterly Journal of Medicine**, 92:175–176
7. Howorka K, Pumpral J, Gabriel M *et al.* 2001 Normalisation of pregnancy outcome in pregestational diabetes through functional insulin treatment and modular out-patient education adapted for pregnancy. **Diabetic Medicine**, 18:965–972

7.5 Gestational Diabetes Mellitus
1. Sermer M, Naylor CD, Gare DJ, *et al.* 1995 Impact of increasing carbohydrate intolerance on maternal-fetal outcomes in 3637 women without gestational diabetes: The Toronto Tri-Hospital Gestational Diabetes Project. **American Journal of Obstetrics and Gynecology**, 173:146–156
2. Crowther CA, Hille JE, Moss JR, *et al.* 2005 The Australian carbohydrate intolerance study in pregnant women (ACHOIS): Trial group – effect of treatment of gestational diabetes mellitus on pregnancy outcomes. **New England Journal of Medicine**, 352:2477–2486
3. Naylor CD, Sermer M, Chen E and Farine D 1997 The Toronto Tri-Hospital Gestational Diabetes Project Investigators. Selective screening for gestational diabetes mellitus. **New England Journal of Medicine**, 337:1591–1596

7.6 Addison's Disease

1. Parker KL and Kovacs WJ 2002 *Addison's disease (adrenal insufficiency)* in Wass JAM and Shalet SM (Eds) **Oxford Textbook of Endocrinology and Diabetes**. Oxford; Oxford University Press 837–844.
2. Molitch ME 1998 Pituitary disease in pregnancy. **Seminars in Perinatology**, 22:157–170

7.7 Prolactinoma

1. Bevan JS 2002 *Prolactinomas* in Wass JAM and Shalet SM (Eds) **Oxford Textbook of Endocrinology and Diabetes**. Oxford; Oxford University Press 172–181

Chapter 8   Neurological Disorders

8.1 Migraine and Headaches

1. Rasmussen B, Jensen R, Schroll *et al*. 1991 Epidemiology of headache in a general population – a prevalence study. **Journal of Clinical Epidemiology**, 44(11):1147–1157
2. Ernst E and Pittler M 2000 The efficacy and safety of Feverfew (*Tanacetum parthenium L*): An update of a systematic review. **Public Health Nutrition**, 3(4A):500–514
3. Nelson-Piercy C 2002 **Handbook of Obstetric Medicine**, 2nd Ed. London; Martin Dunitz 164–167
4. Carhuapoma J, Tomlinson M and Levine S 2006 *Neurologic disorders* in James DK, Steer PJ, Weiner CP and Gonik B (Eds) **High Risk Pregnancy: Management Options**, 3rd Ed. London; Elsevier 1067–1074
5. Lowe A and Sen R 2005 Neurological disease in pregnancy. **Current Obstetrics and Gynaecology**, 15:166–173
6. BNF 2007 **British National Formulary**. Issue53 http://bnf.org/bnf/ [accessed 05-04-2007]
7. Silberstein S 2004 *Migraine, Pregnancy and Lactation* in Washington J (Ed) **Neurologic Disorders in Pregnancy**. London; Parthenon

8.2 Epilepsy

1. Morrow J, Russell A, Guthrie E, Parsons L, Robertson I, Waddell R, Irwin B, McGivern R, Morrison P and Craig J 2006 Malformation risks of epileptic drugs in pregnancy: a prospective study from the UK Epilepsy and Pregnancy Register. **Journal of Neurology, Neurosurgery and Psychiatry**, 77: 193–198
2. Nelson-Piercy C 2002 **Handbook of Obstetric Medicine**. 2nd Ed. London; Martin Dunitz 156–164
3. Martin A (Ed) 1994 **Concise Oxford Medical Dictionary**. Oxford; Oxford University Press
4. Cavazoz J 2005 **Seizures and Epilepsy: An Overview**. http://www.emedicine.com/neuro/topic415.htm
5. Nashef L 1997 SUDEP: terminology and definitions. **Epilepsia**, (38):56–58
6. Crawford P, Appleton R, Betts T, Guthrie E and Morrow J 1999 Best practice guidelines for the management of women with epilepsy. **Seizure**, 8(4):201–217
7. Rosa F 1991 Spina bifida in infants treated with carbemazapine during pregnancy. **New England Journal of Medicine**, 324: 674–677
8. Lindhout D, Omzigt J and Cornel M 1992 Spectrum of neural tube defects in 34 infants prenatally exposed to antiepileptic drugs. **Neurology**, 42(Suppl. 5):111–118
9. NICE 2004 **Clinical Guideline 20 The Epilepsies – The Diagnosis and Management of the Epilepsies in Adults and Children in Primary and Secondary Care Settings**. London; National Institute for Clinical Excellence
10. Schmidt D, Canger R, Avanzini G, *et al*. 1983 Change of seizure frequency in pregnant epileptic women. **Journal of Neurology, Neurosurgery and Psychiatry**, 46:751–755
11. Barron W and Lindheimer M 2000 **Medical Disorders During Pregnancy**. London; Mosby 529–533
12. Lewis G and Drife J 2002 **CEMACH 6th report: Why Mothers Die 2000–2002. Confidential Enquiries into Maternal and Child Health**. London; RCOG Press

13. Adab N and Chadwick D 2006 Management of women with epilepsy during pregnancy. **The Obstetrician and Gynaecologist**, 8(1):20–25
14. Cornelissen M, Steegers-Theunissen R, Kollee L, Eskes T, Vogels-Mentink G, Motohara K, De Abreu R and Monnens L 1993 Increased incidence of neonatal vitamin K deficiency resulting from maternal anticonvulsant therapy. **American Journal of Obstetrics and Gynaecology**, 168(3):923–928
15. Delgardo-Escute AV and Jantz D 1992 Consensus guidelines: preconceptual counselling, management and care of the pregnant woman with epilepsy. **Neurology** 42:149–160
16. BNF 2007 **British National Formulary**. Issue 53 http://www.bnf.org/bnf/ [accessed 05–04–2007]
17. Carhuapoma J, Tomlinson M and Levine S 2006 *Neurologic Disorders* in James DK, Steer PJ, Weiner CP and Gonik B (Eds) **High Risk Pregnancy: Management Options**, 3rd Ed. London; Elsevier
18. Epilepsy Action 2005 **Mothers in Mind** (Booklet) http://www.epilepsy.org.uk/downloads/pdf/epilepsyaction_mothersin mind.pdf

8.3 Cerebrovascular Disease and Stroke

1. Barron W and Lindheimer M 2000 **Medical Disorders during Pregnancy**. London; Mosby 517–520
2. Carroll JD, Leek D and Lee HA 1966 Cerebral thrombophlebitis in pregnancy and the puerperium. **Quarterly Journal of Medicine**, 139:347–368
3. Lowe SA and Sen R 2005 Neurological disease in pregnancy. **Current Obstetrics and Gynaecology**, 15:166–173
4. Tortora GJ and Grabowski SR 1996 **Principles of Anatomy and Physiology**, 8th Ed. New York; HarperCollins 424–425
5. Department of Health 2006 **What is a stroke?** www.dh.gov.uk/PolicyAndGuidance/HealthAndSocialCareTopics/Stroke/StokeArticle [accessed 03–03–2006]
6. Lowe SA and Sen R 2005 Neurological disease in pregnancy. **Current Obstetrics and Gynaecology**, 15:166–173
7. Carbuapoma JR, Tomlinson MW and Levine SR 2006 *Neurologic disorders* in James DK, Steer PJ, Weiner CP and Gonik B (Eds) **High Risk Pregnancy: Management Options**. 3rd Ed. London; Saunders/Elsevier 1067–1074
8. Nelson-Piercy C 2002 **Handbook of Obstetric Medicine**, 2nd Ed. London; Martin Dunitz 174–178
9. Qureshi AI, Giles WH, Croft JB, *et al*. 1997 Number of pregnancies and risk for stroke and stroke subtypes **Archives of Neurology**, 54:203–206
10. Dias M and Sekhar L 1990 Intracranial hemorrhage from aneurysms and arteriovenous malformations during pregnancy and puerperium. **Neurology**, 27:855–866
11. Carbuapoma JR, Tomlinson MW and Levine SR 2006 *Neurologic disorders* in James DK, Steer PJ, Weiner CP and Gonik B (Eds) **High Risk Pregnancy: Management Options**, 3rd Ed. London; Saunders Elsevier 1067–1074
12. Lewis G and Drife J 2002 **CEMACH 6th report: Why Mothers Die 2000–2002. Confidential Enquiries into Maternal and Child Health**. London; RCOG Press

8.4 Other neuropathies

1. Falco NA and Eriksson E 1989 Idiopathic facial palsy in pregnancy and puerperium. **Surgery Gynaecology and Obstetrics**, 169(4):337–340
2. Viotk AJ, Mueller JC, Farlinger DE and Johnston RU 1983 Carpal tunnel syndrome in pregnancy. **Canadian Medical Association Journal**, 128(3):277–281
3. Carbuapoma JR, Tomlinson MW and Levine SR 2006 *Neurologic disorders* in James DK, Steer PJ, Weiner CP and Gonik B (Eds) **High Risk Pregnancy: Management Options**, 3rd Ed. London; Saunders Elsevier 1081
4. Barron W and Lindheimer M 2000 **Medical Disorders During Pregnancy**. London; Mosby 520–521
5. Lowe SA and Sen R 2005 Neurological disease in pregnancy. **Current Obstetrics and Gynaecology**, 15:170–171
6. Rozette C and Houghton-Clemmey R 2003 A review of carpal tunnel syndrome in pregnancy. **British Journal of Midwifery**, 11(3):136–139

7. Tortora GJ and Grabowski SR 1996 **Principles of Anatomy and Physiology**, 8th Ed. New York; HarperCollins 380.
8. Medinfo 2007 **Carpel Tunnel Syndrome.** www.medinfo.co.uk/conditions/carpaltunnel.html [accessed 10–4–2007]
9. British National Formulary 2007 **Aciclovir** www.bnf.org/bnf/bnf/53/126543.htm [accessed 10–4–2007]
10. Sweet BR (Ed) 1997 **Mayes' Midwifery A Textbook for Midwives,** 12th Edition. London; Baillière Tindall 241–242
11. British National Formulary 2007 **Prednisolone** www.bnf.org/bnf/bnf/53/100060.htm [accessed 10–4–2007]
12. British National Formulary 2007 **Corticosteroids** www.bnf.org/bnf/bnf/53/100037.htm [accessed 10–4–2007]

8.5 Multiple Sclerosis
1. NICE 2003 **Clinical Guideline 8 – Multiple Sclerosis: Management of Multiple Sclerosis in Primary and Secondary Care.** London; National Institute for Clinical Excellence
2. Neild C 2006 **MS Essentials: Women's issues – Pregnancy, Menstruation, Contraception and Menopause.** London; Multiple Sclerosis Society www.mssociety.org.uk [accessed 22–3–2007]
3. BBC News 2007 **MS Vaccine Testing To Start in US.** http://news.bbc.co.uk/1/hi/health/4787430.stm [accessed 10–4–2007]
4. Poser CM, Paty DW, Scheinberg L, et al. 1983 New diagnostic criteria for multiple sclerosis: Guidelines for research protocols. **Annals of Neurology,** 13:227–231
5. Tortora GJ and Grabowski SR 1996 **Principles of Anatomy and Physiology**, 8th Ed. New York, USA; HarperCollins 336
6. Carbuapoma JR, Tomlinson MW and Levine SR 2006 *Neurologic disorders* in James DK, Steer PJ, Weiner CP and Gonik B (Eds) **High Risk Pregnancy: Management Options**, 3rd Ed. London; Saunders Elsevier 1085
7. Barron W and Lindheimer M 2000 **Medical Disorders during Pregnancy.** London; Mosby 527–528
8. Nelson-Piercy C 2002 **Handbook of Obstetric Medicine,** 2nd Ed. London; Martin Dunitz 167–168
9. Yentis S, Brighouse P, May A, Bogod D and Elton C 2001 **Analgesia, Anaesthesia and Pregnancy – A Practical Guide.** London; Saunders 278
10. NICE 2002 **Technology Appraisal Guidance 32 – Beta Interferon and Glatiramer Acetate for the Treatment of Multiple Sclerosis.** London; National Institute for Clinical Excellence
11. Bennett KA 2005 Pregnancy and multiple sclerosis. **Clinical Obstetrics and Gynecology,** 48(1):38–47
12. Hughes M 2004 Multiple sclerosis and pregnancy. **Neurologic Clinics,** 22(4):757–769
13. Compston A and Coles A 2002 Multiple sclerosis. **The Lancet,** 359:1221–1231
14. Lowe SA and Sen R 2005 Neurological disease in pregnancy. **Current Obstetrics and Gynaecology,** 15:166–173

8.6 Myasthenia Gravis
1. Flint Porter T and Ware Branch D 2006 *Autoimmune disease* in James DK, Steer PJ, Weiner CP and Gonik B (Eds) **High Risk Pregnancy: Management Options**, 3rd Ed. London; Saunders Elsevier 949–985
2. Nelson-Piercy C 2002 **Handbook of Obstetric Medicine,** 2nd Ed. London; Martin Dunitz 169–173
3. Shah A 2006 **Myasthenia Gravis** http://www.emedicine.com/neuro
4. Idan S 2005 **Myasthenia Gravis and Pregnancy** http://www.emedicine.com/neuro
5. Ciafaloni E and Massey J 2004 *Myasthenia Gravis and Pregnancy* in Washington J (Ed) **Neurologic Disorders in Pregnancy.** London; Parthenon
6. Buckley C and Newsom-Davis J 2007 **Myasthenia Gravis** http://www.netdoctor.co.uk/diseases/facts/myastheniagravis.htm
7. Barron W and Lindheimer M 2000 **Medical Disorders During Pregnancy.** London; Mosby 523–524
8. Yentis S, Brighouse D, May A, Bogod D and Elton C 2001 **Analgesia, Anaesthesia and Pregnancy: A Practical Guide.** London; W.B. Saunders

Chapter 9 Musculoskeletal Disorders

9.1 Back and Pelvic Pain
1. Young G and Jewell D 2002 Interventions for preventing and treating pelvic and back pain in pregnancy. **Cochrane Database Systemic Review** (1):CD1139. Oxford; Update Software
2. Brayshaw E 2003 **Exercises for Pregnancy and Childbirth: A Practical Guide for Educators**. London; Books for Midwives/Elsevier 27–28
3. Henderson C and Macdonald S 2004 **Mayes' Midwifery. A Textbook for Midwives**. London; Baillière Tindall 270
4. Mantle J, Haslam J and Barton S 2003 **Physiotherapy in Obstetrics and Gynaecology**, 2nd Ed. Oxford; Butterworth/Heinemann
5. Bastiaanssen JM, Bie RA and Bastiaenen CGH 2005 A historical perspective on pregnancy related low back and/or girdle pain. **European Journal of Obstetrics and Gynaecology,** 120:3–14
6. Ostgaard HC, Zetherstrom G, Roos-Hansson E, et al. 1994 Reduction of back and posterior pelvic pain in pregnancy. **Spine,** 19:894–900
7. Ostgaard HC 1996 Assessment and treatment of low back pain in working pregnant women. **Seminars in Perinatology,** 20(1):61–69
8. Perkins J, Hammer RL and Loubert PV 1998 Identification and management of pregnancy-related low back pain. **Journal of Nurse-Midwifery,** 43(5):331–340
9. Roche S and Hughes EW 1999 Pain problems associated with pregnancy and their management. **Pain Reviews,** 6:239–261
10. Polden M and Mantle J 1990 **Physiotherapy in Obstetrics and Gynaecology**. Oxford; Butterworth Heinemann
11. Macpherson G 2004 **Black's Student Medical Dictionary**. London; A and C Black
12. Lennard F 2003 Physiotherapy for back and pelvic pain. **British Journal of Midwifery,** 11(2):97–102
13. De Torrente del la Jara G, Pecoud A and Favrat B 2004 Musculoskeletal pain in female asylum seekers and hypovitaminosis D. **British Medical Journal,** 329:156–157
14. Boissonnault JS 2002 Positioning in labour and delivery for women with pre-existing spine or pelvic girdle dysfunction. **Journal of the Association of Chartered Physiotherapists in Women's Health,** 90:3–5
15. Brynhilsden J, Hansson A, Persson A and Hammar M 1998 Follow-up of patients with low back pain during pregnancy. **Obstetrics and Gynaecology,** 91(2):182–186
16. Brayshaw E 2002 Pregnancy associated osteoporosis. **Journal of the Chartered Physiotherapists in Women's Health,** 91:3–9
17. Garshasbi A and Zadeh SF 2005 The effect of exercise on the intensity of low back pain in pregnant women. **International Journal of Obstetrics and Gynaecology,** 88; 271–275
18. Mens JMA, Damen L and Snijders CJ 2005 The mechanical effect of a pelvic belt in patients with pregnancy-related pelvic pain. **Clinical Biochemics,** 21:122–127
19. Carr CA 2003 Use of a maternity support binder for relief of pregnancy related back pain. **Journal of Obstetric, Gynecologic and Neonatal Nursing,** 32(4):495–502

9.2 Diastasis Recti Abdominis
1. Boissonault J and Blaschak M 1988 Incidence of diastasis recti abdominis during the childbearing year. **Physical Therapy,** 68(7):1082–1086
2. Noble E 1988 **Essential Exercises for the Childbearing Year**, 3rd Ed. USA; Houghton Mifflin
3. Polden M and Mantle J 1990 **Physiotherapy in Obstetrics and Gynaecology**. Oxford; Butterworth Heinnemann
4. Mantle J, Haslam J and Barton S 2004 **Physiotherapy in Obstetrics and Gynaecology**, 2nd Ed. Oxford; Butterworth Heinemann
5. Sheppard S 1996 Part I: Management of postpartum gross divarication recti. **Journal of the Association of Chartered Physiotherapists in Women's Health,** 79(August):22–24
6. Sheppard S 1996 Part II: The role of transversus abdominus in post-partum correction of gross divarication recti. **Journal of the**

Association of Chartered Physiotherapists in Women's Health, 79(August):24–26

7. Candido G, Lo T and Janssen PA 2005 Risk factors for diastasis of the recti abdominis. **Journal of the Association of Chartered Physiotherapists in Women's Health,** 97(Autumn):49–54

8. Das S and Jones S 2002 **Abdominal Muscle Performance in Women Who Are 12 To 22 Weeks Post Partum.** www.physiotherapy.curtin.e...onours/99_honours_abstracts.shtm. [accessed 4–6–2006]

9. Hsia M and Jones S 2000 Natural resolution of rectus abdominis diastasis: Two single case studies. **Australian Journal of Physiotherapy,** 46:301–307

10. Brayshaw E 2003 **Exercises for Pregnancy and Childbirth: A Practical Guide for Educators.** London; Books for Midwives/Elsevier 31–34

9.3 Symphysis Pubis Dysfunction

1. Owens K, Pearson A and Mason G 2002 Symphysis pubis dysfunction – a cause of significant obstetric morbidity. **European Journal of Obstetrics, Gynecology and Reproductive Biology,** 105:143–146

2. Snow RE and Neubert AG 1997 Peripartum pubic symphysis separation: a case series and review of the literature. **Obstetrical and Gynecological Survey,** 52(7):438–443

3. Fry D, Hay-Smith J, Hough J, McIntosh J, Polden M, Shepherd J and Watkins Y 1997 Symphysis pubis dysfunction – a guideline. **Physiotherapy,** 83(1):41–42 (Currently under review and available from The Association of Chartered Physiotherapists in Women's Health)

4. Leadbetter RE, Mawer D and Lindow SW 2004 Symphysis pubis dysfunction: a review of the literature. **The Journal of Maternal-Fetal and Neonatal Medicine,** 16(6):349–354

5. Leadbetter RE, Mawer D and Lindow SW 2006 The development of a scoring system for symphysis pubis dysfunction. **Journal of Obstetrics and Gynaecology,** 26(1):20–23

6. Henderson C and Macdonald S 2004 **Mayes' Midwifery. A Textbook for Midwives.** London; Baillière Tindall 274–281

7. Albert H, Godskegen M and Westergaard J 2001 Prognosis in four syndromes of pregnancy-related pelvic pain. **Acta Obsterica et Gynecologica Scandinavia,** 80:505–510

8. Coldron Y 2005 'Mind the Gap!' Symphysis pubis dysfunction revisited. **Journal of the Association of Chartered Physiotherapists in Women's Health,** 96:3–15

9. Hagen R 1974 Pelvic girdle relaxation from an orthopaedic point of view. **Acta Orthopaedica Scandinavica,** 45:550–563

10. Bjorklund K, Bergstrom S, Nordstrom ML and Ulmsten U 2000 Symphyseal distention in relation to serum relaxin levels and pelvic pain in pregnancy. **Acta Obstetricia et Gynecologica Scandinavica,** 79(4):269–275

11. Beischer NA and Mackay EV 1997 **Obstetrics and the Newborn: An Illustrated Textbook.** Saunders 221

12. Shepherd J and Fry D 1996 Symphysis pubis pain. **Midwives,** 109(1302):199–201

13. Culligan P, Hill S and Heit M 2002 Rupture of the symphysis pubis during vaginal delivery followed by two successful uneventful pregnancies. **Obstetrics and Gynaecology,** 100(5):1114–1117

14. Scicluna J, Alderson J, Webster V and Whiting P 2004 Epidural analgesia for acute symphysis pubis dysfunction in the second trimester. **International Journal of Obstetric Anesthesia,** 13(1):50–52

15. Depledge J, McNair P, Smith C and Williams M 2005 Management of symphysis pubis dysfunction during pregnancy using exercise and support belts. **Physical Therapy,** (12 December):1290–1300

16. Ostgaard HC, Zetherstrom GG, Roos–Hansson E and Svanberg B 1994 Reduction of back and posterior pelvic pain in pregnancy. **Spine,** 19(8):894–900

17. Wellock V 2002 The ever widening gap – symphysis pubis dysfunction. **British Journal of Midwifery,** 10(6):348–353

18. Jain S, Eedarapalli P, Jamjute P and Sawdy R 2006 Review – Symphysis pubis dysfunction: a practical approach to management. **The Obstetrician and Gynaecologist,** 6:153–156

19. Davidson MR 1996 Examining separated symphysis pubis. **Journal of Nurse-Midwifery,** 41(3):259–262

9.4 Hypovitaminosis D and Osteomalacia

1. Hollick MF 2002 Vitamin D, the under-appreciated D-lightful hormone that is important in skeletal and cellular health. **Current Opinion in Endocrinology, Diabetes and Obesity,** 9:87–98

2. Pitterick M and Cross HS 2005 Vitamin D and calcium deficit predisposed to multiple chronic diseases. **European Journal of Clinical Investigation,** 35:290–306

3. Garland CF, Garland ED, Lipkin M, et al. 2006 The role of vitamin D in cancer prevention. **American Journal of Public Health,** 96(2):252–261

4. Wilkinson RJ, Llewellyn M, Toossiz, et al. 2000 Influences of vitamin D deficiency and vitamin D receptor polymorphisms on tuberculosis among Gujurati Asians in West London; A case control study. **The Lancet,** 355:618–621

5. Bischoff-Ferrari HA, Dawson-Hughes B, Willett WC, et al. 2004 Effect of vitamin D on falls. A meta-analysis. **Journal of the American Medical Association,** 291(16):1999–2006

6. Bischoff-Ferrari HA, Willett WC, Wong JB, et al. 2005 Fracture prevention with vitamin D supplementation. A meta-analysis of randomized controlled trials. **Journal of the American Medical Association,** 293(18):2257–2264

7. Glerup H, Middelsen K, Poulsen L, et al. 2000 Commonly recommended daily intake of vitamin D is not sufficient if sunlight exposure is limited. **Journal of Internal Medicine,** 247:260–268

8. Hollick MF 1998 Vitamin D requirements for humans of all ages; new increased requirements for women and men 50 years and older. **Osteoporosis International,** Suppl. 8:S24–29

9. Henderson L, Gregory J and Swan G 2003 **The nutrition and diet survey adults age 19–64 years. Vitamin and mineral intake and urinary analyses.** www.food.gov.uk/multimedia/pdf/ndnsv3.pdf

10. Department of Health 1998 Report on health and social subjects: Nutrition and bone health with particular reference to calcium and vitamin D. Report No. 49 of the sub-group on bone health. Working Groups on the nutrition status of the population, of the Committee on Medical Aspects of Food and Nutrition Policy. London; HMSO

11. Iqbal SJ 1994 Vitamin D metabolism and clinical aspects of measuring metabolites. **Annals of Clinical Biochemistry,** 34:109–124

12. Clements MR and Fraser DR 1998 Vitamin D supply to the rat fetus and neonate. **Journal of Clinical Investigation,** 81:1768–73

13. Ford L, Graham V, Wall A and Berg J 2006 Vitamin D concentration in a UK city with multicultural outpatient population. **Annals of Clinical Biochemistry,** 43:468–475

14. Boucher BJ 2006 *Evidence of deficiency and insufficiency of vitamin D in the UK; national diet and nutrition data survey 1994–2004* in Gillie O (Ed) 2006 **Sunlight Vitamin D and Health; Health Research Forum Report No. 2.** London; White Hall Park

15. Iqbal SJ, Kaddam IMS, Wassif W, Walls J and Nichol F 1994 Continuing clinically severe vitamin D deficiency in Asians in the UK (Leicester). **Postgraduate Medical Journal,** 70:708

16. Finch PJ, Ang L, Eastwood JE and Maxwell JD 1992 Clinical and histological spectrum of osteomalacia among Asians in South London. **Quarterly Journal of Medicine,** 302:439–448

17. Dunnigan MG, Patton JPG, Hass ES, McNichol GW and Smith GM 1962 Late rickets and osteomalacia in the Pakistani community in Glasgow. **Scottish Medical Journal,** 7:159–167

18. Allgrove J 2004 Is nutritional rickets returning? **Archives of Diseases of Childhood,** 89:699–701

19. Shaw NJ and Pal BR 2002 Vitamin D deficiency in UK Asian families: activating a new concern. **Archives of Diseases of Childhood,** 86:147–149

20. Lakhani S, Srinivasen L, Buchanan C and Allgrove J 2004 Presentation of vitamin D deficiency. **Archives of Diseases of Childhood,** 89(8):781–784

21. Sehra E, Newton P, Ali H, et al. 1999 Prevalence of hypovitaminosis D in Indo-Asian patients attending a rheumatology clinic. **Bone,** 25:609–611

22. Pal BR, Marshal T, James C and Shaw N 2003 Distribution analysis of vitamin D highlights – differences in population sub-groups;

preliminary observations from a pilot study in UK adults. **Journal of Endocrinology**, 179:119–129

23. Henriksen C, Brunvard L, Stoltenberg C, *et al*. 1995 Diet and vitamin D status among pregnant Pakistani women in Oslo. **European Journal of Clinical Nutrition** 49:211–218

24. Brunvand L, Henriken C and Haug E 1996 Vitamin D deficiency among pregnant women from Pakistan. How best to prevent it? **Tidsskr Nor Laegeforen**, 116:1585–1587

25. Grover SR and Morely R 2001 Vitamin D deficiency in veiled or dark skinned pregnant women. **Medical Journal of Australia**, 175(5):251–252

26. Nozza JM and Rozza CP 2001 Vitamin D deficiency in mothers of infants with rickets. **Medical Journal of Australia**, 175:253–255

27. Smith R and Wordsworth P 2005 **Clinical and Biochemical Disorders of the Skeleton**. Oxford; Oxford University Press 173–200

28. Francis R and Selby P 1997 Osteomalacia. **Baillière's Clinical Endocrinology and Metabolism**, 11:1454–1463

29. Behrman RE, Kliegman R and Jenson HB (Eds) 2000 *Rickets of vitamin D deficiency* in Nelson, **Textbook of Pediatrics**, 16th Ed. Philadelphia; Saunders (sec 44.10) 184–187

30. Carlton-Conway D, Tulloh R, Wood L and Kanabar D 2004 Vitamin D deficiency and cardiac failure in infancy. **Journal of the Royal Society of Medicine**, 97(5):238–239

31. Avery PG, Arnold IR, Hubner PJB and Iqbal SJ 1992 Cardiac failure secondary to hypocalcaemia of nutritional osteomalacia. **European Heart Journal**, 34:426–427

32. Henry A and Bowyer L 2003 Fracture of the neck of femur and Osteomalacia in pregnancy. **British Journal of Obstetrics and Gynaecology**, 110:329–330

33. Dane C, Dane B and Kural C 2005 A rare case of severe dyspareunia: Post-osteomalacia contracted pelvic outlet. **Acta Obstetrica et Gynecologica Scandinavica**, 84(4):407–408

34. Hollingworth J, Howley JH, Davidson AC and Iqbal SJ 1994 Severe vitamin D deficiency in pregnancy. **Journal of Obstetrics and Gynaecology**, 14:430–434

35. Innis AM, Seshi MM, Prasad C, El Syeth S, *et al*. 2002 Congenital rickets caused by maternal vitamin D deficiency. **Paediatrics and Child Health**, 7:455–458

36. Blonde MH, Gould F, Pierre F and Burger C 1997 Nutritional foetal rickets: one case report. **Journal de la Gynecologie Obstetrique et Biologie de la Reproduction**, 26:834–836

37. Mughal MZ, Selma H, Greenway T, *et al*. 1999 Florid rickets associated with prolonged breastfeeding without vitamin D supplementation. **British Medical Journal**, 318:39–40

38. Alfaham M, Woodhead S, Pask G and Davies D 1995 Vitamin D deficiency: a concern in pregnant Asian women. **British Journal of Nutrition**, 73:881–887

39. Iqbal SJ, Walker C and Swift PG 2001 The continuing problem of vitamin D deficiency in pregnant Asian women and their offspring, an interface audit as a prelude to action. **Archives of Diseases of Childhood**, 1:84, Suppl. A36

40. Casey M, West J, Shannon R, Iqbal SJ, Madira W and Simpson H. 1994 Persistent vitamin D deficiency in Asian children in the UK (Leicester). **Proceedings of 9th Workshop on Vitamin D**, Orlando, Florida 148

41. Shenoy SD, Cody D, Swift P and Iqbal SJ 2005 Maternal vitamin D deficiency, refractory neonatal hypocalcaemia and nutritional rickets. **Archives of Diseases of Childhood**, 90:437–443

42. De Torrente del la Jara G, Pecoud A and Favrat B 2004 Musculoskeletal pain in female asylum seekers and hypovitaminosis D. **British Medical Journal**, 329(7458):156–157

43. Brooke OG, Brown IR and Bone CD 1980 Vitamin D supplements in pregnant Asian women: effects on calcium status and fetal growth. **British Medical Journal**, 280(6216):751–754

44. Hellouin de Menibus C, Mallet E, Henocq A, *et al*. 1990 Neonatal hypocalcemia. Results of vitamin D supplement in the mother. Study on 13,377 newborn infants. **Bulletin of the Academy of National Medicine**, 174:1051–1060

45. Tytgat GN, Heading RC, Muller-Lissner, *et al*. 2003 Contemporary understanding and management of reflux and constipation in

the general population and pregnancy: a consensus meeting. **Alimentary Pharmacology and Therapeutics**, 18:291–301

46. Henderson C and Macdonald S 2004 **Mayes' Midwifery**, 13th Ed. London; Elsevier 74

9.5 Osteoporosis

1. Compston JE and Rosen CJ 2004 **Fast Facts – Osteoporosis**, 5th Ed. Oxford; Health Press

2. Smith R and Wordsworth P 2005 **Clinical and Biochemical Disorders of the Skeleton**. Oxford; Oxford University Press 109–172

3. Smith R, Athenasou NA, Ostlere SJ, *et al*. 1995 Pregnancy associated osteoporosis. **QJM**, 88:865–878

4. NOS 2003 **Osteoporosis Associated With Pregnancy**. Bath; National Osteoporosis Society

5. Briggs GG, Freeman RK and Yaffe SJ 2005 **Drugs in Pregnancy and Lactation**, 7th Ed. Philadelphia, USA; Lippincott

6. Lasseter KC, Porras AG, Denker A, Santhanagopal A and Daifotis A 2005 Pharmacokinetic considerations in determining the terminal elimination half-lives of bisphosphonates. **Clinical Drug Investigation**, 25(2):107–114(8): online as www.ingentaconnect.com/content/adis/cdi/2005/00000025/00000002/art00003;jsessionid=u0b26u0md6gg.alice?format=print

Chapter 10 Gastrointestinal Disorders

10.1 Gastro-oesophageal Reflux

1. Spechler SJ 1992 Epidemiology and natural history of gastro-oesophageal reflux disease. **Digestion**, 51(supplement 1):24–29

2. Welsh A 2005 Hyperemesis, gastrointestinal and liver disorders in pregnancy. **Current Obstetrics and Gynaecology**, 15, 123–131

3. Loffeld RJLF and Van Der Putten ABMM 2002 Newly developing hiatus hernia: A survey in patients undergoing upper gastrointestinal endoscopy. **Journal of Gastroenterology and Hepatology**, 17(5):542–544

4. Macpherson G 2004 **Black's Student Medical Dictionary**. London; A and C Black Publishers 251

5. Tytgat GN, Heading RC, Muller–Lissner, *et al*. 2003 Contemporary understanding and management of reflux and constipation in the general population and pregnancy: a consensus meeting. **Alimentary Pharmacology and Therapeutics**, 18:291–301

6. Coad J and Dunstall M 2002 **Anatomy and Physiology for Midwives**. London; Mosby 243

7. Boon NA, Colledge NR, Walker BR and Hunter JAA 2006 **Davidson's Principles and Practice of Medicine**, 20th Ed. London; Churchill Livingstone/Elsevier 878–881

8. Rubenstein D, Wayne D and Bradley J 2003 **Lecture Notes on Clinical Medicine**, 6th Ed. Oxford; Blackwell/Wiley 219–220

9. Wilson LJ, Ma W and Hirschowitz BI 1999 Association of obesity with hiatus hernia and esophagitis. **American Journal of Gastroenterology**, 94(10):2840–2844

10. Sloan S and Kahrilas PJ 1991 Impairment of esophageal emptying with hiatus hernia. **Gastroenterology**, 100(3):596–605

11. Kumar P and Clarke M 2004 **Clinical Medicine**, 5th Ed. London; Saunders 263–266

12. Smith ML 2004 Chap.1: *Gastro-oesophageal Reflux(GORD)*: in **A General Practice Guide to Gastrointestinal Problems**. Dartford; Magister Consulting Ltd 8–20

13. MIMS 2007 **Monthly Index of Medical Specialities**. May.

14. Vakil N 2007 The role of surgery in gastro-oesophageal reflux disease. **Alimentary Pharmacology and Therapeutics**, 25(12):1365–1372

15. Richter JE 2005 Review article: The management of heartburn. **Alimentary Pharmacology and Therapeutics**, 22: 749–757

16. Henderson C and Macdonald S 2004 **Mayes' Midwifery: A textbook for Midwives**, 13th Ed. London; Baillière Tindall/Elsevier 271–272

17. De Swiet M 2002 **Medical Disorders in Obstetric Practice**. Oxford; Blackwell Scientific 350–351

18. Nikfar S, Abdollahi M, Morettti ME, *et al*. 2002 Use of proton pump inhibitors during pregnancy and rates of major malformations. A meta-analysis. **Digestive Diseases Sciences**, 47:1526

10.2 Coeliac Disease

1. Lancaster Smith M 2004 Chap.8 *Coeliac disease* in **Gastrointestinal Problems**. Kent; Magister Consulting

2. Smith G and Watson R 2005 **Gastrointestinal Nursing**. Oxford; Blackwell Publishing

3. Unsworth DJ and Brown DL 1994 Serological screening suggests that adult celiac disease is under diagnosed in the United Kingdom and increases the incidence by up to 12%. **Gut**, 35:61–64

4. Alaedini A and Green PHR 2005 Narrative review: Celiac disease: understanding a complex autoimmune disorder. **Annals of Internal Medicine** 142(4):289–298

5. Eliakim R and Sherer DM 2001 Celiac disease: fertility and pregnancy. **Gynecologic and Obstetric Investigation**, 51(1):3–7

6. Nash S 2003 Does exclusive breastfeeding reduce the risk of coeliac disease in children? **British Journal of Community Nursing**, 8(3):127–132

7. Akobeng AK, Ramanan AV, Buchan I and Heller RF 2006 Effect of breast feeding on risk of coeliac disease: a systemic review and meta-analysis of observational studies. **Archives of Diseases of Childhood**, 91:39–43

8. Raisler J, Alexander C and O'Campo P 1999 Breast-feeding and infant illness: a dose-response relationship? **American Journal of Public Health** 89:25–30

10.3 Ulcerative Colitis

1. NACC 2004 **Ulcerative Colitis** http://www.nacc.org.uk/ontent/ibd/ucBG.asp

2. Kornbluth A and Sachar D 2004 Ulcerative colitis practice guidelines in adults(update): American College of Gastroenterology, Practice Parameters Committee. **American Journal of Gastroenterology**

3. Carter MJ, Lob AJ and Travis SPL 2004 Guidelines for the management of inflammatory bowel disease in adults. **Gut**, 53: 1–16

4. Truelove S 1992 *Medical management of ulcerative colitis and indications for colectomy*, in Jarnerot G, Lennard-Jones J and Truelove S (Eds) **Inflammatory Bowel Disease** Sweden; Corona

5. Reddy S and Wolf J 2001 Management issues in women with inflammatory bowel disease. **Journal of the American Osteopathic Association**, 101(12):s17–s22

6. Alstead EM 2002 Inflammatory bowel disease in pregnancy. **Postgraduate Medical Journal**, 78:23–26

7. Moody G, Probert G, Srivasta E, *et al.* 1992 Sexual dysfunction in women with Crohn's disease, a hidden problem. **Digestion**, 52:179–183

8. Hudson M, Flett G, *et al.* 1997 Fertility and pregnancy in inflammatory bowel disease. **International Journal of Gynaecology and Obstetrics**, 58:229–237

9. Kornfeld D, Cnattingius S, *et al.* 1997 Pregnancy outcomes in women with inflammatory bowel disease – a population-based cohort study. **American Journal of Obstetrics and Gynaecology**, 177:942–946

10. Khare M, Lott J, Currie A and Howarth E 2003 Is it safe to continue azathioprine in a breastfeeding mother? **Journal of Obstetrics and Gynaecology**, 23(supplement 1):S53

11. Sau A, Clarke S, Bass J, Kaiser A, Marinaki A and Nelson-Piercy C. 2007 Azathioprine and breastfeeding – is it safe? **British Journal of Obstetrics and Gynaecology**, 114:498–501

10.4 Crohn's Disease

1. NACC 2004 **Crohns Disease**. http://www.nacc.org.uk/content/ibd/ucBG.asp

2. Carter MJ, Lobo AJ and Travis SPL 2004 Guidelines for the management of inflammatory bowel disease in adults. **Gut**, 53:1–16

3. Alstead EM 2002 Inflammatory bowel disease in pregnancy. **Postgraduate Medical Journal**, 78:23–26

4. Bruno M 2004 Irritable bowel syndrome and inflammatory bowel disease in pregnancy. **Journal of Perinatal and Neonatal Nursing**, 18(4):341–350

5. Irvine J, Feagan B, Rochon J, *et al.* 1994 Quality of life: a valid and reliable measure of therapeutic efficacy in the treatment of inflammatory bowel disease. **Gastroenterology**, 106:287–296

6. Hudson M, Flett G, *et al.* 1997 Fertility and pregnancy in inflammatory bowel disease. **International Journal of Gynaecology and Obstetrics**, 58:229–237

7. Alstead E and Nelson-Piercy C 2003 Inflammatory bowel disease in pregnancy. **Gut**, 52:159–161

8. Caprilli R, Gassull M A, Escher J C, *et al.* 2006 European evidence based consensus on the diagnosis and management of Crohn's disease: special situations. **Gut**, 55:36–58

9. Brandt L, Estabrook S and Reinus J 1995 Results of a survey to evaluate whether vaginal delivery and episiotomy lead to perineal involvement in women with Crohn's disease. **American Journal of Gastroenterology**, 90(11):1918–1922

10. Ilnyckyj A, Blanchard J, Rawsthorne P and Bernstein C 1999 Perianal Crohn's disease and pregnancy: role of the mode of delivery. **American Journal of Gastroenterology**, 94(11): 3274–3278

11. Khare M, Lott J, Currie A and Howarth E 2003 Is it safe to continue azathioprine in a breastfeeding mother? **Journal of Obstetrics and Gynaecology**, 23(supplement 1):S53

12. Sau A, Clarke S, Bass J, Kaiser A, Marinaki A and Nelson-Piercy C. 2007 Azathioprine and breastfeeding – is it safe? **British Journal of Obstetrics and Gynaecology**, 114:498–501

10.5 Irritable Bowel Syndrome

1. Agrawal A and Whorwell P 2006 Irritable bowel syndrome: diagnosis and management. **British Medical Journal**, 332(7536): 280–283

2. Thompson W and Heaton K 2003 **Fast Facts: Irritable Bowel Syndrome**, 2nd Ed. Oxford; Health Press Ltd

3. Bruno M 2004 Irritable bowel syndrome and inflammatory bowel disease in pregnancy. **Journal of Perinatal and Neonatal Nursing**, 18(4):341–350

4. Douglas A and Drossman M 1999 The criteria process: Diagnosis and legitimisation of irritable bowel syndrome. **American Journal of Gastroenterology**, 94(10):2803–2807

5. Bennett E, Tennant C, Piesse C, Badcock C and Kellow J 1998 Level of chronic life stress predicts clinical outcome in irritable bowel syndrome. **Gut**, 43:256–261

6. Grundfast M and Komar M 2001 Irritable bowel syndrome. **Journal of American Osteopathic Association**, 101(4) April supplement:S1–S5

7. Gaynes BN and Drossman DA 1999 The role of psychosocial factors in irritable bowel syndrome. **Baillière's Clinical Gastroenterology**, 13(3):437–452

8. Emarson A, Mastroiacovo P, Arnon J, *et al.* 2000 Prospective, controlled multicentre study of loperamide in pregnancy. **Canadian Journal of Gastroenterology**, 14:185–187

10.6 Haemorrhoids

1. Nisar P and Schofield J 2003 Managing haemorrhoids. **British Medical Journal**, 327(7419):847–851

2. Simon C, Everitt H, Birtwistle J and Stevenson B 2002 **Oxford Handbook of General Practice**. Oxford; Oxford University Press 528–529

3. Bruck C, Lubowski D and King D 1988 Do patients with haemorrhoids have pelvic floor denervation? **International Journal of Colorectal Disease**, 3(4):10–14

4. Prodigy Guidance – Haemorrhoids. UK Department of Health. **Prodigy**. www.prodigy.nhs.uk [accessed 12/06/06]

5. Brisinda G 2000 How to treat haemorrhoids. **British Medical Journal**, 321(7261):582–583

6. McLatchie GR and Leaper DJ 2002 **Oxford Handbook of Clinical Surgery**, 2nd Ed. Oxford; Oxford University Press 293–294

7. NICE 2003 Circular stapled haemorrhoidectomy. **National Institute for Clinical Excellence**. www.nice.org.uk [accessed 12/06/06]

8. Quijano C and Abalso E 2005 Conservative management of symptomatic and/or complicated haemorrhoids in pregnancy and the puerperium. **The Cochrane Database for Systematic Reviews**, July 20, No. 3:CD04077

9. Alonso-Coello P, Guyatt G, Heel-Andsell D, Johanson J, Lopez-Yarto M, Mills E and Zhou Q 2005 Laxatives for the treatment of

haemorrhoids. **The Cochrane Database for Systematic Reviews**. Issue 4, Art. No:CD004649. DOI:10.1002/14651858.CD004649.pub2

10. Abramowitz L, Sobhani I, Benifla J, Vuagnat A, Darai E, Mignon M and Madelenat P 2002 Anal fissure and thrombosed external haemorrhoids before and after delivery. **Diseases of the Colon and Rectum**, 45(5):650–655

10.7 Anal Sphincter Disorders

1. Perry S, Shaw C, McGrother C, Matthews R, Assassa R, Dallosso H, Williams K, Brittain K, Azam U, Clarke M, Jagger C, Mayne C, Castelden C and the Leicestershire MRC Incontinence Study Team 2002 Prevalence of faecal incontinence in adults aged 40 years or more living in the community. **Gut**, 50(4)480–484
2. RCOG 2001 **Greentop Guidelines No. 29: Management of Third and Fourth Degree Perineal Tears Following Vaginal Delivery**. London; Royal College of Obstetricians and Gynaecologists
3. Cook and Mortensen N 1998 Management of faecal incontinence following obstetric injury. **British Journal of Surgery**, 85(3): 293–299
4. Vaizey C, Kamm M and Bartrum C 1997 Primary degeneration of the internal anal sphincter as a cause of passive faecal incontinence. **The Lancet**, 349:612–615
5. O'Herlihy C 2003 Obstetric perineal injury: risk factors and strategies for prevention. **Seminars in Perinatology**, 27(1):13–19
6. Eogan M, Daly L, O'Connell P and O'Herlihy C 2006 Does the angle of the episiotomy affect the incidence of anal sphincter injury? **British Journal of Obstetrics and Gynaecology: An International Journal of Obstetrics and Gynaecology**, 113(2):190
7. Faltin D, Sangali M, Roche B, Floris L, Boulvain M and Weil A 2001 Does a second delivery increase the risk of anal incontinence? **British Journal of Obstetrics and Gynaecology: An International Journal of Obstetrics and Gynaecology**, 108(7):684
8. Fernando R, Sultan A, Radley S, Jones P and Johanson R 2002 Management of obstetric anal sphincter injury: a systematic review and national practice survey. **BMC Health Services Research**, l2(9)
9. Sultan A, Kamm M and Hudson C 1995 Obstetric perineal trauma: an audit of training. **Journal of Obstetrics and Gynaecology**, 15:19–23
10. Cheetham M, Kamm M and Phillips R 2001 Topical phenylephrine increases anal canal resting pressure in patients with faecal incontinence. **Gut**, 48(3):356–359
11. Kamm M 2000 How to treat: faecal incontinence. **Student British Medical Journal**, 11:437–480 December ISSN 0966-6494
12. Malouf A, Norton C, Engel A, Nicholls and Kamm M 2000 Long term results of overlapping anterior anal sphincter repair for obstetric trauma, **The Lancet**, 355:260–265
13. Norton C and Kamm M 2001 Anal sphincter biofeedback and pelvic floor exercises for faecal incontinence in adults – a systematic review. **Alimentary Pharmacology and Therapeutics**, 15(8):1147–1154
14. Kenefick N, Vaizey C, Cohen R, Nicholls R and Kamm M 2002 Medium-term results of permanent sacral nerve stimulation for faecal incontinence. **British Journal of Surgery**, 89(7):896–901
15. Fitzpatrick M and O'Herlihy, C 2005 Short-term and long-term effects of obstetric anal sphincter injury. **Current Opinion in Obstetrics and Gynaecology**, 17:605–610
16. Faradi A, Willis S, Schelzig P, Siggelkow W, Schumpelick V and Rath W 2002 Anal sphincter injury during vaginal delivery – an argument for caesarean section on request? **Journal of Perinatal Medicine**, 30(5):379–387
17. Power D, Fitzpatrick M and O'Herlihy C 2006 Obstetric anal sphincter injury: how to avoid, how to repair: a literature review. **Journal of Family Practitioners**, 55(3):193–200
18. De Souza Caroci da Costa A and Gonzalez Riesco M 2006 A comparison of 'hands off' versus 'hands on' techniques for decreasing perineal laceration during birth. **Journal of Midwifery and Women's Health**, 51(2):106–111
19. De Parades V, Etienney I, Thabut D, *et al.* 2004 Anal sphincter injury after forceps delivery: Myth or reality? A prospective ultrasound study of 93 females. **Diseases of the Colon and Rectum**, 47(1):24–34

10.8 Obstetric Cholestasis

1. Kenyon AP, Girling J, Nelson-Piercy C, Williamson C, Seed PT and Poston L 2002 Pruritus in pregnancy and the identification of obstetric cholestasis risk: a prospective prevalence study of 6531 women. **Journal of Obstetrics and Gynaecology**, 22(supplement 1):S15
2. Abedin P, Weaver JB, Eggintin E 1999 Intrahepatic cholestasis of pregnancy: prevalence and ethnic distribution. **Ethnic Health**, 4:35–37
3. Raine-Fenning N and Kilby N 1997 Obstetric Cholestasis. **Fetal Maternal Medicine**, 9:1–17
4. Turner A 2000 Obstetric cholestasis: symptoms, causes and treatments. **British Journal of Midwifery**, 8(8):530
5. British Liver Trust 2004 **Obstetric Cholestasis: A Liver Disease in Pregnancy**. Ringwood; British Liver Trust
6. Milkiewicz P, Elias E and Williamson C 2002 Obstetric cholestasis. **British Medical Journal**, 324(7330):123–124
7. Fagan EA 1994 Intrahepatic cholestasis of pregnancy: timely intervention reduces perinatal mortality. **British Medical Journal**, 309(6964):1243–1244
8. Chambers J 1996 Obstetric cholestasis – a cause of unexplained stillbirth? **Changing Childbirth Update**, 5:4
9. Redfearn J 1994 Obstetric Cholestasis. **Midwifery Matters**, 62:14
10. Waine C 1995 Beware of itching during late pregnancy. **Practitioner**, 239:97–99
11. Coombes J 2000 Cholestasis in pregnancy: a challenging disorder. **British Journal of Midwifery**, 8(9):565–570
12. Reyes H, Gonzalez M and Ribalta J 1978 Prevalence of ICP in Chile. **Annals of Internal Medicine**, 88:487–493
13. Reyes H 1992 The spectrum of liver and gastrointestinal disease seen in cholestasis of pregnancy. **Gastroenterology Clinics of North America**, 21:905–921
14. RCOG 2006 **Guideline No. 43 Obstetric Cholestasis**. London; Royal College of Obstetricians and Gynaecologists 1–10
15. Axten S 1996 Obstetric cholestasis. **Modern Midwife**, 6(4):32–33
16. Roncaglia N, Arreghini A, Locatelli A, 2002 Obstetric cholestasis: outcome with active management. **European Journal of Obstetrics and Gynaecology and Reproductive Biology**, 100:167–170
17. Williamson C, Hems LM and Goulis DG 2004 Clinical outcome in a series of cases of obstetric cholestasis – identified via a patient support group. **British Journal of Obstetrics and Gynaecology**, 111:676–681
18. Chin GY 2003 Dermatoses of pregnancy. **Journal of Paediatrics, Obstetrics and Gynaecology**, 29(2):22–27
19. Welsh A 2005 Hyperemesis, gastrointestinal and liver disorders in pregnancy. **Current Obstetrics and Gynaecology** 15:123–131
20. Fagan EA 2002 *Disorders of the liver, biliary system and pancreas* in Swiet MD (Ed) **Medical Disorders in Obstetric Practice**, 4th Ed. Oxford; Blackwell 282–345
21. Palmer DG and Eads J 2000 Intrahepatic cholestasis of pregnancy: a critical review. **Journal of Perinatal and Neonatal Nursing**, 14:39–51
22. Rioseco AJ, Ivankovic MB and Manzur A 1994 Intrahepatic cholestasis of pregnancy: a retrospective case–control study of perinatal outcome. **American Journal of Obstetrics and Gynecology**, 170(3):890–895
23. Williamson C and Girling J 2005 *Hepatic and gastrointestinal disease* in James DK, Steer PJ, Weimer CP and Gonik B (Eds) **High Risk Pregnancy: Management Options**, 3rd Ed. Pennsylvania; Saunders Elsevier 1032–1060
24. David AL, Kotecha M and Girling JC 2000 Factors influencing postnatal liver function tests. **British Journal of Obstetrics and Gynaecology**, 107:1421–26
25. British Liver Trust 2004 **Obstetric Cholestasis**. Ringwood; British Liver Trust

10.9 Gall Bladder and Pancreatic Disease

1. Landon MB 2004 *Diseases of the liver, biliary system and pancreas* in Creasy RK and Resnik R (Eds) **Maternal-Fetal Medicine, Principles and Practice**, 5th Ed. Pennsylvania; Saunders Elsevier 1127–1145

2. Summerfield JA 2000 *Diseases of the gallbladder and biliary tree* in Leadingham JGG and Worrell DA (Eds) **Concise Oxford Textbook of Medicine**. Oxford; Oxford University Press 609–613
3. Smith G and Watson R (2005) **Gastrointestinal Nursing**. Oxford; Blackwell Publishing
4. Ramin KD, Ramin SM, Richey SD and Cunningham FG 1995 Acute pancreatitis in pregnancy. **American Journal of Obstetrics and Gynaecology**, 173(1):187–191
5. Maringhini A, Ciambra M, Baccelliere P, *et al.* 1993 Biliary sludge and gallstones in pregnancy: incidence, risk factors and natural history. **Annals of Internal Medicine**, 119:116
6. Yates MR and Baron TH 1999 Biliary tract disease in pregnancy. **Clinical Liver Disease**, 3:131–146
7. Chang T and Lepanto L 1992 Ultrasonography in the emergency setting. **Emergency Medicine Clinics of North America** 10:1–25
8. Angelini DJ 2002 Gallbladder and pancreatic disease during pregnancy. **Journal of Perinatal and Neonatal Nursing**, 15(4): 1–12

Chapter 11   Autoimmune Disorders

11.1   Rheumatoid Arthritis

1. Symmons DP 2005 Looking back – aetiology, occurrence and mortality. **Rheumatology (**Oxford), 44(Suppl.4):iv 14–17
2. Kumar P and Clarke M 2004 **Clinical Medicine**, 5th Ed. London; Saunders 537–548
3. Isaacs JD and Moreland L W 2002 **Fast Facts – Rheumatoid Arthritis**. Oxford; Health Press Ltd 21–29
4. Rubenstein D, Wayne D and Bradley J 2003 **Lecture Notes on Clinical Medicine**, 6th Ed. Oxford; Blackwell 130–134
5. Moots R and Jones N 2004 **Your Questions Answered – Rheumatoid Arthritis**. London; Churchill Livingstone – Elsevier 4–6
6. Hakim A, Clunie G and Haq I 2006 **Oxford Handbook of Rheumatology**, 2nd Ed. Oxford; Oxford University Press 256
7. Symmons DP 2002 Epidemiology of rheumatoid arthritis: determinants of onset, persistence and outcome. **Best Practice and Research Clinical Epidemiology**, 16(5):707–722
8. Silman AJ and Pearson JE 2002 Epidemiology and genetics of rheumatoid arthritis. **Arthritis Research and Therapy**, 4(Suppl.3):265–272
9. Symmons D and Harrison B 2000 Early Inflammatory Polyarthritis: results from the Norfolk Arthritis Register with a review of the literature. 1: Risk factors for the development of inflammatory polyarthritis and rheumatoid arthritis. **Rheumatology**, 39:835–843
10. Kinder AJ 2006 Consultant rheumatologist at University Hospitals of Leicester – Personal communication on 16 May
11. Scott DL 2002 The diagnosis and prognosis of early arthritis: rationale for new prognostic criteria. **Arthritis and Rheumatism**, 46(2):286–290
12. Packham JC and Hall MA 2002 Long-term follow-up of 246 juvenile idiopathic arthritis: social function, relationships and sexual activity. **Rheumatology** (Oxford), 41(12):1440–1443
13. Nell VP, Machold KP, Eberi G, Stamm TA, Uffmann M and Smolen 2004 Benefit of very early referral and very early therapy with disease-modifying anti-rheumatic drugs in patients with early rheumatoid arthritis. **Rheumatology**, 43(7):906–914
14. Wise EM and Issacs JD 2005 Management of rheumatoid arthritis in primary care – an educational need. **Rheumatology**, 44(11): 1337–1338
15. Ernst E 2004 Musculoskeletal conditions and complementary/ alternative medicine. **Best Practice and Research: Clinical Rheumatology** 18(4):539–556
16. Burrow GN, Duffy GN and Copel JA 2004 **Medical Complications During Pregnancy**, 6th Ed. USA; Philadelphia; Elsevier Saunders 430–432
17. De Swiet M 2002 **Medical Disorders in Obstetric Practice**. Oxford; Blackwell Scientific 275–276
18. MIMS 2007 **Monthly Index of Medical Specialities**. May. 296
19. Silman A 2006 **Pregnancy and Arthritis: An information booklet**. Arthritis and Rheumatism Campaign www.arc.org.uk/ about_arth/booklets/6060/6060.htm [accessed on 26–2–06]
20. Kinder AJ, Edwards J, Samanta A and Nichol F 2004 Pregnancy in a rheumatoid arthritis patient on infliximab and methotrexate. **Rheumatology** (Oxford) 43(9):1195–1196
21. Barron WM and Lindheimer MD 2000 **Medical Disorders During Pregnancy**, 3rd Ed. London; Mosby-Harcourt 375–376
22. Silman A 2004 **Rheumatoid Arthritis and Pregnancy**. www. rheumatoid.org.uk/1/medinfo_280904_pregnancy.ph[accessed on 26–2–06]
23. Shepherd AA 2006 Nutrition and rheumatoid arthritis. **Complete Nutrition**, 6(3):16–18

11.2   Raynaud's Phenomenon

1. Black C 2005 **Raynaud's and Scleroderma: An update for the GP**. Alsagar; Raynaud's and Scleroderma Association
2. http://www.surgical–tutor.org.uk/default–home.htm?system/ vascular/raynauds.htm~right [accessed 18–5–2005]
3. http://www.whonamedit.com/doctor.cfm/2508.html [accessed 18–5–2005]
4. Minerva 2000 Review. **British Medical Journal** (321):60
5. Macpherson G 2004 **Black's Student Medical Dictionary**. London; A and C Black Publishers
6. http://www.gpnotebook.co.uk/simplepage.cfm?ID=–2046427123 [accessed 18–5–2005]
7. Anon 2004 **Raynaud's Phenomenon**. Chesterfield; Arthritis and Rheumatism Campaign
8. http://www.bbc.c.uk/health/conditions/raynauds1.shtml [accessed 18–5–2005]
9. Denton CP and Black C 2004 Chap.17 *Raynaud's phenomenon and scleroderma* in Snaith ML (Ed) **ABC of Rheumatology**. Oxford; Blackwell – BMJ Books 87–91
10. http://www.prodigy.nhs.uk/pk.uk/raynauds_phenomenon [accessed 16–05–2006]
11. http://www.raynauds.org/uk [accessed 18–5–05]
12. Block JA and Sequeira W 2001 Raynaud's phenomenon. **The Lancet**, 357(9273):2042–2048
13. Barron WM and Lindheimer MD 2000 **Medical Disorders During Pregnancy**, 3rd Ed. London; Mosby 376
14. De Swiet M 2002 **Medical Disorders in Obstetric Practice**. Oxford; Blackwell 214
15. BNF 51 2006 **British National Formulary**. London; BMA and RPSGB
16. http://emc.medicines.org.uk/emc/industry/default.asp?page= displaydoc.asp and documentid=2301 [accessed 18–5–2005]
17. Nelson-Piercy C 2002 **Handbook of Obstetric Medicine**. London; Martin Dunitz 151–153
18. Coad J 2001 **Anatomy and Physiology for Midwives**. London; Mosby 233
19. Hardwick JCR, McMurtrie F and Melrose EB 2002 Raynaud's syndrome of the nipple in pregnancy. **European Journal of Obstetrics and Reproductive Biology** 102(2):217–218
20. Lawlor-Smith L and Lawlor-Smith C 1997 Vasospasm of the nipple – a manifestation of Raynaud's phenomenon: case reports. **British Medical Journal** (314):644(1 March)
21. Hey E 1997 Vasospasm of the nipple was described in 1970. **British Medical Journal** (314):1625
22. Muir A, Robb R, McLaren M, Daly F and Belch J 2004 The use of *Gingko biloba* in Raynaud's disease: a double-blind placebo-controlled trial. **Vascular Medicine**, 7(4):265–267
23. Anderson JE, Held N and Wright K 2004 Raynaud's phenomenon of the nipple: a treatable cause of painful breastfeeding. **Pediatrics**, 113(4):360–364
24. Kone-Paut I, Olivar E, Elbhar C, Garnier JM and Berbis P 2002 Syndrome de Raynaud chez l'enfant. Etude de 23 cas. **Archives de Pediatrie** 9(4):365–370
25. Nigrovic P, Fuhlbrigge R and Sundel R 2003 Raynaud's phenomenon in children: a retrospective review of 123 patients. **Pediatrics**, 111(4):715–723
26. Hakim A, Clunie G and Haq I 2006 **Oxford Handbook of Rheumatology**. Oxford; Oxford University Press 358

27. BSSA 2003 **Sjogren's Syndrome – A Concise Guide to Diagnosis and Management for Health Care Professionals**. British Sjogren's Association

11.3 Systemic Lupus Erythematosus

1. Mackay IR 2000 Tolerance and autoimmunity. **British Medical Journal**, 321:93–96(8 July)
2. Tsui-Yee Lian and Gordon G 2004 Chap.16 *Systemic lupus erythematosus, antiphospholipid antibody syndrome, and other lupus-like syndromes* in Snaith ML (Ed) **ABC of Rheumatology**, 3rd Ed. Oxford; Blackwell – BMJ Books 50–60
3. Macpherson G 2004 **Black's Student Medical Dictionary**. London; A and C Black Publishers
4. Jessop S, Whitelaw D and Jordaan F 2000 Drugs for discoid lupus erythematosus. **The Cochrane Database of Systematic Reviews**. Issue 2. Art.No.:CD002954.DOI:10.1002/14651858
5. Rubenstein D, Wayne D and Bradley J 2003 **Lecture Notes on Clinical Medicine**, 6th Ed. Oxford; Blackwell 122–124
6. Hughes GRV 2006 **Is it Lupus?** www.lupus.org.uk/article.php?i=66 and v=pf [accessed 29–6–2006]
7. Higgins C 2000 **Understanding Laboratory Investigations**. Oxford; Blackwell
8. Kumar P and Clarke M 2004 **Clinical Medicine**, 5th Ed. London; Saunders 557–560
9. Hakim A, Clunie G and Haq I 2006 **Oxford Handbook of Rheumatology**. Oxford; Oxford University Press 322–340
10. Sofat N, Malik O and Higgens CS 2006 Neurological involvement in patients with rheumatic disease. **Quarterly Journal of Medicine**, 99(2):69–79
11. Puandare KN, Wagle AC and Parker SR 1999 Psychiatric morbidity in patients with systemic lupus erythematosus. **Quarterly Journal of Medicine**, 92(5):283–286
12. Burrow GN, Duffy GN and Copel JA 2004 **Medical Complications During Pregnancy**, 6th Ed. USA; Philadelphia 432–438
13. Nelson-Piercy C 2002 **Handbook of Obstetric Medicine**. London; Martin Dunitz 140–145
14. Norton Y 2000 **Lupus: A GP guide to Diagnosis**. Romford: Lupus UK 84–87
15. Ruiz–Irastoraz G, Khamashta MA, Castinellio G and Hughes GRV 2001 Systemic lupus Erythematosus. **The Lancet**, 357(9261):1027–1032
16. Preidt R 2005 **Lupus, Rheumatoid Arthritis Raise Pregnancy Risks**. American College of Rheumatology – news release 13–11–2005 www.medicinenet.com/script/main/art.asp?articlekey=55334 [accessed 18–5–06]
17. De Swiet M 2002 **Medical Disorders in Obstetric Practice**. Oxford; Blackwell Scientific 271–275
18. Rodriguez IH, Moreno MJ, Morano LE and Benavente JL 1994 Systemic lupus erythematosus presenting as psuedocyesis. **British Journal of Rheumatology**, 33(4):400–402
19. Jeanty P 2004 Answer to case of the week #133 http://thefetus.net/case.php?id=1401 and answers=1
20. Barron WM and Lindheimer MD 2000 **Medical Disorders During Pregnancy**, 3rd Ed. London; Mosby 360–374
21. D'Cruz DP and Hughes GRV 2005 The treatment of lupus nephritis. **British Medical Journal** 330:377–8
22. Shonohara K, Miyagawa S, Fujita T, *et al.* 1999 Neonatal lupus erythematosus: results of maternal corticosteroid therapy. **Obstetrics and Gynaecology**, 93(6):952–957
23. Costedoat-Chalumeau N, Amoura Z, Thi Hong DL, *et al.* 2003 Questions about dexamethasone use for prevention of anti-SSA related congenital heart block. **Annals of Rheumatic Diseases**, 62:1010–1012

11.4 Antiphospholipid (Hughes) Syndrome

1. Gezer S 2003 Antiphospholipid syndrome. **Disease-a-month**, 49(12):696–741
2. McMahon MA 2006 The prevalence of antiphospholipid antibody syndrome among systemic lupus erythematosus patients. **Irish Medical Journal**, 99(10) on line as http://www.imj.ie//Issue_detail.aspx?issueid=+ and pid=1502 and type=Papers
3. RCOG 2003 **Guideline No.17: The Investigation and Treatment of Couples with Recurrent Miscarriage**. London; Royal College of Obstetricians and Gynaecologists. 4.5.2
4. Hughes 1984 Autoantibodies in lupus and its variants: experience in 1000 patients. **British Medical Journal**, 289(6441):339–342
5. Sanna G, Bertolaccini ML and Khamashta MA 2003 Central nervous system involvement in the antiphospholipid (Hughes) syndrome. **Rheumatology**, 42:200–213
6. Khare M and Nelson-Piercy C 2003 Acquired thrombophilias and pregnancy. **Best Practice and Research in Obstetrics and Gynaecology**, 17(3):491–507
7. Branch DW and Khamashata MA 2003 Antiphospholipid syndrome: obstetric diagnosis, management and controversies. **Obstetrics and Gynaecology**, 101(6):1333–1344
8. Sanna G, Bertolaccini ML and Khamashta MA 2006 Unusual clinical manifestations of the antiphospholipid syndrome. **Current Rheumatology Reviews**, 2(4):387–394
9. NHS 2007 Hughes Syndrome: www.nhsdirect.nhs.uk/articles/article.aspx?printPage=1 and articleId=662 [accessed 15–6–2006]
10. Nimmo MC and Carter CJ 2003 The antiphospholipid syndrome: a riddle wrapped in a mystery inside an enigma. **Clinical and Applied Immunology Reviews**, 4(2003):125–140
11. Greaves M, Cohen, Machin SJ and Mackie I 2000 Guidelines on the investigation and management of the antiphospholipid syndrome. **British Journal of Haematology**, 109:704–715
12. James DK, Steer PJ, Weiner CP and Gonik B 2006 **High Risk Pregnancy: Management Options**, 3rd Ed. USA; Elsevier 908
13. Bidot CJ, Wenche J, Lawrence L, *et al.* 2004 Antiphospholipid antibodies in immune thrombocytopenic purpura tend to emerge in exacerbation and decline in remission. **British Journal of Haematology**, 128:366–371
14. Asherson RA 2006 New subsets of the antiphospholipid syndrome in 2006: Pre-APS (probable APS) microangiopathic antiphospholipid syndrome (MAPS). **Rheumatologia**, 20(3):119–129
15. Gomez-Puerta JA, Cervera R, Espinosa G, Bucciarelli S and Font J 2006 Pregnancy and puerperium are high susceptibility periods for development of catastrophic antiphospholipid syndrome. **Autoimmunity Reviews**, 6(2):85–88
16. Tenedios F, Erkan D and Lockshin MD 2006 Cardiac manifestations in the antiphospholipid syndrome. **Rheumatic Disease Clinics of North America**, 32(3):491–507
17. McMillan E, Martin WL, Waugh J, *et al.* 2002 Management of pregnancy in women with pulmonary hypertension secondary to SLE and anti-phospholipid syndrome. **Lupus**, 11(6):392–398
18. Vials J 2001 A literature review on the antiphospholipid syndrome and the effect on childbearing. **Midwifery**, 17:142–149
19. Fakhouri F, Noel L, Zuber J, *et al.* 2003 The expanding spectrum of renal diseases associated with antiphospholipid syndrome. **American Journal of Kidney Diseases**, 41(6):1205–1211
20. Asherson RA, Frances C, Iaccarino L, *et al.* 2006 The antiphospholipid syndrome: diagnosis, skin manifestations and current therapy. **Clinical and Experimental Rheumatology**, 24(suppl.40):s46–251
21. Miesbach W, Glizinger A, Gokpinar B, Claus D and Scharrer I 2006 Prevalence of antiphospholipid antibodies in patients with neurological symptoms. **Clinical Neurology and Neurosurgery**, 108(2):135–142
22. Tincani A, Branch W, Piette JC, Carp H, Rai RS, Khamashata MA and Shoenfield Y 2003 Treatment of pregnant patients with antiphospholipid syndrome. **Lupus**, 12:524–529
23. Nelson-Piercy C 2002 **Handbook of Obstetric Medicine**. London; Martin Dunitz 146–151
24. Carbillon L, Sauvet M, Fain O and Aurousseau 2005 Letter. **Journal of Reproductive Immunology**, 65(1):89–90
25. Shehata HA and Nelson-Piercy C 2001 Connective tissue diseases in pregnancy. **Current Obstetrics and Gynaecology**, 11:329–335
26. Cimez R and Descloux E 2006 Pediatric antiphospholipid syndrome. **Rheumatic Disease Clinics of North America**, 32(3):553–573
27. Motta M, Tincani A, Locjacono A, *et al.* 2004 Neonatal outcome in patients with rheumatic disease. **Lupus**, 13:718–723

28. Girardi G, Redecha P and Salmon JE 2004 Heparin prevents anti-phospholipid syndrome antibody-induced fetal loss by inhibiting complement activation. **Nature Medicine**, 10(11):1222–1226
29. Lakasing L and Khamashta M 2001 Contraceptive practices in women with systemic lupus erythematosus and/or antiphospholipid syndrome: what advice should we be giving? **British Journal of Family Planning**, 27(1):7–12

Chapter 12 Infectious Conditions

12.1 Viral Hepatitis

1. Kane M 1995 Global programme for the control of hepatitis B infection. **Vaccine**, 13(Suppl. 1):S47–49
2. Department of Health 2002 **Getting Ahead of the Curve: A Strategy for Combating Infectious Diseases**. London; DH
3. Hill JB, Sheffield JS, Kim MJ, *et al.* 2002 Risk of hepatitis B transmission in breast–fed infants of chronic hepatitis B carriers. **Obstetrics and Gynaecology**, 99:1049–1052
4. Hoofnagle JH 1990 Chronic hepatitis B. **New England Journal Medicine**, 323:337–339
5. Hoofnagle JH 1997 Hepatitis C: the clinical spectrum of disease. **Hepatology**, 26(Suppl. 1):15S–20S
6. Seeff LB 1997 Natural history of hepatitis C. **Hepatology**, 26(Suppl. 1):21S–28S
7. Vento S, Garfano T, Renzeni C, *et al.* 1998 Fulminant hepatitis associated with hepatitis A virus superinfection in patients with hepatitis C. **New England Journal of Medicine**, 338:286–290
8. Salisbury TM and Begg N (Eds) 1996 *Hepatitis B* in **Immunisation Against Infectious Disease**. London; HMSO 95–108
9. Brook MG, Lever AM, Griffiths P, *et al.* 1989 Antenatal screening for hepatitis B is medically and economically effective in the prevention of vertical transmission: three years experience in a London hospital. **Quarterly Journal of Medicine**, 264:313–317
10. Giacchino R, Tasso L, Timitilli A, *et al.* 1998 Vertical transmission of hepatitis C virus infection: usefulness of viraemia detection in HIV-seronegative hepatitis C virus-seropositive mothers. **Journal of Pediatrics**, 132:167–169
11. Department of Health 2004 **Hepatitis C: Essential Information for Professionals and Guidance on Testing**. London; DH
12. Seow HF 1999 Hepatitis B and C in pregnancy. **Current Obstetrics and Gynaecology**, 9:216–223
13. Andre FE, Zuckerman AJ 1994 Review: protective efficacy of hepatitis B vaccines in neonates. **Journal of Medical Virology**, 44: 144–151

12.2 Human Immunodeficiency Virus

1. Health Protection Agency 2005 **Mapping the Issues: HIV and other Sexually Transmitted Infections in the United Kingdom**. Available at: www.hpa.org.uk/publications/2005/hiv–sti–2005/default.htm
2. British HIV Association 2005 **Guidelines for the Treatment of HIV Infected Adults with Antiretroviral Therapy**, BHIVA. Available at: http://www.bhiva.org/guidelines/2005/HIV/guidelines2005.pdf
3. Brocklehurst P and French R 1998 The association between maternal HIV infection and perinatal outcome: a systematic review of the literature and meta-analysis. **British Journal of Obstetrics and Gynaecology**, 105:836–848
4. European Collaborative Study, Swiss Mother and Child HIV Cohort Study. Combination antiretroviral therapy and duration of pregnancy. **AIDS**, 14: 2913–2930
5. Serraino D, Carrieri P, Pradier C, *et al.* 1999 Risk of invasive cervical cancer among women with, or at risk for, HIV infection. **International Journal of Cancer**, 82(3):334–337
6. Gilling-Smith C and Almeida P 2003 HIV, hepatitis B and hepatitis C and infertility: reducing risk. Educational bulletin sponsored by the practice and policy committee of the BFS. **Human Fertility**, 6:106–122
7. Madge S, Phillips AN, Griffioen A, *et al.* 1998 Demographic, clinical and social factors associated with human immunodeficiency virus infection and other sexually transmitted diseases in a cohort of women from the United Kingdom and Ireland. MRC Collaborative Study of women with HIV. **International Journal of Epidemiology**, 27:1068–1071
8. Leroy V, De Clerq A, Ladner J, *et al.* 1995 Should screening of genital infections be part of antenatal care in areas of high HIV prevalence? A prospective cohort study from Kigali, Rwanda, 1992–1993. The Pregnancy and HIV (EGE) Group. **Genitourinary Medicine**, 71:207–211
9. Hillier SL, Martius J, Krohn M, *et al.* 1988 A case-control study of chorioamnionic infection and histologic chorioamnionitis in prematurity. **New England Journal of Medicine**, 319:972–978
10. Goldenberg RL, Hauth JC and Andrews WW 2000 Intrauterine infection and preterm delivery. **New England Journal of Medicine**, 342:1500–1507
11. Hillier SL, Nugent RP, Eschenbach DA, *et al.* 1995 Association between bacterial vaginosis and preterm delivery of a low-birth weight infant. **New England Journal of Medicine** 333: 1737–1742

12.3 Malaria

1. http://w3.whosea.org/en/section10/section21/section334.htm [accessed 02–02–2006]
2. Martens P and Hall L 2000 Malaria on the Move: Human Population Movement and Malaria Transmission. www.cdc.gov/ncidod/eid/vol6no2/martens.htm [accessed 22–02–2006]
3. Wyler DJ 1992 *Plasmodium and Babesia* in Gorbach SL, Bartlett JG, Blacklow NR (Eds). **Infectious Diseases**. Philadelphia; WB Saunders Company 1967–1975
4. Wellcome Trust 2006 Sickle Cell Trait Offers Malaria Immunity to Children www.wellcome.ac.uk/doc%5Fwtx025264.html5 [accessed 02–02–2006]
5. www.cdc.gov/malaria/disease.htm [accessed 03–03–2006]
6. www.prodigy.nhs.uk/ProdigyKnowledge [accessed 03–03–2006]
7. Stephen L and Hoffman DM 1992 Diagnosis, treatment, and prevention of malaria. **Medical Clinics of North America**, 76(6):1327–1355
8. Ernest JM 2006 *Parasitic Infections* in James DK, Steer PJ, Weiner CP and Gonik B (Eds) **High Risk Pregnancy: Management Options**, 3rd Ed. London; W.B Saunders 697–717
9. http://www.cdc.gov/malaria/faq.htm [accessed 04–03–2006]
10. BNF 52 2006 **British National Formulary**. London; British Medical Association and Royal Pharmaceutical Society of Great Britain
11. Bradley DJ and Bannister B on behalf of Health Protection Agency Advisory Committee on Malaria Prevention for UK Travellers. 2003 Guidelines for malaria prevention in travellers from the United Kingdom for 2003. **Communicable Disease and Public Health**, 6(3):180–199
12. Hughes C, Tucker R, Bannister B and Bradley DJ on behalf of Health Protection Agency Advisory Committee on Malaria Prevention for UK Travellers (ACMP) 2003 Malaria prophylaxis for long-term travellers. **Communicable Disease and Public Health**, 6(3):200–208
13. WHO 2003 **The Africa Report – Malaria During Pregnancy**. Geneva; World Health Organization 38–45
14. http://www.planetwire.org/files.fcgi/3438_BPmal–Ma02e.pdf [accessed 03–03–2006]
15. Whitty CJ, Edmonds S and Mutabingwa TK 2005 Malaria in pregnancy. **British Journal of Obstetrics and Gynaecology**, 112(9):1189–1195 Review
16. http://www.cdc.gov/malaria/pdf/clinicalguidance.pdf[accessed 25–02–2006]
17. WHO 2000 **Management of Severe Malaria: A Practical Handbook**, 2nd Ed. Geneva; World Health Organization. Available: http://www.who.int/malaria/docs/hbsm.pdf[accessed 04–03–2006]
18. http://malariasite.com/malaria/pregnancy.htm [accessed 25–02–2006]
19. Hashemzadeh A and Heydarian F 2005 Congenital malaria in a neonate. **Archives of Iranian Medicine**, 8(3):226–228
20. http://www.hpa.org.uk/srmd/malaria/FAQs_malaria.pdf [accessed 25–02–2006]

12.4 Listeriosis
1. de Valk H, Goulet V, Vaillant V, Perra A, Simon F, Desenclos JC and Martin P 2005 Surveillance of *Listeria* infections in Europe. **Eurosurveillance**, 10(10):251–255
2. www.hpa.org.uk/infections/topics_az/listeria/data_ew.htm [accessed 12–03–2006]
3. www.hps.scot.nhs.uk/index.htm [accessed 12–03–2006]
4. Braden C R 2003 Listeriosis. **Paediatric Infectious Disease Journal**, 22(8):745–746
5. www.amm.co.uk/newamm/files/factsabout/f9_list.htm [accessed 12–03–2006]
6. Hawker J, Begg N, Blair I, Reintjes R and Weinberg J 2005 **Communicable Disease Control Handbook**. Oxford; Blackwell Science 148–150
7. Benenson AS (Ed) 1995 **Control of Communicable Diseases Manual**, 16th Ed. Washington DC; American Public Health Association 270–273
8. Lundén J, Tolvanen R and Korkeala H 2004 Human listeriosis linked to dairy products in Europe. **Journal of Dairy Science**, 87:E6–E12
9. Nelson KE, Warren D, Tomasi AM, Raju TN and Vidyasagar D 1985 Transmission of neonatal listeriosis in a delivery room. **American Journal of Diseases of Children**, 139(9):903–905
10. Hanssler L, Rosenthal E and Fitza B 1990 Listeriosis in newborn infants. **Klinical Padiatric** 202(6):379–382
11. www.merc.com/mrkshared/mmanual/section19/chapter260/260m.jsp [accessed 14–03–2006]
12. www.cdc.gov/ncidod/dbmd/diseaseinfo/listeriosis_g.htm [accessed 26–02–2006]
13. Sweet RL and Gibbs RS 2002 **Infectious Diseases of the Female Genital Tract**. Philadelphia; Lippincott Williams and Wilkins 474–477
14. Silver HM 1998 Listeriosis during pregnancy. **Obstetrical and Gynecological Survey**, 53(12):737–740
15. Nolla-Salas J, Bosch J, Gasser I, Vinas L, de Simon M, Almela M, Latorre C, Coll P and Ferrer MD 1999 Perinatal listeriosis: a population-based multicenter study in Barcelona, Spain (1990–1996). **Obstetrical and Gynecological Survey**, 54(6):358–360
16. Mylonakis E, Paliou M, Hohmann EL, Calderwood S and Wing EJ 2002 Listeriosis during pregnancy: a case series and review of 222 cases. **Medicine**, 81(4):260–269
17. Freitag BC and Gravett MG 2006 *Other infectious conditions* in James DK, Steer JS, Weiner CP and Gonik B (Eds) **High Risk Pregnancy: Management Options**, 3rd Ed. London; WB Saunders 671–696
18. Temple ME, Nahata MC 2000 Treatment of listeriosis. **The Annals of Pharmacotherapy**, 34(5):656–661
19. American Academy of Pediatrics 2005 Breastfeeding and the use of human milk. **Pediatrics**, 115(2):496–506

12.5 Toxoplasmosis
1. Hawker J, Begg N, Blair I, Reintjes R and Weinberg J 2005 **Communicable Disease Control Handbook**. Oxford; Blackwell Science 215–217
2. www.amm.co.uk/newamm/files/factsabout/fa_toxo.htm [accessed 25–03–2006]
3. www.dh.gov.uk/PolicyAndGuidance/HealthAndSocialCare Topics/Toxoplasmosis/fs/en [accessed 25–03–2006]
4. Remington J, McLeod R, Thulliez P, and Desmonts G 2001 *Toxoplasmosis* in Remington J and Klein J (Eds) **Infectious Diseases of the Fetus and Newborn Infant**, 5th Ed. Philadelphia; Saunders 205–346
5. Benenson, AS (Ed) 1995 **Control of Communicable Diseases Manual**, 16th Ed. Washington DC; American Public Health Association 468–471
6. Kravetz JD and Federman DG 2005 Toxoplasmosis in pregnancy. **The American Journal of Medicine**, 118, 212–216
7. Ernest JM 2006 *Parasitic Infections* in James DK, Steer PJ, Weiner CP, Gonik B (Eds) **High Risk Pregnancy: Management Options**, 3rd Ed. London; W.B Saunders 697–717
8. BNF 52, 2006 **British National Formulary**. London; British Medical Association and Royal Pharmaceutical Society of Great Britain

9. Miron D, Raz R and Luder A 2002 Congenital toxoplasmosis in Israel: to screen or not to screen. **Israel Medical Association Journal**, 4:119–122
10. Personal View 1991 Controversy breeds ignorance. **British Medical Journal**, 302:973
11. Naessens A, Jenum PA, Pollak A, Decoster A, Lappalainen M, Villena I, Lebech M, Stray-Pedersen B, Hayde M, Pinon J-M, Petersen E and Foulton W 1999 Diagnosis of congenital toxoplasmosis in the neonatal period: a multicenter evaluation. **The Journal of Pediatrics**, 135(6):714–719

12.6 Chickenpox
1. Miller E, Marshall R, Vurdien JE 1993 Epidemiology, outcome and control of *Varicella zoster* virus infection. **Reviews in Medical Microbiology**, 4:222–230
2. Smego RA, Asperilla MO 1991 Use of acyclovir for varicella pneumonia during pregnancy. **Obstetrics and Gynaecology**, 78:1112–1116
3. O'Riordan M, O'Gorman C, Morgan C, *et al.* 2000 Sera prevalence of *Varicella zoster* virus in pregnant women in Dublin. **Irish Journal of Medical Science**, 169:288
4. McGregor JA, Mark S, Crawford GP and Levin MJ 1987 *Varicella zoster* antibody testing in the care of pregnant women exposed to varicella. **American Journal of Obstetrics and Gynecology**, 157:281–284
5. Paryani SG and Arvin AM 1986 Intrauterine infection with *Varicella zoster* virus after maternal varicella. **New England Journal of Medicine**, 314:1542–1546
6. Pastuszak Al, Levy M, Schick RN, Zuber C, Feldkamp M, Gladstone J, *et al.* 1994 Outcome after maternal varicella infection in the first 20 weeks of pregnancy. **New England Journal of Medicine**, 330:901–905
7. Enders G, Miller E, Cradock-Watson J, Bolley I and Ridehalgh MK 1994 Consequences of varicella and *Herpes zoster* in pregnancy: prospective study of 1739 cases. **Lancet**, 343:1548–1551
8. Pretorrius DH, Hayward I, Jones KL, Stamm E 1992 Sonographic evaluation of pregnancies with maternal varicella infection. **Journal of Ultrasound Medicine**, 11:459–463
9. Anon 2005 Chickenpox, pregnancy and the newborn: a follow-up. **Drugs and Therapeutics Bulletin**, 43:94–95
10. Miller E, Cradock-Watson JE and Ridehalgh MK 1989 Outcome in newborn babies given anti-*Varicella zoster* immunoglobulin after perinatal maternal infection with *Varicella zoster* virus. **Lancet**, 2:371–373
11. BNF 49 2005 **British National Formulary**. London; British Medical Association and Royal Pharmaceutical Society of Great Britain
12. RCOG 2001 **Clinical Guideline No.13, Chickenpox in Pregnancy**. London; Royal College of Obstetricians and Gynaecologists
13. Nathwani D, Maclean A, Conway S and Carrington D 1998 Varicella infections in pregnancy and the newborn. **Journal of Infection**, 36(Suppl.1):59–71
14. Anon 2005 Chickenpox, pregnancy and the newborn. **Drugs and Therapeutics Bulletin**, 43:69–72

12.7 Herpes Simplex Virus
1. HPA 2004 Epidemiological data – genital herpes. **Health Protection Agency** www.hpa.org.uk [accessed: 22–04–2006]
2. Tookey P and Peckham CS 1996 Neonatal *Herpes simplex* virus infection in the British Isles. **Paediatric Perinatal Epidemiology**, 10:432–442
3. Brown ZA, Selke S, Zeh J, Kopelman J, Maslow A, Ashley RL, *et al.* 1997 The acquisition of *Herpes simplex* virus during pregnancy. **New England Journal of Medicine**, 337:509–515
4. Clinical Effectiveness Group 2001 National guideline on the management of genital herpes. Clinical Effectiveness Group – **Association for Genitourinary Medicine and the Medical Society for the Study of Venereal Diseases**
5. Nelson-Piercy C 2002 **Handbook of Obstetric Medicine**, 2nd Ed. London; Taylor and Francis
6. RCOG 2002 **Guideline No. 30 Management of Genital Herpes in Pregnancy**. Royal College of Obstetricians and Gynaecology

7. BNF 49 2005 **British National Formulary**. London; British Medical Association and Royal Pharmaceutical Society of Great Britain

8. Mertz GJ, Benedetti J, Ashley R, Selke SA and Corey L 1992 Risk factors for the sexual transmission of genital herpes, **Annals of Internal Medicine**, 116:197–202

9. Qutub M, Klapper P, Vallely P and Cleator G 2001 Genital herpes in pregnancy: is screening cost-effective? **International Journal of Sexually Transmitted Disease and AIDS**, 12:14–16

10. Sheffield JS, Hollier LM, Hill JB, Stuart GS and Wendel GD 2003 Acyclovir prophylaxis to prevent *Herpes simplex* virus recurrence at delivery: a systematic review. **Obstetrics and Gynaecology**, 102:1396–1403

11. Prober CG, Sullender WM, Yasukawa LL, Au DS, Yeager AS and Arvin AM 1987 Low risk of *Herpes simplex* virus infections in neonates exposed to the virus at the time of vaginal delivery to mothers with recurrent genital *Herpes simplex* virus infections. **New England Journal of Medicine**, 316: 240–244

12. Brown ZA, Benedetti J, Ashley R, Burchett S, Selke S, Berry S, *et al.* 1991 Neonatal herpes simplex virus infection in relation to asymptomatic maternal infection at the time of labor. **New England Journal of Medicine**, 324:1247–1252

Chapter 13 Metabolic Disorders

13.1 Obesity

1. Kanagalingam MG, Forouhi NG, Greer IA, *et al.* 2005 Changes in booking body mass index over a decade: retrospective analysis from a Glasgow maternity hospital. **British Journal of Obstetrics and Gynaecology**, 112(10):1431–1433

2. Lewis G (Ed) 2007 **Saving Mothers' Lives: Reviewing Maternal Deaths to Make Motherhood Safer. 7th Report of the Confidential Enquiries into Maternal and Child Health**. London; CEMACH 25–29

3. Irvine L and Shaw R 2006 The impact of obesity on obstetric outcomes. **Current Obstetrics and Gynaecology**, 16(4):242–246

4. Soltani H and Fraser R 2002 Pregnancy as a cause of obesity – myth or reality? **RCM Midwives Journal**, 5(5):193–195

5. Forsen T, Eriksson JG, Toumilehto J, *et al.* 1997 Mother's weight in pregnancy and coronary heart disease in a cohort of Finnish men: follow up study. **British Medical Journal**, 315(7112):837–840

6. Shaw K, O'Rouke P, Kenardy C 2005 Psychological interventions for overweight or obesity. **The Cochrane Database of Systematic Reviews**, Issue 1

7. NICE 2006 Clinical Guideline – Obesity – guidance on the prevention, identification, assessment and management of overweight and obesity in adults and children www.nice.org.uk/guidance/CG43/guidance/pdf/English/download.dspx

8. Mulders A, Laven J, Eijkemans M, Hughes E, *et al.* 2003 Patients predictors for outcome of gonadotrophin ovulation induction in women with normogonadotrophic anovulatory infertility: a mega-analysis. **Human Reproduction Update**, 9(5):429–449

9. Andreasen K, Anderson M and Schantz A 2004 Obesity in pregnancy. **Acta Obstetrica et Gynecologica Scandinavica**, 83(11):1022–1029

10. Duckitt K and Harrington D 2005 Risk factors for pre-eclampsia at antenatal booking: systematic review of controlled studies. **British Medical Journal**, 330(7491):565

11. Erez-Weiss I, Erez O, Shoham-Vaedi I, *et al.* 2005 The association between maternal obesity, glucose intolerance and hypertensive disorders of pregnancy in non-diabetic pregnant women. **Hypertensive Pregnancy**, 25(2):125–136

12. Shaw G, Todoroff K, Schaffer D, *et al.* 2000 Maternal height and pre-pregnancy body mass index as risk factors for selected congenital anomalies. **Paediatric and Perinatal Epidemiology**, 14:234–239

13. Kristensen J, Vestergaard M, Wisborg K, *et al.* 2005 Pre-pregnancy weight and the risk of stillbirth and neonatal death. **British Journal of Obstetrics and Gynaecology**, 112:403–408

14. Yogev Y, Langar O, Xenakis E, *et al.* 2005 The association between glucose challenge test, obesity and pregnancy outcome in 6390 non-diabetic women. **The Journal of Maternal-Fetal and Neonatal Medicine**, 17(1):29–34

15. Farrell T, Holmes R and Stone P 2002 The effect of body mass index on three methods of fetal weight estimation. **British Journal of Obstetrics and Gynaecology**, 109:651–657

16. Martinez–Frias ML, Frias JP, Bermejo E *et al.* 2005 Pre-gestational Body Mass Index predicts an increased risk of congenital malformations in infants of mothers with gestational diabetes. **Diabetes Medicine** 22(6):775–781

17. Vahratian A, Zhang J, Troendle J, *et al.* 2004 Maternal pre-pregnancy overweight and obesity and the pattern of labour progression in term nulliparous women. **American College of Obstetricians and Gynecologists**, 104(5):943–951

18. Fraser RB 2006 Obesity complicating pregnancy. **Current Obstetrics and Gynaecology**, 16:295–298

19. Dempsey J, Ashiny Z, Qui C, *et al.* 2005 Maternal pre-pregnancy overweight status and obesity as risk factors for caesarean delivery. **The Journal of Maternal-Fetal and Neonatal Medicine**, 17(3):179–185

20. RCOG 2006 Statement No. 4 **Exercise in Pregnancy**. London; Royal College of Obstetricians and Gynaecologists

21. Gates S, Brocklehurst P and Davis L 2002 Prophylaxis for venous thromboembolic disease in pregnancy and the early postnatal period. **The Cochrane Database of Systematic Reviews 2006**, Issue 1

22. RCOG 2004 **Clinical Guideline No.37 Thromboprophylaxis During Pregnancy, Labour and After Vaginal Delivery**. London; Royal College of Obstetricians and Gynaecologists

23. Walker L, Sterling B, Timmerman G 2004 Retention of pregnancy-related weight in the early postpartum period: implications for women's health services. **Journal of Obstetric, Gynecologic and Neonatal Nursing**, 34(4):418–427

13.2 Phenylketonuria

1. UK Newborn Screening Programme 2005 Why are newborn babies screened for phenylketonuria? www.newbornscreening-bloodspot.org.uk

2. Levy H 2003 Historical background for the maternal PKU syndrome. **Paediatrics**, 112(6):1516–1517

3. National Society for Phenylketonuria (UK) 2005 Pregnancy in women with phenylketonuria (PKU) www.nspku.org

4. Politt R, Green A and McCabe A, *et al.* 1997 Neonatal screening for inborn errors of metabolism: cost, yield and outcome. **Health Technology Assessment**, 1:1–203

5. Antshel K and Waisbren S 2003 Developmental timing of exposure to elevated levels of phenylalanine is associated with ADHD symptom expression. **Journal of Abnormal Child Psychology**, 31(6):565–574

6. Poustie V J and Rutherford P 1999 Dietary interventions for phenylketonuria. **The Cochrane Database of Systematic Reviews**, Issue 3 2006

7. Weetch E and McDonald A 2006 The determination of phenylalanine content of foods suitable for phenylketonuria. **Journal of Human Nutrition and Dietetics**, 19:229

8. Rohr F, Munier A, Sullivan D, Bailey I, *et al.* 2004 The resource mothers study of maternal phenylketonuria: preliminary findings. **Journal of Inherited Metabolic Disorders**, 27(2):145–155

9. Duig Z, Georgieu P and Thony B 2006 Administration-route and gender-independent long-term therapeutic correction of PKU in a mouse model by recombinant adeno-associated virus 8 pseudo-typed vector-mediated gene transfer. **Gene Therapy**, 13(7):587–593

10. Lee P, Ridout D, Walker J, *et al.* 2005 Maternal PKU: a report from the UK Registry 1978–1997. **Archives of Disease in Childhood**, 90:143–146

11. Matalon K, Acosta P and Azen C 2003 Role of nutrition in pregnancy with PKU and birth defects. **Pediatrics**, 112(6 part 2):1534–1536

12. Waisbren S and Azen C 2003 Cognitive and behavioural development in maternal PKU offspring. **Pediatrics**, 112(6):P2 1544–1547

13. Levy H, Guldberg P, Guttlerr F, *et al.* 2001 Congenital heart disease in maternal PKU: report from the maternal phenylketonuria collaborative study. **Pediatric Research**, 49(5):636–642

14. Acosta P, Matalon K, Castiglioni L, *et al.* 2001 Intake of major nutrients by women in the maternal PKU (MPKU): study and effects on plasma phenylalanine concentrations. **American Journal of Clinical Nutrition,** 73:792–796

15. Geelhoed E, Lewis B, Hounsome D, *et al.* 2005 Economic evaluation of neonatal screening for PKU and congenital hypothyroidism. **Journal of Paediatrics and Child Health,** 41(11):575–579

16. MacDonald A and Asplin D 2006 Phenylketonuria: practical dietary management. **Journal of Family Health Care,** 16(3): 83–85

17. Van Rijn M, Bekhof J and Dijkstra T 2003 A different approach to breastfeeding for the infant with PKU. **European Journal of Paediatrics,** 162(5):323–326

Chapter 14 Haematological Disorders

14.1 Iron Deficiency Anaemia

1. Mahomed K 2001 Iron and folate supplementation in pregnancy. **Cochrane Database of Systematic Reviews,** issue 3. Oxford; Update Software

2. WHO/UNICEF/UNU 2001 Iron deficiency anaemia: assessment, prevention and control. A guide for programme managers. Geneva; World Health Organization 15 (WHO/NHD/01.3) http//.www.who.int/nutrition/publications/en/ida_assessment_prevention_control.pdf [accessed 22-11-2006]

3. Skikne B and Baynes RD 1994 *Iron absorption* in Brock JH, Halliday JW, Pippard MJ, Powell LW (Eds). **Iron Metabolism in Health and Disease.** London; W.B. Saunders 151–187

4. Murphy JF, O'Riordan J and Newcombe RG 1986 Relation of haemoglobin levels in first and second trimesters to outcomes of pregnancy. **The Lancet,** 1:992–995

5. Milman N, Bergholt T, Eriksen L, Byg K-E, Graudal N, Pedersen P and Hertz J 2005 Iron prophylaxis during pregnancy – how much iron is needed? A randomized dose-response study of 20–80 mg ferrous iron daily in pregnant women. **Acta Obstetricia et Gynecologica Scandinavica,** 84:238–247

6. National Collaborating Centre for Women's Health 2003 **Antenatal Care: Routine Care for Healthy Women.** London; National Institute for Clinical Excellence

7. Lumley J, Watson L, Watson M, *et al.* 2001 Periconceptional supplementation with folate and/or vitamins for preventing neural tube defects. **Cochrane Database of Systematic Reviews, Issue 3.** Oxford; Update Software

8. Siegenberg D, Baynes RD and Bothwell TH 1994 Ascorbic acid prevents the dose-dependent inhibitory effects of polyphenols and phytates on nonheme-iron absorption. **American Journal of Clinical Nutrition,** 53:537–541

9. James DK, Steer PJ, Weiner CP and Gonik B 2006 **High Risk Pregnancy: Management Options,** 3rd Ed. USA, Philadelphia; Elsevier 865–872

10. Barron WM and Lindheimer MD 2000 **Medical Disorders During Pregnancy,** 3rd Ed. Missouri, USA; Mosby Inc. 267–272

11. Hemminki E and Merilainen J 1995 Long-term follow-up of mothers and their infants in a randomized trial on iron prophylaxis during pregnancy. **American Journal of Obstetrics and Gynecology,** 173(1):205–209

12. National Health Service 2006 Healthy Start – Pregnancy www.healthystart.nhs.uk

13. NICE 2003 **Clinical Guideline: Antenatal care.** London; National Institute for Clinical Excellence www.nice.org.uk/guidance/CG6

14. WHO 2006 **Standards for Maternal and Neonatal Care 1.8 – Iron and Folate Supplementation – Integrated Management of Pregnancy and Childbirth.** Geneva; World Health Organization www.who.int/making_pregnancy_safer/publications/Standards1.8N.pdf

15. Simmons WK, Cook JD and Bingham KC 1993 Evaluation of a gastric delivery system for iron supplementation in pregnancy. **American Journal of Clinical Nutrition,** 58:622–626

14.2 Megaloblastic Anaemia

1. Chanarin I 1990 *Folate deficiency in pregnancy* in Chanarin I (Ed) **The Megaloblastic Anaemias,** 3rd Ed. Oxford; Blackwell 140–148

2. Letsky EA 2002 *Blood volume, haematinics, anaemia* in de Swiet M (Ed) **Medical Disorders in Obstetric Practice,** 4th Ed. Oxford; Blackwell 29–60

3. Barron WM and Lindheimer MD 2000 **Medical Disorders During Pregnancy,** 3rd Ed. Missouri, USA; Mosby Inc. 274–275

4. Clark P and Greer IA 2006 **Practical Obstetrical Haematology.** London; Taylor Francis 48–53

5. MRC Vitamin Study Research Group 1991 Prevention of neural tube defects: results of the medical research council vitamin study. **The Lancet,** 228:131–137

6. Mahomed K 2001 Iron and folate supplementation in pregnancy. **Cochrane Database of Systematic Reviews,** issue 3. Oxford; Update Software

7. Langley-Evans SC and Langley-Evans AJ 2002 Use of folic acid supplements in the first trimester of pregnancy. **Journal of the Royal Society of Health,** 122:181–186

8. Lumley J, Watson M, *et al.* 2001 Periconceptual supplementation with folate and or multivitamins for preventing neural tube defects. **Cochrane Database of Systematic Reviews,** issue 3. Oxford; Update Software

9. National Institute for Clinical Excellence 2003 **Antenatal Care: Routine Care for the Healthy Pregnant Woman.** London; National Institute for Clinical Excellence http://www.nice.org.uk/guidance/CG6

10. Department of Health 2000 **Folic Acid and the Prevention of Disease: Report of the Committee on Medical Aspects of Food and Nutrition Policy.** London; The Stationery Office

14.3 Thalassaemia

1. NHS Sickle Cell and Thalassaemia Screening Programme 2006 **NHS Sickle Cell and Thalassaemia Screening Programme Information for Midwives.** Kings College London www.kcl–phs.org.uk/haemscreening

2. Atkin K and Ahmad W 1998 Genetic screening and haemoglobinopathies; ethics, politics and practice. **Social Science and Medicine,** 46(3):445–458

3. Modell B, Harris R, Lane B, Khan M, Darlinson M, Petrou M, *et al.* 2000 Informed choice in genetic screening for thalassaemia during pregnancy: audit from a national confidential inquiry. **British Medical Journal,** 320:337–341

4. Weatheral D and Clegg J 2001 **The Thalassaemia Syndromes,** 4th Ed. Oxford; Blackwell Scientific Publications

5. Weatherall D and Letsky E 1999 *Genetic haematological disorders* in Wald N (Ed). **Antenatal and Neonatal Screening,** 2nd Ed. Oxford; Oxford University Press

6. Letsky E 2002 *Anaemia* in James D, Steer P, Weiner D and Gonik B (Eds). **High Risk Pregnancy: Management Options,** 2nd Ed. London; WB Saunders 729–747

7. James DK, Steer PJ, Weiner CP and Gonik B 2006 **High Risk Pregnancy: Management Options,** 3rd Ed. USA, Philadelphia; Elsevier 878–881

8. Billington M and Stephenson M 2006 **Critical Care in Childbearing for Midwives.** Oxford; Blackwell 78–83

9. National Institute for Clinical Excellence 2003 **Clinical Guideline 6 Antenatal care: Routine care for the healthy pregnant woman.** London; National Institute for Clinical Excellence

14.4 Sickle Cell Disorders

1. Oteng-Ntim E, Cottee C, Bewley S, Anionwu E 2006 Sickle cell disease in pregnancy. **Current Obstetrics and Gynaecology,** London; Elsevier

2. Atkin K and Ahmad W 1998 Genetic screening and haemoglobinopathies; ethics, politics and practice. **Social Science and Medicine,** 46(3):445–458

3. Serjeant GR 2001 Historical review. The emerging understanding of sickle cell disease. **British Journal of Haematology,** 12:3–18

4. Vichinksy EP, Neumayr LD and Ealres AN 2000 Causes and outcomes of the acute chest syndrome in sickle cell disease: National Acute Chest Syndrome Study Group. **New England Journal of Medicine**, 342:1855–1865

5. NHS 2006 Sickle cell and thalassaemia screening programme – screening for sickle cell and thalassaemia in pregnancy. www.kcl–phs.org.uk/haemscreening

6. Streetly A 2006 Sickle cell screening makes genetic counselling everybody's business. **British Medical Journal**, 332:570–572

7. Billington M and Stephenson M 2006 **Critical Care in Childbearing for Midwives**. Oxford; Blackwell 72–78

8. Howard RJ, Lillis C and Tuck SM 1995 Contraceptives counselling and pregnancy in women with sickle cell disease. **British Journal of Obstetrics and Gynaecology**, 102: 945–951

9. Charache S, Terrin ML and Moore RD 1995 Effect of hydroxyurea on the frequency of painful crises in sickle cell anaemia. **New England Journal of Medicine**, 332:1317–1322

10. James DK, Steer PJ, Weiner CP and Gonik B 2006 **High Risk Pregnancy: Management Options**, 3rd Ed. USA, Philadelphia; Elsevier 874–878

14.5 Thrombocytopenia in Pregnancy

1. Kam PC, Thompson SA and Liew AC 2004 Thrombocytopenia in the parturient. **Anaesthesia**, 59(3):255–264

2. Stamilio DM and Macones GA 1999 Selection of delivery method in pregnancies complicated by autoimmune thrombocytopenic purpura. **Obstetrics and Gynaecology**, 94(1):41–47

3. Macpherson G 2004 **Black's Student Medical Dictionary**. London; Black Publishers

4. Strong J 2003 Bleeding disorders in pregnancy. **Current Obstetrics and Gynaecology**, 13:1–6

5. McFadden TM, Lerrieri L and Settler RW 1998 Immune thrombocytopenic purpura in pregnancy: the ongoing debate surrounding obstetric management. **Primary Care Update for Ob/Gyns**, 5(6):300–305

6. Nelson-Piercy C 2002 **Handbook of Obstetric Medicine**. London; Martin Dunitz 259–264

7. Kumar P and Clarke M 2004 **Clinical Medicine**, 5th Ed. London; Saunders 458–459

8. Frederickson H and Schmidt K 1999 The incidence of idiopathic thrombocytopenic purpura in adults increases with age. **Blood**, 94(3):909–913

9. Higgins C 2000 **Understanding Laboratory Investigations**. Oxford; Blackwell 243

10. Fisher M, Peters B, McBride M and Kitchen V 1994 Consider HIV infection in thrombocytopenia. **British Medical Journal**, 308(6921):133–136

11. Webert KE, Mittal R, Sigouin C, Heddle NM and Kelton JG 2003 A retrospective analysis of obstetric patients with idiopathic thrombocytopenic purpura. **Blood**, 102(13):4306–4311

12. Parnas M, Sheiner E, Shoham-Vardi I, Burstein E, Yermiahu T, Levi I, Holcberg G and Yerushalmi R 2006 Moderate to severe thrombocytopenia during pregnancy. **European Journal of Obstetrics and Gynaecology**, 127(1–2):163–168

13. Cines DB 2003 ITP and pregnancy. **Blood**, 102(13):4250–4251

14. Horn EH and Kean L 2006 in James DK, Steer PJ, Weiner CP and Gonik B 2006 **High Risk Pregnancy: Management Options**, 3rd Ed. USA, Philadelphia; Elsevier 901–908

15. British Committee for Standards in Haematology General Haematology Task Force 2003 Guidelines for the investigation and management of idiopathic thrombocytopenic purpura in adults, children and pregnancy. **British Journal of Haematology**, 120:570–596

16. Burrow GN, Duffy GN and Copel JA 2004 **Medical Complications During Pregnancy**, 6th Ed. USA, Philadelphia; Saunders/Elsevier 78–80

17. Gottlieb P, Axelson O, Bakos O and Rastad J 1999 Splenectomy during pregnancy: an option in the treatment of autoimmune thrombocytopenic purpura. **British Journal of Obstetrics and Gynaecology**, 106:373–377

14.6 Von Willebrand's Disease and Other Bleeding Disorders

1. Haemophilia Society 2003 **Fact Sheet – Von Willebrand's: General Information**. London; The Haemophilia Society www.womenbleedtoo.org.uk/User_Files/vwillebrandsgeneral.pdf

2. Kouides PA 2001 Obstetric and gynaecological aspects of von Willebrand's disease. **Best Practice and Research in Clinical Haematology**, 14(2):381–399

3. Lee CA and Abdul-Kadir R 2005 Von Willebrand's disease and women's health. **Seminars in Haematology**, 42(1):42–48

4. Kujovich JL 2005 von Willebrand's and pregnancy. **Journal of Thrombosis and Haemostasis**, 3:246–253

5. Green D and Ludham CA 2006 **Fast Facts: Bleeding Disorders**. Oxford; Health Press 63–69

6. Kadir RA, Lee CA, Sabin CA, et al. 1998 Pregnancy in women with von Willebrand's disease or factor XI deficiency. **British Journal of Obstetrics and Gynaecology**, 105:314–321

7. Lee CA, Chi C and Pavord S, et al. 2006 The obstetrical and gynaecological management of women with inherited bleeding disorders: review with guidelines by a taskforce of UK Haemophilia Centre Doctors' Organisation. **Haemophilia**, 12:311–336

8. Strong J 2006 von Willebrand's disease and pregnancy. **Current Obstetrics and Gynaecology**, 16:1–5

9. Edland M, Blomback M, von Schoulz B and Andersson O 1996 On the value of menorrhagia as a predictor for coagulation disorders. **American Journal of Haematology**, 53:234–238

10. NICE 2007 **Clinical Guideline No.44 Heavy Menstrual Bleeding**. London; National Institute for Clinical Excellence www.nice.org.uk/guidance/CG44

11. James DK, Steer PJ, Weiner CP and Gonik B 2006 **High Risk Pregnancy: Management Options**, 3rd Ed. USA, Philadelphia; Elsevier 911–913

14.7 Disseminated Intravascular Coagulation

1. Mattar F and Sibai BM 2000 Risk factors for maternal mortality. **American Journal of Obstetrics and Gynaecology**, 182:307–312

2. Treacher DF and Grant IS 2006 Chap.8 Major organ failure in Boon NB, Colledge NR and Walker BR (Eds) **Davidson's Principles and Practice of Medicine**, 20th Ed. London; Elsevier 190

3. Craig JIO, McLelland DBL and Ludlam CA 2006 Chap.24 Blood disorders in Boon NB, Colledge NR and Walker BR (Eds) **Davidson's Principles and Practice of Medicine**, 20th Ed. London; Elsevier 1060–1061

4. Bick RL 2000 Syndromes of disseminated intravascular coagulation in obstetrics, pregnancy and gynaecology. **Hematology/Oncology Clinics of North America**, 14(5):999–1044

5. Kumar P and Clarke M 2004 **Clinical Medicine**, 5th Ed. London; Saunders 463–464

6. Stables D 1999 **Physiology in Childbearing: With Anatomy and Related Biosciences**. London; Elsevier 398–399

7. Baglin T 1996 Fortnightly Review: Disseminated intravascular coagulation: diagnosis and treatment. **British Medical Journal**, 312:683–686

8. Steele D 2006 Chap.7 Haemorrhagic disorders in Billington M and Stevenson M (Eds) **Critical Care in Childbearing for Midwives**. Oxford; Blackwell Scientific 118–139

9. James DK, Steer PJ, Weiner CP and Gonik B 2006 **High Risk Pregnancy: Management Options**, 3rd Ed. USA, Philadelphia; Elsevier 1617–1620

10. Letsky EA 2001 Disseminated intravascular coagulation. **Best Practice and Research in Clinical Obstetrics and Gynaecology**, 15(4):623–644

11. Nelson-Piercy C 2002 **Handbook of Obstetric Medicine**. London; Martin Dunitz 264–265

12. Burrow GN, Duffy GN and Copel JA 2004 **Medical Complications During Pregnancy**, 6th Ed. USA; Philadelphia; Saunders/Elsevier 82

13. Green D and Ludham CA 2006 **Fast Facts: Bleeding Disorders**. Oxford; Health Press 90–92

14. Sood M, Juneja Y and Goyal U 1995 Maternal mortality associated with clandestine abortions. **Journal of the Indian Medical Association**, 93(2):77–79

Chapter 15 Thrombo-embolic Disorders

15.1 Deep Vein Thrombosis

1. Walker ID 1993 Guidelines on the prevention, investigation and management of thrombosis associated with pregnancy. Maternal and Neonatal Haemostasis Working Party of the Haemostasis and Thrombosis Task Force. **Journal of Clinical Pathology**, 46(6), 489–496
2. Ginsberg JS, Brill-Edwards P, Burrows RF, Bona R, Prandoni P, Buller HR and Lensing A 1992 Venous thrombosis during pregnancy: leg and trimester of presentation. **Thrombosis and Haemostasis**, 67:519–520
3. Ikard RW, Ueland K, and Folse R. 1971 Lower limb venous dynamics in pregnant women. **Surgery, Gynecology and Obstetrics**, 132:483–488
4. Beyth RJ, Cohen AM, Landefeld CS 1995 Long-term outcomes of deep vein thrombosis. **Archives of Internal Medicine**, 155(10):1031–1037
5. Prandoni P, Lensing AW, Cogo A, Cuppini S, Villalta S, Carta M, Cattelan AM, Polistena P, Bernadi E and Prins MH 1996 The long term clinical course of acute deep vein thrombosis. **Annals of Internal Medicine**, 125(1):1–7
6. Brandejes DP, Buller HR, Heijboer H, *et al*. 1997 Randomised trial of effect of compression stockings in patients with symptomatic proximal-vein thrombosis. **The Lancet, 349**(9054):759–762
7. Gorman WP, Davis KR and Donnelly R 2000 ABC of arterial and venous disease. Swollen lower limb – 1: general assessment and deep vein thrombosis. **British Medical Journal**, 320(7247): 1453–1456
8. Wells PS, Anderson DR, Rodger M, Forgie M, Kearon C, Dreyer J, Kovacs G, Mitchell M, Lewandowski B and Kovacs MJ 2003 Evaluation of D-dimer in the diagnosis of suspected deep-vein thrombosis. **New England Journal of Medicine**, 349:1227–1235
9. SIGN 1999 Report No.36 – **Antithrombotic Therapy**. Edinburgh; Scottish Intercollegiate Guidelines Network
10. McColl MD, Ramsay JE, Tait RC, Walker ID, McCall F, Conkie JA, Carty MJ and Greer IA 1997 Risk factors for pregnancy associated venous thromboembolism. **Journal of Thrombosis and Haemostasis**, 78:1183–1188
11. RCOG 2007 **Clinical Guideline No.28 – Thromboembolic Disease in Pregnancy and the Puerperium: Acute Management**. London; Royal College of Obstetricians and Gynaecologists
12. Bick RL and Haas SK 1998 International consensus recommendations. Summary statement and additional suggested guidelines. **Medical Clinics of North America**, 82(3):613–633
13. British Committee for standards in haematology 1998 Guidelines on oral anticoagulation, 3rd Ed. **British Journal of Haematology**, 101(20)374–387
14. Lewis G and Drife J 2002 Confidential enquiries into maternal and child health. **CEMACH 6th report: Why Mothers Die 2000–2002**. London; RCOG Press
15. Weitz JI 1997 Low-molecular-weight heparins. **New England Journal of Medicine**, 337:688–698
16. Warkentin TE, Levine MN, Hirsh J, Horsewood P, Roberts RS, Gent MN and Kelton JG 1995 Heparin induced thrombocytopenia in patients treated with low molecular weight heparin or unfractionated heparin. **New England Journal of Medicine**, 332: 1330–1335
17. Wutschert R, Piletta P and Bounameaux H 1999 Adverse skin reactions to low molecular weight heparins: frequency, management and prevention. **Drug Safety**, 20(6):515–525
18. McCollum C 1998 Avoiding the consequence of deep vein thrombosis. Elevation and compression are important and too often forgotten. **British Medical Journal**, 317(7160):696
19. Ginsberg JS, Greer I and Hirsh J 2001 Use of antithrombotic agents during pregnancy. **Chest**, 119:122s–131s

15.2 Pulmonary Embolism

1. Barrit DW and Jordan SC 1960 Anticoagulant drugs in the treatment of pulmonary embolism: a controlled trial. **The Lancet**, 1:1309–1312

2. Lewis G and Drife J 2002 **CEMACH 6th report: Why Mothers Die 2000–2002**. London; RCOG/Confidential Enquiries into Maternal and Child Health
3. McColl MD, Ramsay JE, Tait RC, Walker ID, McCall F, Conkie JA, Carty MJ and Greer IA 1997 Risk factors for pregnancy associated venous thromboembolism. **Journal of Thrombosis and Haemostasis**, 78:1183–1188
4. RCOG 2004 **Greentop Clinical Guideline No.37 – Thromboprophylaxis during Pregnancy, Labour and after Vaginal Delivery**. London; Royal College of Obstetricians and Gynaecologists
5. RCOG 2007 **Greentop Clinical Guideline No.28 – Thromboembolic Disease in Pregnancy and the Puerperium: Acute Management**. London; Royal College of Obstetricians and Gynaecologists
6. Cook JV and Kyriou J 2005 Radiation from CT and perfusion scanning in pregnancy. **British Medical Journal**, 331:350
7. Remy-Jardin M. Remy J and Spiral CT 1999 Angiography of the pulmonary circulation. **Radiology**, 212:615–636
8. Checketts MR and Wildsmith J 1999 Central nerve block and thromboprophylaxis: is there a problem? **British Journal of Anaesthesia**, 82:164–167
9. Ginsberg JS, Greer I and Hirsh J 2001 Use of antithrombotic agents during pregnancy. **Chest**, 119:122s–131s

15.3 Thrombophilia

1. RCOG 2004 **Clinical Guideline No.37 – Thromboprophylaxis during Pregnancy, Labour and after Vaginal Delivery**. London; Royal College of Obstetricians and Gynaecologists
2. Khamashata MA, Guadrado MJ, Mujic F, Taub NA, Hunt BJ and Hughes GR 1995 The management of thrombosis in the antiphospholipid-antibody syndrome. **New England Journal of Medicine**, 332:993–997
3. Pattison NS, Chamley LW, Birdsall M, Zanderigo AM, Liddel HS, McDougal J 2000 Does aspirin have a role in improving pregnancy outcome for women with the antiphospholipid syndrome? A randomised controlled trial. **American Journal of Obstetrics and Gynecology**, 183:1008–1012
4. Rai R 2000 Obstetric management of antiphospholipid syndrome. **Journal of Autoimmune Diseases**, 15(2):203–207
5. SIGN 1999 Report No.36 **Antithrombotic Therapy.** Edinburgh; Scottish Intercollegiate Guidelines Network

Chapter 16 Addictive Disorders

16.1 Alcohol Addiction

1. Gerada C and Ashworth M 1997 ABC of mental health: addiction and dependence – illicit drugs. **British Medical Journal**, 315: 297–300
2. Han S 1999 Demographic and psychosocial characteristics of substance-abusing pregnant women. **Clinics in Perinatology**, 26:55–74
3. Department of Health 1999 **Drug Misuse and Dependence – Guidelines on Clinical Management**. London; The Stationery Office www.dh.gov.uk/prod_consum_dh/groups/dh_digitalassets/@dh/@en/documents/digitalasset/dh_4078198.pdf
4. Royal College of Obstetricians and Gynaecologists 2006 **Statement No.5: Alcohol Consumption and the Outcomes of Pregnancy** www.rcog.org.uk/index.asp?PageID=1477 [accessed March 2006]
5. Cabinet Office 1998 **Tackling Drugs to Build a Better Britain. The Government's Ten-Year Strategy for Tackling Drugs Misuse**. London; The Stationery Office
6. Keen J and Alison L 2001 Drug misusing parents: key points for health professionals. **Archives of Diseases in Childhood**, 85:296–299
7. Institute for the Study of Drug Dependence 1999 **Drug Situation in the UK – Trends and Update**. Report to the European Monitoring Centre for Drugs and Drug Addiction www.doh.gov.uk/drugs/drugreport.pdf

8. Food Standards Agency 2007 **Eat Well, Be Well. Helping You Make Healthier Choices** www.eatwell.gov.uk
9. Fetal Alcohol Syndrome Information 2007 **Alcohol and Pregnancy** http://fas–info.uwe.ac.uk
10. Home Office 2004 **Drug Use among Vulnerable Groups of Young People: Findings from the Crime and Justice Survey 2003**. London; The Stationery Office
11. Little B 2006 **Drugs and Pregnancy: A Handbook**. USA; Hodder Arnold
12. Alcohol Concern 2002 **100% Proof. Research for Action on Alcohol**. UK; Alcohol Concern

16.2 Cannabis Use
1. Little B 2006 **Drugs and Pregnancy: A Handbook**. USA; Hodder Arnold
2. Home Office 2007 **Tackling Drugs, Saving Lives: Turning Strategy into Reality**. Home Office
3. Keen J and Alison L 2001 Drug misusing parents: key points for health professionals. **Archives of Diseases in Childhood**, 85:296–299
4. Institute for the Study of Drug Dependence 1999 **Drug situation in the UK – Trends and Update. Report to the European Monitoring Centre for Drugs and Drug Addiction** www.doh.gov.uk/drugs/drugreport.pdf
5. Hawksley J 1990 **Teen Guide to Pregnancy, Drugs and Smoking**. London; Franklin Watts
6. Fergusson D, Horwood L and Northstone K 2002 Maternal use of cannabis and pregnancy outcome. **British Journal of Obstetrics and Gynaecology**, 109:21–27
7. Standing Conference on Drug Abuse and Local Government Forum 1998 **Drug Using Parents: Policy Guidelines for Interagency Working.** London; Local Government
8. Siney C 1995 **The Pregnant Drug Addict**. Oxford; Butterworth-Heinemann
9. Department of Health 1999 **National Service Framework for Mental Health** www.doh.gov.uk/pub/docs/doh/mhmain.pdf
10. Office for National Statistics 1998 **Statistics on Young People and Drug Misuse: England**. London; Office for National Statistics www.statistics.gov.uk/

16.3 Cocaine Addiction
1. Little B 2006 **Drugs and Pregnancy: A Handbook**. USA; Hodder Arnold
2. Siney C 1995 **The Pregnant Drug Addict**. London; Books for Midwives Press/Elsevier
3. Harcapos A, Dennis D, Turnbull PJ and Hough M 2003 **On the Rocks: A Follow-Up Study of Crack Users in London**. London; Criminal Policy Research Unit South Bank University
4. Harvey JA and Kosofsky BE (Eds) 2000 **Cocaine: Effects on the Developing Brain**. USA; Annals of the New York Academy of Sciences
5. Humphries D 1999 **Crack Mothers: Pregnancy, Drugs and the Media**. USA; Ohio State University Press
6. Department of Health 2002 **Tackling Crack Cocaine – A National Plan**. London; Department of Health
7. Hulse GK, Milne E, English DR, *et al.* 1998 Assessing the relationship between maternal opiate use and antepartum haemorrhage. **Addiction**, 93:1553–1558
8. Gillogley KM, Evans AT, Hansen RL, *et al.* 1990 The perinatal impact of cocaine, amphetamine, and opiate use detected by universal intrapartum screening. **American Journal of Obstetrics and Gynecology**, 163, 1535–1542
9. Sherwood RA, Keating J, Kavvadia V, *et al.* 1999 Substance misuse in early pregnancy and relationship to fetal outcome. **European Journal of Pediatrics**, 158:488–492
10. Laegried L, Olegard R and Walstrom JNC 1989 Teratogenic effects of benzodiazepine use during pregnancy. **The Journal of Pediatrics**, 114(1):126–131
11. NHS Northern and Yorkshire Regional Drug and Therapeutic Centre 2000 **National Teratology Information Service. Cocaine – Use in Pregnancy** www.spib.axl.co.uk/Toxbase/Exposures

12. Hancock J 1997 The passive effects of addiction: how maternal substance abuse affects the health and development of the child. **Journal of Neonatal Nursing**, 3(3):14–18
13. National Institute on Drug Abuse 1998 Drug addiction research and the health effects on women. Executive Summary from the 1994 Conference **Drug Addiction Research and the Health Effects of Women**

16.4 Heroin Addiction
1. Siney C, Kidd M, Walkinshaw S, Morrison C and Manasse P 1995 Opiate dependency in pregnancy. **British Journal of Midwifery**, 3(2):63–73
2. WHO 1993 **Expert Committee on Drug Dependence**, 28th Report. Geneva; World Health Organization
3. National Institute on Drug Abuse 1998 Drug addiction research and the health effects of women. Executive Summary from the 1994 Conference **Drug Addiction Research and the Health Effects on Women**
4. Department of Health 1999 **Drug Misuse and Dependence – Guidelines on Clinical Management**. London; The Stationery Office www.doh.gov.uk/drugs/dmfull.pdf
5. Department of Health 2002 **Model of Care for Substance Misuse Treatment**. London; Stationery Office www.doh.gov.uk/nta/models.htm
6. Cabinet Office 1998 **Tackling Drugs to Build a Better Britain. The Government's Ten-Year Strategy for Tackling Drugs Misuse**. London; The Stationery Office
7. Standing Conference on Drug Abuse and Local Government Forum 1998 **Drug Using Parents: Policy Guidelines for Interagency Working**. London; Local Government
8. NHS Executive 1998 **Screening of Pregnant Women for Hepatitis B and Immunisation of Babies at Risk**. Health Service Circular; 1998/127
9. Department of Health 1988 **AIDS and Drug Misuse Part 1: Report by the Advisory Council on the Misuse of Drugs**. London; HMSO
10. Ward J, Hall W and Mattick R 1999 Role of maintenance treatment in opioid dependence. **The Lancet**, 353:221–226
11. Gibbs J, Newson T, Williams J and Davidson DC 1989 Naloxone hazard in infants of opioid abusers. **The Lancet**, 19;2(8660):446
12. Franck RN and Vilardi J 1995 Assessment and management of opioid withdrawal in ill neonates. **Neonatal Network**, 14(2):39–45
13. Hulatt J 2000 Neonatal abstinence syndrome: How and where should babies with the condition be cared for? **Journal of Neonatal Nursing**, 6(5):159–164
14. Richards B and Drennan B 2000 **Helping Hands: Caregivers' Guide for Drug-Exposed Infants**, USA; Idaho RADAR Network Center; Perinatal Videos http://hs.boisestate.edu/RADAR/videos/PerinatalVideos2007.pdf

16.5 Amphetamine Addiction
1. Han S 1999 Demographic and psychosocial characteristics of substance-abusing pregnant women. **Clinics in Perinatology**, 26:55–74
2. Department of Health 1999 **Drug Misuse and Dependence – Guidelines on Clinical Management**. London; The Stationery Office www.doh.gov.uk/drugs/dmfull.pdf
3. Little B 2006 **Drugs and Pregnancy: A Handbook**. USA; Hodder Arnold
4. Siney C 1995 **The Pregnant Drug Addict**. London; Books for Midwives Press/Elsevier
5. NHS Northern and Yorkshire Regional Drug and Therapeutic Centre 2000 **National Teratology Information Service: Cocaine Use in Pregnancy** www.spib.axl.co.uk/Toxbase/Exposures
6. Sherwood RA, Keating J, Kavvadia V, *et al.* 1999 Substance misuse in early pregnancy and relationship to fetal outcome. **European Journal of Pediatrics**, 158:488–492
7. National Institute on Drug Abuse 1998 Drug addiction research and the health effects on women. Executive Summary from the 1994 Conference **Drug Addiction Research and the Health Effects of Women**

8. NHS Executive 1998 **Screening of Pregnant Women for Hepatitis B and Immunisation of Babies at Risk**. Health Service Circular; 1998/127
9. Department of Health 1988 **AIDS and Drug Misuse Part 1: Report by the Advisory Council on the Misuse of Drugs**. London; HMSO
10. Home Office 2007 **Tackling Drugs, Saving Lives: Turning Strategy into Reality**. London; Home Office
11. Department of Health 2005 **Every Child Matters – Young People and Drugs**. London; The Stationery Office
12. White R 2000 Dexamphetamine Substitution in the Treatment of Amphetamine Abuse: an initial investigation. **Addiction** Feb; 95(2): 229–238
13. Hulatt J 2000 Neonatal abstinence syndrome: How and where should babies with the condition be cared for? **Journal of Neonatal Nursing**, 6(5):159–164
14. Richards B and Drennan B 2000 **Helping Hands: Caregivers' Guide for Drug-Exposed Infants**. USA; Idaho RADAR Network Center; Perinatal Videos http://hs.boisestate.edu/RADAR/videos/PerinatalVideos2007.pdf
15. Winyard R (Ed) 2005 **Substance Misuse in Primary Care**. Oxford; Radcliffe Press

Chapter 17 Psychiatric Disorders

17.1 Antenatal Psychiatric Disorders

1. Watson JP, Elliott SA, Rugg AJ, Brough DI 1984 Psychiatric disorders in pregnancy and the first postnatal year. **British Journal of Psychiatry**, 144:453–462
2. Appleby L 1991 Suicide during pregnancy and the first postnatal year. **British Medical Journal**, 302:137–140
3. Evans J, Heron J, Oke S and Golding J 2001 Cohort study of depressed mood during pregnancy and after childbirth. **British Medical Journal**, 323:257–260
4. Lewis G and Drife J 2002 **CEMACH 6th report: Why Mothers Die 2000–2002 Confidential Enquiries into Maternal and Child Health**. London; RCOG Press
5. Cantwell R and Cox JL 2003 Psychiatric disorders in pregnancy and the puerperium. **Current Obstetrics and Gynaecology**, 13:7–13
6. Oates M 2003 perinatal psychiatric syndromes. **Psychiatry**, 2:2(4–8) The Medicine Publishing Company Ltd
7. NICE 2007 **Clinical Guideline 45 – Antenatal and Postnatal Mental Health**. London; National Institute for Clinical Excellence
8. Royal College of Psychiatrists 2000 **Perinatal Maternal Mental Health Services** (Council Report CR88)
9. Wilson LM, Reid AJ, Midmer DK, Bringer A, Carroll JC and Stewart DE 1996 Antenatal psychosocial risk factors associated with adverse postnatal family outcomes. **Canadian Medical Association**, 154:785–799
10. Hedegaard M, Henriksen TB, Sabroe S, Secher NJ 1993 Psychological distress in pregnancy and preterm delivery. **British Medical Journal**, 307:234–239
11. Teixeira JMA, Fisk NM and Glover V 1999 Association between maternal anxiety in pregnancy and increased uterine artery resistance index: cohort based study. **British Medical Journal**, 318:153–157
12. O'Connor TG, Heron J, Golding G, Beverdige M and Glover V 2002 Maternal antenatal anxiety and children's behavioural/emotional problems at 4 years: Report from the Avon Longitudinal Study of Parents and Children. **British Journal of Psychiatry**, 180: 502–508

17.2 Postnatal Psychiatric Disorders

1. Cox JL, Holden JM and Sagovsky R 1987 Detection of postnatal depression. Development of the 10-item Edinburgh postnatal depression scale. **British Journal of Psychiatry**, 150:782–786
2. O'Hara MW and Swain AM 1996 Rates and risk of postnatal depression – a meta-analysis. **International Review of Psychiatry**, 8:37–54
3. Royal College of Psychiatrists 2000 **Perinatal Maternal Mental Health Services** (Council Report CR88)
4. Lewis G and Drife J 2002 **CEMACH 6th report: Why Mothers Die 2000–2002 Confidential Enquiries into Maternal and Child Health**. London; RCOG Press
5. SIGN 2002 **Postnatal Depression and Puerperal Psychosis** – A national clinical guideline. Edinburgh; Scottish Intercollegiate Guidelines Network
6. Cantwell R and Cox JL 2003 Psychiatric disorders in pregnancy and the puerperium. **Current Obstetrics and Gynaecology**, 13:7–13
7. Raynor M 2003 Pregnancy and the Puerperium: the social and psychological context. **Psychiatry**, 2:2(1–3) The Medicine Publishing Company
8. NICE 2007 **Clinical Guideline 45 – Antenatal and Postnatal Mental Health**. London; National Institute for Clinical Excellence
9. Blackmore E, Jones I, Doshi M, Haque S, Holder R, Brockington I and Craddock N 2006 Obstetric variables associated with bipolar affective puerperal psychosis. **British Journal of Psychiatry**, 188: 32–36
10. Jones I and Craddock N 2005 Editorial: Bipolar disorder and childbirth: the importance of recognising risk. **British Journal of Psychiatry**, 186:453–454
11. Martins, C and Gaffan EA 2000 Effects of early maternal depression on patterns of infant–mother attachment: a meta-analytical investigation. **Journal of Child Psychology and Psychiatry**, 41:737–746
12. NICE 2004 Clinical guideline 23: **Depression – Management of depression in primary and secondary care**. London; National Institute for Clinical Excellence

Chapter 18 Neoplasia

18.1 Breast Cancer

1. http://info.cancerresearchuk.org/cancerandresearch/cancers/breast/?a=5441 [accessed 16-06-2007]
2. James DK, Steer PJ, Weiner CP and Gonik B 1994 **High Risk Pregnancy: Management Options**, 2nd Ed. USA; Elsevier 949–950
3. www.breastcancercare.org.uk/content.php?page_id=70[accessed 28-06-2007]
4. Williams SF and Schilsky RL 2000 *Neoplastic disorders – breast cancer* in Barron WM and Lindheimer MD (Eds) **Medical Disorders During Pregnancy**, 3rd Ed. London; Mosby/Elsevier 400–401
5. Burstein H and Winer E 2000 Primary care for survivors of breast cancer. **New England Journal of Medicine**, 343:1086–1094
6. de la Rochefordiere A, Asselain B, Campana F, *et al.* 1993 Age as prognostic factor in premenopausal breast carcinoma. **The Lancet**, 341(8852):1039–1043
7. RCOG 2004 **Guideline No.12 – Pregnancy and Breast Cancer**. London; Royal College of Obstetricians and Gynaecologists
8. Velentgas P, Daling JR, Malone KE, *et al.* 1999 Pregnancy after breast carcinoma: outcomes and influence on mortality. **Cancer**, 85:2424–2432
9. Guinee VF, Olsson H, Moller T, *et al.* 1994 Effect of pregnancy on prognosis for young women with breast cancer. **The Lancet**, 343(8913):1587–1589
10. Petrek JA, Dukoff R and Rogatko A 1991 Prognosis of pregnancy-associated breast cancer. **Cancer**, 67(4):869–872
11. Karim SA and Shafti MI 2005 Malignancy in pregnancy. **Current Obstetrics and Gynaecology**, 15:414–416
12. Bernik SF, Bernik TR, Whooley BP, *et al.* 1998 Carcinoma of the breast during pregnancy: a review and update on treatment options. **Journal of Surgical Oncology**, 7:45–49
13. National Cancer Institute www.cancer.gov/cancertopics/pdq/treatment/breast–cancer–and–pregnancy/healthprofessional [accessed 15-06-2007]
14. Barthelmes L, Davidson LA, Gaffney C, *et al.* 2005 Pregnancy and breast cancer. **British Medical Journal**, 330:1375–1378
15. McEwan A 2005 Cancer in pregnancy. **Current Obstetrics and Gynaecology**, 15:402–408

18.2 Malignant Melanoma

1. **Cancer Research UK** http://info.cancerresearchuk.org/cancer-stats/types/melanoma/ [accessed 17-06-2007]
2. Elwood J and Koh H 1994 Etiology, epidemiology, risk factors and public health issues of melanoma. **Current Opinion in Oncology**, 6:179–187
3. Buchan J and Roberts D 2000 **Pocket Guide to Malignant Melanoma**. Oxford; Blackwell
4. Roberts DLL, Anstey AV, Barlow RJ, *et al.* 2002 UK guidelines for the management of cutaneous melanoma. **British Journal of Dermatology**, 146:7–17
5. Kumar P and Clark M 2005 **Clinical Medicine**, 6th Ed. London; Saunders/Elsevier 1352
6. NICE 2006 **Guidance on Cancer Services: Improving Outcomes for People with Skin Tumours including Melanoma – The Manual**. London; National Institute for Clinical Excellence
7. James DK, Steer PJ, Weiner CP and Gonik B (Eds) 1994 **High Risk Pregnancy: Management Options**, 3rd Ed. USA, Elsevier 950–951
8. Johnston SRD, Broadley K, Henson G, *et al.* 1998 A difficult case: management of metastatic melanoma during pregnancy. **British Medical Journal**, 316:848
9. MacKie RM, Bufalino R, Morabito A, *et al.* 1991 Lack of effect of pregnancy on outcome of melanoma. For The World Health Organisation Melanoma Programme. The **Lancet**, 337(8742): 653–655
10. Shanklin, DR 1990 **Tumours of the Placenta and Umbilical Cord**. Philadelphia; Marcel Decker 154–159
11. Anderson JF, Kent S and Machin GA 1989 Maternal malignant melanoma with placental metastases: a case report with literature review. **Pediatric Pathology**, 9:35–52

18.3 Hodgkin's Lymphoma

1. www.lymphoma.org.uk [accessed 14-06-2007]
2. www.cancerbackup.org.uk [accessed 14-06-2007]
3. Kumar P and Clark M 2005 **Clinical Medicine**, 6th Ed. London; Saunders/Elsevier 508–512
4. Underwood JCE 2004 **General and Systematic Pathology**, 4th Ed. London; Churchill Livingstone/Elsevier 597–601
5. NICE 2005 **Clinical Guideline 27: Referral Guidelines for Suspected Cancer**. London; National Institute for Health and Clinical Excellence
6. Diehl V, Thomas RK, RE, D 2005 Hodgkin's lymphoma: diagnosis and treatment. **The Lancet**, **Oncology** 5(1):19–26
7. National Cancer Institute www.nci.nih.gov/cancertopics/pdq/treatment/hodgkins–during–pregnancy/HealthProfessional/page2 [accessed 15-06-2007]

8. Fisher PM and Hancock BW 1996 Hodgkin's disease in the pregnant patient. **British Journal of Hospital Medicine**, 56(10):529–532

18.4 Gestational Trophoblastic Disease

1. Tham BW, Everard JE, Tidy JA, *et al.* 2003 Gestational trophoblastic disease in the Asian population of Northern England and North Wales. **British Journal of Obstetrics and Gynaecology**, 110(6):555–559
2. www.hmole-horio.org.uk/medics_information_gtt.html [accessed 10-06-2007]
3. Hassadia A, Gillespie A, Tidy J, *et al.* 2005 Placental site trophoblastic tumour: clinical features and management. **Gynecologic Oncology**, 99(3):603–607
4. Soto-Wright V, Bernstein M, Goldstein DP, *et al.* 1995 The changing clinical presentation of complete molar pregnancy. **Obstetrics and Gynecology**, 86(5):775–779
5. RCOG 2004 **Guideline 38: The management of gestational neoplasia**. London; Royal College of Obstetricians and Gynaecologists
6. Tidy JA, Gillespie AM, Bright N *et al.* 2000 Gestational trophoblastic disease: a study of mode of evacuation and subsequent need for treatment with chemotherapy. **Gynecologic Oncology**, 78:309–312
7. RCOG 2000 **Clinical Guideline 25: The management of Early Pregnancy Loss**. London; Royal College of Obstetricians and Gynaecologists
8. Pezeshki M, Hancock BW, Silcocks P, *et al.* 2004 The role of repeat uterine evacuation in the management of persistent gestational trophoblastic disease. **Gynecologic Oncology**, 95(3):421–422 www.chorio.group.shef.ac.uk [accessed 10-06-2007]
9. Tidy JA, Rustin GJ, Newlands ES, *et al.* 1995 Presentation and management of choriocarcinoma after non-molar pregnancy. **British Journal of Obstetrics and Gynaecology**, 102(9):715–719
10. Mace K 1995 Hidden misery of hydatidiform mole **Modern Midwife**, 5(10):15–17
11. Thorstensen KA 2000 Midwifery management of first trimester bleeding and early pregnancy loss. **Journal of Midwifery and Women's Health**, 45(6):481–497
12. Sebire MD, Foskett MA, Paradinas FJ, *et al.* 2002 Outcome of twin pregnancies with complete hydatidiform mole and healthy co-twin. **The Lancet**, 359: 2165–2166
13. Lindsay P 2004 Chap.44 *Bleeding in pregnancy* in Henderson C and Macdonald S (Eds) **Mayes' Midwifery: A Textbook for Midwives**, 13th Ed. London; Baillière Tindall 765–766

Index